PRINCIPLES AND PRACTICE OF
Child and Adolescent Forensic Mental Health

PRINCIPLES AND PRACTICE OF
Child and Adolescent Forensic Mental Health

Edited by

Elissa P. Benedek, M.D.
Peter Ash, M.D.
Charles L. Scott, M.D.

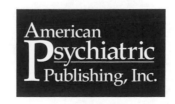

American Psychiatric Publishing, Inc.

Washington, DC
London, England

If you would like to buy between 25 and 99 copies of this or any other APPI title, you are eligible for a 20% discount; please contact APPI Customer Service at appi@psych.org or 800-368-5777. If you wish to buy 100 or more copies of the same title, please e-mail us at bulksales@psych.org for a price quote.

Manufactured in the United States of America on acid-free paper
13   12   11   10   09   5   4   3   2   1
First Edition

Typeset in Kuenst480 BT and Flareserif 821 BT.

American Psychiatric Publishing, Inc.
1000 Wilson Boulevard
Arlington, VA 22209-3901
www.appi.org

Library of Congress Cataloging-in-Publication Data
Principles and practice of child and adolescent forensic mental health / edited by Elissa P. Benedek, Peter Ash, Charles L. Scott. — 1st ed.
      p. ; cm.
   Rev. ed. of: Principles and practice of child and adolescent forensic psychiatry / edited by Diane H. Schetky, Elissa P. Benedek. c2002.
   Includes bibliographical references and index.
   ISBN 978-1-58562-336-5 (alk. paper)
   1. Forensic psychiatry.   2. Child psychiatry.   3. Adolescent psychiatry.   I. Benedek, Elissa P.   II. Ash, Peter, 1947–   III. Scott, Charles L., 1960–   IV. Principles and practice of child and adolescent forensic psychiatry.
   [DNLM: 1. Forensic Psychiatry—methods.   2. Adolescent.   3. Child.   W 740 P9565 2010]
   RA1151.P6736 2010
   614′.1—dc22

                                                                                2009024764

British Library Cataloguing in Publication Data
A CIP record is available from the British Library.

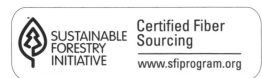

To the vulnerable children and adolescents
who face a complex system of justice

Contents

PART I

Basics

Elissa P. Benedek, M.D.

PART II

Legal Regulation of Practice

Peter Ash, M.D.

PART III

Child Custody

Elissa P. Benedek, M.D.

PART IV

Child Abuse

Charles L. Scott, M.D.

PART V

Youth Violence

Peter Ash, M.D.

PART VI

Juvenile Offenders

Charles L. Scott, M.D.

PART VII

Civil Litigation

Peter Ash, M.D.

Contributors

Diana K. Antia, M.D.
Chief Resident, Division of Child and Adolescent Psychiatry, Jackson Memorial Hospital, Miami, Florida

Peter Ash, M.D.
Associate Professor, Department of Psychiatry and Behavioral Sciences; Director, Psychiatry and the Law Service; Chief, Child and Adolescent Psychiatry, Emory University, Atlanta, Georgia

Catherine C. Ayoub, R.N., Ed.D.
Associate Professor of Psychiatry, Harvard Medical School, Children and the Law Program, Massachusetts General Hospital, Boston, Massachusetts

Sharmila Bandyopadhyay, M.Ed.
Doctoral Candidate, Programs in Clinical and School Psychology, Curry School of Education, University of Virginia, Charlottesville, Virginia

Eraka P.J. Bath, M.D.
Assistant Professor, Department of Psychiatry, and Director, Child Forensic Services, University of California–Los Angeles (UCLA) Neuropsychiatric Institute, David Geffen School of Medicine, Los Angeles, California

Elissa P. Benedek, M.D.
Adjunct Professor of Psychiatry, University of Michigan Medical School, Ann Arbor, Michigan

Stephen Bates Billick, M.D.
Clinical Professor of Psychiatry, New York Medical College, New York, New York

R. James R. Blair, Ph.D.
Chief, Unit on Affective Cognitive Neuroscience, Mood and Anxiety Program, National Institute of Mental Health, Bethesda, Maryland

Randy Borum, Psy.D., ABPP
Professor, College of Behavioral and Community Sciences, University of South Florida, Tampa, Florida

Brenda Bursch, Ph.D.
Clinical Director, Pediatric Psychiatry Consultation Liaison; Professor of Clinical Psychiatry and Biobehavioral Sciences, and Pediatrics, David Geffen School of Medicine, University of California Los Angeles, Los Angeles, California

Charles R. Clark, Ph.D., ABPP
Private Practice, Forensic Psychology, Ann Arbor, Michigan

Emil F. Coccaro, M.D.
Ellen C. Manning Professor and Chairman, Department of Psychiatry and Behavioral Neuroscience, Pritzker School of Medicine, The University of Chicago, Chicago, Illinois

Dewey G. Cornell, Ph.D.
Professor of Education, Programs in Clinical and School Psychology, Curry School of Education, University of Virginia, Charlottesville, Virginia

Debra K. DePrato, M.D.
Associate Professor, Louisiana State University Health Sciences Center, New Orleans, Louisiana

Megan Eliot, M.Ed.
Doctoral Candidate, Programs in Clinical and School Psychology, Curry School of Education, University of Virginia, Charlottesville, Virginia

Todd S. Elwyn, J.D., M.D.
Assistant Clinical Professor, Department of Psychiatry, The University of Hawaii, John A. Burns School of Medicine, Honolulu, Hawaii

James B. Gale, M.S.
Director, Bureau of Children and Adult Licensing, Michigan Department of Human Services, Lansing, Michigan

Marisa A. Giggie, M.D., M.P.Aff.
Pediatric, Forensic, and Adult Psychiatrist; Clinical Assistant Professor of Psychiatry, University of Alabama at Birmingham (UAB) School of Medicine, Birmingham, and University of Alabama School of Medicine, Tuscaloosa Campus, Tuscaloosa, Alabama

Tracy D. Gunter, M.D.
Associate Professor of Psychiatry, Department of Neurology and Psychiatry, St. Louis University School of Medicine, St. Louis, Missouri

Melvin J. Guyer, J.D., Ph.D.
Professor of Psychology, Department of Psychiatry; Adjunct Professor of Psychology, Department of Psychology, University of Michigan, Ann Arbor, Michigan

James C. Harris, M.D.
Director, Developmental Neuropsychiatry; and Professor of Psychiatry and Behavioral Sciences, Pediatrics and Mental Hygiene, Department of Psychiatry and Behavioral Sciences, Johns Hopkins University School of Medicine, Baltimore, Maryland

Jack P. Haynes, Ph.D.
Forensic Psychologist, Private Practice, Bloomfield Hills, Michigan

Thomas M. Horner, Ph.D.
Clinical Psychologist, Private Practice, Ann Arbor, Michigan

Praveen Kambam, M.D.
Fellow in Forensic Psychiatry, University Hospitals Case Medical Center, Cleveland, Ohio

Niranjan S. Karnik, M.D., Ph.D.
Assistant Professor, Department of Psychiatry and Behavioral Neuroscience, Pritzker School of Medicine, The University of Chicago, Chicago, Illinois

Sarah Kulkofsky, Ph.D.
Assistant Professor, Department of Human Development and Family Studies, Texas Tech University, Lubbock, Texas

Robert J. Levy, J.D.
William L. Prosser Professor of Law, University of Minnesota, Minneapolis, Minnesota

Kamala London, Ph.D.
Assistant Professor, Department of Psychology, University of Toledo, Toledo, Ohio

Pamela S. Ludolph, Ph.D.
Clinical and Forensic Psychologist, Adjunct Faculty, The University of Michigan, Ann Arbor, Michigan

JoAnn E. Macbeth, J.D.
Washington, DC

Daryl Matthews, M.D., Ph.D.
Clinical Professor of Psychiatry; Director Emeritus, Forensic Psychiatry Program, The University of Hawaii, John A. Burns School of Medicine, Honolulu, Hawaii

Stephen W. Phillippi, Ph.D.
Assistant Professor, Louisiana State University Health Sciences Center, New Orleans, Louisiana

Kathleen M. Quinn, M.D.
Director of Training in Child and Adolescent Psychiatry, Cleveland Clinic, Cleveland, Ohio

Vivek S. Sankaran, J.D.
Clinical Assistant Professor of Law, Child Advocacy Law Clinic, University of Michigan Law School, Ann Arbor, Michigan

Robert B. Sanoshy, LCSW
Clinical Therapist, Center for Contextual Change, Chicago, Illinois

Diane H. Schetky, M.D.
Clinical Professor of Psychiatry, University of Vermont College of Medicine at Maine Medical Center, Portland, Maine

Herbert A. Schreier, M.D.
Chief, Department of Psychiatry, Children's Hospital and Research Center, Oakland, California

Charles L. Scott, M.D.
Professor of Clinical Psychiatry; Chief, Division of Psychiatry and the Law; Director, Forensic Psychiatry Fellowship, University of California Davis Medical Center, Sacramento, California

Jon A. Shaw, M.D.
Professor of Psychiatry and Pediatrics and Director, Division of Child and Adolescent Psychiatry, Department of Psychiatry and Behavioral Sciences, University of Miami Miller School of Medicine, Jackson Memorial Medical Center, Miami, Florida

Matthew F. Soulier, M.D.
Assistant Professor of Clinical Psychiatry, Division of Psychiatry and the Law, Department of Psychiatry and Behavioral Sciences, University of California Davis Medical Center, Sacramento, California

Mary F. Spence, Ph.D.
School Psychologist, Ann Arbor Schools, Ann Arbor, Michigan

Hans Steiner, M.D.
Professor Emeritus, Department of Psychiatry and Behavioral Sciences, Stanford University School of Medicine, Stanford, California

Humberto Temporini, M.D.
Assistant Clinical Professor of Psychiatry, University of California Davis Medical Center, Sacramento, California

Wen Shing Tseng, M.D.
Professor of Psychiatry, The University of Hawaii, John A. Burns School of Medicine, Honolulu, Hawaii

Frank E. Vandervort, J.D.
Clinical Assistant Professor of Law, University of Michigan Law School, Ann Arbor, Michigan

Jerry Wishner, Ph.D.
Director of Special Education and Related Services, Chappaqua Central School District, Chappaqua, New York; Psychologist, Private Practice, Valhalla, New York

Disclosure of Interests

The following contributors to this textbook have indicated a financial interest in or other affiliation with a commercial supporter, manufacturer of a commercial product, and/or provider of a commercial service as listed below:

Dewey G. Cornell, Ph.D. Lead author, *Guidelines for Responding to Student Threats of Violence* (Sopris West).

Emil F. Coccaro, M.D. *Consultant:* Alexza and Pfizer; *Scientific advisory board:* Azevan.

Randy Borum, Psy.D., ABPP *Royalties:* Co-author, *Structured Assessment of Violence Risk in Youth* (risk assessment instrument published by PAR) and *Assessing and Managing Violence Risk in Juveniles* (Guilford).

The following contributors stated that they had no competing interests during the year preceding manuscript submission:

Diana K. Antia, M.D.; Catherine C. Ayoub, R.N., Ed.D.; R. James R. Blair, M.D.; Sharmila Bandyopadhyay, M.Ed.; Charles R. Clark, Ph.D., ABPP; Debra K. DePrato, M.D.; Megan Eliot, M.Ed.; Todd S. Elwyn, J.D., M.D.; James B. Gale, M.S.; Marisa A. Giggie, M.D., M.P.Aff.; Tracy D. Gunter, M.D.; Melvin J. Guyer, J.D., Ph.D.; James C. Harris, M.D.; Jack P. Haynes, Ph.D.; Praveen Kambam, M.D.; Niranjan S. Karnik, M.D., Ph.D.; Sarah Kulkofsky, Ph.D.; Kamala London, Ph.D.; Pamela S. Ludolph, Ph.D.; Daryl Matthews, M.D., Ph.D.; Stephen W. Phillippi, Ph.D.; Kathleen M. Quinn, M.D.; Jon A. Shaw, M.D.; Robert B. Sanoshy, LCSW; Vivek S. Sankaran, J.D.; Diane H. Schetky, M.D.; Herbert A. Schreier, M.D.; Matthew F. Soulier, M.D.; Mary F. Spence, Ph.D.; Humberto Temporini, M.D.; Frank E. Vandervort, J.D.

Preface

This volume replaces the previous *Principles and Practice of Child and Adolescent Forensic Psychiatry*. It is intended to be a textbook not only for psychiatrists but also for psychologists, social workers, and other mental health clinicians, as well as attorneys and judges. An additional goal of this book is to serve as an important resource for both clinicians and forensic experts who are faced with an ever-increasing number of child and adolescent mental health issues that interface with the law. To address these varied perspectives, we include chapters written by child psychiatrists, psychologists, and attorneys. Although it has been only 7 years since the last textbook was published, it seems much longer as many new content areas have emerged, in both the theory and practice of forensic psychiatry, psychology, and social work. These new areas affect the daily work of mental health clinicians and attorneys and judges. Because some issues only change slowly, the basic issues addressed in previous textbooks in the field of child and adolescent forensic mental health are revisited in this volume. For example, the chapters dealing with forensic evaluations and testifying discuss the basic issues of prac-

tice that are of import to both the novice and experienced practitioner. We have expanded the areas previously covered to deal with new information on those topics. Other completely new topic areas have long been of interest to clinicians but have assumed increasing importance in the twenty-first century. For example, a chapter on forensic telepsychiatry introduces the reader to the use of telepsychiatry in contemporary forensic practice. The Internet has assumed increasing importance in understanding the world of children and adolescents and in forensic evaluations. A chapter dealing with cultural competence addresses special issues involved in evaluating children and adolescents who come from diverse and different cultures.

We have tried to follow a similar format in this book to that used in the previous book. Authors have been encouraged to include tables in their chapters and to end each chapter with key points that they believe are most useful to the reader.

Elissa P. Benedek, M.D.
Peter Ash, M.D.
Charles L. Scott, M.D.

Acknowledgments

Drs. Benedek, Ash, and Scott wish to acknowledge their families for their encouragement and patience and Tina Coltri-Marshall for her ongoing work in organizing us and keeping us on track.

Special appreciation is also extended to the book's authors not only for providing their contributions but also for adhering to deadlines and for communicating in a timely fashion about any problems that they encountered.

Finally, the editors would like to thank Bob Hales and the administration of American Psychiatric Publishing, Inc., for recognizing the importance of the topics we cover to the fields of child psychiatry and child and adolescent forensic mental health.

PART I

Basics

Elissa P. Benedek, M.D.

Chapter 1

Introduction to the Legal System

Melvin J. Guyer, J.D., Ph.D.
Robert J. Levy, J.D.

We address this chapter to those with no formal training in law or the legal system. But most of you read the newspaper; have watched *The Practice, Boston Legal*, or *Law and Order*; and occasionally indulge in a novel about lawyers. Moreover, you are probably acquainted with at least some legal proceedings: impeachment, to be sure, and rules of evidence—*Daubert* and *Frye* admissibility rules, perhaps. Some of you may have had experience with criminal procedure: "Mirandizing" suspects or the "not guilty by reason of insanity" defense. However, such contacts with the legal system must have been ambiguous at best.

We will assume, with your permission, that you know little about the topic. We set out the legal system's basic framework in a sort of basic civics course style to help you as mental health clinicians in your many and various interactions with the courts, legal agencies, legal actors of several kinds, and, especially, with your patients who are also lawyers' clients. The concepts and definitions to which we introduce you may well make your professional contacts more comfortable and your contributions more useful.

We address the following topics: structure of the court system; types of legal proceedings; pretrial proceedings; and a potpourri of important (and sometimes arcane) legal niceties and doctrines, such as appeals and appellate courts' roles in the legal system (and how such cases are "cited," i.e., found in judicial reports), judicial treatment of clinicians (e.g., are you always considered an expert?), judicial decision making, and evidence doctrine dynamics.

Structure of Courts

History

The origins of the American legal system may be traced to ancient English principles and the emergence of modern nation-states from their medieval antecedents close to a millennium ago. Over the centuries, "the King's" (or "national") courts replaced the local magistrates, and national legal codes—the "common law"—replaced the idiosyncratic doctrines previously imposed by all-powerful nobles on serfs and renters in their fiefdoms. These historical roots eventually produced the doctrines controlling the contracts you now sign with your employers and employees and the law determining whether you can sue or be sued by the angry therapy patient who rear-ended your car in the parking lot. More importantly, from these roots grew the foundations of the system of courts in which you will testify, the formal substantive rules for adjudication of the civil disputes for which you will provide clinical expertise, and the "adversary" procedures that favor jury decision in civil and criminal cases and permit a lawyer for litigants opposed to your patient's or client's claim or defense to cross-examine. This adversarial system is governed both in procedure and substantive doctrine by adherence under most circumstances to established principles determined by previous, sometimes even ancient, decisions (called *precedents*). The policy of such adherence is described by an ancient term, *stare decisis*.

The same ancient tradition tracing to the emergence of nation-states contains the roots of modern American criminal procedure, shaping and sometimes controlling several of the frequently controversial constitutional rights afforded criminals. These include the right to be presumed innocent until proved guilty, trial by a jury of peers, the right to confront and cross-examine witnesses, and protection from self-incrimination.

Hierarchies

State Courts

State court systems are arranged as hierarchies: the "lower" courts functioning as trial courts and "higher" courts providing appellate review, a supervisory function for trial court decisions. Such review typically includes the trial court's procedure, as well as the merits of substantive decisions. With some exceptions, trial courts exercise general jurisdiction—the authority to hear and decide all types of cases, civil and criminal, that the state legislature, the ultimate source of all judicial jurisdiction, has authorized. The one exception to this rule of state legislative hegemony derives from the U.S. Constitution's decree that the "Great Writ," the writ of habeas corpus, which frees any person from illegal imprisonment, "shall not be suspended except in cases of invasion or rebellion." This provision governs the states because of the Constitution's supremacy clause, designed to prevent the states from evading constitutional principles. Every state legislature also provides a system of specialized courts, or courts of limited jurisdiction, for cases of less importance (e.g., misdemeanors rather than felonies, small monetary claims) and cases in which special training for judges is thought to be necessary (e.g., juvenile delinquency and neglect, housing, commitment of those who cannot take care of themselves, decedents' estates and wills).

Federal Courts

The U.S. Constitution authorizes and Congress has provided a parallel system of federal trial and appellate courts to decide cases arising under the Constitution and specifically enacted federal statutes. Congress has also authorized federal court jurisdiction of civil cases if the parties are residents of different states. Appeals from federal trial courts are heard by one of nine Courts of Appeal. And, of course, the nine justices of the U.S. Supreme Court may exercise their appellate jurisdiction and review any decision by one of the courts of appeal. The often arcane rules governing federal jurisdiction lie far beyond the intended scope of this chapter. Because of the centrality of federal-state relations in the American judicial and political system, the United States Constitution specifically authorized U.S. Supreme Court appellate jurisdiction to review any final state judicial decision. This review most often occurs when a state supreme court holds that a state statute passes federal constitutional muster and when a citizen's constitutionally protected rights may have been abridged by a state statute or some state official. U.S. Supreme Court decisions of appeals of such state action cases occur in criminal proceedings when defendants claim some denial of the individual protections afforded by the Constitution's Bill of Rights.

Specialized Courts

As we have indicated, some state courts are specialized and exercise jurisdiction constrained by subject matter or by the special character of particular cases. The example most of you will recognize is the juvenile court, which usually has authority over matters relating to minors: delinquency (any act which if committed by an adult could be prosecuted as a criminal offense) and dependency and neglect (any child who is at risk due to caretaker inability, dangerous inattention, abuse, or abandonment). These sources of judicial jurisdiction, if proved, allow supposedly specially trained or assigned judges to exercise authority over the problematic behavior of minors and the care of such minors by their parents, even if the behavior of the minor and the care of the parent are not criminal. Suppose a child regularly refuses to obey the reasonable demands and instructions of his or her parent or a parent refuses to provide his or her child with essential food or medical care. The child could be adjudicated neglected or dependent, the judge could order the child removed from the family and placed in foster care, the family could be ordered to provide the needed services, the child could be ordered to obey his or her parents, or the parents' parental rights could be terminated. In short, under this legal regime, at least during the child's minority, judges are given enormous power to determine the circumstances of the child's family relationships and upbringing.

Surrogate, probate, and orphans' courts are different names for another type of specialized tribunal, exercising authority over such matters as the financial affairs of persons who are legally or otherwise vulnerable, the young and the aged, the infirm, and the mentally ill. These courts conduct civil commitment and guardianship proceedings, grant adoptions, supervise the administration of estates and trusts and their trustees, and decide contested wills. From ancient times, such courts, acting as *parens patriae* (the community's parent, originally the king), have exercised authority and responsibility to protect those who cannot protect themselves. These specialized courts often call on clinical professionals for advice and testimony. A probate court might ask for mental health professional testimony as to the ability of a patient with Alzheimer's disease to handle his own finances; parents whose parental rights the state is seeking to terminate may ask a child clinician for an opinion that they are capable in the future of taking adequate care of their children despite one parent's drug addiction or mental illness. The litigation contexts in which requests for clinical advice and testimony may be requested are multifarious, and the roles of the professional will vary with the client and the context. The clinician must understand how these variations affect his or her role and responsibility. The bulk of this book focuses on these contextual and role variations and the professional and ethical double binds these variations can cause the unwary.

Types of Legal Proceedings

Courts of general jurisdiction hear both civil and criminal cases. For civil cases, a forum is provided to resolve the enormous variety of disputes that can arise between two litigants, plaintiff or defendant, third-party intervenors, called cross-plaintiffs, and cross-defendants. Each of these legal actors is called a party, the generic label for any entity asserting a legal claim. A party may be an individual, a corporation, or indeed even a large class of individuals who share a common legal grievance or defense. An example of such a class is all women with silicon breast implants who claim injury and illness caused by the implants; another such class is all patients who develop tardive dyskinesia after years of compelled psychiatric medication.

Dynamics of Legal Proof

The essence of most cases can be explored by asking and answering three fairly simple questions:

1. **What must be proven?** Each type of civil lawsuit requires, if the plaintiff is to prevail, that specific assertions, known as the elements of the cause of action, be proved (similarly with a defendant's defenses, such as self-defense as a response to a lawsuit for assault and battery).

2. **Who must prove the elements?** In a civil suit, the plaintiff, that is, the person lodging the legal complaint, must prove the elements of the cause of action. This duty is expressed, in legal jargon, as the burden of proof. In criminal cases, because of the presumption of innocence (remember the old saw, "It's better that ten guilty defendants go free than that one innocent defendant be convicted," that goes back to the Old Testament's Book of Genesis), the state has the burden of proving the elements of the crime charged against the defendant. Despite these cautions designed to protect defendants in criminal cases, burdens of proof can and do shift for strategic and efficiency reasons. For example, if a criminal defendant claims the defense of not guilty by reason of insanity, in at least some states the defendant must carry the burden of introducing sufficient evidence of insanity to make a *prima facie* case (one that has offered evidence sufficient to allow a jury verdict favorable to the plaintiff)—and only then does the burden of proof shift and require the prosecution to prove that the defendant is not insane.

3. **How much proof must be offered?** In most civil cases, the plaintiff, who has the burden of proof, must prove his or her case by a "preponderance of the evidence." But in some cases, again for practical or efficiency or fairness reasons, the more stringent "clear and convincing evidence" is required. This burden is imposed in some cases where the state is plaintiff or where the case involves some measure of punishment or stigma for the defendant. Paternity suits, terminations of parental rights, and commitments to mental hospitals have all been identified (occasionally by constitutional decree) as situations in which the more onerous burden of proof is required. In criminal cases, for reasons we have already mentioned, the burden of proof required is the even more stringent "beyond a reasonable doubt."

Civil Cases

Civil disputes are usually categorized generically: contract claims; property and financial disputes; *torts*, including such subtypes as negligence, medical malpractice, libel, and slander; and various nonphysical invasions of the plaintiff's person or interests claimed to cause mental or physical injury and/or financial loss. An example of the last category is a claim by a child's parent or other relative for pain and suffering caused when the defendant killed or seriously injured the child.

Civil disputes typically involve a plaintiff asserting a financial loss because of the defendant's behavior and a request for a legal remedy for the loss—either a financial recovery or an injunction that the defendant must cease and desist from continuing the behavior causing the plaintiff injury. A contract claim, for example, must assert the legal elements of the cause of action; these include that one of the parties made an offer to the other, that the offeree made a valid acceptance of the offer, that the resulting agreement contained adequate consideration (the financial inducement for acceptance of the agreement), and that the defendant had breached the agreement to the plaintiff's financial disadvantage. Contract claims are typically set in the world of business dealings, but many contract lawsuits involve personal relationships in which finances are secondary considerations. For centuries marriages were considered contracts, and their validity (in annulment proceedings) was determined, and is still assessed, as business contracts; divorce was considered the remedy for breach of the marriage contract, with damages assessed against the breaching party. This is only one small way in which ancient concepts and the elements of causes of action conceived hundreds of years ago, under very different social and legal conditions, continue to affect social relationships and the development of legal remedies.

Indeed, many legal scholars avouch the law's attachment to historical tradition, where change occurs with reluctance and only when changed conditions demand change. The doctrine of this respect for tradition, *stare decisis*, gives stability to the law and so to society.

Tort actions are probably the most common form of civil action and the one most familiar to nonlawyers. A plaintiff asserts that the defendant owed her a *duty of care* and acted in a negligent manner, causing the plaintiff a foreseeable harm, loss, or injury. Personal injuries from car accidents, medical malpractice, and product liability claims are all examples. That the defendant owes the plaintiff a duty of care is sometimes clear and settled from statutes or judicial precedents: the physician's responsibility to a patient, for example, or the landlord's to a tenant. In some instances, however, especially when a novel cause of action is being asserted, the duty issue may be doubtful. The action for damages filed by many states, once

against the tobacco companies and now against some pharmaceutical companies, affords timely examples. Another is the spate of suits by parents of adult patients against therapists for assisting patients to recover "memories" of childhood abuse. The duty of care issue is whether a therapist whose patient's relatives have been injured by the patient's false allegations can be liable to the relatives for negligent therapy. Courts have reached different conclusions about the issue.

Procedure and Evidence in Civil Cases

Civil suits follow a fairly standard course, governed by formal rules of civil procedure and codified rules of evidence. These rules provide in specific detail for every aspect of a lawsuit; where the suit can be filed, time deadlines for filing (called statutes of limitations), and methods of serving notice of the suit to the defendant are all specified in rules. Deviations may result in dismissal of the suit before the merits are reached.

Pretrial and Discovery in Civil Cases

Rules of civil procedure, unique to each state but everywhere closely following the rules adopted in federal courts, allow and encourage full pretrial (i.e., preliminary to court hearings) exploration by each party of the opposing party's legal claims or defenses. The rules typically require full disclosure by each party of facts that conceivably bear on the cause of action or defenses to it. The parties are permitted to seek and obtain information through a variety of specified methods. The process is called discovery. It can include a variety of techniques.

Depositions. Depositions involve the taking of sworn testimony of the opposing party and any other person thought by the deposing party to have some knowledge of facts pertaining to the issues in the lawsuit. Depositions of clinicians are often taken if they have examined a child during the period preceding filing of a divorce or custody case.

Interrogatories. This technique involves a written deposition, usually questions requiring a written answer under oath, submitted to a party by the opposing litigant. The information sought can be far reaching and extensive. In a suit claiming personal injury, for example, the plaintiff may be asked to set out the name and location of every health care provider ever visited, the reason for the visit, and any diagnosis or treatment received.

Subpoenas. A subpoena is a court order (prepared and served by a lawyer) requiring the appearance of a witness for deposition or trial. A demand for the appearance of a witness or party with his or her records is known as a *subpoena duces tecum* (the Latin persists because lawyers, unlike clinicians, dislike giving up any of their ancient, mystifying vernacular). A request for record production may be very broad and general, such as when a company is asked to produce all phone logs, e-mails, and interoffice memos having any bearing on a case. Such requests for documents are open-ended and deemed continuing at least during the discovery phase of the case. The party seeking records or testimony does not need to know what the records contain before making a blanket request for production.

Examination of evidence. The rules of discovery permit examination and testing, where appropriate, of evidence produced. Documents may be analyzed and tested for authenticity, origin, and age. Similarly, plaintiffs who seek damages for physical and/or emotional loss—as well as any person, such as a custody contestant, whose mental state is "in issue"—may be required to submit to an independent medical [and/or psychological] examination (IME), conducted by an examiner of the demanding litigant's choosing. In damage actions, the defendant is permitted to test the claims of loss or injury made by the plaintiff before the case proceeds to trial. The expert conducting an IME may be deposed by the opposing party concerning background, training, experience, and values. Typical deposition questions might include: "Doctor, have you ever done an IME of a defendant, or do you restrict your practice to testifying against injured plaintiffs?" "Isn't it true that the child psychiatry training program at [your university] has been suspended by the American Academy of Child and Adolescent Psychiatry?" "Isn't it true, Doctor, that you wrote an article for the *Psychological Bulletin* arguing that children [here fill in anything awful]?" Of course, the expert's opinions can also be explored and questioned. If a trial occurs, the IME examiner may expect to be called as an expert witness and to be examined and cross-examined by the litigants, and reference can be made to the expert's prior deposition for purposes of impeachment (i.e., to cast doubt on the reliability of the testimony).

Evidence disclosure. The parties may be required, before trial, to disclose the witnesses whom they intend to call, the nature of the witnesses' testimony, as well as any documents or physical evidence that might be introduced in evidence at trial. Expert witnesses' claimed expertise, education, and experience and the nature of their opinions must be disclosed so that the opposing party can prepare a defense, can perform a *voir dire* of the expert (an examination to prove, if the

opponent wants to and can, that the expert is not in fact qualified as an expert), and can prepare to rebut the expert's testimony by calling an opposing expert as a witness.

Free discovery. Free discovery was introduced into the rules of procedure as a way of guaranteeing that the parties to a civil suit would approach trial knowing what evidence their opponent would introduce and be prepared to rebut it. Most observers believe that liberal pretrial discovery has produced earlier and fairer settlements and trials based on the merits rather than "surprise" and "ambush." But it has also made it possible for wealthier litigants to intimidate their less-well-off opponents through extensive discovery, raising their opponents' legal costs to sometimes unbearable amounts.

Civil Trials

If a civil case goes to trial, it may be heard by a jury, or if both parties agree, by the judge, acting as the fact finder. Some cases, those that traditionally were considered equity (or injunction) causes of action, are heard and decided only by a judge. The first element of a trial by jury is for the litigants, with the judge's supervision, to impanel a jury after the voir dire of a jury panel. This exercise, consisting of questioning of jurors either individually or in groups by either the lawyers or the judge (depending on the jurisdiction), is designed to ensure that no juror biased about a particular litigant or a particular cause of action will be permitted to sit in judgment. Thus a juror who has been robbed at gunpoint would be excused from a prosecution for armed robbery, as would a relative of one of the case's parties.

At trial, the plaintiff puts his or her case on initially, setting out the facts that support the claim. Evidence is presented in the form of witness testimony and exhibits, which may include documents, photographs, charts, and so forth. The introduction of evidence is governed by formal rules of evidence. These are complex and codified rules applied by the judge to proffered testimony—but only at the request of the party against whose interest the testimony is proffered. These rules and the judge's application of them determine what the jury will be permitted to know about the case. When an objection is made to a proffer of evidence, the judge must rule on admissibility. These trial objections, always sharpening interest in dramatized trials or *Court TV*, are obviously attempts by one party to influence the fact finder's view of the evidence and the case by precluding attention to some bit of evidence. "Speculation," "hearsay," "irrelevant," "repetitious," and "no foundation" are among the many objections you are likely to find familiar.

Each of the party's witnesses can be cross-examined by the opposing party. When the plaintiff's presentation of her case is complete (she "rests"), the defendant will usually make a motion to dismiss on grounds that the plaintiff has not proved a prima facie case. If this motion is denied, the defendant will then proceed to introduce his defenses and rebuttals to the plaintiff's witnesses. The trial now proceeds for the defendant as it did for the plaintiff. Then, before closing argument and the judge's "charge" to the jury, the plaintiff has a chance to introduce witnesses in rebuttal of the defendant's case. Rebuttal witnesses are often used against expert witnesses; they may challenge the opposing expert's knowledge, experience, or training or simply testify that the expert's testimony is based on some kind of factual or theoretical error.

The rules of evidence provide for the use of expert witnesses if it can be shown that by reason of scientific training, educational experience, or specialized knowledge, the expert has an understanding that ordinary persons do not possess and if the expert's testimony can be shown to aid the jury's deliberation in any fashion. As this phrasing indicates, the rules of evidence are generally oriented toward admissibility of expert testimony, subject to cross-examination and rebuttal "for what it's worth." In many states, though, expert testimony is still frowned on when the testimony "usurps the role of the jury"—for example, is directed to the ultimate issue, that is, answers the question that is the jury's responsibility to decide, as in "I believe the defendant was not guilty by reason of insanity" or "I conclude that the child was sexually abused." Once qualified by the court as an "expert," the expert witness may offer learned opinions and explanations derived from his or her special knowledge. Lay witnesses are usually restricted to testimony about what they have directly experienced.

After completion of the case presentations, the judge instructs ("charges") the jury on the law to be applied to the facts the jury finds proved from the testimony presented. The jury is told that it can make credibility judgments about the testimony of the various witnesses but that it is bound by the facts as presented and may not seek additional or external data to resolve its uncertainties. The jury is also instructed on the burden of proof, a topic we discussed earlier.

The judge's charge informs jurors of the legal elements of the cause of action and reminds them to ignore any testimony they heard to which proper objection was made. Although such testimony is typically struck from the record, it remains both in the transcript and, many contend, in the memories of jurors. Indeed, some social psychologists' laboratory research with mock jurors has shown that objections only call evidence more dramatically to jurors' attention and make the objectionable evidence more salient than at least some of the testimony to which no objection was made. Because of this fact, many trial attorneys try to find ways to object in advance and exclude from the trial testimony that would harm their client's case. Jury instructions these days are generally standard text material, prepared by professional groups and called JIGs and CrimJIGs (jury instruction guides and criminal jury instruction guides).

It is interesting to note that jurors quizzed on judges' instructions often display little understanding of the law they have applied or even recollection of what they have been told. Jurors do know that they have to decide who wins, and if it is the plaintiff, how much money must be awarded to provide compensation for the losses they have found the plaintiff incurred. In recent years, efforts to compel jurors to follow the law more—rather than only their rough sense of justice—in particular cases have led many jurisdictions to adopt the practice of requiring *special verdicts*. These are verdict forms delivered when the jury begins its deliberations that require the jurors collectively to answer specific questions. The notion is that jurors' discretion will be constrained by compelling greater adherence to the legal elements of the case; in the event that special verdict forms show that the jury wanted the plaintiff or the defendant to win despite contrary factual findings (an inconsistent verdict), the judge is in a better position to correct the jury's error.

Juries can award plaintiffs their actual losses, of course, and, in some instances, punitive damages as well. Excessive punitive damage awards in some recent highly publicized civil actions have led to a new legislative and even constitutional movement, approved by the U.S. Supreme Court, to constrain the imposition of punitive damages.

Criminal Cases

Criminal cases invoke the community's direct and vital interest in protecting the safety of its citizens and their values and community order (and, sometimes, what legislators believe should be their morals). Forbidden behaviors are legislatively codified in criminal statutes, providing citizens with advance notice of what acts by individuals are subject to societal sanction. Criminal sanctions can be imposed on behavior of minor significance, such as traffic infractions, or on behavior of substantial consequence and taboo, such as intentional homicide. As a consequence of this enormous variety in rule-breaking behavior, sanctions imposed on persons convicted of a crime can vary enormously, from small fines and community service to capital punishment, with great discretion left to judges to address the individual circumstances of individual defendants. In recent years, however, at least for major crimes, there has been a movement to adopt sentencing guidelines, designed to lessen judicial discretion and to equalize punishment for similar crimes and for similarly situated defendants. Sentences, and the proper method of punishing those who commit criminal acts, have become highly emotional issues. Sentencing guidelines have lessened the importance of clinical analysis and prediction by probation officers and clinicians in individual cases; they have also led to enormous increases in public costs and populations of prisons. Crime and the punishment for crimes will be among the major social and political issues in the next decades.

Procedure in Criminal Cases

Criminal justice is characterized by the constitutional and legislative imposition of a variety of formal procedures intended to protect a defendant from the vast powers the state has at its disposal in prosecuting defendants. Defendants' procedural rights usually derive from ancient English law, some of it codified in England in the Magna Carta, centuries of parliamentary statutes and judicial decrees, and other concepts derived from colonial reactions to the abuses of power of the Inquisition and the "Star Chamber." Many of the most well-known criminal procedural protections were codified in the Bill of Rights (the first ten amendments to the U.S. Constitution). These rights include: protection from compelled self-incriminating testimony, prohibition of illegal searches and seizures of evidence, a right to help from an attorney and a free attorney for the indigent, trial by jury, ability to confront and cross-examine opposing witnesses, a right to call witnesses in defense, and a bar against cruel and unusual punishment on conviction. The rights enumerated in the Bill of Rights now apply to state criminal prosecutions by virtue of the due process clause of the Fourteenth Amendment. The general trend of decisions over time has expanded defendants' procedural rights—but the course has been neither smooth nor always in the same direction. For example, it took 40 years after the U.S. Supreme Court first declared that indigent criminal defendants are entitled to a free at-

torney before the Court held that all such defendants are entitled to counsel in both state and federal courts, and even today, indigent defendants are entitled to assigned counsel only if they are threatened with imprisonment rather than financial sanction alone. In short, constitutional protections for criminal defendants are controversial and subject to continuing shaping and trimming by state and federal courts.

Pretrial proceedings. After a suspected criminal is arrested, a series of formal steps, some of them imposed by constitutional decree, must follow. The person arrested must be advised of his or her legal rights (Miranda warnings); the defendant must be formally notified of the charges and must be given an opportunity to plead to the charges and, with a few exceptions in cases of violent crimes, offered an opportunity to be released under conditions that provide some assurance (usually money, called bail) that the defendant will appear at subsequent proceedings.

The next stage requires the prosecutor to make some formal showing, either to a grand jury, which can issue an indictment, or, in some jurisdictions, to a judge in a preliminary hearing requested by the defendant after an "information" has been filed alleging the crime, that there is a threshold measure of evidence (probable cause to believe) that a crime has been committed and that the defendant committed it. The prosecutor need not put on the full measure of evidence available on these occasions, only enough to convince the grand jury or the preliminary hearing judge that probable cause exists. If the defendant is "bound over" for trial (and the defendant almost always is), security arrangements to assure the defendant's attendance are reviewed.

In most states the prosecutor is obligated to share his or her file on the case with the defense, allowing the defendant to peruse reports from the police, witnesses' statements, and physical and other evidence. Constitutional precedents require the prosecutor to make available to the defendant any exculpatory evidence known to the prosecutor. The U.S. Supreme Court has ruled that if the prosecutor fails to disclose exculpatory evidence, the prosecution must be dismissed.

Pleas and jury verdicts in criminal cases. If a criminal case does not settle, the trial is governed by formal rules of procedure and the usual rules of evidence with some special intricacies adapted to the criminal context. Most prosecutions do not reach trial because defendants and their lawyers justifiably believe that a negotiated agreement, a plea bargain, is likely to get the defendant a better deal—for example, conviction of a lesser offense with a less onerous penalty—than the defendant might obtain if he or she "rolls the dice" by going to trial. The Constitution requires that the defendant be allowed a jury trial, which can be waived. The defendant is not required to take the stand in his or her own defense (a requirement that would violate the self-incrimination prohibition). Conviction of the defendant leads to a sentencing hearing and imposition of a sentence by the judge.

Trial Advocacy

As we have already indicated (and occasionally illustrated), the legal system posits that "truth" will most likely emerge when factual matters are disputed, and that justice will most likely be served, in general and between litigants, if decisions (both factual and legal) are the product of adversarial contests where the disputants have skilled champions who can present their claims and dispute contradictory claims as effectively as possible. That means, at a minimum, that "fact finders," the judges, will be neutral and will consider only evidence (properly presented and allowable under the rules of evidence) presented by the parties and in the proper form. It also means that the litigants will be bound by assertions under oath made by the witnesses their lawyers present to the fact finder, that the honesty, ability to understand context, observational skills, and opportunities to observe facts relevant to the dispute of witnesses must be tested by the legal opponent's lawyer's cross-examination. It is this feature of the adversarial system's method that has drawn most attention (and criticism if not hatred) from critics of the legal system, especially mental health experts who are subjected as witnesses to the system without much indoctrination about its purposes or the utility of its techniques. Needless to say, criticism often comes from witnesses who are subjected to aggressive and unskilled applications of cross-examination as well as from witnesses whose lack of preparation, inadequacies of training, or poor reasoning in the matter at hand leads to painful exposure during cross-examination. It is important for nonlawyers to understand that, as is the case with empirical research and scientific study generally—although mistakes can be made in individual cases that, for a variety of reasons, particular cross-examiners can be rude, wrong, biased, even ignorant—in general the adversarial system has proved over the centuries to provide the best and most certain way to get to the truth where factual and legal issues are in dispute.

Summary

This account of a vital and dynamic legal system, whose edges (if not its underlying principles) are under continuing examination and reflection, is necessarily elementary. When you come into contact with lawyers and the legal system, you will discover many idiosyncrasies of law and practice (and often many idiosyncratic practices of lawyers and judges) that might make you wonder about the accuracy of this account. Nonetheless, one lesson we hope you will not doubt: Lawyers, judges, and court systems all have one great (but not always attainable) goal—to do justice in individual cases without disrupting the orderliness and fairness of the legal system and of the community the system seeks to serve.

Appendix: Legal Citations

Clinicians are often confronted, either in the courtroom while testifying or in consultations with lawyers, with questions such as: "Well, Doctor (occasionally pronounced with slight, forensic scorn), isn't it true that in the *Jones* case (alternatively, in *Jones v. Smith*), the court rejected your theory in a case identical to this one? You can find the case at 21 Ark [Arkansas Supreme Court Reports] 496, 375 SW2d [West's Southwest Reporter Second Series] 1025." Needless to say, such questions are designed, at least in part, to intimidate the forensic mental health expert, who usually doesn't have his or her own lawyer nor does the expert's client's lawyer care in the slightest about the expert's comfort level. And the lawyer is often successful because the expert doesn't know the case or how to distinguish it from the case at hand and has no clue as to the meaning of the numbers or the books to which the lawyer is referring.

The following short description is not designed to give clinicians law library research skills. Indeed, it seems sensible initially to warn readers that when situations of the kind described in the previous paragraph occur, they should seek legal help rather than relying on their own case-finding or, even more important, case-reading skills. Nonetheless, some awareness of what judges and lawyers mean when they talk such numbers mumbo jumbo may help experts to keep their cool. Appellate (but not trial court) decisions in every state are recorded and retrieved according to a volume-numbering system originally conceived and currently maintained by the West Group, a large and dominant legal publishing house. (Today, all cases can also be retrieved electronically either through Lexis, a system maintained by a West Group competitor, or through WestLaw, a computerized service of the West Group.) At one time, every state maintained official reports of all decisions by its supreme court (and sometimes of decisions of its intermediate courts of appeal). For cases reported officially as well as by the West service, the citations are typically reported in a parallel fashion. Therefore, a decision's citation in a brief might look like this:

Jones v. Smith, 225 Mass 75, 410 NE2d 513 (1994)

In ordinary language, this citation means that a reader who wants to read the *Jones v. Smith* case can find it in volume 225 of the official *Massachusetts Reporter* at page 75 or in volume 410 of the *Northeast Reporter,* second series, at page 513, and that the case was decided in 1994.

If the case had been in the Massachusetts intermediate appellate court, the citation would have looked like this:

225 Mass App 75, 410 NE2d 513 (1994)

To an ever-increasing extent, state judicial systems are forgoing their own official publications and relying solely on the West system. Thus the citations for the cases referred to would look like this:

410 NE2d 513 (Mass 1994) (the Massachusetts Supreme Court decision)

or

410 NE2d 513 (Mass App 1994) (the intermediate appellate court decision)

For decision-reporting purposes, the West system arbitrarily divides the country into seven areas: Atlantic (A and A2d—including Pennsylvania, Delaware, etc.), Northeast (NE and NE2d—including New York, Massachusetts, etc.), Southeast (SE and SE2d—including Virginia, North Carolina, etc.), Southern (So and So2d—including Mississippi, Kentucky, etc.), Southwestern (SW and SW2d—including Texas, Oklahoma, etc.), Northwestern (NW and NW2d—includ-

ing Minnesota, Iowa, etc.), and Pacific (Pac, P2d and P3rd—including California, Oregon, etc.).

There are additional mystifying idiosyncrasies with which we can bore you. Some state courts are known by unusual names, and sometimes (but not always) the names affect citation forms. For example, the highest court in New York is known as the New York Court of Appeals, but the citation form is not affected; on the other hand, unlike court designations in any other state, the New York trial court is known as the supreme court, and official citations to its decisions, for reasons unknown to your otherwise expert authors, come in the form 27 Misc 424,525 NY Supp (or NYS2d) 1002; the New York intermediate appellate court is known as the Supreme Court, Appellate Division.

The federal courts have their own designations and citation forms. The U.S. Supreme Court cites its own decisions in three different citation styles, although commentators usually refer only to one official set of reports and one unofficial set. We could go on—but those of you who are not bored must be bewildered—and here your education into (some of the easier to understand) legal research intricacies must pause.

We have not tried to provide an exhaustive (and certainly not complete) introduction to the legal system. Indeed, many readers with substantial experience as expert witnesses will find our effort somewhat superficial. Our intention within the page confines of this chapter has been to provide a broad survey of "lawyer talk" and a brief overview of the legal universe for the mental health professionals who have yet had only a limited exposure to legal concepts.

Supplemental Reading

Burnham W: Introduction to the Law and Legal System of the United States, 2nd Edition. St. Paul, MN, West Group, 1999

Friedman LM: American Law: An Introduction, 2nd Edition. New York, WW Norton, 1998

Llewellyn KL: The Common Law Tradition: Deciding Appeals. Boston, MA, Little, Brown, 1960

Mauet TM: Trial Techniques, 4th Edition. Boston, MA, Little, Brown, 1996

Chapter 2

Ethics of Child and Adolescent Forensic Psychiatry

Matthew F. Soulier, M.D.

Basic Tenets of Medical Ethics

Society has imbued physicians with a special responsibility and privilege to heal the sick. Although it is an exhilarating experience to participate in the healing process, the physician's role and stature are founded and sustained by a tradition of ethics dating back to Hippocrates in the fourth century B.C. Ethics reflect the moral values, principles, beliefs, and standards of conduct in the practice of medicine. Ethics relate to a consideration of what is right and what is wrong. The ethics of medicine generally attempt to balance a patient's best interest with societal good, while maintaining substantial respect for the patient's rights as a person (Dingle and Stuber 2008).

Ethics evolve with standards of society and are the source of vigorous debate because they fail to concretely address every situation, but the Hippocratic Oath has remained the bedrock of medical ethics. Many medical schools initiate their students with a recitation of the Hippocratic Oath, whose core tenet is for the physician to do no harm. Nonmaleficence is assumed by a trusting and often vulnerable patient and is essential for a physician to effect positive change.

The counterpart to do no harm is beneficence, an affirmative duty to do good, and forms the basis of many physicians' selection of medicine. Physicians who sense that they are not doing good in their practice of medicine will feel some dissonance from their original aspirations as medical students. Although the Hippocratic Oath makes no mention of autonomy, it has superseded beneficence as central to modern medical codes of ethics (Adshead and Sarkar 2005). Patients want to control their medical care and make informed decisions about their care and treatment. Medicine respects this autonomy, assuming that patients can make competent decisions or lack capacity for only discrete periods.

The fourth central principle in medical ethics is justice, which traditionally refers to equal and fair access to services and resources (Taylor and Buchanan 1998). In addition to resource allocation, justice can include the legal rights of patients, particularly to prevent the exploitation of susceptible patients such as the incarcerated and mentally ill (Sen et al. 2007). Psychiatrists can do much to ensure that the mentally ill have an equal voice and claim to justice as the rest of society. The four principles of traditional medical ethics are summarized in Table 2–1.

Many Hats to Wear

Do no harm, beneficence, autonomy, and justice form a useful and proven structure for medical practice within the traditional dyadic doctor–patient relation-

TABLE 2–1.   Four principles of traditional medical ethics

- Do no harm
- Beneficence
- Autonomy
- Justice

ship. However, child forensic psychiatrists will quickly find conflict and dilemmas with these principles in everyday practice. Child forensic clinicians complete multiple steps in training, with each specialization adding a new identity and set of moral complexities. For instance, a psychiatrist is charged with protecting patients from harming themselves. Involuntarily hospitalizing a suicidal patient after a risk assessment in an emergency department overrides the principle of autonomy, but such a psychiatrist may argue that he or she is doing good by attending to the safety and welfare of society. However, this situation only invites more moral dilemmas: Did the patient have the capacity to be autonomous? Did the patient benefit, and what should be the definition of benefit: feeling better or behaving better? A psychiatrist has numerous conflicts with the four traditional principles of medical ethics.

When a psychiatrist wears the additional hat of a forensic expert, the ethical dilemmas seem to multiply. Forensic psychiatrists do not operate within a dyadic relationship with a patient, but rather balance serving a patient with duties to a third party such as the judicial system. Forensic psychiatry is not patient-centered, and it does not represent a doctor–patient relationship. Even though forensic psychiatrists are trained as therapists to understand and accept patients' narratives as internal reality, they strive to ascertain a more objective truth from their evaluees. Forensic psychiatrists use the same tools of psychiatric interview and mental status evaluation, but they also search for corroborating and contradictory data to consider and factor into their assessments. The "patient" may or may not perceive benefit from the forensic evaluation.

Some have contended that forensic psychiatry is unique such that it needs its own code of ethics. Forensic psychiatry cannot find harmony and theoretical backing attempting to adhere to the four basic principles of medical ethics. As I discuss later in this chapter, forensic psychiatry has leapt forward in this regard and found more ethical solace in arguing that justice should be paramount (Sen et al. 2007) instead of embracing core medical values. These arguments may be

applicable to the added specialty of child forensic psychiatry, but the framework will not be sufficient to apply in all situations. Just as every pediatrician knows that children are not little adults, child forensic clinicians are discovering their own distinctive dilemmas.

From the first juvenile court developed in 1899 in Chicago, Illinois, it was assumed that children were less mature and thus less culpable for delinquent behavior (Grisso et al. 2003). The birth of the juvenile court was intended to rehabilitate troubled children and put a strong emphasis on the disposition of youth that would best reform the deviant behavior (Ainsworth 1996). The state was supposed to act in place of the parent for the child's best interest, with the judge acting as a benevolent parent. It is debatable if the juvenile system has succeeded in its original goal of rehabilitation and if society still supports this goal politically as laws are enacted that further criminalize juvenile courts. With such ambiguity, child forensic clinicians must ask what their role should be if the goal of juveniles is treatment and promoting healthy development and what their role should be if the juvenile judicial system departs from these ideals? Is the role of child forensic psychiatrist specialized enough that it too will require its own principles for ethical analysis? The primacy of justice in adult forensic psychiatry may not be sufficient to tackle the moral dilemmas of a child forensic psychiatrist.

The scope and goals between adult and juvenile criminal systems can vary widely. In many cases involving children, the focus is more prospective and future oriented. Future disposition can be the critical question in cases of custody, child protection, and other juvenile matters. Rather than the more typical retrospective inquiry that attempts to ascertain the "truth" about a past event, the focus in a child case may concern who will be the better parent. Child forensic experts' opinions regarding issues of character and personality become very important and influential. Maintaining objectivity remains critical for the credibility and ethical standing of a child forensic clinician. Evaluations that involve questions such as custody are highly charged emotionally, and the outcome profoundly affects many lives.

"There Is No Such Thing as a Baby"

The British pediatrician and psychiatrist D.W. Winnicott (1965) posited, "There is no such thing as a baby," with the implication that a child cannot develop or exist in the absence of a mother. It would be further futile to consider an infant's internal psyche in the absence of the inseparable link to his or her mother. The link between children and their custodians is equally important for a child forensic psychiatrist in the consideration of governing ethical principles. Child forensic ethics struggles with the fundamental distinction between children and adults as autonomous persons.

Children are often presumed to be too young, immature, and cognitively underdeveloped to entrust making critical decisions afforded to an adult. Children have fixed ages for the legal right to drive, vote, and drink alcohol. Children will never have the same political clout as adults who write laws supported by adults. Most of these age distinctions stem from legislative sensibilities rather than grounding in child development theory. The law tends to treat children the same, regardless of individual maturity (Horowitz 2002). Child forensic clinicians must respect the bounds of the laws, but they are trained to know how children move through a wide range of cognitive, physical, and emotional changes. Chronological age is not necessarily congruent with maturational age. Child forensic clinicians can be helpful in the example of a court weighing the transfer of a juvenile to adult court in elucidating these developmental distinctions. Experts can also provide the court with developmentally appropriate recommendations about rehabilitation to meet a youth's needs (Beyer 2006). The individual determination of a child's maturity is not always administratively convenient but ethically preferred to strict age requirements (Horowitz 2002).

Children have custodians to make decisions on their behalf. Unless legally emancipated through a demonstration of financial and residential independence from their parents, children depend on their parents to make most legal decisions. Custodians are believed to act in their children's best interest, and courts have a history of deferring to parents' judgment. In *Parham v. J.R.* (1979), the Supreme Court decided that the commitment of children to psychiatric hospitals by parents was legal, assuming idealistically that parents would uphold their child's welfare. Society hopes for this ideal, yet parents sometimes betray their children's best interest, and children's rights can be jeopardized by a proxy decision maker they usually never chose (Morrison 1986).

Parents can frankly abuse and neglect children, or the rights of the child may be infringed by a parent whose unconscious agenda may not favor the welfare of the child. For example, parents sometimes seek peer-like friendship, abdicating their responsibility to set limits and provide appropriate oversight to a juvenile in trouble (Koocher 2008). Parents also may lack an understanding of development and attachment or fail to advocate on their children's behalf. A child forensic clinician often has to work with parents, seek their permission, and assess their effect on the child's case. Concurrently, the child forensic psychiatrist must consider the developmental potential for a child to participate and understand the decision-making process. The interests of the parent and child do not always coincide, and their rights may conflict. Child forensic ethics must address the developmental distinction between a child and an adult and how much a child can participate and contribute to a legal process autonomously from a parent (Sondheimer and Klykylo 2008).

The Search for Ethical Consensus

The child forensic psychiatry literature lacks a clear articulation of its own ethical principles. As discussed further later in this chapter, the American Psychiatric Association (APA) and American Academy of Child and Adolescent Psychiatry (AACAP) ethics guidelines and the AACAP practice parameters for child custody evaluation speak little about child forensic ethics issues.

However, the general field of forensic psychiatry has continued to have a spirited discussion about its own ethical underpinnings. Forensic psychiatrists have long recognized that working in a legal system creates a tension between two different codes of behavior and ethical frameworks. The law is concerned with justice, retribution, and maintaining social order, whereas forensic psychiatrists come from a helping profession. Forensic psychiatrists generally have been found to consider core medical values important to their practice (Weinstock et al. 1991). Western law presumes people rationally control their own actions, but psychiatry finds explanations based on childhood and environmental influence, creating further philosophical differences.

This tension between the law and psychiatry is relevant to child forensic psychiatry, and the debate particularly ignited in 1982 when Alan Stone, Touroff-Glueck Professor of Law and Psychiatry, Harvard University, gave a lecture to the American Academy of Psychiatry and the Law (AAPL): "The Ethics of Forensic Psychiatry: A View from the Ivory Tower" (Stone 1984/2008). His address came at a vulnerable time when forensic psychiatry was still struggling for recognition as a subspecialty of psychiatry (Bloom 2008). Dr. Stone argued that it was ethically incoherent for psychiatrists to testify in the courtroom as disinterested neutral experts when they would inevitably be drawn to advocate as partisans for the hired side. He was concerned about forensic psychiatrists testifying with certainty based on uncertain knowledge and the potential to help or harm the evaluee. Stone concluded that the ethics of forensic psychiatry were untenable because a forensic psychiatrist would violate medical ethical boundaries, attempting to combine the traditional goal of beneficence while serving the interests of justice (Miller 2008).

Forensic psychiatrists responded to Dr. Stone's challenge to their ethical standing through multiple contributions that reconsidered, postulated, and articulated new theories for forensic ethical principles. Throughout this discussion, forensic psychiatrists ultimately separated themselves ethically from clinical psychiatrists. The fracture was articulated by Dr. Appelbaum (1997, 2008), whose formulation became widely accepted by current forensic psychiatrists and is often referred to as the "standard position." Dr. Appelbaum believes that forensic psychiatry requires a different ethical analysis than traditional medicine and clinical psychiatry. He believes that a forensic psychiatrist's duty is to present the truth, with less emphasis on beneficence in favor of justice. However, the definition and representation of "truth" remain controversial among forensic psychiatrists. Dr. Morse (2008) agrees with Dr. Appelbaum's formulation of a psychiatrist as a truth-teller but is even more restrictive in his belief that experts' testimony should be limited to only description of mental states that will allow the fact finders to make informed decisions. Dr. Morse recommends that psychiatrists avoid ultimate legal opinions, diagnoses, and unqualified jargon.

The ethical debate among forensic psychiatrists continues, but the clinical foundation of the field has remained honesty and striving for objectivity (Ash and Derdeyn 1997). Forensic psychiatrists have their own biases, values, and experiences that affect consciously or unconsciously the evaluation. Thus, forensic psychiatrists can only strive for objectivity rather than the illusion of complete indifference (Martinez and Candilis 2005). It remains debatable what constitutes sufficient "striving." Although some have expressed concern that forensic psychiatrists can have such varying

opinions for the same case, it is not a limitation exclusive to psychiatry (Dike 2008). Other specialties such as oncology have varying opinions about how to treat a particular cancer. The fact finders of the court benefit from expert opinion and do not disqualify expert testimony because the views of a specialty may widely diverge. The adversarial court must weigh and consider the forensic psychiatrist's opinion in the light of the expert's potential for partisan advocacy.

A forensic psychiatrist should respect the individual in the process by performing the evaluation in an honest and confidential manner (Norko 2005), but there is no pretense of necessarily doing good or helping the evaluee. However, a psychiatrist does not typically know before beginning an evaluation if it is going to cause harm. Ratner (2002) argues that the forensic psychiatrist is only an agent for the party paying him or her to do the work. The maintenance of a more therapeutic role separate from the patient both explicitly and implicitly is critical for an ethical forensic psychiatrist.

It is not within the scope of this chapter to discuss fully all of the scholars that have added to the study of ethics in forensic psychiatry, but there have been other notable ideas in this debate. Dr. Griffith (2005) argues that the truth should be sought with a cultural formulation that reflects history and political knowledge (see also Chapter 8, "Cultural Competence in Child and Adolescent Forensic Mental Health"). Especially in the legal system, in which a dominant culture presides over the court, nondominant groups have a unique experience sometimes at odds with the dominant culture. A forensic psychiatrist must be attuned to this perspective and consider questions, such as whether an accused person can find justice when he or she perceives the legal system to be racist (Griffith 1998). Child forensic psychiatrists must consider the fact that African American and Hispanic persons are overrepresented in the juvenile population—up to 60% of those detained (Abram et al. 2003). In one study, African American and Latino juveniles and those with more system experience expected greater injustice. Such anticipatory injustice increased with age among African American participants. It also predicted choices about police interrogations, attorney consultations, and plea agreements. Individuals who do not believe that they will be treated fairly are less likely to confess or take a plea and are more likely to distrust authorities and have less acceptance of court decisions (Woolard et al. 2008).

Ethical Guidelines and Professional Organizations

Besides theories of ethical principles, codes of ethics are part of what distinguishes professions. Ethics provide the moral compass and bedrock to any vocational group. They define the rules, principles, and ideals for the organization. However, ethical guidelines in medicine are not designed as absolutes or laws but rather to serve as standards of conduct.

Psychiatrists began addressing their evolving ethical dilemmas systematically in 1944 with the creation of the APA ethics committee. The ethics committee of the APA currently consists of six voting members, including an APA past president. This committee is charged with the regulation of ethics complaints and the creation of educational materials for the general membership. This subsequently led to the publication of the APA Code of Ethics in 1973. It is based on *The Principles of Medical Ethics* of the American Medical Association (AMA), first published in 1847 and last revised in 2001 (American Medical Association 2001). The AMA *Principles of Medical Ethics* stresses core medical tenets of ethics: autonomy; beneficence; justice. The AMA *Principles of Medical Ethics* emphasizes the foremost responsibility a physician has to the patient. The APA Code of Ethics embraces the AMA principles but adds its own *Annotations Especially Applicable to Psychiatry,* the most recent edition of which was published in 2009.

Examples of APA annotations relevant to forensic psychiatry include the following:

1. *AMA Section 1, APA Annotation 1:* "A psychiatrist shall not gratify his or her own needs by exploiting the patient. The psychiatrist shall be ever vigilant about the impact that his or her conduct has upon the boundaries of the doctor–patient relationship, and thus upon the well-being of the patient." A forensic psychiatrist should clarify and maintain professional boundaries throughout the evaluation. A forensic psychiatrist does not serve as a "hired gun" or passionate advocate that fails to consider contradictory information. Forensic clinicians should use their skills to elicit information and conduct an interview, but they should remain mindful of an evaluee who is "forgetting" the boundary and never exploit a misunderstanding of their role. For instance, forensic psychiatrists should not seek or report incriminating information from an evaluee.

2. *AMA Section 2, APA Annotation 3:* "A psychiatrist who regularly practices outside his or her area of professional competence should be considered unethical." Child forensic psychiatrists should receive specialized training, ongoing medical education, and supervision as necessary to competently perform a specific type of evaluation. For instance, a child psychiatrist may have assessed many children but lack competence to perform a custody evaluation.

3. *AMA Section 4, APA Annotation 5:* "Ethically, the psychiatrist may disclose only that information which is relevant to a given situation. He or she should avoid offering speculation as fact." A forensic psychiatrist may acquire a significant amount of information about a person, but the dispersal of this information should be deliberate and may not necessitate the revelation of sensitive information such as a person's sexual orientation.

4. *AMA Section 4, APA Annotation 6:* "The psychiatrist must fully describe the nature and purpose and lack of confidentiality of the examination to the examinee at the beginning of the examination." Treating another person respectfully includes the preceding disclosure prior to beginning an examination. The psychiatrist should document this disclosure and the evaluee's demonstrated understanding.

5. *AMA Section 4, APA Annotation 13:* "Ethical considerations in medical practice preclude the psychiatric evaluation of any person charged with criminal acts prior to access to, or availability of, legal counsel. The only exception is the rendering of care to the person for the sole purpose of medical treatment." Evaluees should be reminded of the availability of their legal counsel, and the psychiatrist must contact that legal counsel before he or she begins an evaluation. This principle is of particular importance before beginning insanity evaluations in which a person will be asked for an account of the alleged crime.

6. *AMA Section 7, APA Annotation 3:* "However, it is unethical for a psychiatrist to offer a professional opinion unless he or she has conducted an examination and has been granted proper authorization for such a statement." Forensic psychiatrists must base opinions on evaluations, or the opinion should include a disclaimer that it is without a conducted evaluation.

In 1975, the AACAP responded to their experiences in clinical situations with the formation of a five-member ethics committee. In contrast to the APA committee, the AACAP committee is not charged with a regulatory role. Complainants are referred to the APA and/or state licensing boards. Both committees are charged with educating their members about ethical matters (Sondheimer and Klykylo 2008). A code of ethics was drafted in 1980 that provided principles and guidelines, specifically relevant to the needs of children. The AACAP code endorsed the AMA and APA codes of ethics, and there are no systemic conflicts between the codes (Ratner 2002). The AACAP *Preamble to the Code of Ethics* emphasizes the unique relationship between children and parents because parents usually seek the psychiatric evaluation (American Academy of Child and Adolescent Psychiatry 1995).

Examples of AACAP principles relevant to forensic psychiatry include the following:

1. *Principle V:* "The evaluation and treatment of a child, adolescent, or family...focus on the uniqueness of the individuals involved, their developmental potentials." Children are unique developmentally and should be evaluated within their social, racial, ethnic, and economic context. Child forensic clinicians should be cautious about their own biases in these domains. An additional implication of Principle V is that "rating scales alone cannot take into account all of the variables in a child's situation." As child forensic actuarial tools improve, the evaluator must never completely abandon good clinical judgment. Rating scales are important, but they must not be the sole data in a forensic evaluation.
2. *Principle VI:* "Regardless of the locus of decision, the psychiatrist should seek to develop with the child(ren) or adolescent(s) as thorough an understanding of the professional judgments, opinions, and actions as possible." Even if custodians are making the legal decisions, the forensic evaluator should still respect the evaluees and attempt to educate them about the purpose and scope of an evaluation.
3. *Principle X:* "The release of any information regarding a minor to persons outside the family (including the noncustodial parent) requires the agreement of parents or guardians." Forensic psychiatrists should guard private information and release information only in accordance with the written agreement of parents or a court.

The American Psychological Association has published both a code of ethics—*Ethical Principles of Psychologists* (American Psychological Association 2002)—and additional guidance pertaining to forensic psychologists—*Specialty Guidelines for Forensic Psychologists* (Committee on Ethical Guidelines for Forensic Psychologists 1991). Although the *Specialty Guidelines* does not represent an official statement of the American Psychological Association, it does not contradict the *Ethical Principles*. The *Specialty Guidelines* emphasizes basic ethical principles of confidentiality, professional competence, and consent. These guidelines add the recommendations that all data that form the basis of psychologists' evidence should be available, and professional integrity will be maintained through examining the issue from all reasonable perspectives, minimizing hearsay for the basis of opinion, and acknowledging the difference between corroborated and uncorroborated data. The *Specialty Guidelines* states that judicial testimony should be fair but can be "forceful" and emphasize that the critical role for the expert is to assist the trier of fact. The 2002 revision of the *Ethical Principles of Psychologists* of the American Psychological Association removed a section about forensic evaluations that had been included in the previous code and instead focused on more general principles applicable to all psychologists.

The AAPL adopted ethical guidelines for the practice of forensic psychiatry in 1989 and last updated its ethical guidelines in 2005 (American Academy of Psychiatry and the Law 2005). These guidelines supplement the *Annotations Especially Applicable to Psychiatry* of the APA and the *Principles of Medical Ethics* of the AMA. AAPL guidelines highlight the tension between legal and medical ethics in the Preamble: "Forensic psychiatrists practice at the interface of law and psychiatry, each of which has developed its own institutions, policies, procedures, values, and vocabulary. As a consequence, the practice of forensic psychiatry entails inherent potentials for complications, conflicts, misunderstandings and abuses." The most unique section of the AAPL code of ethics is

> *Honesty and Striving for Objectivity:* When psychiatrists function as experts within the legal process, they should adhere to the principle of honesty and should strive for objectivity. Although they may be retained by one party to a civil or criminal matter, psychiatrists should adhere to these principles when conducting evaluations, applying clinical data to legal criteria, and expressing opinions.

AAPL is transparent by not demanding its members be completely objective and disconnected from the evaluation, but the organization does encourage forensic psychiatrists to recognize and resist unethical pressures from attorneys and self-biases. It does not recognize the presence of an absolute truth, encouraging forensic psychiatrists to state the limitations in their opinions. Pertinent to child forensic psychiatrists, the AAPL guidelines recommend interviewing all parties in custody disputes.

Perhaps in the future, additional ethical guidelines addressing the specific needs of child forensic psychiatrists will be drafted and adopted. For now, child clinicians are bound by the guidelines of their member organizations.

Complaints of Unethical Professional Conduct

If an evaluation falls below professional standards, forensic clinicians are generally immune from a malpractice action because of the lack of a doctor–patient relationship (see Chapter 30, "Malpractice and Professional Liability," for exceptions), but they are not shielded from ethics complaints.

Forensic psychiatry is considered by the AMA to be the practice of medicine. It is subject to peer review and potential disciplinary action (American Medical Association 1998). Should a complainant file an ethics complaint, the AAPL ethics committee does not serve as a regulatory body. Although AAPL contends that the ethics of forensic practice are substantially different from clinical practice to demand its own ethics, AAPL has no means of addressing an ethics complaint. Instead, a complainant is referred to the APA and/or state medical board. The APA ethics committee handles complaints in accordance with pertinent APA bylaws and the *Principles of Medical Ethics With Annotations Especially Applicable to Psychiatry*. Complaints are usually first addressed by the ethics committees of district branches. The committee can act only on complaints against members of the organiza-

tion. The APA *Principles* outlines details regarding the procedures, enforcement, and sanctions in response to a complaint against an APA member. It can be an emotionally taxing and costly process for the respondent, and it is usually recommended that the psychiatrist seek independent legal representation. The national committee reviews district findings and recommendations. Sanctions recommended by the committee may include reprimand, censure, expulsion, or suspension from the APA. The respondent may be required to have education, supervision, or other corrective actions as directed by the ethics committee (American Psychiatric Association 2008). The frequency of child forensic complaints is not published, but expulsions and resignations during the process of ethics investigations are rare (Sondheimer and Klykylo 2008). Ethics committees of medical professional organizations are required by law ([Health Care Quality Improvement Act of 1986]) to report expulsions and prolonged suspensions to the National Practitioners Data Bank.

Ethical Issues in Child Forensic Evaluations

Attorney Interactions

Child forensic psychiatrists can be very beneficial to attorneys in multiple capacities. It is ethical to interview an evaluee, prepare a child to testify, assist in the development of cross-examination questions for an opposing expert witness, or serve as an educational consultant (Leavitt and Armitage 2002). In each of these roles, the child expert will maintain sound standing if the psychiatrist remains an objective consultant to the attorney. Essential considerations when interacting with attorneys are summarized in Table 2–2.

TABLE 2–2. Essential considerations when interacting with attorneys

- Forensic experts should serve as objective consultants to attorneys.
- The referral questions and parameters of the evaluation should be clarified with the attorney.
- The evaluation belongs to the hiring attorney or court, if court-ordered.
- It is customary to ask for a retainer fee, but contingency fees are unethical.
- Prior to beginning an evaluation, forensic psychiatrists should ensure that they have the time and sufficient competency to complete the evaluation.
- Evaluations should be avoided if any of the parties are already known.
- It is unethical to alter reports or opinions at the request of an attorney.

Prior to agreeing to serve any function for an attorney, terms should be set with the referring attorney, including the attorney's expectations and specific referral question. The legal question and parameters of the evaluation should be clarified with the attorney, not with self-referred patients who lack legal representation, unless the referred patients are attempting to represent themselves. The evaluation belongs to the hiring attorney or the court, and the expert serves as a consultant. In the case of children, multiple attorneys are often involved, including separate attorneys for the children and parents. A forensic psychiatrist should be clear about the role, scope, and responsibility of each attorney to his or her client. If hired by a specific attorney, care should be exercised about disclosure of information or *ex parte* communications with the other attorneys. All parties should be treated equitably and respectfully.

The forensic fees for evaluation, report writing, travel, and testimony should be presented explicitly to the hiring attorney who agrees to be responsible for the final bill. It is ethical to charge higher fees for forensic time according to expertise and experience because it can be highly disruptive to a clinical practice. It is customary to ask for a retainer fee. A forensic psychiatrist also should ensure that sufficient time is available to complete the evaluation and be available for potential depositions or testimony.

After review of the referring question, forensic psychiatrists should review their own competencies and biases in the requested area to ensure they can be objective and helpful to a court. Psychiatrists should avoid evaluations when one of the parties is known or if other potential conflicts of interest arise. Materials, school records, court records, police records, past testing, and previous mental health evaluations should be requested from the attorney. If the attorney is unethical, withholds critical information, or suggests unethical behavior such as demanding a contingency fee, a forensic expert should withdraw. If the attorney chooses not to use the evaluation, it is generally unethical to testify for the opposing attorney because parties are not notified of this possibility prior to interviews. Attorneys may request the alteration of reports. It is ethical to make grammatical changes or correct facts such as birth dates, but it is not appropriate to alter an opinion or "spin" a conclusion in favor of one side by omitting or altering contradictory evidence. A forensic psychiatrist is never paid for an opinion and should not become overinvested in a particular outcome (see also Chapter 1, "Introduction to the Legal System").

Informed Consent and Assent

Before beginning an evaluation, all parties should be informed of the purpose and scope of the interview. If the custody is ambiguous, the forensic clinician should ask for a copy of the custody document that grants legal decision-making power to a particular parent.

Informed consent involves informing a patient or parents, confirming that the parents understand, and achieving voluntary agreement to proceed. Informed consent reflects the principle of autonomy. The purpose of the examination should be reviewed with the child and custodian, even though minors cannot consent to treatment or a forensic evaluation. Minors can consent in some states to receive contraceptives or treatment for pregnancy and drug dependence (Vernick 2002), but a clinician can only seek assent, or a verbal agreement to proceed, from a minor for the purpose of a forensic evaluation. Exceptions to required parental consent may include minors who have been waived to adult court and evaluations sought by the defense for criminal cases in many jurisdictions. Federal regulations now mandate that children's assent, in addition to parents' consent, is necessary before a child can be a research subject. Although assent is not mandated in most forensic situations, it should be sought out of respect for a child's capacity, rights, and vested interest in the outcome. If an evaluee is not adequately warned before the evaluation of the purpose, the gathered information may not be usable.

Explaining the rationale of an examination and determining an evaluee's understanding of the notice of nonconfidentiality can sometimes be difficult, particularly when evaluating children and adolescents. Evaluees should understand that the evaluation does not involve treatment, and the judge makes the ultimate decisions. Children may be incapable of giving meaningful consent. Before age 14 years, and before the formal operations stage, children tend to reason more concretely. In these situations, the use of guardians ad litem can be considered to provide adequate advocacy to a child.

Similar to a clinician reviewing the potential side effects of a medication with a patient, forensic psychiatrists may consider how much time and information are needed for adequate consent. If too much effort is spent on formally informing a patient, the rapport will be limited, and the evaluee may not be forthright. However, if the evaluee does not understand the warning, and the evaluation proceeds without any documentation of this limitation, it may create a worse situation than if no protection were legally presumed.

Some have suggested that the amount of information and level of demonstrated understanding should correspond to the stakes of the legal matter. A juvenile's waiver to adult court should require strict procedural and substantive protections, but a status offense may be less stringent (Barnum et al. 1987).

Confidentiality

Despite the locus of decision making, children should be aware of the limits of confidentiality. Limits of confidentiality must be explained to all involved parties. Confidentiality is more likely to be broken for children than for adults. Similar to informed consent, determining a child's appreciation of the limits of confidentiality can be complex. Very young or developmentally immature children may not be able to appreciate confidentiality or conceptualize that adults keep secrets from one another (Koocher 2003). For children and adolescents, there is no such thing as absolute confidence. In most jurisdictions, parents have the right to access the minor's health records. Although most parents will respect bounds of confidentiality if properly outlined before an evaluation, children are generally allowed to keep secrets as much as the parents will permit. In forensic evaluations, children should be aware that what they say will be written in a report that parents can read. As in clinical situations, forensic clinicians also should warn children and adolescents that they are obligated to report any statements minors make that endanger themselves or others. Forensic clinicians remain mandated reporters in forensic settings, and any reasonable suspicion of child abuse or neglect may need to be reported to state authorities regardless of the source or context of the information.

Child Mental Health Records

In forensic evaluations, clinicians are highly invested in examining the utmost pertinent data regarding an evaluee. More information has the potential to formulate a more objective and balanced opinion. However, the pursuit of data can often create a tension with an individual's rights to privacy and against self-incrimination. In most situations, the privilege to keep mental health records confidential belongs to the patient, and only he or she can waive it.

For children, only the legal custodian can waive the privilege of confidentiality. Forensic evaluators should ask parents to sign and date documents that formally release their children's records. Therapists should be cautious about the release of any mental health records. Therapists should discuss the request for records with the custodian and parents. If obligated to release information, only essential information should be divulged. In particularly sensitive evaluations such as custody, the evaluator or treating therapist could consider asking the judge to appoint a guardian ad litem to review the records and determine their relevance and potential risk of harming the future therapist-patient relationship (Coates et al. 2004). The same guardian ad litem may be empowered to oversee the child's privacy and exercise the child's privilege (such authority is not routine in many jurisdictions).

In limited situations, privilege is negated. In a malpractice suit, a plaintiff waives control over the medical record. The full medical record and corresponding clinicians are accessible to the defendant. In many jurisdictions, medical records are similarly accessible when a defendant makes his mental status a legal question such as in matters of competency and insanity.

Competency and Insanity Evaluations

Children are not permitted legally to drive a car, vote, or enter into a contract. Society assumes that children have social, cognitive, and emotional limitations that render them unable to have the same rights and privileges as adults. These jurisdictional boundaries based on age are supported by little empirical evidence (Jones and Cauffman 2008). Even though incompetent in all of these areas, children and adolescents are presumed competent in juvenile courts until the issue is raised, and only some states require juveniles to be competent to stand trial in juvenile court. The child forensic psychiatrist must be proficient in assessing the developmental needs of a child and the ability of the child to work with legal counsel and become involved in the decision-making process (Morrison 1986). Parental involvement does not guarantee the protection of incompetent juvenile defendants in the legal process (Pierce and Brodsky 2002), and a significant percentage of juveniles do not receive effective legal representation. Many adolescents waive their right to counsel and neglect further afforded procedures (Ainsworth 1996).

The case of *In re Gault* (1967) heralded the beginning of the legal status and due process of children such as the right to counsel, the right to cross-examine witnesses, and the privilege against self-incrimination. However, juvenile courts have varied regarding the need for competency to proceed. The importance of competence is often diminished by the polarizing view of holding a child accountable for violent crimes (Baranoski 2003). As courts responded to increased juvenile violent crimes by criminalizing the courts, some wondered if children were still viewed as less culpable and more amenable to rehabilitation (Grisso et al. 2003).

A child forensic psychiatrist has the developmental expertise to assess competence. There are many types of competencies throughout a legal process. Each competency needs to be carefully assessed on an individual basis. Because a juvenile can competently waive Miranda rights, he or she is not automatically competent to stand trial (Redlich et al. 2003). In *Godinez v. Moran* (1993), the court decided that a defendant's waiver to proceed to trial pro se was no higher than the competence standard (Fitch 2007). Although the standards may be equal, it would be unethical to assign a general competency to adolescents given their rapidly changing developmental course.

To punish a person, *mens rea* (a guilty mind) is required. Very little literature is available regarding the insanity defense in the juvenile justice system. Criminal responsibility will become increasingly important in a more retributional system (Newman et al. 2007). An evaluator should notify a defense attorney before engaging a minor in a self-report of an alleged crime. Furthermore, an ethical forensic psychiatrist should ensure that a child appreciates the purpose and potential consequences of recounting the offense by sufficiently disclosing the parameters of the evaluation and actively seeking to ascertain the child's developmental understanding before proceeding. Should the expert determine that the evaluee does not adequately comprehend the purpose and scope of the evaluation, these findings should be explicitly reported in the evaluation.

Juvenile Waiver to Adult Courts

Even though juveniles have gained many legal rights, they still lack significant procedural process. Juveniles are not afforded a jury trial, and they can be held in preventive detention without bail. Consequences of delinquency can include detention in juvenile correctional facilities until age 21 and waiver to diversion programs or the adult criminal court system. The consequences of adult court include the loss of the right to vote, longer sentences, and criminal records that can be used against the juvenile at a later date (Horowitz 2002). Children are more likely to be victimized in adult correctional settings, and fewer services exist to focus on their developmental needs (Zerby and Thomas 2006).

The Supreme Court in *Kent v. United States* (1966) rejected the arbitrary transfer of a juvenile to criminal court without due process (Quinn 2002; Zerby and Thomas 2006). (See Chapter 26, "Juvenile Waiver and State-of-Mind Assessments," for more detailed information about juvenile waiver.) Experts can give the court developmentally sound recommendations regarding rehabilitation and treatability (Zerby and Thomas 2006). Given the potential consequences of adult court compared with juvenile court, the juvenile should have the opportunity to consult with a parent and/or counsel before the clinical examination. The juvenile should participate with demonstrated understanding of the purpose of the evaluation (Barnum et al. 1987).

Correctional Setting/ Juvenile Facilities

Forensic psychiatrists are often employed at correctional settings, caring for the mentally ill among the juvenile population. Juvenile detainees have a higher incidence of mental illness, even after conduct disorder is excluded (Abram et al. 2003). Compared with the community, juveniles have higher rates of disabilities, trauma, and posttraumatic stress disorder (PTSD). Studies have confirmed incidence rates of PTSD among juveniles in custody to range from 11.2% to 48.9% (Abram et al. 2004). The problems should be addressed through advocacy, and forensic psychiatrists can play an important role in the care and treatment of juveniles.

However, psychiatrists must not become entangled in the problems of dual agency, attempting to simultaneously serve the masters of a patient and the judicial system. The roles of clinician and forensic evaluator must be clearly demarcated and clarified for the patient, staff, and psychiatrist. Dual roles should be avoided except when absolutely necessary, such as geographic areas that have a shortage of providers. Clinicians emphasize advocacy and patient-focused care and may be called to testify as fact witnesses. As the treatment provider, it is ethical to testify regarding the patient's diagnosis and treatment if obligated to comply, but the clinical provider should avoid opinions and judgments that are more reserved for the role of an expert witness.

Sexual Abuse Allegations

Forensic evaluations that assess sexual abuse allegations can be emotionally charged and have the risk of enticing a forensic evaluator away from the role of neutral, objective fact finder to an advocate for a particular position. Important ethical principles regarding sexual abuse allegations are summarized in Table 2–3. As an advocate, questions have a higher likelihood of confirming the bias. Before psychiatrists agree to such an evaluation, they must have training and competence in child development, child interviewing techniques, attachment, and trauma. All opinions should be based on empirically established relations between data and the behavior of interest rather than subjective observations.

It is not within the scope of this chapter to review the effect of questions and interview techniques on children's suggestibility and report of allegations, which are discussed in more detail in Chapter 17 ("Interviewing Children for Suspected Sexual Abuse"), but an evaluator should understand the risks of inappropriate questioning before embarking on this inquiry. If qualified, the expert must maintain a fact-finding role, consider multiple hypotheses, seek multiple sources to test the validity of these hypotheses, and avoid conclusions based on insufficient evidence (Kuehnle 1998). As the standardization of the conduct of sexual abuse evaluations has increased, the reliability of expert opinion about whether abuse occurred has not necessarily improved (Ash and Derdeyn 1997). The forensic clinician is ethically bound to stay current on the relevant literature. In the process of this evaluation, if the forensic expert suspects abuse, state authorities must be notified.

Child Custody and Parental Termination of Custodial Rights

Case Example

Dr. A has been a 9-year-old girl's therapist for 2 years. After initial improvement, her depression slowly worsened in the last 2 months. Dr. A asks for some time with her mother, who has faithfully brought her daughter to all of her appointments. Her mother shares that she has recently separated from her husband after she discovered that he was abusing cocaine on the weekends with friends and recounts examples of poor parenting on his part. The mother believes that her daughter's depression has worsened because of her father's erratic behavior. She asks Dr. A for help in an upcoming custody dispute: "A letter explaining the problems for a young girl with a drug-abusing father would be extremely helpful. I just want what is best for her."

Evaluations that involve the custody of children have the potential to permanently affect the relationships of multiple people. They are matters that require a high level of ethical behavior from the evaluator. If a forensic expert does not remain vigilant, these evaluations can expose personal biases and prejudices. It is not atypical to identify with a particular patient and to have biases about custody arrangements, the role of the father, or homosexual parents (Schetky 1998). Other biases may concern the economic conditions of a parent and the ability to provide for a child. According to the AACAP practice parameters for custody evaluations, the evaluator should be aware of biases and seek objective evidence to provide to a court. An expert should be adequately trained to conduct these evaluations, and a clinician involved in the treatment of any of the parties should avoid opinions or speculation about custody. Parties on both sides should be equitably interviewed (Herman 1997). In custody matters, the best interest of the child is the legal standard, but this usually translates to the least detrimental alternative.

Cases that involve the termination of parental rights have extremely high stakes, and procedures regarding confidentiality and consent should reflect the highest standards.

The warnings should be more thorough and formal (Barnum et al. 1987). The legal standard for terminating parental rights is determining that a parent's care is not minimally adequate; however, many parents' capacities are just above this line (Quinn 2002). In these situations, forensic experts may feel a tension between representing an opinion in what they consider to be best for the child and telling the objective truth. Rescue fantasies and educational and class biases have the potential to further jade a forensic evaluation. For instance, restoring custody to an impoverished mother in recovery from drug abuse from affluent parents whose foster child is thriving under their care may pull a clinician to make questionable ethical compromises (Schetky 1992).

Case Example Epilogue

After considering the issues and best interest of the patient, Dr. A respectfully declines to involve himself in the parents' custody dispute. He explains that participating in the custody litigation would be potentially damaging to his therapeutic relationship with their daughter. Furthermore, Dr. A empathically tells the mother that he appreciates her concern about the

TABLE 2–3.   Ethical principles regarding sexual abuse allegations

- Evaluations that assess sexual abuse allegations are highly specialized and require sufficient training, supervision, competency, and ongoing education.
- Evaluators should remain neutral, objective fact finders.
- Opinions should be founded on supportive objective data.
- Multiple hypotheses must be considered, including contradictory and supportive data.
- If a forensic expert suspects abuse, state authorities must be notified.

father's alleged drug abuse, but it would be inappropriate to write an opinion to the court regarding their daughter without interviewing both parties. Dr. A suggests that the parents seek an independent guardian ad litem or custody evaluator who can assess the needs of their daughter. Meanwhile, Dr. A will further explore if the father is endangering his daughter's life by his alleged drug abuse. If Dr. A has such a suspicion, he will report this to state authorities.

Expert Witness

At the conclusion of an evaluation, forensic experts may be called to testify regarding their opinions in a legal matter. Expert witnesses are permitted to opine in judicial settings when they have special knowledge that will be useful to inform the fact finder. Psychiatrists strive to be honest and objective in this process. One can tell the subjective truth by saying what one believes to be true, and one can tell the objective truth by acknowledging the limitations of the testimony (Appelbaum 1997). For instance, it is important to state that an opinion is based on only records if the evaluee was never personally interviewed.

Lawyers may attempt to shape expert testimony through an examination that elicits truthful data but still does not represent the entire truth. The courts can further impose limits on testimony about the whole truth. Experts are instructed to answer attorneys' questions responsively and not argue. They have little control over the judicial process, and they must comply with the legal rules. The court will consider whether the testimony was presented in a fair, thorough, and objective manner. Forensic psychiatrists must tolerate the tension between the legal goal of justice and their commitment to presenting the truth and defending their opinions against misrepresentation. Experts can often rely on the retaining attorney to correct and sharpen their opinion for the fact finder. An expert plays a role only in the larger workings of the court. Ethical psychiatrists should concede the limits of testimony, make clear the parameters of the opinion, speak truthfully, and remain alert to actions that distort their opinions such as inaccurate summations or misleading questions (Gutheil et al. 2003). An expert can be vigorous and forceful in the courtroom but strive for honesty and objectivity.

—Key Points

The definition, professional consensus, and enforcement of ethical principles are essential to the practice of medicine. These rules and standards are not absolute because they cannot anticipate every future clinical dilemma, but they serve as the foundation and theoretical framework to analyze behavior and decisions. Child forensic psychiatry is a unique and highly specialized field that frequently confronts moral dilemmas. Attention to ethics will assist the child expert navigating through these complexities. Key ethical considerations include the following:

— Child forensic psychiatrists' clinical dilemmas often conflict with traditional medical ethical principles: beneficence, do no harm, autonomy, and justice.

— Adult forensic psychiatrists have struggled over their own ethical basis for more than two decades, ultimately recognizing justice as the foremost governing principle.

— Although several ethical codes and theories apply to child and adolescent forensic mental health work, many controversies remain regarding key ethical principles in these areas.

— The "standard" ethical position for most adult forensic psychiatrists is to seek justice by striving for honesty and objectivity while respecting individuals. However, the meaning of "striving" and "objectivity" remain controversial.

— An area that differentiates adult and child forensic work is the lack of a child's capacity to consent to a forensic evaluation, which then implicates ethical issues that are centered on autonomy.

— Child forensic psychiatrists have not articulated their own ethical framework through guidelines or principles.

— Child forensic experts are currently bound by the ethical principles of their professional organizations.

— The ethics committees of the district (or state, depending on the organization) branches of professional organizations handle ethics complaints.

— Given the original rehabilitation goals of the juvenile system, justice may not sufficiently address the moral dilemmas of a child forensic expert.

— Children are uniquely tied to their custodians, and child forensic ethics are challenged by the distinction between children and adults as autonomous persons.

— Children should be considered as rapidly developing individuals. Experts can serve an important role by assessing children in forensic settings and educating courts.

— Given the high emotional valence of many child evaluations, such as determinations of custody, maintaining objectivity and minimizing personal biases are essential.

References

Abram KM, Teplin LA, McClelland GM, et al: Comorbid psychiatric disorders in youth in juvenile detention. Arch Gen Psychiatry 60:1097–1108, 2003

Abram KM, Teplin LA, Charles DR, et al: Posttraumatic stress disorder and trauma in youth in juvenile detention. Arch Gen Psychiatry 61:403–410, 2004

Adshead G, Sarkar SP: Justice and welfare: two ethical paradigms in forensic psychiatry. Aust N Z J Psychiatry 39:1011–1017, 2005

Ainsworth JE: The court's effectiveness in protecting the rights of juveniles in delinquency cases. Future Child 6(3):64–74, 1996

American Academy of Child and Adolescent Psychiatry: Code of Ethics With Annotations, 1995. Available at: http://www.aacap.org/galleries/AboutUs/CodeOfEthics.pdf. Accessed December 14, 2008.

American Academy of Psychiatry and the Law: Ethics Guidelines for the Practice of Forensic Psychiatry, 2005. Available at: http://www.aapl.org/pdf/ethicsgdlns.pdf. Accessed December 14, 2008.

American Medical Association: AMA Policy Compendium 1998: Policy H-265.993. Chicago, IL, AMA Press, 1998

American Medical Association: Principles of Medical Ethics, 2001. Available at: http://www.ama-assn.org/ama/pub/category/2512.html. Accessed December 14, 2008.

American Psychiatric Association: The Principles of Medical Ethics With Annotations Especially Applicable to Psychiatry, 2009. Available at: http://www.psych.org/MainMenu/PsychiatricPractice/Ethics/ResourcesStandards/PrinciplesofMedicalEthics.aspx. Accessed June 10, 2009.

American Psychological Association: Ethical Principles of Psychologists and Code of Conduct, 2002. Available at: http://www.apa.org/ethics/code2002.pdf. Accessed June 10, 2009.

Appelbaum PS: A theory of ethics for forensic psychiatry. J Am Acad Psychiatry Law 25:233–247, 1997

Appelbaum PS: Ethics and Forensic Psychiatry: Translating Principles Into Practice. J Am Acad Psychiatry Law 36:195–200, 2008

Ash P, Derdeyn AP: Forensic child and adolescent psychiatry: a review of the past 10 years. J Am Acad Child Adolesc Psychiatry 36:1493–1502, 1997

Baranoski MV: Commentary: Children's minds and adult statutes. J Am Acad Psychiatry Law 31:321–326, 2003

Barnum R, Silverberg J, Nied D: Patient warnings in court-ordered evaluations of children and families. Bull Am Acad Psychiatry Law 15:283–300, 1987

Beyer M: Fifty delinquents in juvenile and adult court. Am J Orthopsychiatry 76:206–214, 2006

Bloom JD, Dick DW: Commentary: 1982 was AAPL's year of living dangerously. J Am Acad Psychiatry Law 36:175–180, 2008

Coates CA, Deutsch R, Starnes HH, et al: Parenting coordination for high-conflict families. Family Court Review 42:246–262, 2004

Committee on Ethical Guidelines for Forensic Psychologists: Specialty guidelines for forensic psychologists. Law and Human Behavior 15:655–665, 1991

Dike C: Is Ethical Forensic Psychiatry an Oxymoron? J Am Acad Psychiatry Law 36:181–184, 2008

Dingle AD, Stuber ML: Ethics education. Child Adolesc Psychiatr Clin N Am 17:187–207, xi, 2008

Fitch WL: AAPL Practice Guideline for the Forensic Psychiatric Evaluation of Competence to Stand Trial: an American legal perspective. J Am Acad Psychiatry Law 35:509–513, 2007

Godinez v Moran, 509 US 389 (1993)

Griffith EE: Ethics in forensic psychiatry: a cultural response to Stone and Appelbaum. J Am Acad Psychiatry Law 26:171–184, 1998

Griffith EE: Personal narrative and an African-American perspective on medical ethics. J Am Acad Psychiatry Law 33:371–381, 2005

Grisso T, Steinberg L, Woolard J, et al: Juveniles' competence to stand trial: a comparison of adolescents' and adults' capacities as trial defendants. Law Hum Behav 27:333–363, 2003

Gutheil TG, Hauser M, White MS, et al: "The whole truth" versus "the admissible truth": an ethics dilemma for expert witnesses. J Am Acad Psychiatry Law 31:422–427, 2003

Herman SP: Practice parameters for child custody evaluation. American Academy of Child and Adolescent Psychiatry. J Am Acad Child Adolesc Psychiatry 36 (10 suppl):57S–68S, 1997

Horowitz R: Legal rights of children. Child Adolesc Psychiatr Clin N Am 11:705–717, 2002

In re Gault, 387 US 1 (1967)

Jones S, Cauffman E: Juvenile psychopathy and judicial decision making: an empirical analysis of an ethical dilemma. Behav Sci Law 26:151–165, 2008

Kent v United States, 383 US 541, 556 (1966)

Koocher GP: Ethical issues in psychotherapy with adolescents. J Clin Psychol 59:1247–1256, 2003

Koocher GP: Ethical challenges in mental health services to children and families. J Clin Psychol 64:601–612, 2008

Kuehnle K: Ethics and the forensic expert: a case study of child custody involving allegations of child sexual abuse. Ethics Behav 8:1–18, 1998

Leavitt WT, Armitage DT: The forensic role of the child psychiatrist in child abuse and neglect cases. Child Adolesc Psychiatr Clin N Am 11:767–779, 2002

Martinez R, Candilis PJ: Commentary: toward a unified theory of personal and professional ethics. J Am Acad Psychiatry Law 33:382–385, 2005

Miller GH: Alan Stone and the ethics of forensic psychiatry: an overview. J Am Acad Psychiatry Law 36:191–194, 2008

Morrison HL: The forensic evaluation and treatment of children: ethics and values. Bull Am Acad Psychiatry Law 14:353–359, 1986

Morse SJ: The ethics of forensic practice: reclaiming the wasteland. J Am Acad Psychiatry Law 36:206–217, 2008

Newman SS, Buckley MC, Newman SP, et al: Oregon's Juvenile Psychiatric Security Review Board. J Am Acad Psychiatry Law 35:247–252, 2007

Norko MA: Commentary: Compassion at the Core of Forensic Ethics. J Am Acad Psychiatry Law 33:386–389, 2005

Parham v J.R., 442 US 584 (1979)

Pierce CS, Brodsky SL: Trust and understanding in the attorney-juvenile relationship. Behav Sci Law 20:89–107, 2002

Quinn KM: Juveniles on trial. Child Adolesc Psychiatr Clin N Am 11:719–730, 2002

Ratner RA: Ethics in child and adolescent forensic psychiatry. Child Adolesc Psychiatr Clin N Am 11:887–904, ix, 2002

Redlich AD, Silverman M, Steiner H: Pre-adjudicative and adjudicative competence in juveniles and young adults. Behav Sci Law 21:393–410, 2003

Schetky DH: Ethical issues in forensic child and adolescent psychiatry. J Am Acad Child Adolesc Psychiatry 31:403–407, 1992

Schetky DH: Ethics and the clinician in custody disputes. Child Adolesc Psychiatr Clin N Am 7:455–463, ix, 1998

Sen P, Gordon H, Adshead G, et al: Ethical dilemmas in forensic psychiatry: two illustrative cases. J Med Ethics 33:337–341, 2007

Sondheimer AN, Klykylo WM: The Ethics Committees of the American Academy of Child and Adolescent Psychiatry and the American Psychiatric Association: history, process, education, and advocacy. Child Adolesc Psychiatr Clin N Am 17:225–236, xi–xii, 2008

Stone AA: The ethical boundaries of forensic psychiatry: a view from the ivory tower (Bull Am Acad Psychiatry Law 12:209–219, 1984). J Am Acad Psychiatry Law 36:167–174, 2008

Taylor RW, Buchanan A: Ethical problems in forensic psychiatry. Curr Opin Psychiatry 11:695–702, 1998

Vernick AE: Forensic aspects of everyday practice: legal issues that every practitioner must know. Child Adolesc Psychiatr Clin N Am 11:905–928, 2002

Weinstock R, Leong GB, Silva JA: Opinions by AAPL forensic psychiatrists on controversial ethical guidelines. Bull Am Acad Psychiatry Law 19:237–248, 1991

Winnicott DW: The theory of the parent–infant relationship, in The Maturational Processes and the Facilitating Environment. London, England, Hogarth Press, 1965, pp 37–55

Woolard JL, Harvell S, Graham S: Anticipatory injustice among adolescents: age and racial/ethnic differences in perceived unfairness of the justice system. Behav Sci Law 26:207–226, 2008

Zerby SA, Thomas CR: Legal issues, rights, and ethics for mental health in juvenile justice. Child Adolesc Psychiatr Clin N Am 15:373–390, viii, 2006

Chapter 3

Introduction to Forensic Evaluations

Diane H. Schetky, M.D.

Case Example 1

Dr. A is doing a custody evaluation on a family with three children. The father has agreed to pay for the evaluation in installments, with the final payment due prior to the release of her report. The court date is approaching, and Dr. A, being compulsive and conscientious, has her report ready to release pending the final payment. She receives a telephone call from the father saying that he and his wife have decided to reconcile and do not need her report.

Case Example 2

An attorney refers his client to a child and adolescent psychiatry clinic for a forensic evaluation of her parenting skills. The state has filed a petition to terminate her parental rights, and he is requesting an independent evaluation. The attorney insists his main concern is with what is in the best interests of his client's children. Dr. B, a resident, is assigned the case and reviews records, meets with the mother, and observes her with her young children. He produces a very comprehensive report in which he raises serious concerns about the mother's parenting skills. He is irate because the attorney does not like his findings and chooses not to use his evaluation.

Case Example 3

An attorney calls Dr. C requesting an urgent evaluation of her client's two children, who are refusing to return to their mother after a 2-month summer visitation with their father, the client. The children are

alleging physical abuse by their mother and verbal abuse by their stepfather.

Legal Issues

Dealing With Attorneys

Initial Involvement With a Case

Attorneys contact forensic examiners because of mental health– or disability-related issues in their cases, which, according to one survey of attorneys and judges, arose in one-seventh of their cases and in one-third of juvenile cases (Mossman and Kapp 1998). The same survey found that the most important factors attorneys consider in selecting expert witnesses are their knowledge, ability to communicate, and local reputation. The importance of obtaining a favorable opinion from the expert ranked only fifth above previous experience with the expert. Attorneys are also interested in the integrity of a potential witness and whether he or she will stand by his or her opinion.

Most often, forensic referrals come directly from an attorney or the guardian ad litem for the child, or the expert is appointed by the court. Requests for parenting assessments may also come from protective services. Those requests that come directly from parties involved in a legal matter always should be funneled through their attorneys to clarify legal issues and determine that they, in fact, have legal representation. It is wise to ascertain whether a psychiatric or psychological examination is being requested because some attorneys and judges do not understand the difference.

In the initial contact, the attorney will want to know something about the forensic examiner's background. It is customary for the expert to send his or her curriculum vitae; however, this alone does not reflect forensic experience. The latter may be kept in a separate file and should include the names of the cases in which the forensic examiner has testified or been deposed, docket numbers, court jurisdiction, dates of cases, types of cases, places of testimony, and names of retaining attorneys. A computer database is a good way of keeping track of forensic cases. The retaining attorney may request this list, as may the attorney for the other side once the examiner's name has been produced as a potential witness. The forensic examiner should be aware that attorneys also have ready access to any prior testimony he or she has given through computer databases such as WestLaw and Lexis-Nexis, and they may read any relevant publications authored by the forensic examiner.

It is important to clarify which party the contracting attorney represents, and it is useful to know who the parties and other attorneys are to rule out any possible conflicts of interest. For instance, I was once requested to do a visitation assessment by an attorney representing a father who lived in Alaska who said that the children in question lived "somewhere in the midcoast area of Maine." Somewhere in midcoast Maine turned out to be a block away from my home, which was too close for comfort, and I withdrew from the case.

Determining the Purpose of the Evaluation

Because the legal issue at hand will be the focus of the evaluation, it is critical to know what it is and what the pertinent legal standard is; the forensic examiner must be certain that he or she understands the meaning of the wording. Attorneys may not always be sure at the onset of a case how they plan to defend it. They may be seeking the views of an expert to determine whether, for instance, mental illness provides grounds for an insanity defense or in civil cases whether damages have ensued as a result of psychic trauma. It is useful to request a cover letter in which attorneys articulate their particular questions about the case.

In child and adolescent forensic psychiatry, cases typically involve issues of child custody, personal injury, criminal issues, presentencing evaluations, occa-

sional malpractice cases, and, rarely, the insanity defense. These issues are discussed in subsequent chapters (see Chapter 11, "Child Custody Evaluation"; Chapter 12, "Parenting Assessment in Abuse, Neglect, and Permanent Wardship Cases"; Chapter 13, "Children in Foster Care"; and Chapter 29, "Civil Litigation and Psychic Trauma"). The distinctions between civil and criminal cases are major. Civil cases that involve money typically have a lower standard of proof (preponderance of evidence), and abuse or neglect cases usually have clear and convincing evidence as the standard. Criminal cases that involve potential loss of liberty generally require a higher standard of proof (beyond a reasonable doubt). In practical terms, civil and custody cases often take years to settle. Criminal cases are settled more swiftly and are usually heard on a trailing docket, which means that the expert may be called to testify on short notice.

Spelling Out Ground Rules

Forensic examiners should never give premature assurances about the nature of their potential testimony until they have had a chance to complete their evaluation. It is advisable for the forensic examiner to tell the referring attorney that he or she will call the case as he or she sees it, which may not necessarily be to his or her liking. Examiners should make it clear from the onset that their ethics and objectivity will not be compromised. It is generally not possible, nor is it ethical, to offer diagnostic opinions on a particular party one has not personally evaluated. However, experts may be retained for other purposes such as critiquing prior evaluations, testifying about theoretical issues, or advising the attorney on trial strategy.

Deciding Whether to Accept a Case

Expert's Qualifications

The expert needs to ask whether he or she has sufficient expertise in the area in question, because credentials will be reviewed in court as part of qualifying the expert. If he or she has doubts, these should be shared with the referring attorney, and he or she might even suggest a more experienced colleague. Neophytes should not be embarrassed by paucity of credentials; inexperience may often counter the image of being a hired gun. For instance, knowledge of forensic principles and the ability to do a thorough, objective assessment may be more important than being able to boast of having seen two dozen juvenile arsonists. It is always appropriate to seek consultation on difficult cases at any stage in one's career.

The expert also needs to be open regarding any skeletons in his or her closet that might preclude his or her involvement in a case, such as a pending malpractice suit, prior ethical complaints, or even a recent arrest for speeding or driving under the influence, if relevant to the case.

Merits of the Case

Considering the time and energy that go into a forensic evaluation, it is useful at the onset to ask whether the case merits such an investment on your part. Is this an issue about which the expert feels strongly? Are there enough data available to permit an in-depth evaluation? If a party is claiming false allegations of abuse, is there sufficient doubt to warrant examining the records or parties?

Time and Distance Limitations

It is almost always ill advised to accept a case on short notice. Rarely is there time in which to do adequate preparation, and such referrals often indicate that a witness has backed out of the case at the last minute or that the attorney is poorly organized.

Given the paucity of child and adolescent forensic examiners, requests for evaluations from out of state are not uncommon, particularly if the expert has a national reputation or area of special expertise. One needs to weigh the effect of time lost to travel on one's practice and family.

Trials may not proceed on schedule, and the expert may spend many long hours waiting to testify or stuck in airports. Travel time need not be lost time and can be put to good use reviewing the case, reading, or enjoying audiobooks. Geographic desirability and novelty-seeking genes also enter into the equation. A word of caution: accepting a case in Florida in the depths of winter may be appealing, but the case is likely to come to trial in the heat of summer.

Conflicts of Interest

Dual agency occurs if one has a duty to two different parties, such as the therapist who tries to simultaneously act as forensic examiner, as was discussed in Chapter 2, "Ethics of Child and Adolescent Forensic Psychiatry." With forethought, such duality can be avoided in most situations.

Sometimes the opposing side may contact an expert after he or she has already discussed the case with the other side's attorney. This is almost always grounds for refusing to become involved, even if the side that first contacted the expert did not hire the expert because he or she is now tainted and privy to confidential information and considered part of the first attorney's team. If this situation arises, the forensic examiner should cite a conflict of interest without going into details. Unfortunately, some attorneys engage in what Berger (1997) refers to as preventive contracting, in which they contact a potential witness with no intention of using his or her information, merely to prevent the other side from retaining that person.

Another conflict of interest might involve a vested interest in the outcome. For example, the forensic examiner might happen to hold stock in a discount department store that is being sued by the parents of a 5-year-old who was injured when a large, poorly stacked box fell from a shelf and landed on her head.

Any prejudices the examiner holds that could be related to the case also should be shared, such as strong feelings about sexual preference or custody arrangements.

Is the Attorney Someone With Whom the Forensic Examiner Can Work?

It may not be possible to determine whether the expert can work with the attorney until the expert has begun the evaluation. In some instances, the examiner can ask around about the attorney's reputation and speak to others who might have worked with him or her. Qualities to look for include legal acumen, ethical conduct, respect for clients, organizational skills, and good communication skills. It is important that attorneys be accessible, maintain good lines of communication with their experts, and not withhold important information. Attorneys who are unduly familiar or attempt to seduce you with flattery or money should give you reason to think twice about accepting referrals from them.

Liability of the Expert Witness

Can an expert witness be sued for what that witness says in his or her report or on the witness stand? In most jurisdictions, if the expert is court appointed, he or she is considered to be acting in a quasi-judicial capacity and accordingly is entitled to the protection of absolute immunity. Courts have expanded the doctrine of absolute judicial immunity to include those persons involved in an integral part of the judicial process. This enables them to act freely without the threat of a lawsuit and encourages them to act with disinterested objectivity. Less clear is the liability of the expert who is acting without a court order. Liability of experts is discussed in more detail in Chapter 30, "Malpractice and Professional Liability."

Out-of-State Cases

In 1998, the American Medical Association passed a resolution stating, "expert witness testimony is the practice of medicine." This has raised the unresolved question of whether licensing should be required in each state in which the expert testifies. If the expert is asked to perform a forensic evaluation in a state where he or she is not licensed, then the expert must ascertain that the laws of that state permit him or her to perform an evaluation and/or testify there. If not, the expert might be disqualified to testify and could face civil or criminal actions as well as disciplinary actions (Simon and Shuman 1999). Reid (2000) provides a useful list of state licensure requirements for out-of-state forensic psychiatric examinations. Yet another issue to be aware of is that the examiner may not be covered by liability insurance if he or she is conducting an evaluation in a state where he or she does not hold a license and that state requires licensure for forensic evaluation. Alternatively, the evaluee could come to a state where the expert is licensed to perform the evaluation.

It is important to become familiar with the legal standards of the examinee's state and the interpretation of these standards, particularly if they differ from those in the state in which the forensic examiner works. For instance, within the United States, there are three different standards for the insanity defense, and the wording of the standards varies from state to state.

Clinical Evaluations

Structuring the Evaluation

Fees

Fees should be discussed at the onset. Rates vary regionally and by experience and are customarily much higher than the reimbursement one would receive for psychotherapy. Justification for higher rates includes added training and skills, the demanding nature of the work, and the often-disruptive effect these cases have on one's practice and life. Most experts charge by the hour. Gutheil (1998) recommends choosing a fee that you would not be embarrassed to state in court. Exorbitant fees may alienate jurors and lead them to believe

your opinion has been bought. Flat fees are not a good idea because one can never anticipate exactly how much time might be involved in a case. The amount of material to be reviewed in civil cases often mushrooms as the cases mature and as parties and their experts are deposed; the expert may be asked to review hundreds of pages of depositions.

In out-of-state cases, it is customary to request a per diem rate in addition to reimbursement for travel, lodging, and meals. It is not proper to bill for time spent sleeping. When possible, a retainer fee should be requested at the onset, which covers estimated time to be spent reviewing records, interviewing parties and collaterals, conferring with the attorney, and preparing a report. Retainers are not possible when doing defense cases for the state, that is, for a public defender or protective services, and often there is a cap on what they are willing to pay. Reimbursement in state cases is usually lower, but the cases are often of interest and good for the learning curve.

Some forensic experts charge more for time spent testifying. The amount of time spent in court is but a small fraction of the time devoted to the case, and jurors may raise eyebrows at what they view as excessively high fees for courtroom testimony.

Contract With the Attorney

It is advisable to develop a service agreement with the retaining attorney. This should cover the nature of the services to be provided, the expert's hourly rate, and policies on billing for telephone calls, missed appointments, or appointments canceled at the last minute. In addition, it should cover per diem rates, travel policies, and expectations of reimbursement for portal-to-portal travel and waiting time when called to testify. A statement that failure of the party to pay the attorney does not relieve that attorney of obligation to pay fees related to the referral should be included. The attorney should sign the agreement and return a copy to the examiner. The expert should provide the attorney with his or her tax identification number to expedite payment.

Access to Parties and Information

Having agreed to participate in the case, the examiner should state which parties he or she wishes to see, discuss which records to review, and anticipate approximately how much time will be involved. Attorneys can be very helpful in amassing and even indexing discovery material such as school records, prior psychiatric evaluations, medical records, and hospitalizations. Physicians are not the best judges of what material is legally relevant, nor are attorneys the best judges of what materials are clinically relevant. Therefore, it is often necessary to sift through a great deal of information, some of which may not be relevant. The other rationale for reviewing all of the material is to make sure the attorney has not withheld records unfavorable to his or her client. However, there may be cases in which it would be prohibitively expensive to expect the expert to read all of the documents that do not appear to be relevant to the forensic issue in question.

Deadlines

Attorneys, in contrast to psychiatrists, work under a variety of deadlines. Discovery dates refer to the deadline for listing one's experts and allows each side time in which to review data, depose experts, and explore strategies prior to trial. Written reports need to be submitted prior to trial in time to allow both sides to review them. It is important to inquire whether the referring attorney wants a written report and, if so, by what date.

Determination of Need for Further Consultation

Early into the evaluation, it is usually apparent what additional consultations will be needed. For instance, psychological testing often helps bolster the examiner's opinions and may be useful in ruling out "faking good" in parenting assessments or "faking bad" in tort litigation. Neurological or other medical assessments may be indicated in some children, and these should be obtained in time to incorporate results into the expert's report.

Scheduling

Berger (1997) recommends that referring attorneys schedule the evaluation and offers a twofold rationale for this: 1) if the patient fails to show or arrives late, this becomes the attorney's problem, and he or she is liable for paying for the scheduled time; and 2) it avoids the problem of prior contact with the examinee, which might affect the examiner's objectivity. However, direct contact with the parties might ensure that they know how to find the examiner's office, and some of these early interchanges may be quite telling and could be considered part of the evaluation.

Obtaining Consent

At the onset, the examiner must clarify with the parties to be examined who retained him or her and for what purpose. The fact that the examination is not therapy should be stated and may need to be reiterated in the course of the evaluation. Examinees must be apprised of the limited confidentiality and told who will have access to the report. The previous discussion provides the basis for informed consent to the forensic evaluation. Forms should be signed indicating consent to the evaluation and waivers for release of information.

If there is any question about capacity to give consent, the examiner should refer to the court or counsel and have a guardian appointed. For instance, I was once asked to do a parenting assessment regarding possible termination of parental rights on a blatantly psychotic woman who denied giving birth to the child in question.

Meeting With the Parents

In ordinary diagnostic evaluations, one assumes that parents are being straightforward and acting out of concern for the child. In contrast, in forensic evaluations, parents' presentations may be colored by the nature of the legal issue, skewed memories, and other motives. In custody or visitation disputes, parents will often offer information that is self-serving and withhold information that might put them in a bad light. Parents in the throes of crisis or divorce may show regressive behavior that is not representative of their usual level of functioning. Occasionally, parents will reveal extremely damaging information about themselves that may raise concerns about their motivation for custody and their judgment. Forensic examiners need to be more aggressive than therapists in looking for contradictions and inconsistencies and probing for more detail.

If parents are not living together, it may be necessary to obtain their respective accounts of the child's history and current functioning. Contradictions may abound and leave examiners feeling as if they are on a seesaw. It is critical to hear both sides to obtain a balanced picture of what is going on and to treat them with parity. This involves spending approximately equal amounts of time with each parent and asking them similar questions. The forensic examiner is not expected to play detective, and many areas of disparity will have to be resolved by the court. Assessment of parental capacity is covered separately in Chapter 11, "Child Custody Evaluation," and Chapter 12, "Parenting Assessment in Abuse, Neglect, and Permanent Wardship Cases."

Meeting With the Child or Adolescent

It is always interesting to ask a child or an adolescent what his or her understanding of the purpose of the evaluation is and whether anyone has told him or her what to say. The child or adolescent needs to be told at the onset the purpose of the interview, with whom it will be shared, and that it is the judge or jury, not the examiner, who is the ultimate decision maker. With young children, the examiner might say that his or her job is to help the judge understand how the child is doing, how he or she has been affected by something, such as divorce or trauma, and what his or her needs are. Most evaluations of a child can be accomplished within 2–4 hours over several visits, depending on the nature and complexity of the case. If the visits are lengthy, as may occur if the child is coming from a great distance, he or she should be offered a break. The risk of extended evaluations is that the child or adolescent may perceive them as a demand for more information and begin to confabulate either for attention or to appease the examiner. In addition, the more involved the examiner becomes, the easier it is to slip into a therapeutic stance.

The interview should be tailored to the legal questions at hand. With young children, the examiner can use standard playroom tools such as puppets, drawing, and a dollhouse. However, it is also necessary to take a more structured approach that includes assessment of cognitive functioning, reality testing, ability to differentiate pretend from fantasy, and memory for past and current events in their lives. As is discussed in Chapter 16, "Reliability and Suggestibility of Children's Statements," and Chapter 17, "Interviewing Children for Suspected Sexual Abuse," the use of narrative recall will yield the most accurate statements from children, and multiple-choice, either/or, and leading questions should be avoided whenever possible. With very young children or those lacking in cognitive maturity, it may be impossible to avoid using some leading questions.

The interview should be recorded in some form, and there is no problem-free way of doing this. Audiotapes do not capture nonverbal behavior and may not always be audible. Videotapes are excellent as teaching tools and for the examiner to review what has transpired. However, it is difficult to keep young children in one place, they may feel intimidated by the camera, and if they have been subjects of child pornography, there is a risk of retraumatizing them. Other concerns about videotapes include the risk that they may be shown in court out of context, be used to coach a witness, or fall into the wrong hands. Taking notes during the interview may distract the child but is an effective way of recording if one's handwriting is legible. It is important to record not only the child's responses to questions but also how the question was phrased. The examiner should be aware that the opposing attorney may request to see these notes, and if they are illegible, he or she may request that they be dictated. Handwritten notes should not be discarded; it is perfectly acceptable for the opposing attorney to request to examine them.

At closure, the child should be praised for effort or cooperation but not for content of what is disclosed. It is important not to give the child any premature assurances about the outcome of the case.

Rarely, a third-party parent, guardian, or attorney may request to sit in on the evaluation. This is usually awkward, and the third party may influence or inhibit the evaluee or, by his or her very presence, imply that the examiner is not to be trusted. This practice should be discouraged unless the examinee is a very young child with separation problems or terrified of the evaluation and needs a support person, or an interpreter is needed. The examiner might want to check state laws applicable to this situation.

Observing the Parent–Child Relationship

Observing children with their parents is an important part of any evaluation involving custody or visitation. Exceptions might be an infant removed at birth who has no relationship with the parent or children who are not having ongoing visitation with their parents. Observing interactions between parent and child is an excellent tool for assessing attachment and parenting skills, which are discussed further in Chapter 11, "Child Custody Evaluation," and Chapter 12, "Parenting Assessment in Abuse, Neglect, and Permanent Wardship Cases." These observations may be made through a one-way mirror, with the examiner sitting in but not participating in the visit in his or her office, or during home visits. These evaluations are also useful for the unconscious material that emerges that a parent does not ordinarily volunteer, such as seductive, intimidating, or overly controlling behavior.

Corroborating Information

Much more effort goes into corroborating information in forensic evaluations than in diagnostic evaluations. If the clinician errs in the initial diagnosis of a patient he or she is treating, then the clinician has the opportunity to reassess and make adjustments in the treatment plan, and usually no serious harm ensues. In contrast, experts do not have the luxury of extended time in forensic evaluations, and much more is at stake concerning the outcome of legal proceedings. For instance, if a father is wrongfully acquitted of child sexual abuse, the victim and other potential victims remain at risk. On the other hand, if a father is erroneously convicted of sexual abuse, irreparable harm is done to his child's relationship with him, not to mention his reputation, career, and the possibility of incarceration.

Because credibility is often an issue in forensic evaluations, care needs to be taken in cross-checking what the child has said to others, when possible. Police reports obtained immediately after disclosures are helpful. Although children's descriptions of abuse may shift over time, the core features usually remain consistent. Results of physical examinations are helpful in determining whether injuries are consistent with allegations. However, the examiner should heed the dictum that absence of physical findings does not mean absence of sexual abuse. Verbal reports from teachers, day care providers, and babysitters help complete the picture of how a child is functioning.

Other sources of valuable data include school reports, past psychological testing, and previous psychiatric evaluations. These may be used to document prior levels of functioning relevant to a particular trauma or event. They also provide cross-checks on the reliability of the history given by parents. Not uncommonly, parents may ascribe all of a child's symptoms to a particular event, but a review of the records indicates similar behaviors prior to the trauma being litigated or other traumas not volunteered by the parents.

Covering Housekeeping Issues

Keeping track of all the discovery material that accompanies a case is challenging. Attorneys will often want to know at what point materials were received and whether they were read before or after the forensic examination. In civil cases, documents may arrive with each page already numbered (e.g., Bates numbers) by the attorneys for their use and the court's use in referring to documents. For unnumbered pages, Berger (1997) offers a useful system for labeling documents, in which the first packet is labeled A, with the date on it, and lowercase letters are used for the individual documents, followed by numbers, indicating the number of pages in the document; for example, Ab 1–3.

The next packet received would be Ba 1–5, Bb 1–10, and so on. Mailings are usually accompanied by cover letters listing the enclosures. It is important to cross-check to ensure that no pages are missing.

Sometimes material arrives nicely indexed in a binder. At other times, there may be no apparent order. It is helpful to begin by reviewing the complaint, then the police or the medical and psychiatric reports in chronological order, saving the opinions of other experts or professionals until the end so as not to be biased by them. It is tempting to use highlighting markers in reviewing documents, but the risk is that the other side may request to see the materials you reviewed and question the meaning of highlighted material. Alternatively, you can make notations on a separate piece of paper or a laptop computer as you go along, indicating the pages to which you are referring. It is very useful to construct a timeline of significant events, which will help to organize the chronology of the case and also may accentuate inconsistencies in the history.

It is not unusual to end up with several crates of materials on a case, and storage soon becomes a problem. Records need to be kept until a case has settled, and it is prudent to hold onto your own report until the statute of limitations has expired. With juveniles, this does not begin to toll until they have reached the age of majority. It is best to check with the attorney before disposing of other documents related to the case. Disposal of records should be done in such a way that there is no risk of them falling into the wrong hands or flying around the town dump on a windy day. Burning or shredding works well, and the latter may be composted or disposed of with trash. Alternatively, services are available that will destroy records on location.

The Written Report

Function of the Report

The well-written report often becomes a bargaining chip in reaching an out-of-court settlement. Should the case go to court, the report becomes the basis for the expert's testimony and will serve to refresh his or her memory. The cross-examining attorney will attempt to discredit the report, and it is useful to anticipate the weaknesses of the report at the time of writing and rectify them if possible. The report is also the expert's work product and should not contain anything that might embarrass him or her in years to come. Usually attorneys want a preliminary verbal report, and if it is not favorable, they may not want a written report. Sometimes attorneys may request that a report be modified. This is ethically permissible if changes have to do with errors of fact, misinterpretations, rewording of the conclusion to be consistent with statutes, or shortening or elaborating the report. It would be unethical to comply with requests to alter facts or change the expert's opinion.

The report should be directed toward the legal question at issue. The length of the report will depend on the complexity of the issues and sometimes the age of the child. The report should contain the building blocks that provide the foundation for the expert's opinion. It should confirm that the examiner has attempted to rule out other possible causes for the evaluee's behaviors or symptoms. Psychodynamic formulations and speculations should be kept to a minimum because they are difficult to prove in court. A carefully documented history of child neglect, its effect on the child, and a mother's failure to avail herself of services will provide more ammunition for terminating parental rights than will psychoanalytic interpretations about her ambivalence toward her child.

Diagnoses usually are not included in custody evaluations. In contrast, they are more relevant in parenting assessments for protective services and tort litigation that focuses on damages.

Language of the Report

The report is likely to be read by attorneys from both sides, their clients, the judge, and experts hired by the opposing side. It should be free of psychiatric jargon and intelligible to a layperson.

Tact is required, and pejoratives or judgmental statements should be avoided. For example, it is easy to substitute "he states" for "he claims" and "he was suspicious and mistrustful" for "he was paranoid." The report should strive for balance, addressing strengths and weaknesses. Direct quotes are very helpful for bringing the report to life and allowing the parties to speak for themselves. A mother's statement that she is a good mother because her "kids ain't torched the house yet" tells a lot about her concept of parenting. Vague or speculative statements should be avoided along with terms such as *obviously* or *clearly*, which may not be so to others reading the report.

The examiner should proofread the report ever so carefully for typos and content. Computer spell checks are wonderful but do not pick up on transposed names, wrong numbers, and homonyms. Finally, the envelope in which the report is sent should not be overlooked. I once used a new typist who sent a report to "The Horrible Judge Gil." Fortunately, Judge Gil had a sense of humor.

Organization of the Report

The report should bear the examiner's letterhead, and the title of the report should reflect that it is a forensic evaluation. It is useful to have the evaluee's birth date among identifying information so that when the expert goes to court months or years later, he or she can remember how old the child was when examined. It also helps to orient the reader. The report might be organized as follows:

- *Circumstance of the evaluation.* This indicates who retained the forensic examiner and for what purposes.
- *Sources of information.* This section includes both firsthand and secondhand information that was relied on in reaching a conclusion and recommendations. The report should reflect where, when, and for how long the examiner saw the parties. If records were requested but never received, this should be stated.
- *Purpose of evaluation.* This section should state the legal issue and what was requested of the forensic examiner.
- *Informed consent.* This part of the report should begin with comments that the purpose of the evaluation has been discussed with the evaluee along with discussion regarding who might have access to the report.
- *History.* In relating the history, it should be clear from whose perspective it is coming—that is, "according to the mother"—rather than presenting data as factual. History that is not relative to the issue may be excluded or abbreviated.
- *Observations and foundations for opinions.* Direct observations provide a strong bulwark for opinions and should be carefully detailed. The evaluee's manner should be described in terms of degree of cooperation, defensiveness, and rapport that may have bearing on the material elicited. Whether to include a formal mental status examination will depend on the nature of the legal question being asked. In custody evaluations, which parent brought the child may have bearing on that session. Children's drawings may be amended to reports, but caution should be exerted in how much interpretation to offer. Often they will speak for themselves. Inasmuch as they may be admitted

into evidence, the examiner should make a copy so as not to be left empty-handed.

- *Other sources of information.* Those sources of information relied on in forming the opinion may be summarized and may include police, school, medical and psychiatric records, and other collateral parties with whom the expert has spoken.
- *Formulation and recommendations.* Any conclusions must be supported by data in the report, including the history, direct observations, and records reviewed. Courts are likely to ask whether opinions are fair and reasonable and whether recommendations are feasible. In some cases, it may not be possible to arrive at an opinion; for example, whether a child's allegations of sexual abuse are credible. In such cases, one can state the pros and cons; the limiting factors that made it difficult to resolve the questions, such as young age of child at time of alleged abuse; or contaminated interviews. The examiner can still be helpful to the court by coming up with recommendations to safeguard the child.

Pitfalls

Forensic Examiner–Related Pitfalls

Myopia

The expert may be overly focused and, for instance, only see the world through the lens of child sexual abuse. He or she is not troubled by the nonspecificity of the sexually abused child syndrome and fails to consider that enuresis in a child of divorcing parents might just be stress-related. Such an expert tends to cling to his or her views, is not open to other interpretations for a child's behavior changes, and fails to do an in-depth evaluation.

Bias

Closely related to myopia is the problem of bias. As noted in Chapter 2, "Ethics of Child and Adolescent Forensic Psychiatry," the examiner may not even be aware of it. Perhaps the worst sort of bias is the expert's conviction that he or she is not biased. Judge Bazelon (1974) noted: "Like any other man, a physician acquires an emotional identification with an opinion that comes down on one side of a conflict: he has an inescapable, prideful conviction in the accuracy of his own findings."

Dual Agency

It is very easy to fall into the trap of dual agency if the expert is not vigilant about his or her role. The examiner cannot wear two hats and cannot serve two masters.

Inadequate or Faulty Database

Taking shortcuts usually backfires and may end up embarrassing the evaluator. For instance, a guardian ad litem wrote off a father based on information obtained solely from the mother. She went through a cursory home visit, spending a total of 15 minutes with him, and had nothing good to say about him in her report. She was quite embarrassed in court when a neutral child development specialist who had spent ample time observing both parents with their toddler countered many of her negative assertions.

Nonmedical clinicians may misinterpret physical findings; for example, equating yeast infections or urinary tract infections with child sexual abuse. If in doubt, they should confer with the physician who treated the child in question.

Quoting the Literature

It is tempting to bolster one's opinions by citing the literature. This is usually a losing gambit, because the other side will come up with tomes countering the expert's opinion and will make the expert look foolish when forced to admit that he or she has not heard of the impressive texts from which they are quoting. If the other side happens to quote something written by the expert, the expert should ensure that it is in context and ask to see it.

The Need to Please

Forensic psychiatrists may succumb to the need to please the referring attorney. This may occur out of the wish to be liked or from fear of turning off a good referral source.

Inflation of Credentials

The examiner should not try to inflate a meager curriculum vitae with courses taken, lectures attended, or media interviews given. The examiner should not imply that he or she is board certified if the examiner is only board eligible. The examiner should not be apologetic about his or her status, but should draw on any cumulative learning and training and remember that even the most respected forensic psychiatrists once stood in his or her shoes.

Evaluee-Related Pitfalls

Noncompliance

If an evaluee fails to appear or appears but refuses to participate in the evaluation, the evaluee's attorney should be notified. In some cases, a limited report may be submitted on the basis of record review alone. Failure of the evaluee to cooperate should be noted.

"You've Been Had"

Getting taken in by a con artist or skilled psychopath is a learning experience. Such a person may be very charming, use the right buzzwords, and even feign sincerity and remorse. However, the charm is usually only skin deep, and when the individual does not get his or her way, he or she can become intimidating and threatening. History usually points to externalizing behaviors, lack of conflict about his or her behavior, and antisocial behaviors.

Harassment

Harassment may occur in the form of threats to one's person, obscene telephone calls, or calls in the middle of the night with no one on the other end. Such calls should be reported, although the telephone company is not always helpful. A female psychiatrist complained about obscene telephone calls she was getting at her office and was told to get an unlisted number. She solved the problem on her own by getting caller ID. Stalking behaviors should be reported to the police. A more likely form of harassment is the filing of complaints without merit against the expert with licensing boards or ethics committees. Some examinees arrive with a long history of litigious behavior, which should put the forensic examiner on notice.

Attorney-Related Pitfalls

Coercive Tactics

A lawyer may have trouble hearing no and may try to convince the expert to alter his or her report or testimony. If the attorney is behaving unethically, this is reason to withdraw from the case (Gutheil and Simon 1999).

Withholding of Information

Lawyers need not send the forensic examiner all of the relevant discovery material they have. If they withhold critical pieces of information, such as the fact that a

mother has lost custody of two previous children, this is a problem. The lawyer may attempt to defend his or her actions, stating that he or she did not want to bias the examiner. However, if the lawyer is not being honest with the examiner, it will be difficult to work with him or her. Furthermore, it is preferable to hear damaging information from the lawyer than to be confronted with it for the first time while being cross-examined.

Boundary Violations

Attorneys, like mental health professionals, are not immune to boundary violations. They may occur with clients, expert witnesses, or both. If an attorney who has never met the forensic examiner calls the examiner at home on the weekend, addresses him or her by first name, and is unduly familiar, this should raise red flags. The examiner might do well to avoid contracting with this attorney.

Unpreparedness

An unprepared attorney often requests an expert "under the wire," sounds disorganized and inarticulate, and is not entirely clear about what he or she wants from the examiner. If the attorney acts this way with the examiner, the examine should wonder how the attorney will present himself or herself in court.

Poor Communication

If an attorney is too busy to return calls from the examiner, the examiner should wonder if the case is important to the attorney and whether he or she will devote adequate time to it. Mental health professionals also can be faulted for not returning calls. However, with answering machines, fax machines, e-mail, and cell phones, there is no excuse for notifying an expert, just before he or she was scheduled to testify, that a case had settled when the attorney had known this for a week. Experts also appreciate follow-ups on the outcome of court cases and feedback, both good and bad, on their testimony.

Case Example Epilogues

Case Example 1

Not only is Dr. A's report not needed, but the father refuses to pay for the time she spent preparing it, stating that the lawyers in the case have depleted his funds. Dr. A is left with the options of taking the father to small claims court, paying for her attorney to write him a letter, handing the account over to a collection agency, or overlooking the bill. She resolves to work only on retainer in future custody cases and to have a formal contract regarding payment with the retaining attorney.

Case Example 2

Dr. B has become too invested in his evaluation and the outcome. He has forgotten that he did the evaluation for the attorney, not the children, and that it is protected as the attorney's work product. The attorney ethically is bound to represent his client's interests and wishes, despite telling Dr. B that he only wants what is best for the children.

Case Example 3

Dr. C, who is a seasoned forensic psychologist, immediately asks what the custody arrangement is and learns that the mother has sole custody of the boys. He informs the attorney that he cannot see the children without the mother's permission and offers the attorney several suggestions, including 1) getting consent from the mother, 2) contacting protective services, and 3) petitioning the court for an order to change custody.

Action Guidelines

Strive for Honesty and Objectivity

The forensic examiner should not be afraid to admit that he or she does not know something. He or she should take time to self-reflect and examine the basis for his or her opinions. Ethical integrity will help maintain the examiner's reputation and that of the profession.

Maintain Control of the Evaluation

The forensic examiner must be firm about his or her terms and not allow anyone to force him or her into doing something that he or she feels is unethical or against the law.

Learn to Live With Ambiguity

The forensic examiner should avoid premature closure and wait for pieces of the puzzle to fall into place. He or she should try to look at issues from all sides and steer a middle course according to what seems most reasonable. The examiner needs to reconcile himself or herself to not being able to resolve all contradictions.

Learn to Critique the Report From the Other Side

The forensic examiner should ask himself or herself, "How will this statement stand up under cross-examination?" The examine needs to try to anticipate where he or she is vulnerable and consider how to deal with the weaknesses in the case.

Recognize Limitations

The forensic examiner should not overload himself or herself with too many forensic cases or too many cases of one kind. He or she should avoid exceeding the limits of his or her database when offering opinions. The examiner should be cautious about making predictions and recognize that past behavior is usually the best predictor of future behavior. He or she needs to pace himself or herself and take good care of himself or herself.

Seek Consultation

When in doubt, the examiner should turn to a more experienced colleague. He or she may use peer review or ethics committees of professional organizations. Legal consultation may be available from a hospital's attorneys or the expert's liability insurance plan carrier. Effective use of consultation also provides some protection in the event that one is sued.

Keep Current and Stay Involved

The forensic examiner should not allow fears of the legal system or malpractice litigation to restrict his or her practice. He or she must read the forensic literature, take courses, attend annual meetings, stay involved, and learn from each case.

References

American Medical Association: Report of the Board of Trustees on Expert Witness Testimony. Board of Trustees Report 18-1-98. Chicago, IL, American Medical Association, 1998

Bazelon D: Psychiatrists and the adversary process. Sci Am 230:18–23, 1974

Berger S: Establishing a Forensic Psychiatric Practice. New York, WW Norton, 1997

Gutheil T: The Psychiatrist as Expert Witness. Washington, DC, American Psychiatric Press, 1998

Gutheil T, Simon R: Attorneys' pressures on expert witnesses: early warning signs of endangered honesty, objectivity and fair compensation. J Am Acad Psychiatry Law 27:546–553, 1999

Mossman D, Kapp J: Courtroom whores or why do attorneys call us? Findings from a survey on attorney's use of mental health experts. J Am Acad Psychiatry Law 26:27–36, 1998

Reid W: Licensure requirements for out-of-state forensic examinations. J Am Acad Psychiatry Law 28:433–437, 2000

Simon RI, Shuman DW: Conducting forensic examinations on the road: are you practicing your profession without a license? J Am Acad Psychiatry Law 27:75–82, 1999

Chapter 4

Testifying

The Expert Witness in Court

Praveen Kambam, M.D.

Elissa P. Benedek, M.D.

It has been estimated that mental health clinicians participate in up to 1 million legal cases per year. The involvement of psychiatrists, psychologists, social workers, nurses, nurse clinicians, and mental health clinicians in the legal arena continues to grow and remains controversial. Expert testimony by mental health professionals potentially alters many lives—the lives of plaintiffs, defendants, and the experts themselves. The appropriate role of a mental health professional as an expert witness has been debated by numerous authors; while the debate rages, mental health professionals continue to participate as expert witnesses and consultants to attorneys and courts. In this chapter we discuss the broad role of the expert witness from a psychiatrist's point of view.

Legal Issues

Basis of Expert Testimony

A mental health professional may be called to testify as a *fact witness* or as an *expert witness*. A fact witness testifies about matters directly observed and is treated the same way as other witnesses. For example, a treating psychiatrist may be asked to provide information about his or her patient's symptoms, diagnosis, course of treatment, and prognosis. If a patient enters his or her emotional and mental health into the record as a possible cause of damage, the treating psychiatrist is at risk for being called as a fact witness.

The psychiatrist may attempt to dissuade an attorney from calling him or her by suggesting that a review of the patient's psychiatric care and other information may not be helpful to the patient's case. For example, if a patient alleges emotional damages subsequent to sexual harassment during the course of employment, it would not be helpful to the patient if medical records revealed intensive psychotherapy and psychopharmacology 3 years prior to the alleged incidents. This tactic is ordinarily more persuasive to an attorney than suggesting that testifying in court will disrupt the doctor–patient relationship or may be harmful therapeutically to a patient since, unfortunately, for many attorneys the "case" is more important than the patient's mental health. If the patient's attorney insists on the treating psychiatrist's testimony, the psychiatrist may call his or her own attorney for advice. As a final effort, the treating psychiatrist can attempt to contact the judge personally; however, this tactic rarely succeeds.

An expert witness possesses "specialized knowledge" and may opine about facts relevant to his or her area of knowledge and "assist the trier of fact [jury or judge] to understand the evidence or to determine a fact in issue" (Federal Rules of Evidence 2006). One may be "qualified as an expert by knowledge, skill, experience, training, or education" (Federal Rules of Evidence 2006). The expert's testimony must be relevant to the matter in dispute, reliable (have a scientific basis), and based on special expertise not otherwise available to the average layperson. Probative value should be greater than prejudicial value; that is, the testimony must be deemed to do more good than harm. An expert witness may draw conclusions from his or her own database (e.g., examination and knowledge) and others' databases (e.g., medical records). For example, an expert asked to provide an opinion about the psychiatric diagnosis and amenability to treatment of an adolescent brought into the juvenile justice system may examine the patient, review school and medical records, speak with family members, speak with school teachers about the behavior of a patient, and request that psychological testing be done. Additionally, information gathered by others and communicated to the expert (e.g., via depositions, interviews, psychological testing, and other laboratory testing) may be useful in formulating an opinion, and after reviewing the other opinions, the expert may be allowed to formulate an opinion using hearsay material (material not gleaned from a firsthand assessment of the patient).

The underlying theory of the American legal system and the adversarial model of justice requires that each side advocates the causes they represent without perjury or manufactured evidence. The expert's client is the attorney or the court that asks for his or her consultative expertise. Regardless of whether the expert's testimony helps or harms the attorney's client, the expert's job is to inform and educate the judge or jury, not to empathize with, treat, or help a patient.

In many cases, an expert's testimony is helpful; in others, it is essential and required, and a court may even refuse to entertain certain forms of litigation without expert testimony. For example, in Michigan, in a medical malpractice case, without an expert agreeing in a written affidavit that there are legitimate grounds for a suit, the court will not entertain the case. Throughout the United States, in standard of care or medical malpractice cases, only an expert in a particular medical specialty can offer testimony about standard of care (e.g., an obstetrician would not generally be accepted as an expert with regard to depression and suicidal ideation). Moreover, the advent of advanced technology in the mental health field has resulted in increasingly complex litigation and has intensified the use of psychiatrists and psychologists to explain to the court sophisticated tests, procedures, and their meaning—for example, the Millon Clinical Multiaxial Inventory (MCMI) and computed tomography (CT) or magnetic resonance imaging (MRI) scans.

In criminal cases, failure to engage an expert may constitute ineffective assistance of counsel and result in the reversal of a conviction. For example, in death penalty cases in which ingestion of drugs is involved prior to the commission of a crime, failure to call a psychopharmacologist or an addiction specialist may constitute grounds for an appeal and a possible reversal. In *Ake v. Oklahoma* (1985), a murder case that involved possible mental illness, no psychiatrist was called to testify. The U.S. Supreme Court overturned a conviction on the grounds that the defendant, Ake, should have had access to psychiatric assistance in preparing an insanity defense. The court stated, "We note that when the defendant has had a preliminary showing, his insanity of the time of offense is likely to be a significant factor at trial. The Constitution requires the State provide access to a psychiatrist's assistance on this issue if the defendant cannot otherwise afford one."

Tort Reform

One area in which expert mental health testimony is most used is in civil litigation, or torts. A tort is a civil wrong, other than a breach of contract, committed against a person for which the law provides mechanisms for compensation for the resultant injury. In the United States, there has been a movement for tort reform, including attempts to raise burden of proof rules to control the use of professional experts and exclude "hired guns." Gutheil (2009, p. 7) defines a hired gun as "an expert witness who sells testimony instead of time." Hired guns may testify to opinions favorable to an attorney and his or her client regardless of their clinical validity or may be recognized as often testifying in areas beyond their expertise or only for the plaintiff or defense.

In Michigan, for example, in an attempt at tort reform, the state senate passed a bill that required an expert to devote no less than 50% of his or her professional time to active clinical practice in the same specialty as the physician who is identified as a defendant in a medical malpractice action, or to be an instructor in that specialty in a medical school. Mental health professionals are routinely queried during voir dire examinations regarding the amount of time they spend in clinical practice and are disqualified as experts if they no longer practice clinical medicine/psychiatry. For example, during a high-profile trial, one well-known psychiatrist, who testified primarily as a plaintiff's expert, admitted that he had last seen a patient in clinical practice 10 years prior to testifying as an expert with regard to the use of medication in a psychiatric patient. The court opined that his experience was no longer current nor was it applicable.

Exceptions to Expert Testimony

The three most common exceptions to the broad admissibility of expert testimony are 1) eyewitness reliability, 2) truthfulness of a witness, and 3) syndrome or profile testimony. Generally, psychologists are called as experts to testify regarding the reliability of eyewitness testimony. This testimony typically focuses on psychological research describing the fallibility of eyewitness memory and the role of such factors as the effects of stress on the witnesses, problems associated with cross-racial identification, and effects of postevent misinformation (i.e., information learned by an eyewitness after the event in question). The legal arguments that have been offered against expert testimony on eyewitness evidence include the following: 1) mental health professionals do not have special expertise concerning eyewitness behavior; 2) the evaluation of the credibility of witness testimony is a province of the trier of fact and therefore not appropriate testimony for an expert; 3) the findings of eyewitness research have not "gained general acceptance in a particular field to which it belongs" (the *Frye* or *Daubert* standard will be discussed later); 4) the findings of eyewitness researchers are common sense, and therefore, there is no need for an expert to inform the court of results; and 5) an expert opinion may have undue influence on jurors, who can sort out credibility issues for themselves.

In eyewitness identification cases, generally it is the defense who wishes to use an expert. In the United States, legal opinion is divided about the value of expert evidence on eyewitness testimony, with evidence allowed in some jurisdictions and not in others. In most states, it is left to the discretion of the trial court judge.

A second area in which expert testimony is often disputed is the area of truthfulness, or credibility, of other witness testimony, such as that may be offered in cases that with deal child abuse, sexual abuse, malingering, or feigning of mental illness. Traditionally, common law did not permit direct expert testimony on the truthfulness of another witness who has simply been observed in the courtroom and not directly examined. Most courts today do not allow expert testimony with regard to client credibility, believing that it invades the province of the trier of fact. Typically, when attorneys attempt to use clinicians to establish the credibility of their client, legal objections are raised and upheld.

Frye Standard

There is considerable resistance in courts to accept syndromes and diagnoses not included in the DSM-IV-TR (American Psychiatric Association 2000). Such syndrome testimony might include battered woman syndrome, brain trauma syndrome, violent parent syndrome, brainwashing, or syndromes surrounding sexual abuse. In the past, courts have held that these profiles or syndromes do not meet the *Frye* standard. This standard or test is derived from language in *Frye v. United States* (1923), when an opinion provided by the district court of appeals in the murder conviction of James A. Frye was affirmed. In an attempt to prove Mr. Frye had been truthful in his description of events concerning the alleged felony, an expert witness attested that the systolic blood pressure taken during a polygraph exam was a definite way to determine if a subject was lying. According to the expert, if the subject were lying, systolic blood pressure would be elevated; if not, it would remain normal. Both the trial court and the appellate court rejected the expert's testimony.

The *Frye* standard, also known as the general acceptance rule, mandates that any scientific or professional opinion expressed by an expert witness must represent generally accepted thinking by a *significant* membership of that discipline or profession. It is not sufficient that an expert may testify that techniques, procedures, or principles are valid or that a court believes that the evidence is helpful or reliable; testimony must meet a standard of general acceptance in the associated scientific community. The *Frye* standard allowed radar evidence, public opinion surveys, Breathalyzers, psycholinguistics, trace metal detection, bite mark comparisons, and blood spatter analysis in the courtroom. On rare occasions, it has been a mechanism for denying polygraph test results, spectrographic voice identification, voice stress test, and hypnosis as a means of refreshing a witness's memory.

Daubert Standard

In 1993, the U.S. Supreme Court established a new standard for the admissibility of scientific evidence in federal court cases in *Daubert v. Merrell Dow Pharmaceuticals, Inc.* (1993). *Daubert* involved the attempt by a plaintiff in a products liability case to introduce expert testimony that the drug Bendectin could cause birth defects. The district court ruled such testimony inadmissible, because all prior studies had concluded that Bendectin did not cause birth defects, thus indicating that the plaintiff's expert's position was not generally accepted within the scientific community. The court of appeals affirmed the district court's opinion. The U.S. Supreme Court reversed, however, holding that the proper standard for admissibility was contained in the 1975 Federal Rules of Evidence, specifically Rule 702, which superseded *Frye* and which provided: "if scientific, technical, or other specialized knowledge will assist the trier of fact to understand the evidence or to determine a fact or issue, a witness qualified as an expert by knowledge, skill, experience, training, or education may testify thereto in the formative opinion or otherwise." The Court ruled that nothing in the Federal Rules of Evidence indicated general acceptance as a prerequisite to the admissibility of scientific evidence.

The standard adopted by the *Daubert* court appears, at first blush, to be more permissive than the *Frye* standard; however, it has been heralded as an important tool provided to trial judges to prevent the introduction of unsubstantiated conjecture or "junk science" into evidence under the guise of expert scientific testimony. *Daubert* required that when faced with an offer of expert scientific testimony, it was part of the trial judge's role to make a preliminary assessment and determine whether that testimony was both relevant and reliable. These preliminary matters must be established by a preponderance of the evidence prior to the introduction of such testimony before a jury.

Daubert thus places the trial judge in the role of gatekeeper. An anonymous legal commentator observed, "Before *Daubert,* the trial judge had to ask, 'What do the relevant scientists think of this?' The judge had to decide, 'Has the proponent of this evidence shown that scientists agree with her?' After *Daubert,* the trial judge had to decide, 'Is this good science or junk science?'"

The role of the judge as gatekeeper of the trial court is designed to prevent juries from being persuaded by "expert testimony" from an expert whose credentials may seem impressive and whose novel theory may seem plausible, but whose opinion is based on "science" or quasi-science that may be worthless. One commentator on *Daubert,* Judge Kozinski, observed, "Something doesn't become scientific knowledge just because it is uttered by a scientist, nor can an expert's self-serving assertion that his conclusions were derived by the scientific method be deemed conclusive." The court's task, then, is "to analyze not what the experts say but what basis they have for saying it" (43 F3d [9th Cir 1995], pp. 1315–1316).

Unfortunately, the Supreme Court in *Daubert* did not provide the trial judges/gatekeepers with concurrent instructions on how to determine when to open or close the gate. It provided a list of factors for trial courts to consider to help determine reliability and basis in the scientific method, such as whether the expert's methodology could be tested and falsifiable, whether it had been subject to peer review and publication, the known or potential rate of error of methodology, and whether methodology is generally accepted within the relevant scientific community, but it did not weigh these factors nor did it note whether all of them needed to be satisfied in a particular case. Moreover, these factors were referred to as "general observations" and were not intended to be an exact checklist.

Two additional Supreme Court rulings have further honed the *Daubert* standard. Together, these three rulings are referred to as the "*Daubert* trilogy." In *General Electric Co. v. Joiner* (1997), the Supreme Court ruled that an abuse-of-discretion standard be used for appellate courts when reviewing a lower trial court's decision regarding the admissibility of expert testimony. Thus, appellate courts must defer to the trial court unless they are clearly incorrect. In *Kumho Tire Co. v. Carmichael* (1999), the Supreme Court ruled that a judge's gatekeeper role applies to all expert testimony, including that which is not scientific.

The principles in the *Daubert* trilogy were incorporated into amendments to the Federal Rules of Evidence, approved by the Supreme Court in 2000. Rule 702, the rule discussing expert testimony, had provisions added which state that an expert witness may only testify "if (1) the testimony is based upon sufficient facts or data, (2) the testimony is the product of reliable principles and methods, and (3) the witness has applied the principles and methods reliably to the facts of the case" (*Federal Rules of Evidence 2006*).

With regard to the acceptance of expert testimony, these standards may prevent testimony from hired-gun experts who may lack sufficient training and experience in clinical diagnosis of mental illness. Additionally, they may bar testimony from experts who, although possessing the requisite training and experience, fail to employ standard diagnostic techniques or who may testify with little more support than that of conjecture. Finally, they may prevent experts without clinical expertise from basing their opinions solely on academic research that may suggest a causal link between a particular event and a significant psychological injury.

Clinical Issues

Negotiation With Retained Attorney

The process of becoming an expert witness begins the moment one accepts a telephone call from an attorney or court and agrees to review the case material (and to possibly become involved in litigation). It continues through evaluation to report writing and may culminate in testifying in court. Thus, in broader terms, being an expert witness involves evaluation, consultation, and possible testimony, despite the fact that this chapter deals predominately with testifying.

Preparation

Subsequent to a clinical evaluation, discussion with an attorney, and completion of a written report, if a clinician becomes aware that testimony at a deposition or trial or answers to interrogatories will be necessary, the clinician needs considerable preparation to be an effective expert witness. Gutheil (2009) described preparation, planning, practice, pretrial conference, pitfalls, and presentation as the "6 *P*s of trial preparation." *Preparation* includes extensively reviewing the database and opposing expert's opinion. *Planning* involves adjusting one's schedule and commitments to allow for changes in the timing or duration of the trial and such mundane matters as knowing where a courtroom is located, knowing how to get into a courtroom, knowing where to park, and advance planning about clinical coverage when one is unavailable. *Practice* involves rehearsing ways of communicating information, including practicing potential visual aids to be used, such as blackboards, video machines, and projectors (see also Chapter 3, "Introduction to Forensic Evaluations").

A *pretrial conference* is recommended to confer with the attorney regarding answers to interrogatories. It is important to review written reports, conclusions, and their meanings with the referring attorney. This formal meeting allows the attorney and the clinician to define medical terminology and legal standards in nontechnical terms. In this setting, clinicians and attorneys have an opportunity to meet one another and to become apprised of the strengths and weaknesses of each other and the case. Such a meeting is also valuable for understanding the attorney's trial strategy, anticipating questions in a deposition, and anticipating a possible sequence of direction and cross-examination. In a trial setting, there may be additional information, not gleaned from medical records, deposition testimony, or other documents, that has been presented to the court by other witnesses prior to one's trial testimony. It is prudent to get a synopsis of the trial testimony to date before being on the stand. The pretrial conference may be used to emphasize particular points indirectly bearing on a plaintiff/defendant's credibility, by underscoring how the plaintiff/defendant's historical narrative in the evaluation process differs from the narrative he or she has presented during deposition and trial testimony. Finally, a pretrial motion may limit the scope of the proposed expert testimony and an expert may not be allowed to testify in certain areas because of a ruling made by the judge before or during the trial.

Pitfalls refer to reviewing weaknesses in one's opinion and anticipating potential areas of attack. By the time testimony is necessary at a trial, it is apparent to both the attorney and consultants that there are weaknesses in the expert's opinion. Opinion testimony by another expert may have been presented. It is important to discuss possible pitfalls and how these will be handled with counsel.

Lastly, *presentation* involves clarifying methods of communicating one's opinion to the judge or jury. Metaphors, analogies, and references to court's and jurors' everyday experience are helpful in this regard. Presentation also encompasses appearance, demeanor, and speech. One should dress in a conservative, nonflamboyant manner that does not detract from one's testimony. An expert should not lean or slouch back, as this conveys that one is anxious, nervous, or bored. An expert should make proper eye contact with the judge or jury; one strategy is to look at an attorney when a question is asked, then break eye contact, turn, and look at judge or jury when answering. An expert should avoid appearing condescending or disrespectful and should treat both sides with courtesy and dignity. Resnick (2003) discussed that style of speech has significant impacts on credibility and cited studies of mock testimony showing powerful speech (straightforward, using more one-word answers) was more convincing than powerless speech (more frequent use of intensifiers, hedges, overly formal grammar, hesitation forms, gestures, questioning forms, and excessive politeness).

Interrogatories and Depositions

Interrogatories

Interrogatories are a series of standardized questions, from one attorney to the opposing side, required to be answered under oath. Interrogatories are similar to depositions in that their purpose is to discover information about the opposed expert and his or her proposed testimony. In some circumstances, interrogatories may be substituted by a letter or report from the expert. In other cases, either the expert will draft the answers to the interrogatories or the attorney will draft answers and the expert will review and criticize them. Although it may be a temptation to allow an attorney to draft a response to an interrogatory and not review it or simply accept an attorney's summary of one's expert opinion, this is not recommended. Interrogatories are a form of sworn testimony and should be treated as such. As knowledgeable as attorneys are, they may not understand how a specific choice of words or medical terms may affect or change an opinion and may either overstate or understate an expert's qualifications to testify in a specialized area (see also Chapter 1, "Introduction to the Legal System").

Depositions

A deposition is stated witness testimony under oath and recorded for use by the court. A deposition has been described as a "dress rehearsal" for a trial. No judge or jury is present at a deposition; however, attorneys, a court reporter, a plaintiff/defendant, and the plaintiff's/defendant's family and friends may be present. The site for a deposition is the expert's choice, and it can be held in a clinician's office, an attorney's office, or a court reporter's office. The proceedings in a deposition are recorded by a court reporter.

Depositions are taken for discovery purposes to preserve testimony and gather information, or for cross-examination at the time of a trial to impeach the credibility of a witness. Originally, depositions were done solely for the purpose of preserving testimony at a trial in the event a potential witness might be unavailable at the time of a trial because of conflicting obligations or even death. Expert witness depositions are often taken *de bene esse* (conditionally, prior to the trial without judge and jury) and may be videotaped and used at trial; however, in our experience, most attorneys prefer live testimony at a trial, since most witnesses present as more interesting and credible live as compared with on videotape.

The second purpose of a deposition is to gather information about what a potential witness may say at a trial and the style and manner of the witness's presentation. Here, the expert's opinions and the basis for such opinions are explored by the opposing counsel. Opposing counsel also has an opportunity to observe

firsthand how an opposing witness will hold up under the stressful circumstances of cross-examination at a trial. Infrequently, experts change their opinions during the course of questioning during a deposition, for example, when attorneys ask if the expert is familiar with a particular piece of evidence or testimony. A change in opinion or waffling of an opinion is always helpful to opposing counsel. Infrequently, after the rigors of a deposition, an expert may decide not to testify if called at trial.

The third purpose of a deposition is to impeach the credibility of a potential witness. During the trial, an attorney may use material recorded in a deposition to demonstrate differences between an expert's answer in a deposition and opinion expressed at trial or information that the expert had previously published. Statements from a deposition may be quoted out of context to support or bolster opposing counsel's position. The potential expert witness should be aware that, especially since the advent of the Internet, attorneys share old depositions and trial transcripts. It is not unusual to have one's opinions from an old deposition or trial be used to impeach a new opinion in a similar but distinct case.

In preparing for a deposition, an expert must know his or her report intimately and be familiar with all materials that have been previously furnished. The subpoena notes what material should be brought to the deposition and may include a curriculum vitae of the expert, copies of the expert's previously published scientific papers, a text that the expert has relied on in formulating an opinion, and other miscellaneous items. All material requested (except the attorney's work products, such as letters) is open to opposing counsel and may be inspected and attached to the record of the deposition as exhibits. These materials include clinical notes, summaries of the case, notes that the expert has generated on medical records, and even other depositions. An expert should be aware that he or she may be asked to explain why he or she has underlined material in a deposition, made a marginal comment, or used a Sticky Note to find or summarize material.

In preparation for a deposition, it is ethical and wise to discuss with counsel the form of answers he or she prefers. Most counsels will advise experts to always answer "yes," "no," "I don't know," or only report in short narratives, being careful not to volunteer any information not required to answer questions. Some others, however, encourage experts to discourse extensively in answer to queries to frighten opposing counsel, to prepare the grounds for settlement, and to discourage trial. Ultimately, it is the expert's choice with regard to style, but the expert should always remain cool, calm, and collected. Even if attorneys become enraged and act in outrageous fashions, the rule to follow is to remain impartial and objective, projecting the sense of a credible and dispassionate witness.

Because a judge is not present to rule on objections, attorneys exercise more latitude in the range of questions. An attorney may offer an objection to a question posed by the opposing counsel, but many attorneys object infrequently. If the behavior of one attorney is too objectionable to the expert, too hostile, too demeaning, or ranges too far and wide, opposing counsel may choose to terminate the deposition and ask for a ruling from a presiding judge on whether to continue; however, termination of a deposition is rare.

It is important to clarify payment for a deposition prior to the actual deposition. If there is reason to believe opposing counsel will not be responsible for payment, it is both ethical and common practice to ask for payment before the deposition. The firm that deposes the expert generally pays for the deposition, although it is prudent to clarify in advance who is responsible for payment. It is also permissible to charge for time spent proofreading the deposition.

The expert is advised to insist on the opportunity to review and sign the deposition even if told the "usual stipulation" is that the expert is not required to review and sign the deposition. The deposition copy should be read carefully and corrected for typographical errors and errors of content. Possessing a written record of the deposition also allows for preparation and review for trial (see also Chapter 1, "Introduction to the Legal System").

Courtroom Testimony

If a clinician has never visited a courtroom, either as an expert or a defendant, it is helpful to visit a courtroom prior to testifying because a courtroom can be a strange, bewildering, and forbidding place to the un-

initiated. The role and function of courtroom personnel may appear unclear, and the mere atmosphere may feel hostile to a novice. A novice may ask a colleague sophisticated in forensics to critique the content of proposed testimony and observe testimony prior to an actual testifying experience. A more experienced colleague may accompany the novice expert to court to provide a support system and to critique the novice's performance subsequent to actual testimony. Table 4–1 offers additional suggestions for the novice.

Qualification of Experts

The process of examination of an expert witness's qualification is called *voir dire*. When an expert is called, the first step in the testimony process is that the attorney leads a witness through a standard set of questions designed to provide the foundation for the expert's credentials. These questions include relevant aspects of education and training, such as medical school, residency, and fellowships and any special qualifications of a particular expert, including membership and offices held in local and national organizations, publications, presentations, awards, and special consultations.

Following the recital of credentials, the opposing counsel has an opportunity to cross-examine further. Opposing counsel may attempt to discredit the expert witness. Opposing counsel's emphasis may be on the weakest areas of the witness's experience and training, such as lack of board certification or special qualifications, limited contact with a particular population, and short duration of a particular evaluation. Some attorneys often skip cross-examination during voir dire, as it allows the expert once again to reemphasize his or her credentials. Voir dire is generally not particularly difficult or dramatically challenging. On occasion, it may feel like a personal attack, and, in fact, it may be a tactic to embarrass or discomfort the expert witness. Experts should remain calm, composed, and dispassionate.

TABLE 4–1. Courtroom testimony: skill-building suggestions

Go to court before acting as an expert witness and observe a skilled ethical expert in action.

Participate in mock trials at a training institution or law school to improve comfort and critically assess errors. Videotapes of mock trials or real trials are also useful for critique training.

Seek feedback from peers who have observed your testimony with regard to style and accuracy of testimony.

Do not underestimate the value of preparation in being an effective expert witness.

Consider watching *Court TV* as a way of desensitizing yourself to anxiety over the courtroom process.

Direct Examination

During the direct examination portion of the testimony, a witness will be asked first to identify the defendant/plaintiff and to explain the facts and conclusions on which an opinion is based. The expert should present all relevant data in a clear, logical, and coherent fashion. If relevant, it is important to present a balanced picture even if data may include information that is not helpful to a particular plaintiff or defendant. Previously discussed aspects of presentation preparation, with respect to communication, dress, demeanor, and speech, should be employed here. The expert should avoid using technical jargon (e.g., terms such as psychomotor agitation, hallucinations, affect, and loosening of associations) and instead use equivalent nontechnical terms. If a technical term is used, the expert should carefully define what the term means and spell it for the benefit of the court transcriptionist. In addition, any laboratory or psychological tests and their significance must be explained. Judges and jurors have no innate understanding of psychological tests, and they may tend to think of psychological testing as objective and clinical evaluations as subjective. On occasion, it is important to articulate that the interpretation of a particular neuropsychological test is as subjective as the interpretation of a clinical evaluation.

During testimony, an objection may be raised. Once this occurs, the expert must wait and allow counsel to argue the merits of an objection and the court to rule on it. A novice expert may find it difficult to remember that an objection is not a personal objection against the clinician but an objection based on a legal precedent or grounds. Testimony is resumed when the court rules on an objection. When an objection is sustained, if an expert witness does not attempt to modify his or her testimony to comply, he or she may be chastised from the bench, making an unfavorable impression on the jury. For example, a judge may sustain an objection to extensive narrative testimony in an area and insist that the expert reply with a "yes" or "no" answer.

The attorney may decide prior to the onset of a trial whether to use direct examination to elicit material that is unfavorable to a client and may be inconsistent with the expert's findings, such as a patient's prior statement, a patient's medical history, or comments by another expert. If such material does not come out during direct examination, it most likely will come out during cross-examination. The ultimate decision in regard to trial strategy and the conduct of the case is the attorney's responsibility (even when the expert may feel or be significantly more experienced than a particular attorney), and second-guessing an attorney is not advised (see also Chapter 1, "Introduction to the Legal System").

Cross-Examination

The behavior of attorneys that arouses the greatest anger among mental health professionals is that exhibited during cross-examination. Purposes of cross-examination include discrediting or impeaching a witness, mitigating the impact of testimony, and telling a client's story, all for the stated purpose of seeking the truth. In practice, a novice expert witness may perceive cross-examination to be more concerned with embarrassing and humiliating the expert. Some attorneys may go to great lengths to suggest bias or expose uncertainty in a witness's testimony. Some attorneys attempt to malign or distort a witness's testimony or to misconstrue it to a judge or jury. The following are some guiding principles for an expert during cross-examination:

1. *Always be honest.* Mental health professionals not only have an ethical responsibility to be honest but are also under a sworn oath in a courtroom.
2. *Acknowledge limitations and admit when you do not have certain information.* That information may not be in the database or in an expert's fund of knowledge and may include specific information about a patient or literature related to a disputed area in the case. Admitting obvious points helps preserve credibility.
3. *Take time to think.* Pausing before answering allows time for collecting one's thoughts and formulating a response, time for objections, and may strategically break up rapid-fire questions from an attorney. If being pushed to answer a question without sufficient time, a witness can request time from the court.
4. *Just as in deposition and other aspects of testimony, do not talk too much.* Straightforward, concise, jargon-free answers are preferred. An expert can be boring if too pedantic or lose the attention of the judge and jury during lengthy, ponderous, and unnecessary explanations.
5. *Conversely, attempt to give full answers.* If a question cannot be truthfully answered in a "yes" or "no" manner, you may state so. If an attorney appears to limit answers, the jury may perceive this as attempting to hide something.
6. *Do not speak for other experts.* An expert can only provide his or her expert opinion and cannot speculate on what other experts might write or say.

7. *Do not be critical of other experts.* Such criticism is ultimately not valid, because it is impossible to know all the material, data, skills, and experience that another expert took into consideration in formulating an opinion. Criticizing another expert is not looked upon favorably by the bench or jury.

Redirect and Recross

During this stage of the proceedings, the experts, attorney, and opposing counsel have an equal opportunity to elaborate challenge points that may have emerged during direct examination and cross-examination. Only material that has emerged on direct and cross-examinations may be referred to during redirect and recross, and objections related to introduction of new material may occur.

Attorneys and psychiatrists are divided with regard to whether experts should answer the "ultimate issue" question in the case. This would mean directly addressing the legal issue in question, for example, whether a person is incompetent or insane, whether a child has been sexually abused, whether parental rights should be terminated, or which parent serves the best interest of a child. Most commentators suggest experts should only testify with regard to evaluation and diagnosis, treatment, and potential outcome. Still others would allow testimony with regard to the ultimate issue.

When the expert's testimony is completed, the judge will excuse the expert. We recommend the expert leave the courtroom to preserve credibility and avoid appearing excessively interested in the outcome of the trial. On occasion, attorneys may request that an expert sit at a counsel's table and act as a personal coach to that attorney while other witnesses are being questioned. It is much better to prepare the attorney for cross-examination of other witnesses ahead of time or during pretrial conferences because stopping by or sitting at a counsel's table may make the expert appear nonobjective and overly invested in the outcome of the case.

Pitfalls

An expert witness must attempt to remain objective and impartial and strive for accuracy in presenting data and conclusions based on a database. The psychiatric expert witness is not an advocate for the plaintiff or defendant. The following pitfalls should be avoided:

Witness-Related Pitfalls

- *Inadequate database.* One should insist on access to all available materials in the attorney's files.
- *Inadequate literature review.* Although one cannot hope to review all the literature in a given area, it is prudent to review the relevant clinical literature in the area in question by other authors, one's own published literature in the area, and deposition testimony that may have been given in the area.
- *Testifying outside one's area of expertise.* It may be seductive to be called an expert and thus easy to be trapped into testifying outside one's area of expertise. One must consider whether one has the proper qualifications, training, and expertise to be an expert and recognize one's limitations and biases.
- *Hired gun.* The psychiatric witness, who always testifies for the prosecution/plaintiff or defense/defendant, fails to remain impartial, and does not base opinions on sound reasoning and factual data will quickly become known in the local and national community as a hired gun.

Attorney-Related Pitfalls

- *Coercion.* Attorneys, adept at persuasion and prepared to evaluate and attack the opposing side of the case, may attempt, overtly or covertly, to coerce a witness into changing an opinion.
- *Lack of preparation.* Attorneys who come to court without adequate preparation may be disconcerting for the expert. Many skilled attorneys are unfamiliar with mental health issues and materials mental health experts use, such as standard textbooks like the DSM-IV-TR (American Psychiatric Association 2000) and the *Physicians' Desk Reference* (2007). A pretrial conference helps the expert determine the degree of the attorney's preparation and make suggestions regarding mental health areas in which the attorney should be knowledgeable.
- *Communications.* Attorneys may not be skilled in communicating legal standards in a nontechnical way. However, it is important for the expert to clarify the legal standard for the referral question and continue to ask for clarification of relevant issues not understood.

Patient-Related Pitfalls

- *Dual agency.* One cannot assume the roles of forensic expert and treating clinician without falling into the trap of dual agency. As noted in Chapter 2,

"Ethics of Child and Adolescent Forensic Psychiatry," it is difficult, if not impossible, to retain the objectivity necessary to be an expert when treating a patient, and in addition, there are ethical guidelines to avoid this dual agency (American Academy of Psychiatry and the Law 2005).

—Key Points

— When functioning as an expert witness, the typical doctor–patient relationship does not exist. An expert witness's client is the attorney or the court that asks for his or her consultative expertise. Regardless of whether the expert's testimony helps or harms the attorney's client, the expert's job is to inform and educate the judge or jury, not to empathize with, treat, or help a patient.

— The *Frye* standard (also known as the general acceptance rule) requires that an expert witness's scientific or professional opinion must represent generally accepted thinking by a significant membership in the associated scientific community.

— The *Daubert* standard places trial judges in the roles of gatekeepers to determine admissibility of expert witness testimony based on a two-pronged test of relevancy and reliability.

— Rule 702 in the Federal Rules of Evidence, incorporating principles of the "*Daubert* trilogy," states that an expert witness may only testify "if 1) the testimony is based upon sufficient facts or data, 2) the testimony is the product of reliable principles and methods, and 3) the witness has applied the principles and methods reliably to the facts of the case."

— Extensive preparation for testimony is critical to being an effective expert witness.

References

Ake v Oklahoma, 470 US 68 (1985)
American Academy of Psychiatry and the Law: Ethics Guidelines for the Practice of Forensic Psychiatry. May 2005. Available at: https://www.aapl.org/pdf/ETHICS-GDLNS.pdf. Accessed June 2, 2008.
American Psychiatric Association: Diagnostic and Statistical Manual of Mental Disorders, 4th Edition, Text Revision. Washington, DC, American Psychiatric Association, 2000
Daubert v Merrell Dow Pharmaceuticals Inc, 113 S Ct 2786 (1993)
Federal Rules of Evidence (2006), Article VII, Rule 702—Testimony by Experts
Frye v United States, 293F 1013, 34 ALR 145 (DC Cir 1923)
General Electric Co v Joiner, 522 US 136 (1997)
Gutheil TG: The Psychiatrist as Expert Witness, 2nd Edition. Washington, DC, American Psychiatric Press, 2009

Kumho Tire Co v Carmichael, 526 US 137 (1999)
Physicians' Desk Reference 2008: Hospital/Library Version, 62nd Edition. Montvale, NJ, Thompson PDR, 2007
Resnick PJ: Guidelines for courtroom testimony, in Principles and Practice of Forensic Psychiatry. Edited by Rosner R. London, UK, Arnold, 2003, pp 37–44

Supplemental Reading

Appelbaum PS: The role of the mental health professional in court. Hosp Community Psychiatry 36:1043–1046, 1985
Appelbaum PS: Evaluating the admissibility of expert testimony. Hosp Community Psychiatry 45:9–10, 1994
Bank SC, Poythress NG: The elements of persuasion in expert testimony. Psychiatry and Law 10:173–204, 1982
Benedek EP: Testifying in court, in Child and Adolescent Psychiatry: A Comprehensive Textbook. Edited by Lewis M. Baltimore, MD, Williams & Wilkins, 1996, pp 1150–1154

Harrol PA: A new lawyer's guide to expert use: prepare your expert so you don't have to prepare for disaster. The Practical Lawyer 39:55–63, 1993

Poythress NG: Coping on the witness stand: learned responses to learned treatise. Professional Psychology 11:169–179, 1980

Quen JM: The psychiatrist as expert witness, and the psychiatrist in the courtroom, in Selected Papers of Bernard Diamond. Edited by Quen JM. Hillsdale, NJ, Analytic Press, 1994, pp 233–248

Resnick PJ: Perceptions of psychiatric testimony: a historical perspective on the hysterical invective. Bull Am Acad Psychiatry Law 14:203–219, 1986

Strassburger L, Gutheil T, Brodsky A: On wearing two hats: role conflict in serving as both psychotherapist and expert witness. Am J Psychiatry 154:448–456, 1997

Weinstock R, Leong G, Silva A: Opinions by the AAPL forensic psychiatrists on the controversial ethical guidelines: a survey. Bull Am Acad Psychiatry Law 19:237–248, 1991

Ziskin J, Faust D: Coping With Psychiatric and Psychological Testimony. Venice, CA, Law and Psychology Press, 1981

Chapter 5

Special Education

Screening Tools, Rating Scales, and Self-Report Instruments

Mary F. Spence, Ph.D.

History of Education

Since the beginning of recorded history, children learned by watching and imitating adults. This established the use of others' judgments about a particular child's skills and abilities. By the middle of the first century, formal education was established in Oriental societies as written language was developed, a definite curriculum was constructed, and established roles (e.g., master, pupil) were created. Greek, Roman, and European civilizations defined what education was, who had access to it, and what beliefs would guide its development. During the Reformation in the early 1500s, access to education began to be seen as a natural right. Hence, the cornerstone of an all-inclusive public educational system was created (Monroe 1907).

The concept of compulsory education for children dates back to the first century, when Jewish high priest Joshua ben Gamla first required a formal process of educating children by age 6 or 7 years. Public education became mandated in the United States in 1852. Efforts to educate those with special needs predated compulsory education, with the American School for the Deaf in Hartford, Connecticut, established in 1817.

A significant amount of governmental legislation is focused on education, with special education law being one of the fastest growing areas of law (Gerl 2008). The system promotes equal access to all because of society's core belief in the value inherent in the education process. This societal value is grounded in the belief that being allowed to fully access educational opportunities affects a person's lifetime in terms of outcomes—financial, social, and personal—perhaps more than any other facet of government-regulated activity. All industrialized countries show a similar emphasis.

The U.S. Department of Education was established in 1980, consolidating educational matters under one department for the first time. More recently, with the passage of the No Child Left Behind Act of 2001 (NCLB; Public Law 107-110), schools must now conduct annual proficiency testing, use evidence-based practices, ensure their teachers meet standards for "highly qualified," and supplement educational services and school choice. Additionally, NCLB increased the schools' requirements to inform, involve, and empower parents. NCLB is a general education initiative that has been broad reaching, with tremendous impact on how schools are mandated to function.

Development of Current Special Education System

During the Great Society years of the Kennedy/Johnson era, the civil rights movement of the 1960s became a significant force worldwide, with widespread civil unrest and efforts to shape governments toward equality. The inclusion of the handicapped in this movement resulted in a change from the established institutionalization methods of caring for the disabled. In 1975, this resulted in the passage of a seminal piece of legislation referred to as the Education of All Handicapped Children Act (Public Law 94-142). This was the first piece of legislation that required a free appropriate public education (FAPE) to all children with disabilities in order for states to receive federal education funds.

According to the National Center for Education Statistics (2008), rates of identification for special education programs increased from 8.3% during the 1976–1977 school year to 13.5% during the 2006–2007 school year. This represents a 62.7% increase in total public school enrollment that is served under the Individuals With Disabilities Education Act (IDEA) during the preceding 30-year period. As the identification of disabilities has increased within educational settings, so has the sophistication of special education legislation. The increased incidence and extensive legal requirements have caused schools to need the expertise of psychiatry and other health-related areas. However, working within school environments is a dramatically different context than working in clinical settings. Professionals who work within school settings must be knowledgeable about educational environments.

Epidemiological data (Walter et al. 2004) indicate that 9% to 13% of school-age children have a diagnosable mental disorder that creates significant functional impairment. Of those 6–9 million children, only approximately 1.5 million receive any type of mental health intervention. Although it is likely that there is considerable overlap between the similar percentages found in the epidemiological and special education data, it is unlikely that they represent identical data sets. Within the schools, students must meet two requirements to qualify for special education. First is the disability itself, which is defined in the law, with special education categories much broader than specific diagnoses within DSM-IV-TR (American Psychiatric Association 2000). For example, children certi-

fied under autism are likely to include the diagnoses of autism, pervasive developmental disorder not otherwise specified, and Asperger's syndrome. Second, the student's disability must negatively affect the student's educational performance. This means that even if a student has been diagnosed by mental health professionals, he or she may not qualify if the disability is deemed to not have "substantial educational impact." For example, a child who is diagnosed with diabetes or attention-deficit disorder (ADD) may not be identified within the schools. Though the child has a medical diagnosis, the ongoing treatment often ameliorates symptoms, rendering the child capable of receiving "educational benefit" without specialized services. This is a key difference between the mental health and educational systems, which one does well to recognize if working with school-age children.

Legislative Mandates in Special Education

Special education services are housed within the U.S. Department of Education and are tightly regulated. Four overarching pieces of federal legislation now set the parameters for educating children with disabilities: 1) the Individuals With Disabilities Education Improvement Act of 2004 (IDEA 2004); 2) Section 504 of the Rehabilitation Act of 1973; 3) the Americans With Disabilities Act of 1990 (ADA); and 4) the Family Educational Rights and Privacy Act of 1974 (FERPA). Two related pieces of legislation that apply to all children and have had broad-reaching effects are the No Child Left Behind Act of 2001 and the McKinney-Vento Homeless Assistance Act of 1986. Educators today are faced not only with the mandate of ensuring that the legal requirements (which still primarily deal with access to service) are met but also with the more challenging issues of determining how individuals who are experiencing poverty or family crises, along with those who have learning differences and significant disabilities, can best learn so that they may become productive members of society. The latter aspect of the work within the field of education is the more arduous, with educators required to develop interventions to effectively deliver an Individualized Educational Plan (IEP).

Despite the preponderance of legal cases within special education law, the demarcation between general education and special education is far from absolute at the implementation level. Legal experts refer to special education law as "new law," which is a term to denote areas of law that have no longstanding foundation in tradition. Since special education law began in the 1970s, it remains a combination of public policy mixed in with congressional mandates and judicial and administrative decisions (Gerl 2008). Because there was need for extensive compromise to pass the bill, vague language was used to reach a majority vote. This increases the chances for litigation to occur on the basis of varied interpretations. The term *appropriate education* is central to the definition of FAPE and has been a key tenet of much of special education litigation for over 30 years (Wrightslaw and Wrightslaw 2007).

Children who have a documented disability may also qualify for services in the form of accommodations (e.g., extended time on tests, oral presentation of written material) under Section 504 or ADA laws. Section 504 indicates that a person must have a physical or mental impairment that substantially limits at least one major life activity. In relation to education, the parameters of these two pieces of legislation are comparable, and both are enforced by the Office of Civil Rights rather than the Office for Special Education Programs within the federal Department of Education, which implements IDEA 2004 legislation. FERPA legislation provides the foundation for confidentiality rights for children with disabilities and is enforced through the federal court system (Sattler 2008). Significantly more protections are afforded students and their families through the special education system procedural safeguards than through either ADA or Section 504 plans.

Definitions

The specific terms used within the fields of education and special education are too numerous to mention. Additionally, they change and are added to frequently, with some terms affected by social desirability or changes in policy and procedure. The ones that are considered to be most essential to the work of the forensic examiner have been included in the text of this chapter, with references included for a more comprehensive listing of such terminology (see U.S. Department of Education 2008; Wrightslaw and Wrightslaw 2007).

IDEA Programs and Services

Because special education is most regulated by the IDEA legislation, it will be reviewed in detail here. It is important to note both its broad-reaching implications and the dynamic nature of case law on new policy and procedure. For example, IDEA allows for protection from disciplinary action under the statute for children who have not yet been made eligible for services when there is "a basis of knowledge" that the child did have a disability (Wrightslaw and Wrightslaw 2007).

IDEA 2004 mandated provision for services to newborn infants and toddlers, commonly referred to as Part C or early intervention. Congress recognized that this developmental period is thought to be the most significant period of brain development. Regulations for early intervention are similar to those under IDEA, although the Individual Family Support Plan mandates more family-centered services. The focus is on promoting school readiness skills, though services are also mandated for children who have been traumatized by family violence. This program has been significantly affected by the public health concerns such as the early identification of autism initiative launched by the Centers for Disease Control and Prevention (2005).

By age 3 years, any student who is certified with an eligible disability is entitled to FAPE, which is provided through the IEP process. Eligibility is regulated by rules and regulations that have been promulgated in each state, using the framework of IDEA. Additionally, the IDEA statute states that the educational program and related services should be designed to meet the students' "unique needs and prepare them for further education, employment and independent living" (IDEA 2004).

An interdisciplinary team at school evaluates any student suspected of having a disability that impacts his or her education. The IEP process refers both to the document that is written to describe the specifics of the educational program and the actual educational program that is provided to a child with a disability. Key considerations in developing an IEP include the following: 1) assessing student, 2) determining how access to the general curriculum is affected, 3) considering how the student's learning is affected, 4) prioritizing goals and objectives, and 5) choosing a placement, with least restrictive environment (LRE) concept as a driving force in the decision-making process.

Least restrictive environment is a principle directive of IDEA. This principle states that, to the maximum extent appropriate, a child with a disability should be educated in the environment that allows the child to be educated with nondisabled peers while ensuring that the child achieves educational outcomes. The implementation of LRE is frequently referred to by terms such as "mainstreaming," "inclusion," or "push in." The implication of these terms is that the student "belongs" to special education, which continues to be hotly debated within education. Current practice states that all students are general education students first. The interpretation of the LRE standard can result in program decisions that vary greatly between districts. One can clearly envision how interpretation of the term "to the maximum extent appropriate" can lead to widely disparate program decisions and outcomes for individual children.

Eligibility

Rules and regulations for special education are delineated at the federal level. Within IDEA 2004, there are 13 different categories under which a child may potentially be eligible for services:

1. Autism
2. Deaf-blindness
3. Deafness
4. Hearing impairment
5. Mental retardation
6. Multiple disabilities
7. Orthopedic impairment
8. Other health impairment
9. Serious emotional disturbance
10. Specific learning disability
11. Speech or language impairment
12. Traumatic brain injury
13. Visual impairment, including blindness

States follow the federal statues closely. State rules and regulations may always provide more rights than the federal-level regulations but cannot provide fewer than guaranteed by the federal law (Wrightslaw and Wrightslaw 2007).

There are a number of factors that can impact whether a student is found eligible for special education programs and services. Major factors that affect this determination at an aggregate as well as individual level include the following: 1) school reform movements that "back in" more sophisticated intervention techniques to the regular classroom, 2) poor overall schoolwide performance, 3) parent or staff resistance to having a child identified as having a disability, 4) limited staffing to conduct evaluations, and 5) school staff determining that even though a child may be diagnosed with a particular disorder, it does not interfere with the child's ability to profit from general education.

Other Key Areas of Impact

In addition to the concepts of FAPE and LRE within IDEA, the legislation addressed issues of discipline for the first time, using a behavioral analytic paradigm that directs school staff to try and determine the function of a student's behavior and to modify the learning environment to meet the student's underlying needs. If a student who is eligible for special education services has recurring behavioral issues that would normally trigger disciplinary action, the school is charged with developing a Functional Behavioral Analysis (FBA) and Behavior Intervention Plan (BIP) to decrease the aberrant behaviors and encourage the development of skills that are more positive. Schools that suspend students for more than 10 days (cumulative) must convene a Manifestation Determination Review meeting, to determine if the behavior subject to discipline should be considered as having a direct and substantial relationship to the child's disability. If the behavior is found to be a manifestation of the student's disability, schools must develop an appropriate intervention plan rather than enforce the discipline code alone. One of the shortcomings of this aspect of IDEA is that many school personnel have not had sufficient training to adequately meet the standard of care associated with developing an FBA or BIP, nor do most school systems understand or support the principles underlying applied behavioral work. A significant body of case law is defining the parameters of this relatively new aspect of special education law, with a continued emphasis on evidence being required (e.g., data collection) to demonstrate that educators are, in fact, using effective interventions with students who are experiencing behavioral problems.

IDEA prohibits school staff from requiring that a student take a controlled substance in order to attend school or obtain an evaluation or special education services. Some states have also passed laws that do not allow for school staff to indicate that "your child needs to be on medication," commonly referred to as the "gag rule," or make recommendations for medication use as such. The legislation occurred in response to parental complaints that teachers pressured parents to medicate their children and interfered with their parental prerogative to provide appropriate medical care for their children. Physicians have often been drawn into this dilemma, particularly when the child is experiencing attentional issues. In fact, in a statewide survey of more than 1,300 primary care physicians conducted in Michigan in 2003, 55% of physicians endorsed the statement "Teachers pressure me to diagnose ADHD [attention-deficit/hyperactivity disorder]," and 71% endorsed the statement "Teachers expect me to use medication" (Clark and Fant 2004).

Case Examples

The following case vignettes are provided as examples germane to the evaluation concerns that are commonly found in school settings.

Case Example 1: Inappropriate Use of a Screening Tool to Make a Diagnosis

A 4-year-old boy began attending preschool. His parents had recently separated and custody was shared between them, although this was not made known to day care staff. The boy had significant behavioral problems within the day care setting, including selective mutism, lining things up, and having major tantrums when asked to share. The teacher expressed concern to a teacher consultant, who completed the Gilliam Autism Rating Scale with the teacher. Scores indicated that the boy was "highly likely" to have autism. The teacher tells the mother that her son is having terrible problems and that she believes "he's autistic." The mother bursts into tears and screams, "That's it! We won't be back tomorrow!"

Case Example 2: Overreliance on Computerized Scoring

A 15-year-old girl has been referred for special education services because of slipping academic performance. The school social worker administers the Behavior Assessment System for Children but does not interview the student, teacher, or parents because of time constraints. The school social worker hastily reviews the computer score printouts, failing to see that the validity scales indicate there should be significant concerns about the results for three of the four teachers who completed the forms. Cautious interpretation is recommended as the scores indicate that the respondents view the student in an extremely negative light. At the meeting with the girl's parents, the school social worker indicates that teachers find the student to have significant issues with attention and atypicality and recommends that the parents talk to their family doctor about getting their daughter on medication. The parents are stunned by this news and become increasingly angry with school staff, feeling that they discriminated against their daughter.

Case Example 3: Inappropriate Use of a Self-Report Instrument Given Student Reading Level

A seventh-grade Hispanic boy from a migrant family is struggling with his transition to middle school. His parents work at the local farms and do not speak English; Spanish is the primary language spoken in the home. The student is discussed at a Student Study Team meeting, and it is decided that some preliminary screening measures should be administered to determine if he is seriously depressed, which might account for his poor grades. The school psychologist talks to the boy and determines that he "should be able" to complete the Beck Depression Inventory, which is written at a grade 5/6 reading level. The student responds with the highest rating for all items, which classifies him in the severely depressed range.

Case Example 4: Insufficient Input From Parents and Teachers

The parents of a fourth-grade girl have filed a suit against the school system for not providing FAPE to their daughter. The girl was diagnosed with Turner's syndrome, a rare genetic disorder affecting only females that commonly presents with a specific difficulty in perceiving spatial relationships, although more global cognitive delays are possible. She is currently placed in a general education classroom and cannot keep pace with the math instruction. She often needs to be redirected for talking to her classmates, particularly the boys, and she speaks regularly of wanting to have a "boyfriend." She recently was found drawing hearts and writing her name and other male classmates' names inside the hearts on the bathroom stall walls. Parents and school staff were asked to fill out forms about her behavioral and emotional functioning. Parent forms were not returned, and only one of the three staff who worked with the girl regularly completed one.

General Assessment Information

There are four general categories that define the aspects of assessment: norm-referenced tests, interviews, observations, and informal assessment procedures (Sattler 2008). Most of the instruments discussed here are norm-referenced tests and represent one of the cornerstones of assessment. This means that a child's answers or the ratings that an individual makes of a student are compared with normative information that has been developed with respect to age and grade level and, occasionally, gender. Although qualitative descriptions of a student's behavior honed from clinical expertise can be quite useful, norm-referenced information can be used to corroborate such clinical opinions. This type of cross-referencing is well suited for the needs of the forensic examiner who provides an expert opinion within a court of law where rules of evidence favor the use of factual information.

Use of Computer-Based Measurement

It has become increasingly common for the measures discussed herein to be administered, scored, or analyzed by computer programs. In fact, some measures do not allow for hand scoring, which is a significant limitation. Examiners must take sufficient time to ensure that the results of the computer analysis are not only accurately stated but also integrated with other critical elements of an evaluation. The illusion of a higher degree of authority may be given to computer-based measures without sufficient caution as to their limitations. However, computers have allowed for increased standardized administration and thereby have assisted in limiting bias or halo effects that can be factors during administration. This, along with significant analysis, elimination of protocols, and the storage of large amounts of data, can be very useful.

Assessment Instruments Commonly Used in Education

During the past 30 years, there has been extensive development in the use of screening tools and rating scales, including self-report instruments, to assess children. Numerous instruments in each of these categories are developed regularly, so that an exhaustive listing of measures is never possible without frequent updates. Specific texts such as the *Mental Measurements Yearbook* published by the Buros Institute at the University of Nebraska are devoted to this. Various online test reviews are also available to the reader, many with free access. The *Standards for Educational and Psychological Testing* (American Educational Research Association et al. 1999) is also an excellent resource for general testing guidelines. Additionally, Sattler (2008) has provided the most comprehensive text

on the assessment process, titled *Assessment of Children: Cognitive Applications*, 5th Edition, which provides the formative reference for individual test reviews within the field of school psychology. Sattler's (1997) text, *Clinical and Forensic Interviewing of Children and Families*, also provides a wealth of information about specific issues relevant to the interview techniques of the forensic examiner.

Although numerous screening tools, rating scales, and self-report instruments have been developed from a clinical perspective, many lack normative information. Although they may have adequate face validity, which even an experienced clinician may evaluate favorably upon review, they are not recommended for use in forensic work owing to the lack of established psychometric integrity.

Specifically, screening tools, rating scales, and self-report instruments can be used in educational settings to 1) determine whether a full evaluation is required, 2) qualify a student for special education, 3) improve the understanding of factors associated with learning challenges, and 4) inform instruction.

Screening Tools

Screening tools are usually administered within school settings for the purposes of identifying children who may be at risk for academic failure, identified as having special educational needs, or determined to have a specific need for intervention within school settings. Child Find programs, which are required to screen young children during the developmental years prior to formal schooling, represent one such initiative, along with screening English language learners whose English is not sufficient to learn from English-based instruction. Some tools may be administered individually or within a group setting. Children who are identified by such tools may be provided with a different type of intervention or may be referred for more comprehensive evaluation. Typically, the decision as to whether to refer a student for a full evaluation takes into account additional risk factors that suggest the presence of a disability that is likely to impair the student's academic performance. This model is becoming increasingly common with the adoption of educational reforms such as the Response-to-Intervention (RTI) and Instructional Consultation Team (ICT) models.

Examples of currently used screening tools. An example of a screening tool is the Dynamic Indicators of Basic Early Literacy Skills (DIBELS), which is a set of standardized, individually administered measures of early literacy development. DIBELS is identified as a screening measure as well as an instrument that can be used for progress monitoring and determining whether a student has achieved a grade-level mastery in reading (outcome measure). With numerous statistics indicating that only approximately 30%–40% of 4th, 8th, and 12th graders are proficient readers, this is an urgent area of improvement within education (National Reading Panel 2000). The measures themselves have very short administration times (approximately 1 minute) and are used to regularly monitor the development of prereading and early reading skills. Probes are used as a repeated measure to increase reliability. Results of such ongoing progress monitoring may result in increased or different types of reading intervention, or over time they may support a referral for a special education evaluation.

Universal screening is another aspect of education where screening tools are used. Screening tools may require asking a series of standard questions to determine whether an individual appears likely to be at risk for a disorder and may meet the requirements of a specific certification (eligibility) category. In 2006, the American Academy of Pediatrics recommended this type of procedure be done as part of the regular well baby visits in response to both the increased incidence of autism and compelling findings about the significantly better prognosis for children who are identified early in life (Council on Children With Disabilities et al. 2006). The "Learn the Signs. Act Early" campaign launched by the CDC in 2005 has also been developed to support this public health concern. Children who meet a certain established cutoff or range of scores are likely to be referred for a full evaluation for autism spectrum disorder. Screening tools such as these have utility for school professionals who are faced with meeting the needs of all children who are serviced by the school system and yet have limited resources to meet the demand. Other screening tools aim to measure a specific area of content, such as spelling or math, or reading fluency.

Limitations and benefits of screening tools. Screening tools have a distinct advantage in that they are short and typically easy to administer. A number of screening tools can be administered by individuals who are less credentialed, such as an intake worker, with minimal additional training required. They may take the form of an abbreviated version of a more comprehensive measure when previous data are already available or time constraints are present. The cost of shortening the measure to maintain its brevity is that it is likely to severely restrict the item pool. This may affect both its reliability and validity and can lead to

misinterpretations. A general caveat for use of screening tools is that one should always research their psychometric properties, including ensuring that up-to-date norms are available, and be sufficiently careful in remaining within the limits of the data when interpreting their significance.

Screening-level data should be considered preliminary and viewed with caution. Issues related to forensic work should not be determined on the basis of such data alone, due to the data's susceptibility to overidentification. Because the principal goal of forensic work is to provide information that is objective, relevant, and will also hold up in a court of law, measures must have a high level of accuracy. This requires that the test's sensitivity (the percentage of affected people who are identified as having the condition) and its specificity (the percentage of people who are unaffected and also identified as not having the condition) are at higher levels than found in screening tools.

Rating Scales

A rating scale is defined as "any instrument designed to assist in the measurement of subjective evaluations of, or reactions to, a person, object, event, statement, or other item of interest...Rating scale instruments are used in psychological research primarily to assess qualities for which no objective criteria exist" (Strickland and Cengage 2006).

The reliance on others' opinions of a child's ability, attitude, or behavior has been fundamental to the U.S. educational system. Rating scales provide additional structure and quantification to this more informal process. However, rating scale systems have major limitations: ratings can vary widely from person to person and are inherently subjective and may actually be biased. To address this, a system of multiple-informant data is recommended when using rating scale information if at all possible as they have the highest reliability and validity. Second, some systems offer validity scales that allow one to analyze the response profile to determine if the rater may have been biased or may actually be lying. Rating scale systems that provide validity scale information are of great value to forensic proceedings, as one can indicate with a higher level of assurance that the information represents a reliable perceptual set, particularly in areas that are more amorphous, such as a child's temperament or personality.

Personality measures are not typically given in schools, which tend to rely on broader, less clinically oriented measures of functioning. This is a procedural safeguard for students and their families, with the intent of protecting students who come to school from unnecessary evaluation or mental health oversight. Parents or guardians of a child must give express consent for any use of a specific personality measure for this reason. The focus of educational evaluation remains understanding behaviors related to academic performance, even if in the broader social adjustment sense, "How well is the child getting along in school?"

Examples of currently used rating scales. As mentioned earlier, multi-informant measures are preferred for their increased reliability and inclusion of validity scales. The Behavior Assessment System for Children, Second Edition (BASC-2; Reynolds and Kamphaus 2004) is one such measure. This measure is designed to provide comprehensive information about an adolescent's behavioral and emotional functioning. It is frequently used in school evaluations when certifications of emotional impairment, ADD/ADHD, or autism spectrum disorder are being considered. The student would be asked to complete the self-report measure, while several teachers and parents provide their perspectives of the student's behavior. This information can be entered into a computer scoring system that generates T-scores along with cross-correlational data between respondents, which can be exceedingly helpful in describing how the student's behavior changes in relationship to his or her environment.

Rating scales are also used in the area of adaptive behavior. The Vineland Adaptive Behavior Scales–II (Sparrow et al. 2005) is one example of such a comprehensive measure. These scales are criterion-based measures in which respondents rate an individual on specific skills that are ranked developmentally among three or four major categories, including communication, activities of daily living, and social and motor skill development. These types of measures are required for determining eligibility as cognitively impaired and are important to use in a number of other instances. Normative information provides standard scores, and grade/age equivalents can be calculated. Multiple informants are not often used with adaptive functioning measures; however, in some cases where perspectives vary widely, these types of measures can help to document where differences are seen across environments. If properly presented, they can aid discussion about how to improve the generalization of skills that are mastered in one environment but not another or provide caregivers with specific techniques to increase a child's level of independence.

Rating scales for assessing the presence of ADD/ADHD symptomatology are commonly used, with the Conners Rating Scale–3 and Brown ADD Scale having the highest level of psychometric integrity. Individuals familiar with the student are asked to rate the frequency with which the student behaves in certain ways in major attentional issues within the classroom setting. Though these ratings can be helpful, they are not diagnostic in and of themselves, as responses primarily reflect overt behaviors only. In many respects, these scales are screening instruments that should be interpreted in conjunction with a thorough developmental history, behavioral observations, and cognitive and achievement testing. School staff reports, if they are comprehensive and objective, can be quite helpful to a physician who is asked to evaluate a child for ADD/ADHD. Because there are a host of reasons why individuals do not "pay attention" within classroom settings, cross-environment data are essential to ensuring accurate diagnosis. Frustration, boredom, poor instruction, as well as substance abuse, family discord, and personal distress are all possible factors that can result in limited attending within an educational setting and are important to investigate as part of the diagnostic evaluation process.

Self-Report Instruments

Self-report instruments are used to collect information about an individual's perspective relative to his or her emotional or behavioral functioning or specific attitudes toward life circumstances, such as school. Although self-report measures have been criticized for their subjectivity, they are indispensable in evaluation work. However, because there are legitimate concerns about cognitive biases (Razavi 2001), instruments that also have validity scales to determine the integrity of an individual's responses are best suited for forensic work. Additionally, when possible, self-report instruments that allow for multiple-informant data and a cross-informant analysis greatly augment the accuracy of this type of psychological information. Extreme caution should be used when using retrospective self-report data, such as when one asks a person to look back in time and remember details of a behavior or experience. Research indicates that this is the least accurate type of self-report, because it is confounded by both the uncertainty of self-report and the uncertainty of memory reconstruction. Experimental data show that this is a human frailty in memory capacity, so that even individuals who are trying to be completely honest may not be able to differentiate between a distortion and their actual memory (Hanita 2000). Within forensic work, recovered memories are particularly fraught with possible confabulation and the secondary gain that can be associated with filing a suit alleging personal injury.

Examples of currently used self-report instruments. One example of use of a self-report measure would be having a student complete the Beck Depression Inventory–II, which has been thoroughly researched over many years and has a readability level between fifth and sixth grade. This measure has been used in varied populations and could be useful in conjunction with other data in documenting a student's level of depression, assuming it is administered to a child 13 years or older who has a commensurate reading level to the inventory. Though it is permissible to administer this inventory orally, it is likely to be affected by factors such as social desirability that has been well documented in the literature (Loevinger 1958), and interpretations should be provided with that caveat.

Another area in which there is considerable value in obtaining the subjective experience of an individual is trauma. A number of published self-report measures for trauma are now available. Some of the more general emotional/behavioral assessment measures, such as the BASC-2 (Reynolds and Kamphaus 2004), are more useful for differential diagnostic work, as compared with a measure that is more specific to the issue of trauma, such as Children's PTSD Inventory (Saigh et al. 2000). Good diagnostic practice would include both the more broad-based measures and one with a higher level of specificity, in conjunction with a thorough developmental history, a structured clinical interview, and, at minimum, cognitive and memory measures prior to determining an eligibility or making a diagnosis.

Legal Issues Within Special Education

Because students who receive special education are afforded a higher level of legal protection, there are numerous processes in place to allow for disagreement and due process proceedings within the school system. Students who are served under the laws governing special education are provided with the highest level of regulation regarding access to services, modifications to instruction, disciplinary procedures, and support required to be successful in the academic environment, in order to have access to the same opportunities as their same-age peers who are not disabled. The IEP serves as the legal document and contract between the school system and the parents/student as to what is open to litigation. Several legal remedies are afforded parents of a child with a disability when they believe their child is not receiving FAPE.

Typically, once parents believe they cannot effectively dialogue with school personnel or impact change within the school setting, they may file a due process complaint. This is a request of the school system to have their particular case heard by a hearing officer. Procedural safeguards that are specifically delineated within IDEA 2004 provide the basis for the legal proceedings. Schools must provide prior written notice (PRW) for actions that parents raise related to identification, evaluation, or the educational placement of their child. Parents may request an independent educational evaluation at public expense to address the issue of eligibility, along with making recommendation for the child's educational program. If disputes remain between the parents and the school, parents can ask for mediation and work toward resolution. Mediation is offered when a due process complaint is filed, but it is a voluntary program that requires both parties' willingness to engage in the process in order to be successful. Another avenue for legal resolution includes follow-up written settlement agreements after mediation, which can now be assured implementation owing to the authority of a federal court.

Due process hearings are the final aspect of the legal remedies available within the educational system, and very specific timelines, pretrial procedures, and rules for the process are delineated. There is a 2-year statute of limitations in presenting a complaint. In addition, a school must submit a written response to the complaint within 10 days of receiving it, along with PRW of their justification and rationale for proceeding in the manner they did.

Although parents or individual students can file a complaint with the monitoring agent about lack of appropriate education when served under the Section 504 plan or ADA, the law is less stringent and requires a greater degree of evidence to be levied by the parents or individual students as to how their rights to educational services were denied. Students eligible under Section 504 plans do have a written plan that documents the disability and lists the specific accommodations that the school is obligated to provide. Typically, each school has a 504 plan coordinator who is responsible for the development and dissemination of this information to the student's teachers and school personnel on a need-to-know basis. Section 504 and ADA complaints must indicate that the school's practices involved specific discrimination against a student, as protection under these statutes is grounded in discrimination law.

Recent U.S. Supreme Court Rulings in Special Education

Because legal remedies are sought from a variety of avenues, most cases arrive at a settlement or disposition long before reaching a federal-level court. However, key questions include what constitutes FAPE, to what extent a school system must provide medical care, what responsibilities a school system has for intervening with behavioral problems before recommending disciplinary measures, including expulsion, and whether parents are entitled to reimbursement for private placements, as well as procedural questions such as whether parents may represent their case without legal counsel and who pays expert witness fees (Norlin 2007). A brief review of some of these U.S. Supreme Court cases is provided here.

Board of Education v. Rowley (1982)

Ms. Rowley was a deaf child whose parents requested that the school provide a qualified sign language interpreter to assist her communication in her regular education classes. The child was performing better than average in her classes, though the U.S. district court appeal found that she also "understood less than she would if she were not deaf." The Supreme Court found that the schools were providing FAPE by virtue of Ms. Rowley having both access and receiving educational benefit, which the Court interpreted to be the intent of FAPE within IDEA. The decision stated that this did not entitle one to the best program or one that would "maximize their potential."

Honig v. Doe (1985)

This is the first discipline case that was brought before the U.S. Supreme Court. The San Francisco Unified School District expelled indefinitely two students who were labeled emotionally disturbed. This raised the question as to whether FAPE was denied students who faced long-term suspensions or expulsions. The ruling in this case created the "stay-put" requirements that exist today, which states that a student will remain in his or her current placement during any legal proceeding unless an exception of "dangerousness" can be convincingly argued.

Florence County School District IV v. Shannon Carter (1993)

Parents of a ninth-grade student with learning disability objected to specific goals within her IEP that indicated that 4 months' progress was expected during the 10-month school year. They withdrew the student from the school and enrolled her in a private academy, requesting tuition reimbursement. The school had argued that the academy setting did not meet the requirements of least restrictive environment (LRE), which allowed them relief from financial obligation. The Supreme Court clearly stated that if the schools defaulted on their obligation to provide an appropriate education within the public setting, they would be required to either ensure that FAPE was provided within the public sector or pay for services in a private setting of the state's choice. This case set a precedent for litigation for applied behavior analysis (ABA) home-based services for young children with autism.

Schaffer v. Weast (2005)

An eighth-grade boy diagnosed with a learning disability and speech and language impairment attended private school through the end of seventh grade. When his parents approached the local public school, they believed the program the school offered was not sufficiently intensive. The parents enrolled him in a private school and requested a due process hearing. This case raised the question about who has the burden of proof over a child's IEP under IDEA, and the Supreme Court ruled that the party that is seeking relief bears to persuade the Court.

Arlington v. Murphy (2006)

During a due process hearing requested by the parents, an advocate acted as an educational consultant. The parents prevailed in both district court and the U.S. Court of Appeals for the Second Circuit. The issue that was brought before the Supreme Court was the parents' request for reimbursement for both the attorneys' fees and the "costs" of the advocate's time. The Court ruled that parents who prevail in due process are not entitled to be reimbursed for expert witness fees.

Winkelman v. Parma City School District (2007)

The Court of Appeal for the Sixth Circuit ruled that IDEA did not entitle parents of Jacob Winkelman to represent him in federal court in 2005. Circuits split on this issue, and it was appealed by the parents to the U.S. Supreme Court, which ruled that IDEA does in fact grant parents rights of their own, so that they may pursue federal FAPE claims without being required to have counsel.

Clinical Management of School Litigation

The dynamics that are found between research/clinical settings and court proceedings also exist between the school systems and the legal remedies available to students and their families when there is disagreement. At the fundamental level, psychology and mental health disciplines conceptualize behavior in relative terms, looking for the various factors that provide the best plausible explanation for behavior. Moralistic perspectives are discouraged in favor of objective understanding, with the larger goal of promoting good mental health. Court systems are designed to promote justice, looking for absolute answers to moral and legal questions (Sattler 2008). Therein lies the rub.

How is this polarization of philosophical perspectives best dealt with within a forensic situation? There are at minimum three major stakeholders in cases that involve educational law: the school system itself, the parent(s), and the child. Depending on the nature of the case, there may also be a specific individual or set of individuals who is being charged at a civil or criminal level, such as in the case of alleged sexual abuse by a teacher. Parents may have opposing viewpoints, particularly if they have divorced or are experiencing significant marital problems over child management. With a divorce rate of 85% cited for parents of children with severe disability (Gerl 2008), this is quite common. Child discipline issues are often significantly intensified by the presence of a disability both at home and at school, creating an increase in the amount of conflict over how to provide structure and discipline to a child. Schools, whose focus remains on the larger unit of measure (e.g., classroom, school) in conjunction with individual needs, are at odds with the singular focus of special education law and the parents who believe in the primacy of the individual student's—their child's—needs.

Staff working within schools should understand that these opposing views are present in their work, both in terms of their own inherent biases and those of others, in order to work toward compromises that are in the best interest of the specific child in question but that do not create undue concessions that affect the overall functioning of the larger unit. Large doses of reflection and thoughtfulness are recommended to educators who are grappling with this, rather than adopting an authoritarian stance that is easily manufactured in an institutional setting where colleagues and others may support such a view. When children are experiencing major difficulty, particularly when it is chronic in nature, there is a tendency to justify positions that may be diametrically opposed and, ultimately, not lead to a goal of reaching resolution. Parents who harbor resentment or display overt and sometimes intense anger toward school staff who are already frustrated by trying to cope with the child's difficulties increase the likelihood that school staff will not be able to maintain a balanced perspective.

Two major issues are essential within school settings to help resolve disputes involving a child's education. One is how data and perceptions are interpreted and gathered. The other is addressing issues of environmental toxicity. First, assessment data must be reviewed from multiple measures and perspectives, always. The assessment data are most useful when there is an integrated analysis of information from various caregivers and measurement tools, with convergence of the findings creating the most reliable and valid interpretations (Kaplan 2008). Though psychiatric opinion may override other findings, recent case law scrutinized the psychiatrist's methodology to ensure that "all available information was considered" before ruling out a diagnosis of autism (Board of Education of the Croton-Harmon Union Free School District, 49 IDELR 265 [SEA NY 2007]). This becomes increasingly true as a child develops and begins to receive services from a wider array of staff, becoming more independent and opinionated in the process. Because motivation accounts for an increasingly larger proportion of the variance as a child transitions from the younger grades to becoming an adolescent and young adult, managing relationships and relevance within the academic environment becomes critical to academic success. With high school dropout rates at an all-time high and 20% of those who have left school falling in the gifted range (Hyde 2007), schools are faced with reinventing traditional high schools in lieu of the current realities. Individual cases should ensure that schools factor in these larger systemic issues to ensure that they are addressed in a manner that leads to resolution of the dispute and increases the likelihood that effective collaboration can be achieved.

Second, mental health staff should be alert to the possibility of the development of environmental toxicity when individual students or families create significant systemic stress. As mentioned earlier, the confluences of forces can readily create the development of strong, opposing forces that, at best, are difficult to manage and, at worst, create a sense of adversarial relations that can be deleterious to the individual child and the ongoing school–parent connection. The possibility of toxicity can occur at all levels: within the school, among the teaching staff, with and between the parents, as well as at the child level. Students who are experiencing significant stress and academic failure within school can easily develop a sense that no one cares about them within the school setting. Research substantiates that the key school variable for optimizing adolescent health is a sense of connectedness to school. It is particularly important for schools to treat students fairly and encourage closeness between staff and students, with appropriate boundaries when students are the subject of legal conflicts (Blum and Rinehart 1997).

If all parties have been diligent in sincere efforts to mediate disagreements and obtain resolutions that can be mutually beneficial without result, a case is likely to move forward in litigation. Should this occur, the forensic examiner may be involved in the assessment of relevant details and completion of additional testing and may be asked to offer an opinion as to the ultimate questions of fact finding. Purposes of the forensic examination within educational settings include 1) how specific events may have contributed to the medical or psychological problems of an individual, 2) whether a child has been subjected to maltreatment or abuse, or 3) whether procedural safeguards were adequately followed, such as in the event of an arrest of an adolescent on school grounds. Although forensic examiners are also asked to comment on issues of child custody and psychiatric hospitalizations, these types of cases are not typically found within educational arenas.

In preparation for legal proceedings, such as mediation or due process hearing, there is a need to address the dynamic issues that are typically present to ensure that case can move forward in the most objective fashion possible to elucidate fact finding and ultimate resolution based on a balanced view of the evidence. There is an immediate need for decreasing the extent to which the adversarial relationship impacts the child during the proceedings. School staff can assist in reducing their own emotionality by reflecting on the larger picture, obtaining feedback on their objectivity, making data-based statements, and checking their perspective against such data and dealing with issues of environmental toxicity. Though this may alienate some staff who refer to each other to provide validation of why they are "right" and the student or parents "wrong," it is deleterious to any legal proceedings and one's ability to participate in those proceedings.

The needs of parents who are preparing for litigation include creating a safe space for grief, frustration, and sadness and minimizing how much their often legitimate anger affects their ability to participate in the legal proceedings. As mentioned earlier, the additional complicated dynamics of parenting a child with a disability take a large toll on marital relationships, and legal remedies are sometimes inadvertently sought to direct intense loss and anger in a way that feels productive to parents who are suffering greatly. Additional issues such as divorce, abuse/neglect, single parenting, cultural issues, and speaking a different language are factors that should be considered when answering the questions presented in the case.

Children who are required to be part of litigation need to be protected from the adult-level conversations about the case's details and have a sense of constancy and predictability to their daily routine. Interview techniques that do not lead or overexpose them to reliving traumatic events should be used in conjunction with the guidelines that have been established by various professional organizations. Additionally, creating a safe space to allow for the children's viewpoints to be heard and assisting them in the development of meta-cognitive (thinking about their thinking) abilities can significantly augment their coping abilities during this most stressful time. Supporting their growth and validating their perspective will decrease the possibility of the development of dissociative thinking, which can dramatically affect their mental health throughout childhood as well as in adulthood.

—Key Points

- Education has a long history rooted in helping the disabled, grounded in the core belief that there is value inherent in education.

- Education benefits greatly from the expertise of mental health professionals, but it is critical to understand the educational environment when working with school-age children and their families.

— Special education is highly regulated and dynamic in nature, constantly affected by legislative action and case law decisions.

— More than 13% of children and youth ages 3–21 years receive services through the Individuals With Disabilities Education Act, representing a substantial increase in the numbers and types of disabilities served over the past 30 years.

— Expert witnesses should be sure to indicate the limitations of the "evidence" gleaned from psychological testing, for example, self-report measures and rating scales. Don't be pressed by attorneys who attempt to obtain statements that suggest that the information is factual in the absolute sense.

References

American Educational Research Association, American Psychological Association, and National Council on Measurement Evaluation: Standards for Educational and Psychological Tests. Washington, DC, AERA Publications, 1999

American Psychiatric Association: Diagnostic and Statistical Manual of Mental Disorders, 4th Edition, Text Revision. Washington, DC, American Psychiatric Association, 2000

Americans With Disabilities Act of 1990 (ADA) (Public Law 101-336)

Arlington v Murphy, 548 US 291 (2006)

Blum R, Rinehart P: Reducing the Risk: Connections That Make a Difference in the Lives of Youth. Minneapolis, University of Minnesota, Division of General Pediatrics, Adolescent Health, 1997

Board of Education of the Croton-Harmon Union Free School District, 49 IDELR 265 (SEA NY 2007)

Board of Education v Rowley, 458 US 176 (1982)

Centers for Disease Control and Prevention: The "Learn the Signs. Act Early" Campaign. Atlanta, GA, Centers for Disease Control and Prevention, 2005

Clark SJ, Fant KE: Parent perspectives on ADHD care provided by general pediatricians. Paper presented at the annual meeting of the Pediatric Academic Societies, San Francisco, CA, May 2004

Council on Children With Disabilities Section on Developmental Behavioral Pediatrics, Bright Futures Steering Committee, and Medical Home Initiatives for Children With Special Needs Project Advisory Committee: Identifying infants and young children with developmental disorders in the medical home: an algorithm for developmental surveillance and screening. Pediatrics 118:405–420, 2006

Education of All Handicapped Children Act (Public Law 94-142)

Family Educational Rights and Privacy Act of 1974 (FERPA), 20 U.S.C. § 1232g; 34 CFR Part 99

Florence County School District IV v Shannon Carter, 510 US 7 (1993)

Gerl J: ABA special education law blog. May 14, 2008. Available at: http://specialeducationlawblog.blogspot.com/2008/05/tom-f-rides-again.html. Accessed July 8, 2008.

Hanita M: Self-report measures of patient utility: should we trust them? J Clin Epidemiol 53:469–476, 2000

Honig v Doe, 484 US 305 (1985)

Hyde S: Drop Out Rates Soar: Schools Are Still Leaving Many High School Students Behind. Available at: http://curriculalessons.suite101.com/blog.cfm/drop_out_rates_soar. Accessed November 5, 2007.

Individuals With Disabilities Education Act (IDEA) (Public Law 101-476, 104 Stat. 1142, October 30, 1990)

Individuals With Disabilities Education Improvement Act of 2004 (IDEA 2004) (Public Law 108-446, 118 Stat. 2647, December 3, 2004)

Kaplan A: Psychiatric medication guidelines set for preschoolers. Psychiatric Times XXV(3), 2008

Loevinger A: Theory of test response, in Testing Problems in Perspective. Edited by Anastasi A. Washington, DC, American Council on Education, 1958

McKinney-Vento Homeless Assistance Act of 1986 (Public Law 100-77)

Monroe P: A Brief Course in the History of Education. New York, Macmillan, 1907

National Center for Education Statistics: Table 8–1, Number and percentage of children and youth ages 3–21 served under the Individuals With Disabilities Education Act from 1976–77 through 2006–07. 2008. Available at: http://nces.ed.gov/programs/coe/2008/section1/table.asp?tableID= 867. Accessed June 15, 2008.

National Reading Panel: Teaching Children to Read: An Evidenced-Based Assessment of the Scientific Research Literature and Its Implication for Reading Instruction—Reports of the Subgroups. April 13, 2000. Available at: http://www.nationalreadingpanel.org/Publications/subgroups.htm. Accessed March 17, 2008.

No Child Left Behind Act of 2001 (Public Law 107-110)

Norlin JW: From Rowley to Winkelman: 52 Key Court Decisions Special Educators Need to Know. Horsham, PA, LRP Publications, 2007

Razavi T: Self-Report Measures: An Overview of Concerns and Limitations of Questionnaire Use in Occupational Stress Research. Southampton, UK, University of Southampton, 2001. Available at: http://eprints.soton.ac.uk/35712/. Accessed July 21, 2008.

Reynolds C, Kamphaus RW: Behavior Assessment System for Children, 2nd Edition (BASC-2). Circle Pines, MN, AGS Publishing, 2004

Saigh PA, Yasik AE, Oberfield RA, et al: The Children's PTSD Inventory: development and reliability. J Traumatic Stress 13:369–380, 2000

Sattler JM: Clinical and Forensic Interviewing of Children and Families: Guidelines for the Mental Health, Education, Pediatric, and Child Maltreatment Fields. La Mesa, CA, Jerome Sattler Publishers, 1997

Sattler JM: Assessment of Children: Cognitive Applications, 5th Edition. San Diego, CA, Jerome Sattler Publishers, 2008

Schaffer v Weast, 546 US 49 (2005)

Section 504 of the Rehabilitation Act of 1973 (Public Law 93-112)

Sparrow SS, Cicchetti DV, Balla DA: The Vineland Adaptive Behavior Scales–II. Circle Pines, MN, AGS Publishing, 2005

Strickland BR, Cengage C (eds): Rating scale, in Encyclopedia of Psychology.eNotes.com. 2006. Available at: http://www.enotes.com/gale-psychology-encyclopedia/rating-scale. Accessed June 1, 2008.

U.S. Department of Education: Building the Legacy: IDEA 2004, Preamble—Major Changes in the Regulations. Available at: http://idea.ed.gov/explore/view/p/%2Croot%2Cregs%2Cpreamble1%2C. Accessed July 29, 2008.

Walter HJ, Berkovitz IH, Hanson G, et al: Practice Parameters for Psychiatric Consultation to Schools. 2004. Available at: http://www.aacap.org/galleries/Practice Parameters/psychConsSchools.pdf. Accessed February 17, 2008.

Winkelman v Parma City School District, 550 US 516 (2007)

Wrightslaw PWD, Wrightslaw PD: Special Education Law, 2nd Edition. Hartfield, VA, Harbour House Law Press, 2007

Chapter 6

Psychological Testing in Child and Adolescent Forensic Evaluations

Charles R. Clark, Ph.D., ABPP

Case Example 1

A social services department, which has placed two children in foster care for a year because of neglect by their single mother, considers filing a petition to terminate her parental rights and asks for an evaluation of her parental fitness. The children, a boy age 6 years and a girl age 8 years, have had sporadic supervised visits with their mother in the past year. They were described by their foster parents as hyperactive and undersocialized at the time of their initial placement. Although the children have "settled down," the foster parents report that they revert to their old behavior after each visit with their mother. The social service worker who has supervised the visits describes the mother as seeming to be "spaced out," and she wonders if the mother might be "a little crazy." However, she also describes the mother as being attached to the children and eager to get them back.

The psychologist conducts interviews with the mother and the children and observes them together. The mother completes a battery of psychological tests that includes an intelligence test, projective tests, and standardized psychological inventories. She also completes rating scales assessing her perception of her children's adaptation and behavior. The foster parents are interviewed and complete the same rating scales on the children. Both of the children are given intelligence tests, tests of academic achievement, and age-appropriate projective tests. The older child is able to be given a self-report measure assessing emotional and behavioral problems.

The test data indicate that the mother may be impulsive and unable to tolerate stress, and they raise a question about her potential for alcohol or drug abuse. They point to antisocial attitudes and to poor interpersonal skills, along with strong narcissistic needs. The mother's account of her children's behavior on the rating scales is sharply different from those provided by the foster parents, which indicate much more concern than the mother expresses about the children's behavior and adjustment. The children's test results indicate significant intellectual deficits. The older child appears to be well behind her peers in academic skills, and her test results include some alarming indications of disorganized thinking and distortion, particularly of interpersonal relationships. The younger child appears from the testing to be withdrawn from adults, with no expectation that adults can help him. The psychologist compares the test data with information received from the interviews, observations, and external sources; interview data appear to confirm that the mother has a drug problem. The psychologist prepares to write her report.

Case Example 2

Divorcing parents in a bitter custody dispute involving their three children, ages 2, 5, and 7 years, are referred for evaluation. The psychologist has each child draw pictures of his or her family and gives the two older children an intelligence test. The mother and father are tested with a projective test, the Rorschach inkblot test. Because of the mother's complaints about the father, which appear to the psychologist to raise questions of psychopathology or personality disorder, he is asked to complete the Minnesota Multiphasic Personality Inventory–2 (MMPI-2). In the report, the psychologist extensively quotes the computer-generated interpretation of the MMPI-2. The psychologist concludes that the mother is the more nurturing parent because of people-oriented responses to the Rorschach. He also notes that this test shows that she has healthily resolved oedipal conflict. Citing the MMPI-2 results (an unspecified elevation of Scale 4, or Psychopathic Deviate), he notes that the father is not to be trusted and may be sociopathic. He also indicates concern that one of the father's responses to one of the Rorschach cards, Card III, a perception of human figures that have both breasts and penises, indicates sexual identity confusion and fits the profile of a potential sex abuser. He further notes that one of the children drew a picture of a person without hands, which he writes indicates conflict over aggression or sexuality, and perhaps even past sexual victimization. The psychologist recommends that sole custody be awarded to the mother and that parenting time with the father be suspended until he has been further evaluated for sexual abuse potential.

Case Example 3

An 11-year-old boy and his 9-year-old sister are present when the boy's clothing is set on fire by an electric heater. The boy is severely burned on his face and hands. The parents sue the heater manufacturer and distributor, alleging damages that include not only the boy's physical injuries but also the mental trauma he suffered, as well as the psychological trauma his sister sustained from witnessing the fire. A psychiatrist and psychologist evaluate the children and their parents. Each is interviewed. The boy says little about the injuries and seems withdrawn; the parents express concern about his withdrawal but describe him as a child who never talks about his problems. In fact, because of their concerns, the boy was tested in school prior to the fire. The boy's younger sister freely discusses the experience without much difficulty, and she indicates she feels sorry for her brother but is not worried about him in any way. The parents report they have been able to talk to their daughter about the situation at length.

A battery of tests is given to each child. The daughter performs within normal limits on all of the tests. She demonstrates healthy problem-solving abilities and good overall adjustment. The boy's test results, however, suggest pervasive concerns about health and body integrity. Images of fire are repeated in the projective testing, and his projective stories are replete with children who are injured or in grave danger. Additionally, he appears from the test results to be markedly anxious and socially withdrawn.

Legal Issues

Psychologists in the United States have testified in court on a variety of legal issues since the early 1920s, but they have provided information to the courts even earlier on the basis of research findings or the results of psychological testing (Bartol and Bartol 2006). Controversies about the admissibility of psychologists' testimony based on testing have nearly always been resolved in favor of granting broad latitude to psychological expert testimony. A primary issue before the courts in years past was whether medical training and methodology was necessary for expert testimony about mental and emotional conditions; the general response by courts has been that it is not. When psychologists' qualifications have been addressed in appellate decisions concerning the admissibility of testimony based on testing, they have included factors such as the possession of a doctorate, licensing, teaching experience, publication in nonmedical but peer-reviewed professional journals, membership in the American Psychological Association, and board certification by the American Board of Professional Psychology. Medical credentials as such have not been identified as necessary, nor has medical supervision of psychological work.

A secondary controversy regarding the admissibility of testimony based on testing pertains not to credentials but the scientific acceptability of test findings in general and the results of particular test instruments. Indeed, all psychological tests are not created equal with regard to their scientific merit—their reliability and validity—and some valid and reliable instruments are more applicable to particular legal issues than are others. Courts have generally upheld the admissibility of psychological testing, leaving open the question of the weight that might be given to it. Testing in general and certain instruments in particular—such as new tests, old tests with weak research support, and tests administered in nonstandard ways—are always subject to challenge in court, in the *voir dire* or questioning of a proposed expert witness who intends to cite testing or in the witness's cross-examination. This, however, is no different than the challenges any mental health testimony is liable to face.

A related issue, and one that concerns all expert testimony, is the extent to which psychological expert testimony should include opinions on the so-called ultimate issue, the factual and legal question on which the judge or jury must rule, such as the best interests of the child in a custody dispute, the occurrence of negligence, or the presence of damages. Case law and rules of evidence adopted by federal and state courts may impose different limits on the scope of expert testimony, but all such testimony is limited to some extent. Where ultimate issue testimony is permitted—most jurisdictions, in most cases—the adequacy of the claimed bases for those opinions, whether psychological testing or other evaluative data, is always subject to scrutiny and challenge.

Clinical Issues

What Is Psychological Testing?

Any mental health assessment, in forensic or other contexts, with children or adults, involves the identification and observation of behavior, including abilities and disabilities, personality traits and trends, interpersonal and relational strengths and weaknesses, and the signs and symptoms of a range of disorders. Tests are methods for obtaining and weighing behavioral information that have known statistical and empirical properties. Psychological tests are standardized and objective measures of behavior, different in that respect from other means of data gathering such as clinical interview and behavioral observation. Tests are standardized in that they involve uniformity of procedure in obtaining samples or indicators of behavior. Their standardization permits one person to be compared with "normal" individuals similar to the test subject with respect to demographic characteristics such as age, sex, ethnicity, and education, or with clinical populations of individuals with known traits, problems, or diagnoses. Tests are objective insofar as their administration, scoring, and interpretation are prescribed and systematic, independent of the idiosyncratic practices or subjective judgment of any particular examiner.

Not all standardized and objective behavioral sampling techniques or tests are equally useful. The descriptive, predictive, or diagnostic value of a test instrument depends on the extent to which it serves as a real indicator of a significant area of behavior and has demonstrable relevance to the purpose of the assessment. Tests must themselves be tested and objectively evaluated to determine their reliability and their validity in specified situations. A number of projective tests developed in the early part of the last century were introduced into practice and are still in use despite any clear determination of their psychometric characteristics. Tests that have not been subjected to rigorous examination have nothing certain to contribute to an overall assessment: what the results of such tests mean in any particular case is unclear. The examiner considering the use of psychological testing in a forensic examination needs to consider the psychometric properties of the test instruments, namely their reliability and validity.

With reference to psychological testing, the term *reliability* refers rather narrowly to a test's consistency, always involving the statistical computation of correlational coefficients (Anastasi 1988; see Table 6–1 for explanations of selected technical terms used in psychological testing). Not all forms of test reliability apply to particular tests or need to be considered in choosing a test to administer. Test–retest reliability, perhaps the best known, is the correlation between the scores obtained by persons on repeated administrations of the same test after specified periods of time. Important with respect to tests of abilities or traits that are relatively stable, such as intelligence, test–retest reliability is less relevant to tests of behaviors affected by the passage of time or clinical changes, such as symptomatic improvement produced by treatment. Alternate-form reliability and split-half reliability are important consistency measures of some instruments, such as achievement tests. Scorer or interscorer reliability, the consistency of scores assigned by different raters to the same performance, is an especially important consideration with respect to projective tests, structured interviews, and behavioral rating schedules.

Whatever forms of reliability are most pertinent, the computation of test reliability stands as the first and primary means of assessing the test's value and usefulness, in that it permits an estimation of the error rate of the test. This estimate, formulated as the standard error of measurement, indicates the extent to which differences between test scores for different individuals, or between particular test subjects and others in normative or clinical samples, are due to irrelevant or chance factors, also known as error variance.

The *validity* of a test is the degree to which the test actually measures what it is supposed to measure (Anastasi 1988). Like test reliability, test validity takes different forms, not all of which apply to particular tests. Content validity, commonly examined with respect to test of knowledge, skill, or achievement, is the extent to which a test covers or surveys a representative sample of the range or domain of behavior being measured. Criterion validity is the extent to which a test can effectively identify or predict a person's concurrent or future performance in specific activities. In diagnostic testing, criterion validity is the extent to which a test identifies someone likely to meet the diagnostic criteria for particular diagnoses. Criterion-related validity may be understood as the practical

---

TABLE 6–1. Psychological testing: selected technical terms

Test: A standardized and objective measure of a sample of behavior

Standardization: Uniformity of administration and scoring

Objectivity: Freedom from the subjective judgment of an examiner

Reliability: Extent to which a test's results are consistent, for example, internally, across repeated administrations, and across scorers or raters

Standard error of measurement: Statistical computation of the extent to which test scores may vary as a result of chance

Validity: Extent to which a test measures what it is designed to measure

Content validity: Extent to which a test measures a specified domain of information

Construct validity: Extent to which a test accurately assesses a psychological construct

Concurrent validity: Extent to which a test's scores correlate with the results of other measures designed to measure the same content or construct

Criterion validity: Extent to which a test's scores correlate with a measure of interest

Predictive validity: Extent to which a test's scores correlate with behavioral outcomes, such as grades, or future test scores

---

Source. Adapted from Anastasi 1988.

utility of a test for a particular purpose. Whether or to what extent a test's results generalize beyond the purposes originally assessed in validating the test and serve to predict other criteria can never be determined without specific study. Tests designed for one use (e.g., the identification of transitory mood states) cannot be assumed to be valid for other purposes (e.g., the identification of mood disorder).

As Anastasi (1988) indicated, a frequently important issue with respect to validity—what a test measures—is construct validity. This is the extent to which a test measures a theoretical construct or trait, such as intelligence or anxiety, and it is determined by calculating the degree to which the test's scores are equivalent to other measures designed to assess the same construct. This will often involve the statistical techniques of factor analysis, which identify the common factors that account for the correlations between two or more tests of the same construct. Construct validity may be either convergent or divergent—identifying the similarities between measures that ought to produce similar scores if they actually assess the same construct, or the dissimilarity between a test and another measure from which it should differ.

Because tests, even those few created to specifically address forensic issues, were designed to assess relatively broad areas of behavior, and the groups on which normative and validation research was conducted embrace a range of individual differences not all of which can match those of a particular test subject, clinicians may be concerned that tests cannot speak specifically enough to the issues involved in forensic assessment to provide definitive answers to legal questions. In fact, testing should never be used as a stand-alone means of reaching a conclusion on any legal issue, such as custody. The results of testing must always be correlated with other sources of information, including history, observation, and interview, and with previous test results when available. Testing can, however, provide unique information that augments other assessment methods.

In addition to objective information that is open to normative comparison, the use of psychological tests can shed important light on the approach a person takes to the assessment itself. Understanding an individual's set or general approach to the evaluation—candor and insight, guardedness and deception, repression and denial—can be essential to an evaluation of the assessment results as a whole. Close attention to a child's approach to testing can yield indications that the child may have been coached or otherwise influenced by a parent. For example, in a custody dispute, if a child were to give rote answers to every card on the Rorschach (Exner 1995), and these answers all had the theme of a bad man, there is reason to consider whether the child might have been told to make sure that thought was conveyed. Continuation of this set throughout the interview, parental interaction, and observation portions of the evaluation would reinforce such a concern.

Some tests, such as the Minnesota Multiphasic Personality Inventory (MMPI-2 and MMPI-A), used respectively with adults and adolescents (Butcher and Williams 1992), incorporate "validity" measures that provide information about the test subject's behavior in taking the test, for example, whether the subject was underestimating or exaggerating difficulties or was otherwise presenting a distorted picture of current functioning. With tests of ability such as intelligence and memory, internal or external measures of a test subject's response tendencies can provide important indications of attenuated effort, exaggeration of difficulties, or outright malingering. Some external measures, normed on adult populations, examine the likelihood of a particular level of poor performance by an individual considering responses by larger groups of nonimpaired or impaired individuals. Other techniques aimed at assessing effort and malingering, which may be adapted to children as well as adults, rely on so-called symptom validity testing, identifying the statistical likelihood of errors in series of two-option forced choice items. Error rates that are statistically below chance levels indicate that the test taker knew the correct answers but suppressed them, possibly to create a false impression of impairment.

Choice of Tester

The administration and interpretation of psychological tests require specific training, not only in personality theory, psychological development, and psychopathology but also in test construction and quantitative research methodology. Although some tests can be administered by a technician, the interpretation should not be done by anyone other than a psychologist fully trained and experienced in all of the instruments given. Responsibility for the interpretation of testing cannot be left to a computer program alone. The programmed interpretation of tests such as the MMPI can provide important actuarial information, but will not take into account a variety of factors, some involving the integration of the test data (programs cannot include every aspect of test performance that may be relevant to consider) and some involving behavior aside from the test, performance on other tests, history, and interview data. Finally, because of important issues involving role, clinicians who are providing ongoing treatment to a child or a child's family members should usually avoid evaluating and testing those individuals in conjunction with legal proceedings (Greenberg and Shuman 1997).

Indications for Testing

Many, if not most, evaluations of children and adolescents could benefit from psychological testing. Its research base and standardized administration make it particularly useful in forensic settings in which clinicians are called upon to account for and explicate their opinions. The following are the principal forensic issues for which testing of children, adolescents, or family members is commonly indicated.

Abuse and Neglect

Testing can be particularly helpful in three general areas of abuse and neglect. First, with regard to sexual abuse, there are often questions about the reliability of a child's report. Second are questions of the effects of abuse and neglect on the child. Third, there may be questions pertaining to the adult involved, either as an alleged perpetrator of abuse or in terms of parenting ability in the case of neglect. It is important to note that although testing should be used with caution in any forensic setting, like other assessment techniques it should be used with the greatest care and circumspection in the area of sexual abuse, when the focus is often on a question of fact: whether sexual abuse occurred or not. Whatever information it may provide about behavioral traits or conditions, neither testing nor any other clinical assessment technique can provide a definitive answer to a question about a fact in dispute. Case Example 2 illustrated a situation in which testing can be misused to identify something it was never designed to identify and in which it may lead to unsupportable recommendations.

While it cannot identify the truth or even truthfulness, testing can contribute to determinations of the reliability of a child's report. Intelligence tests, for example, can provide information about the child's ability to remember, understand, and coherently report an incident. Knowledge of a child's intellectual functioning, cognitive and developmental level, and view of his or her world can provide a context for the clinician's consideration of the child's report. Specific references to abuse are not commonly encountered in the test situation. However, comparison of less direct themes in the child's test productions with interview data can help in assessing the reliability of reports of abuse. The child's approach to the test situation, as measured by the validity scales available in some rating scales and personality inventories, may also be helpful in this regard. Indications of pervasive defensiveness and reluctance to disclose problems on testing, for instance, may have implications for an examiner's understanding of the denial or recanting of a report by a child of sexual abuse, just as signs of exaggeration or false reports of problems may have implications for complaints of abuse or neglect.

When what happened or failed to happen is not at issue, testing may provide independent information about the effects of abuse and neglect. Physical abuse or neglect can contribute to or produce decrements in intellectual functioning and learning. Testing can elucidate these issues, as well as such effects as trauma- or anxiety-induced problems in attention and concentration. The thematic content of some tests can provide data on the effects of abuse. More stories by a child than the norm on the Roberts Apperception Test for Children, Second Edition (Roberts–2; Roberts 2005), about being physically damaged or terrorized by adults will indicate the need by an evaluator to consider whether serious damage has occurred. Similarly, bland and affectless test responses from a child who suffered abuse may signal maladaptive emotional blunting, internalization, and withdrawal. Information on the coping style and interpersonal skills of a child can add important data to the choice of placement when that becomes necessary.

With respect to cases in which the adult disputes allegations of abuse or neglect, testing of the accused may have value in contributing to a clearer picture of the individual, which may be helpful to the trier of fact. It is important to underscore, however, that psychological testing is not capable of identifying the guilty or the innocent or of establishing the credibility or truthfulness of a person. Any conclusion supposedly demonstrated by test data that an individual is or is not a sexual abuser is a conclusion that goes beyond the test data. As is true for other assessment strategies, there is no reliable test-based profile of offenders or any pattern of test results that would indicate truthfulness. Test indications of intentional distortion of the person's presentation—denial, exaggeration, guardedness, or malingering—may shed light on the individual and that person's approach to the assessment but cannot be brought to bear directly on a question of guilt or innocence (see also Chapter 12, "Parenting Assessment in Abuse, Neglect, and Permanent Wardship Cases").

Termination of Parental Rights

Evaluation of the adults involved in the question of termination of parental rights is as important as evaluation of the children themselves. Although there are often data in social service records on both parents and children, frequently a forensic evaluation is not considered until late in the termination process. Often the available mental health data are from therapists who may be placed in the difficult position of both treating the child or parents and providing evaluative information for the court or social services. An evaluation that includes information from testing regarding the presence or absence of character disorder or frank psychopathology in the parents, their intelligence and cognitive functioning, and their social skills and personality traits can be of great use in court. It can help to generate hypotheses about a parent's insight and ability to use psychotherapeutic or educational and social intervention. Treatment issues, goals, and impediments may be identified by testing, increasing the likelihood of success when a strategy of intervention is implemented.

In addition, testing the children in cases in which termination of parental rights is at issue can provide information on the children's level of functioning and attachment to the parent, which can be woven together with interview, observation, and history to determine whether further contact with the parent would be beneficial or detrimental. The complex question of how the parents' and children's temperaments, strengths, and weaknesses interact can be addressed by considering test results. Case Example 1 involved a situation in which relatively vague speculations by foster parents and social service workers were evaluated in light of testing that provided information on the chronicity of the mother's problems and her intellectual limitations, as well as a complexity in the children's problems that might tax even the most able parent.

Delinquency and Criminal Proceedings

Testing is frequently used in cases of juvenile delinquency commitments to identify psychopathology, personality variables, treatment goals, and academic and social skill levels. Assessments are ordered by courts to determine whether adolescents and even children charged with serious felonies, particularly murder and sexual assaults, ought to be tried not as juveniles but as adults, subject to the full range of adult sentencing provisions. Where the binding over of juvenile defendants to adult jurisdictions is not automatic, that is, simply based on factors such as age, provisions for the waiver of juvenile court jurisdiction to an adult court differ across the states. Many considerations taken into account by the courts, such as the seriousness of the offense, the juvenile's criminal record, or the welfare of the community, are not assessment questions open to psychological or psychiatric assessment. Although in practice frequently outweighed by those considerations, juvenile waiver provisions commonly involve an assessment of the juvenile's character and amenability to treatment or rehabilitation in a juvenile facility. On those issues, psychological testing can serve as another source of information about personality functioning, insight, and treatment motivation.

Often, questions raised with respect to adult defendant of competency to proceed and insanity or state of mind at the time of an offense are raised with respect to juveniles as well. While it is debatable whether adult standards of competency and criminal responsibility are appropriate to juveniles, when juveniles are tried as adults it is usual for the adult standards of competency and insanity to be used. Testing has a recognized place in all such assessments and might focus on cognitive abilities, particularly intelligence and memory, and on psychopathology.

Clinicians are increasingly asked to provide risk assessments of juveniles involved in delinquent activities, especially violent and sexual offenses. Research into risk factors has greatly increased in recent years, and a number of rating procedures developed for use with adult offenders are being researched and adapted for use with juveniles (Borum and Verhaagen 2006). These rating procedures, though not psychological tests as such—their focus is on social, family, criminal, and other history rather than behavioral sampling—hold promise for improving classification and thus effective interventions for youth at risk for violence.

Child Custody

As with termination of parental rights, child custody questions require thorough evaluations of both adults and children, including interview, observation of parent–child interaction, and consideration of testing. When a dispute has reached an impasse that requires a custody evaluation, parental animosity may be expected to be high, together with concern by the parents that their points of view be fully heard. Testing can contribute to the thoroughness of the evaluation as well as add an objective comparative standard to the process. Testing also enhances the clinician's ability to compare and contrast parental strengths and weak-

nesses in relation to those of their children. Parent rating scales can be compared with interview data as a measure of how accurately a parent understands the children. Testing of the children can lend important information about any special needs or problems they have, how children view adult figures, how they perceive the family, and whether and how the divorce process has affected them (see also Chapter 11, "Child Custody Evaluation").

Civil Damages

Civil suits involving children often call for the evaluative services of a forensic clinician. In addition to complaints of physical damages, including neurocognitive impairment, these suits may involve claims of psychological effects of a physical injury, emotional stress caused by disasters or toxic exposure, and psychological trauma resulting from sexual or physical abuse. At times, parents are also named as plaintiffs in these suits. In the case of sexual abuse occurring outside the home (e.g., in school or preschool), a parent may enter the suit because of claims of psychological stress caused by having to deal with the trauma experienced by a child.

In the assessment of psychological damage to plaintiffs, testing may help identify or rule out preexisting conditions, which may have continued unchanged or may have been exacerbated by the events in question. Testing can help answer questions about malingering or about the reliability of plaintiff reports, matters that often need to be considered in situations in which large amounts of money are at stake or in which children may be pressured or influenced by adults who have an interest in the outcome. Comparisons of current and past testing, when available, can point to significant changes or stability in psychological functioning.

The intrusion of the traumatic event into test data may indicate how pervasive the response to the injury is. For example, during testing, the boy in Case Example 3, a burn victim, became anxious and tearful and could not respond to Card IX of the Rorschach, in which perceptions of smoke and fire are frequently seen, illustrating the claims made on his behalf regarding traumatic symptoms. A general picture of personality functioning and coping skills will aid in the difficult task of predicting future effects of the trauma. Research has shown the importance of addressing the aftermath of trauma by adults and institutions (Friedrich 1997). Information on the parents' functioning as well as that of the children provides a systematic picture of the experience of the family unit. Testing of plaintiffs is ordinarily an important part of that information.

Selection of Tests

Most often a battery of tests, rather than a single instrument, is administered. Instead of enlisting a standard collection of tests given to everyone, individual tests should be selected for inclusion in an assessment strategy to provide information about specific problems at issue in the case.

Adults

Intelligence Tests

The most commonly used adult intelligence tests are the Wechsler series: currently the Wechsler Adult Intelligence Scale, Fourth Edition (WAIS-IV; Wechsler 2008). The Stanford-Binet Intelligence Scales, currently in their fifth edition as SB5 (Roid 2003), which have a lower "floor" allowing for more sensitive measurement of impaired intellectual functioning, are also widely used, particularly with adults and children with developmental disabilities. These instruments, the so-called IQ tests, provide measures of a variety of abilities associated with what is commonly referred to as intelligence. They especially assess abilities important to academic and occupational achievement, rather than social skills and creativity. Cognitive impairment of various types can be identified by Wechsler or Stanford-Binet performance, as can areas of strength and comparative skills. Many psychologists tap intelligence test results for useful information regarding personality factors, similar to the information obtained from projective testing. Although these tests can be useful this way, tests of intelligence are usually not administered to adults in the context of assessments of children and adolescents unless there is some concern about the adult having an intellectual deficit or cognitive impairment.

Personality Inventories

Well-researched personality inventories are commonly given to adults in any assessment situation. These inventories have strong reliability as tests and provide quantified results that can be readily interpreted in terms of published norms. Such tests are paper-and-pencil or computer-administered instruments that require endorsement by the subject of various statements pertaining to attitudes, emotions, and behavior. Among the instruments not oriented to diagnosis of clinical disorders but developed for use with nonclinical populations are the California Psychological Inventory (Gough 1987), the Sixteen Personality Factors Questionnaire (Cattell et al. 1993), and the NEO Personality Inventory—Revised (Costa and McCrae 1992). The revised Minnesota Multiphasic Personality Inventory (MMPI-2; Hathaway et al. 1989), for some years the most commonly administered psychological test, is designed to assess significant functional disorders in the neurotic, characterological, and psychotic spectra but is also sensitive to subclinical personality factors or traits. The Personality Assessment Inventory (PAI; Morey 1991) and the Millon Clinical Multiaxial Inventory, Third Edition (MCMI-III; Millon 1994) are briefer and differently constructed self-report measures that are sometimes given along with the MMPI-2.

Although they are often called objective tests, the personality inventories, no less than other tests, require considerable clinical skill to use and are susceptible to subjectivity in interpretation. Undue reliance on the score profiles from such instruments in reaching diagnostic conclusions, much less recommendations on matters such as custody or sexual abuse, without considering the psychometric properties of the instruments together with a variety of data obtained elsewhere, invites costly error. The instruments are objective in the sense that, compared with projective tests, they essentially eliminate subjective variations in administration and scoring and sharply reduce subjective factors in interpretation. Although time-consuming for subjects to complete, these inventories allow for efficient and inexpensive use of examiner time.

It should be noted, with respect to personality inventories, that in the case of adults involved in assessments of children, particularly custody and related evaluations, all adults should be given the same instruments to complete. Because of the sensitivity of tests such as the MMPI-2, the PAI, and the MCMI-III to personality disorder and psychopathology, administering such a test to only one of two or more adults involved with the assessment may cause that person to look worse in some respect than the others who were not tested with the same instrument.

Projective Tests

Projective tests require responses by the subject to ambiguous stimuli. A wide variety of such instruments have been developed, though few are in common use currently. The Rorschach inkblot technique is the best known and most widely used of these instruments. Ten cards are presented in sequence to the subject, who is asked to indicate what the inkblots on the cards might be; inquiry follows as to where on the card the percept was seen and what made it appear to the subject in the way it had. The Rorschach is used to provide information on psychopathology or its absence and to examine subjects' response or coping styles, how they approach ambiguous situations, and how they handle emotions. Comparison of the Rorschach summaries of various family members can help generate hypotheses about how the styles of various members might interact with those of others in the family.

Most clinical psychologists value projective tests as adding otherwise unavailable information to an examination. Because of their ambiguity, projective tests, unlike the objective self-report measures, provide few clues as to what a "good" or desirable response might be, and thus they provide some protection against invalid or distorting response sets. This aspect of projective techniques is particularly useful in forensic settings, in which test subjects cannot be expected to be disinterested in the outcome of the examination and recommendations made on that basis, and in which they may feel strong needs to present themselves in particular ways.

Projective tests vary in the extent to which they have been subjected to empirical studies of their psychometric properties. Generally, when examined, such instruments appear to have, relative to the "objective" personality measures or tests of ability and aptitude, poor reliability and uncertain validity. With some projective tests, these problems are compounded (and stem from) a lack of standardization in administration, scoring, and interpretation. Because of the subjectivity they invite, projective techniques are more vulnerable than other types of testing to examiner error and bias. Used carelessly, they may be more tests of the examiner than of the subject. In the case of the Rorschach, at least, considerable work was done by Exner and his associates (Exner 1995) on improving standardization and reliability, quantifying scoring, and identifying from empirical research personality and behavioral correlates of test data. As a result, Exner's Rorschach shares more in common with objective personality measures than do other projective tests. Tests such as the Thematic Apperception Test (TAT; Murray 1971), Draw-A-Person (Goodenough and Harris 1950), and non-Exner Rorschach techniques, while still popular and possibly useful in some types of assessments, lack the psychometric properties necessary for forensic evaluation and are difficult to recommend for use in testing adults in forensic settings, especially in light of the availability of other, more rigorous measures.

Parenting Inventories

If parental attitudes and abilities are in question, such as in child custody and parental fitness evaluations, there are psychometrically valid instruments available to aid in such assessments (Heinze and Grisso 1996). The Parent–Child Relationship Inventory (Gerard 1994) assesses parental attitudes toward parenting and children. Data are obtained regarding the similarity of the parents' responses to those parents who display attitudes consistent with good parenting. The Parenting Stress Index—Third Edition (Abidin 1995) aids in the identification of potentially stressful parent–child relationships by screening for reported parental stress. The Child Abuse Potential Inventory (Milner 1986) was developed to assess a parent's risk of physically abusing a child. It measures a set of risk factors that are compared on that basis with parents who have physically abused their children.

Children

Intelligence and Adaptive Behavior Tests

Intelligence testing for children can be helpful even if there is no question of serious intellectual difficulties. Such testing can provide significant information about a child's cognitive abilities, especially the ability to understand the current legal or familial situation, to report events accurately, and to interpret events. The Wechsler tests—the Wechsler Preschool and Primary Scales of Intelligence, Third Edition (WPPSI-III; Wechsler 2002), and the Wechsler Intelligence Scale for Children, Fourth Edition (WISC-IV; Wechsler 2003)—as well as the Kaufman Assessment Battery for Children, Second Edition (KABC-II; Kaufman and Kaufman 2004), are the most commonly used. For very young children, the Bayley Scales of Infant Development, Third Edition (Bayley–III; Bayley 2006), and the Miller Assessment for Preschoolers (MAP; Miller 1982) are available. Inventories such as the Vineland Adaptive Behavior Scales, Second Edition (Sparrow et al. 2006), use structured interviews to help determine the functioning level of developmentally disabled children.

Personality Inventories

Several inventories assessing developing personality traits, problematic behaviors, and psychopathology have been developed for use with children. These have similar advantages to adult personality inventories, with validity scales that provide information on the child's approach to the test itself, as well as the ability to compare scores with normative nonclinical and psychiatric populations. The Adolescent Minnesota Multiphasic Personality Inventory (MMPI-A; Butcher and Williams 1992) is available for teens 14 years and older, and the MCMI-III has its counterpart in the Millon Adolescent Clinical Inventory (MACI; Millon 1993). For children 9 years and older, the Personality Inventory for Youth (PIY; Lachar and Gruber 1995), and for children 8 years and older, the Self-Report of Personality form of the Behavior Assessment System for Children, Second Edition (BASC-2; Reynolds and Kamphaus 2004), are available.

As most clinicians are aware, children are not always the most accurate reporters of their emotional states and behaviors. To supplement children's reports, there are a number of instruments available that allow parents and others to report. The PIY has a counterpart, the Personality Inventory for Children, Second Edition (PIC-2; Lachar and Gruber 2007), which is completed by parents or guardians for children age 5 years and older. In addition to parent rating scales, the BASC-2 provides for ratings by teachers; the scales can by integrated to form a comprehensive picture of the child. Although it does not have validity scales, the Child Behavior Checklist (Achenbach 1991) can be useful in making comparisons of the way each parent in a custody dispute, for instance, sees the children and in examining the extent to which either viewpoint addresses the evaluator's hypotheses about the children. Parents in custody disputes may be quite discrepant in their views of the children, and both may underestimate the effect of the dispute on their children. In other situations, such as termination of parental rights, the scales can be compared with those filled out by teachers and other significant adults, such as foster parents. With regard to questions of civil damages, comparisons of ratings by parents or others may shed light on the reliability with which certain features of behavior appear. This type of information about the parents' own assessments of their children and how they relate to those of others can be an asset in making recommendations.

Projective Tests

Discovering how children, especially young children, feel and think about events in their lives is not an easy task. In forensic evaluations, the issue is particularly sensitive. Most would agree that it is not appropriate to directly ask young children about their preference for one parent over another in a custody evaluation, or to ask leading questions in an evaluation of sexual abuse. Most children, no matter what their age, are exquisitely aware of why they are being evaluated and may feel anxious about what they say to an evaluator in light of how it may affect their parents or the decision of a court. Projective testing provides a forum one step removed from direct discourse and can skirt a child's conscious intentions and permit reasonable inferences about the child's needs and fears. Case Example 3 showed how testing can reveal difficulties in a child who is uncomfortable in an interview situation.

Poorly validated child projective tests, such as the Children's Apperception Test (Bellak 1986), should be avoided in forensic evaluations, whatever their value in other situations. An Exner Rorschach, however, can provide information about a child similar to that provided for adults. Validated projective tests, such as the Roberts–2 (Roberts 2005) and the Tell-Me-A-Story (TE-MAS; Costantino et al. 1988), are particularly useful in forensic cases. Both tests have children representing typical situations and possible problems in child and family life. The tests are then quantitatively scored and compared with a normative sample of children.

Projective drawings are sometimes used by clinicians. Great care should be taken in the interpretation of drawings. Tests such as the Draw-A-Person Test (Goodenough and Harris 1950) may be too far removed from the referral question and too indefensible in court to be of much utility. However, the Kinetic Family Drawing (Burns 1982), which asks the child to draw a picture of his or her family engaged in an activity, appears to be quite directly related to the issues involved in much child forensic work. How the child describes the picture and answers questions about it may provide useful clinical information or provoke hypotheses, even if the procedure does not yield test scores that permit normative comparisons. Who is and is not included in the picture, the activity depicted, and the interaction among family members may help generate hypotheses about the child's view of the family. For younger children, there are structured play techniques (e.g., Gardner 1982; Lynn 1959, as found in Palmer 1983) that take the child through a series of vignettes, during which the type of play is observed and recorded. It is important to note that these techniques are not psychological tests as such and might more properly be considered to be clinical observation tools. Inferences from a child's performance on these tasks must be made cautiously and must be integrated with interview and other observational data.

Tests of Academic Functioning

It is often helpful to determine whether and how a child's school performance has been affected by events at issue. The Wide Range Achievement Test, Fourth Edition (WRAT; Wilkinson and Robertson 2007), and the Wechsler Individual Achievement Test, Second Edition (WIAT-II; Wechsler 2001), test basic skills in reading, spelling, and mathematics. For a broader picture of a child's academic abilities, the Woodcock-Johnson Psychoeducational Battery, Third Edition (WJ-III; Woodcock et al. 2001), provides data on a number of skills in relation to the child's age and grade level. With these tests, the evaluator can determine a child's academic rank relative to peers and can use this information in conjunction with the intelligence scales and teacher and parent reports to examine the child's overall adaptation. There are also tests related to specific learning disabilities that can be used if indicated. In some cases, such as personal injury litigation involving head trauma or toxic exposure, tests of children's neuropsychological functioning are indicated. Adult testing methodology has been adapted to pediatric cases, and a number of batteries and tests of specific aspects of neurocognitive functioning, such as memory, are available for use by qualified neuropsychologists (Baron 2004).

Tests Addressing Specific Forensic Issues

There are several specific issues that commonly arise in child forensic evaluations that have been addressed by equally specific tests. The Trauma Symptom Checklist for Children (Briere 1996) is a self-report instrument aimed at assessing posttraumatic stress in children. The Child Sexual Behavior Inventory (Friedrich 1997) and the Trauma Symptom Checklist for Young Children (Briere 2001) are parent or caretaker report measures that compare the behavior of the child with normative behavior of children the same age. While measures such as these are psychometrically sound and even include validity scales, they should be used cautiously in the forensic arena because they involve items with open content—items that clearly pertain to claims of trauma. Unlike tests such as the MMPI or Rorschach, it will be quite obvious what the test purports to measure, and they may be somewhat more vulnerable to exaggeration or to defensiveness by a plaintiff, or a plaintiff's parents, who have an interest in making a certain presentation.

There have been other efforts to develop tests that are designed specifically for use in child custody evaluations. The Bricklin Scales (Bricklin and Elliot 1997) and the Ackerman-Schoendorf Scales for Parent Evaluation of Custody (ASPECT; Ackerman and Schoendorf 1992) are examples of this genre. Although such scales invite strong and even exclusive reliance by examiners and the court on their results, they are not substitutes for a full consideration of the wide variety of data obtained in standard evaluations.

The juvenile and criminal prosecution of children and adolescents continues to be an issue that leads to assessment referrals. In addition to other tests of behavioral pathology, such as the MMPI-A, the Jesness Inventory—Revised (Jesness 2003) can be used to identify and classify delinquent and conduct-disordered youth.

Interpretation of Test Data

The results of psychological tests never stand alone but must be interpreted in light of information obtained in the rest of the evaluation. Test interpretation is inherently inferential, and care must be taken to stay as close to the data as possible. Although it may be interesting to make wide-ranging, dynamically oriented hypotheses about test responses when evaluating a person for treatment planning, it is inappropriate to do so in the forensic arena, where the examiner must be able to account for the basis on which conclusions and recommendations are made. Speculation about unconscious conflict stemming from responses to the Rorschach is much less helpful to the court than clear statements about how such conflicts may be expressed in behavior, personality style, or parenting abilities. Misidentifying remote and speculative inferences from testing as "findings" or "indications" amounts to a misuse of testing and is a disservice to the individuals affected. Opinions and recommendations must be grounded in actual data rather than in speculation.

Integration With Other Evaluation Data

In Case Example 2, the psychologist made an important error in interpretation, taking several isolated responses from the test data and extrapolating evidence of sexual abuse from them. There is no single response on any test that warrants such a conclusion. Test data must be considered together, as a whole, and individual responses have little significance by themselves.

Interpretations of test responses should not go beyond what the tests themselves have been validated as measuring. In a thorough evaluation, each test should be carefully scored and interpreted. The information gained from the tests should be integrated into hypotheses about the individuals and how they interact with one another, if that is relevant to the legal question. These hypotheses can then be considered in light of other data from the evaluation, including documents and records that were reviewed and clinical interviews and observations. Interpretive hypotheses from testing can help objectively confirm or disconfirm what the clinician has learned and can enrich an understanding of otherwise unexplained facts. They serve also to point out discrepancies or other avenues to pursue. In Case Example 1, testing indicated that the mother might have substance abuse problems. This led the psychologist to interview her in depth about drug abuse, which she then acknowledged. Rather than simply reporting an inference from test data, the psychologist was then able to report clear and direct evidence that could be used in her report.

Computer Interpretations

Many psychological tests have computer programs available that not only score the tests but also provide clinical interpretations based on the data. It may be tempting for the clinician not trained in psychometrics and not knowledgeable about a particular test to consider this computer-generated material as a finished interpretation and to incorporate it whole in reports and in testimony, without further investigation. As all manuals for these tests point out, this is not the anticipated use for the automated interpretations. The programmed results may assist the clinician, especially one inexpert in testing, to generate hypotheses, but those will need to be integrated with many other sources of data. Because only the data from a particular test are used in generating the automated report, computer-generated interpretive statements are liable, to some extent, to be inaccurate descriptions of an individual. The program cannot take into account the richness of the full evaluation or even all of the data generated by the test itself. The interpretive statements are derived from aggregate data; each individual's behavior, characteristics, or score occupies a place around a group average or other measure of central tendency. To conclude from an individual's score on a test that he or she is typical or atypical of the normative group, or of a clinical group, neglects the effects of variance.

Without referring to other data, the extent to which a person fits the picture of the group to which he or she is assigned by virtue of a score cannot be known. Computerized interpretations in actuality are more or less accurate for a person depending on a variety of factors.

Reporting of Test Data

In the reporting of test results in the forensic setting, there needs to be attention to accountability. Nothing should be reported as opinion in written work or in testimony that cannot be supported by data and reasoned inference. It should be clear from the written report which data were considered and the way in which conclusions were reached. A treatment of test results that is overly technical mystifies rather than elucidates the basis of opinions and may mask an absence of any adequate basis for an opinion.

Release of Test Data

There has been controversy within psychology over the appropriateness of releasing test data, including score sheets and computer-generated results, directly to attorneys. Psychologists agree that they must protect test security so that the instruments are not invalidated and rendered useless by their exposure to the public. There is also agreement that test results, by thoughtless distribution, not be left open to misuse and misinterpretation by untrained parties. In some cases, clinicians concerned about these issues may seek a protective order or attorney agreement to have the circulation of the test material restricted, or they may agree to release the test data only to another psychologist or qualified mental health professional to assure its appropriate use.

Balanced Reporting

Clinicians who use psychological tests, as well as those who conduct forensic evaluations, sometimes forget that attention needs to be paid to the relative strengths of each person being evaluated, not only their weaknesses. Custody disputes in particular should not ordinarily be battles of pathology, testing which party is the most disturbed. The court needs to know what they can do well. It also needs to know not only how a child has been and might be affected, but also the positive aspects of how the child is coping with a stressful situation. It may be tempting for the clinician, who has already formed some hypotheses about a subject from the interview, to report test findings that support only these hypotheses. In Case Example 2, the psychologist neglected to report his observations of the father and children, which indicated a warm and loving relationship. Further, he neglected to mention that he had never interviewed the children about possible abuse. Instead, he selectively used some test responses to confirm his hypotheses of sexual abuse. Test data that are discrepant with the clinician's overall viewpoint should be reported and explained candidly. In the end, it is left to the court, not the clinician, to determine which of the data are most compelling.

Pitfall: Failure to Administer Tests in a Standard Manner

Psychological tests should be administered in the standardized way prescribed by their manuals. Administering a few subscales of an intelligence test, or a couple of Rorschach cards, is poor practice in general, but never more so than in a forensic setting. Such administration outside the test protocols results in nonvalid findings that have no clear and interpretable relationship to the test's norms.

Anything that might allow the test taker to be influenced by outside sources during test administration must be avoided. For this reason, as well as to protect test security, tests should not be sent home for completion, nor should interested parties or lawyers be present and communicating with the test subject, much less giving assistance, when tests are taken. Failure to observe these basic precautions may result in a contamination of the test results and an inability of the examiner to affirm that it was the test subject, and only the test subject, who completed the assessment. In some forensic settings, attorneys or parents may wish to observe the examination, promising not to interact with a child, and may obtain the permission of the court to do so. This is problematic and should be avoided. Test subjects, especially children, may be affected by the presence of other individuals and alter their responses if they are aware of being observed. For example, a child who knows that his parents are watching may be uncomfortable telling a story in response to the Robert-2 that reflects family conflict

or problematic behavior by a parent. When such monitoring is deemed necessary, unobtrusive audio or video recording, or observation from behind a one-way mirror, while still undesirable, might be preferable to the direct presence of another person during testing.

Case Example Epilogues

Case Example 1

The psychologist prepares an extensive report that includes a separate section on test results and integrates the results with the rest of the information gathered. On the basis of her familiarity with the laws of her state regarding termination of parental rights, she concludes that the children have extensive, serious, and complicated problems that will require intensive attention and monitoring by a parent, as well as long-term treatment. She concludes that the mother's concern about her children seems only to reflect her own needs. Her drug problems and longstanding interpersonal difficulties do not allow her to provide the level of care required by her children, and the psychologist recommends termination of parental rights.

Case Example 2

The psychologist in this case has gone far beyond the test data by making speculative statements that have little grounding in objective data. His use of interpretations of the projective tests and drawings as clearcut signs of an actual occurrence of sexual abuse is inappropriate. On the basis of these insufficient and faulty data, the court moves to cut off the father's access to his children. The children are upset by this and begin to show signs of emotional distress. The father's attorney calls for a new examiner, who does extensive interviewing and observation of the father but who is denied access to the mother or the children now in her custody. The new evaluator concludes that there is an insufficient basis to arrive at a finding of sexual abuse in this case. The judge, having ruled, is not swayed, citing the earlier court-ordered evaluation of all parties. Parenting time with the father is not restored. The father files a complaint against the first psychologist.

Case Example 3

The psychologist carefully reviews the previous test battery given to the son. She notes that there was some concern about the boy's social skills and that his level of anxiety appears to have increased. The concerns about body integrity and danger so prominent in the current assessment were not apparent in the earlier testing. Academic functioning has shown marked impairment. As tests show, the boy has fallen behind his classmates in most areas. The psychologist and the psychiatrist can identify no other life events that may have contributed to this change, and they conclude that what the child is experiencing appears to have occurred after he was burned. Neither interview nor test data support a claim of damage to the daughter, who appears to be dealing successfully with the accident and is functioning normally.

—Key Points

Test Selection and Administration

— Know the law.

— Use a qualified examiner.

— Use tests appropriate to child's age.

— Use tests relevant to legal and other issues in evaluation.

— Administer tests uniformly to all parties.

— Administer tests in standardized fashion within prescribed protocol.

— Avoid tests lacking proved validation.

Interpretation

— Integrate test data with other clinical findings.

— Do not use tests as solitary source of diagnosis or forensic opinion.

— Do not rely solely on computer-generated test interpretations.

— Keep test interpretation close to data, avoiding remote inferences and unsupported generalizations.

Reporting of Results

— Say nothing that would not withstand cross-examination in court by citation of data, research, and inferences.

— Provide balanced view of competing parties.

— Include all relevant data, even data not supporting conclusions and recommendations.

— Assume that test subjects will have access to the report.

References

Abidin RR: Parenting Stress Index, 3rd Edition. Lutz, FL, Psychological Assessment Resources, 1995

Achenbach R: Conceptualizations of developmental psychology, in Handbook of Developmental Psychopathology. Edited by Lewis M, Miller S. New York, Plenum, 1991, pp 3–13

Ackerman MJ, Schoendorf S: Ackerman-Schoendorf Scales for Parent Evaluation of Custody (ASPECT). Los Angeles, CA, Western Psychological Services, 1992

Anastasi A: Psychological Testing, 6th Edition. New York, Macmillan, 1988

Bayley N: Bayley Scales of Infant Development, 3rd Edition. San Antonio, TX, Psychological Corporation, 2006

Baron IS: Neuropsychological Evaluation of the Child. New York, Oxford University Press, 2004

Bartol C, Bartol A: History of forensic psychology, in The Handbook of Forensic Psychology, 3rd Edition. Edited by Hess AK, Weiner IB. New York, Wiley, 2006, pp 3–27

Bellak L: The Thematic Apperception Test, the Children's Apperception Test, and the Senior Apperception Technique in Clinical Use. Orlando, FL, Academic Press, 1986

Borum R, Verhaagen D: Assessing and Managing Violence Risk in Juveniles. New York, Guilford, 2006

Bricklin B, Elliot G: Critical Child Custody Evaluation Issues: Questions and Answers. Test Manual Supplement for the BPS, BORT, PASS, PPCP. Furlong, PA, Village Publishing, 1997

Briere J: Trauma Symptom Checklist for Children. Lutz, FL, Psychological Assessment Resources, 1996

Briere J: Trauma Symptom Checklist for Young Children. Lutz, FL, Psychological Assessment Resources, 2001

Burns RC: Self Growth in Families: Kinetic Family Drawings: Research and Application. New York, Brunner/Mazel, 1982

Butcher JN, Williams CL: Essentials of MMPI-2 and MMPI-A Interpretation. Minneapolis, University of Minnesota Press, 1992

Cattell RB, Cattell AK, Cattell HEP: Sixteen Personality Factors Questionnaire. San Antonio, TX, Psychological Corporation, 1993

Costa PT, McCrae RR: NEO PI Manual. Lutz, FL, Psychological Assessment Resources, 1992

Costantino G, Malgady RG, Rogler LH: Tell-Me-A-Story: Manual. Los Angeles, CA, Western Psychological Services, 1988

Exner JE: The Rorschach: A Comprehensive System, Vols I–III. New York, Wiley, 1995

Friedrich, WN: Psychotherapy of Sexually Abused Children and Their Families. New York, WW Norton, 1997

Gerard AB: Parent-Child Relationship Inventory. Los Angeles, CA, Western Psychologist Services, 1994

Goodenough FL, Harris DB: Studies in the psychology of children's drawings, II. Psychol Bull 47:369–433, 1950

Gough HG: California Psychological Inventory Administrator's Guide. Palo Alto, CA, Consulting Psychologists Press, 1987

Greenberg S, Shuman DW: Irreconcilable conflict between therapeutic and forensic roles. Professional Psychology: Research and Practice 28:50–57, 1997

Hathaway SR, McKinley, JC, Butcher JN, et al: Minnesota Multiphasic Personality Inventory–2 (MMPI-2). Minneapolis, University of Minnesota Press, 1989

Heinze MC, Grisso T: Review of Instruments Assessing Parenting Competencies Used in Child Custody Evaluations. Behavioral Sciences and the Law 14:293–313, 1996

Jesness CF: Jesness Inventory—Revised. North Tonawanda, NY, Multi-Health Systems, 2003

Kaufman AS, Kaufman HL: Kaufman Assessment Battery for Children, 2nd Edition (K-ABC-II). Minneapolis, MN, Pearson Assessments, 2004

Lachar D, Gruber CT: Personality Inventory for Youth. Los Angeles, CA, Western Psychological Services, 1995

Lachar D, Gruber CT: Personality Inventory for Children, 2nd Edition. Los Angeles, CA, Western Psychological Services, 2007

Miller LJ: Miller Assessment for Preschoolers. San Antonio, TX, Psychological Corporation, 1982

Millon T: Millon Adolescent Clinical Inventory (MACI). Minneapolis, MN, National Computer Systems, 1993

Millon T: Millon Clinical Multiaxial Inventory–III (MCMI-III). Minneapolis, MN, National Computer Systems, 1994

Milner JS: The Child Abuse Potential Inventory: Manual. Lutz, FL, Psychological Assessment Resources, 1986

Morey LC: Personality Assessment Inventory (PAI). Lutz, FL, Psychological Assessment Resources, 1991

Murray HA: Thematic Apperception Test Manual. Los Angeles, CA, Western Psychological Services, 1971

Palmer JO: The Psychological Assessment of Children, 2nd Edition. New York, Wiley, 1983

Reynolds CR, Kamphaus RW: Behavioral Assessment System for Children, 2nd Edition (BASC-2). Minneapolis, MN, Pearson Assessment, 2004

Roberts GE: Roberts Apperception Test for Children, 2nd Edition (Roberts–2). Los Angeles, CA, Western Psychological Services, 2005

Roid GH: Stanford-Binet Intelligence Scales, 5th Edition (SB5). Itasca, IL, Riverside Publishing, 2003

Sparrow SS, Balla DA, Cicchetti DV: Vineland Adaptive Behavior Scales, 2nd Edition. Circle Pines, MN, American Guidance Service, 2006

Wechsler D: Wechsler Individual Achievement Test, 2nd Edition (WIAT-II). San Antonio, TX, Harcourt Assessment, 2001

Wechsler D: Wechsler Intelligence Scale for Children, 4th Edition (WISC-IV). San Antonio, TX, Harcourt Assessment, 2003

Wechsler D: Wechsler Adult Intelligence Scale, 4th Edition (WAIS-IV). San Antonio, TX, Harcourt Assessment, 2008

Wilkinson GS, Robertson, GJ: Wide Range Achievement Test 4 (WRAT4). Los Angeles, CA, Western Psychological Services, 2007

Woodcock RW, McGrew, KS, Mather,N: Woodcock-Johnson Psychoeducational Battery, 3rd Edition (WJ-III). Itasca, IL, Riverside Publishing, 2001

Chapter 7

Forensic Telepsychiatry

Tracy D. Gunter, M.D.

The use of technology to deliver mental health services has expanded rapidly in recent years and represents the convergence of readily available cost-effective technology with a recognized need to improve access to quality care (Gibbons 2005; Graeff-Martins et al. 2008; McGinty et al. 2006). In addition to the use of traditional technologies such as telephone and facsimile transmission, modern technologically mediated health care includes the use of Web-based communications, satellite transmission, and wireless systems, in addition to real-time videoconferencing (Ferrante 2005; Hilty et al. 2006; Strecher 2007). There has been much confusion surrounding the nomenclature used to discuss these technologies, and it remains far from standardized (Gunter et al. 2003; Oh et al. 2005). For clarity, the following definitions are offered. This chapter focuses on telepsychiatry, which is narrowly defined as the use of line-based interactive videoconferencing to deliver mental health services. The remainder of modalities previously listed might best be considered as e-health or e-mental health (McGinty et al. 2006; Norman et al. 2007; Strecher 2007). Telemedicine is a more general term that is defined as "the use of telecommunications and information technology to provide health care services to persons at a distance from the provider" (J. Grigsby and Sanders 1998).

The major advantage of using interactive videoconferencing over other forms of distance technology lies in the provider's ability to simultaneously observe physical signs and hear verbal information. In addition to facilitating accurate assessment (S.P. Singh et al. 2007), this ability for communicating both verbal and nonverbal information in a real-time fashion facilitates the communication of authenticity and trustworthiness necessary to the successful formation of the provider–patient relationship in a superior way to asynchronous or unimodal technologically mediated communication (Morgan et al. 2008). The synchronous nature of telepsychiatry is its principal strength, but a number of factors such as line speed and image quality affect the accuracy and utility of this approximation of in-person services (Pesamaa et al. 2004).

While recognizing the potential of telepsychiatry to provide services to patients distant from sites of in-person care, it is not universally successful, and some providers remain ambivalent about its use (Barton et al. 2007; Elford et al. 2000; B. Grigsby et al. 2007; May et al. 2001; Wagnild et al. 2006). Providers have been frustrated by technological innovations in the delivery of health in general because of technical difficulties and the apparent devaluing of the physical presence, which has been so highly valued in traditional paradigms of service delivery. In a broader sense, technology challenges medicine's traditional definition of, and requirement for, physical presence. Once the requirement for physical presence is eliminated, the digitizing of health care enables activities to be outsourced to providers at a considerable distance from the patient. These activities are typically undertaken as a way to ease the burden on local providers and contain costs (Wachter 2006). Now increasingly common in the practices of radiology, pathology, and intensive care monitoring (S.N. Singh and Wachter 2008), there is every reason to believe that these kinds of innovations will expand to include some types of behavioral health interventions. Although international outsourcing may be relatively limited for traditional tele-psychiatry delivered in a line-based fashion, it will increase as costs fall and greater services are delivered over the Internet. In addition to concerns about erosion in the provider–patient relationship and overcoming technical barriers, outsourcing of medical care should encourage more traditional providers to think about cost containment for durable services, advocate for patient safety and privacy, and think creatively about ways to ensure delivery of quality and appropriate services to those in need of them (S.N. Singh and Wachter 2008; Wachter 2006).

Recognizing the rapidly evolving role of this complex technology in the provision of mental health services to children and adolescents, the American Academy of Child and Adolescent Psychiatry has developed a practice parameter that provides a detailed review of the development of telepsychiatry in providing mental health services to children and assists the clinician in developing an effective telepsychiatry service, including detailed discussions of technical, organizational, legal, and ethical considerations that are beyond the scope of this brief overview chapter (Myers and Cain 2008).

Telepsychiatry With Children and Adolescents

Telemedicine consultation has been used in the care of children by a number of specialties worldwide, including ophthalmology, otology, radiology, cardiology, pulmonology, endocrinology, medical genetics, intensive care, surgery, and psychiatry (Smith 2007b). Estimating the specific number of active telemedicine programs providing child and adolescent mental health services at any given point in time is a difficult task. In the mid-1980s there were no active telepsychiatry programs, and by 2000 there were 43 active general telepsychiatry programs (Whitten et al. 2000). In a search of the Telemedicine Information Exchange database (www.telemed.org) in March 2008, there were 90 active programs listed as delivering mental health care and 65 active programs listed as delivering pediatric care, although subspecialty details were not readily available.

Telepsychiatry services have been delivered to children and adolescents in a variety of settings beyond traditional settings such as mental health center and private offices, including correctional facilities (Myers et al. 2006), hospitals (Myers et al. 2008), schools (Khasanshina et al. 2008; Mackert and Whitten 2007),

shelters (Thomas et al. 2005), and postdisaster outreach (Mack et al. 2007). Though not yet routine in the practice of child and adolescent psychiatry, telepsychiatry has been demonstrated by a number of studies (Shore et al. 2007b; Yellowlees et al. 2008) to be an effective component of modern mental health service delivery and has been increasingly used to reach individuals unable to access traditional in-person services (e.g., rural and incarcerated populations).

In considering the use of these services with children, one should pay particular attention to the maturational stage, cognitive abilities, manual dexterity, and distress tolerance of the child as well as the wishes and needs of those responsible for authorizing care for the child (Myers and Cain 2008; Myers et al. 2008). Very young or highly active children may have difficulty focusing on the screen, manipulating the equipment, or remaining relatively still for the interview. Assessments that involve prolonged single-session contact might prove too fatiguing to complete in a relatively small room using interactive videoconferencing. Evaluation types that require multiple observations of the child interacting with multiple care providers in multiple constellations might be difficult for the remote telepsychiatrist to follow using videoconferencing. Despite its apparent limitations, providers using these services for even intensely interactive activities, such as play therapy, note that appropriate modifications can be made to facilitate the provision of this service over videoconferencing, such as having the child interact with a support person locally in a variety of roles (Bryant 2007).

As has been consistently reported for more than 30 years, experiences in rendering and receiving telepsychiatry services are different from in-person services but appear at least satisfactory, and in some cases preferable, in the eyes of patients (Dwyer 1973; Sulzbacher et al. 2006). The use of technology in the delivery of psychiatric services may not be appropriate for all patients or providers, however. Regular reviews of services delivered in this way must therefore be undertaken to ensure that both patients and providers are comfortable with the process.

Forensic issues involving children evaluated via telepsychiatry include risk of dangerous behavior, abuse and neglect, custody disputes, and needs assessments (Keilman 2005). Although Miller and colleagues describe general concepts relevant to telepsychiatry services using the context of a child and adolescent forensic clinic (Miller et al. 2005), and there are occasional anecdotal reports presented at conferences and in the literature, there are currently few published data on the process of using telepsychiatry in forensic practice involving children.

Practice Models

A variety of practice models may be employed in the delivery of telepsychiatry services. Broadly defined, these service delivery practice models will involve either consultation or direct care (Dwyer 1973). The selection of practice model has many implications in assessing and addressing potential difficulties faced in providing services using this technology.

The consultation model is most commonly used and involves a local care team actively caring for the patient and contacting the telepsychiatrist for subspecialty expertise. Under this model, the local team initiates and facilitates the initial evaluation, supports the patient through the process of remote evaluation, and implements any treatment suggestions generated as the result of the consultation. The initial consultation may then be followed by a case presentation or discussion between the remote telepsychiatrist and local team with follow-up as dictated by the needs of the local team. The local team then provides ongoing care, crisis management, and emergency care.

In the direct care model, the telepsychiatrist may conduct an initial evaluation or make intermittent site visits in person, and then use teleconferencing for follow-up treatment and therapy (Sulzbacher et al. 2006). Some authors have described situations in which limited direct care is offered without the use of site visits with satisfactory results. In the direct care scenario, the telepsychiatrist is the primary mental health provider and is therefore responsible for addressing needs that arise between sessions and for emergency intervention, in addition to scheduled sessions. The delivery of emergency services using telepsychiatry is an active area of study at this time (Shore et al. 2007a). While this direct care model has been used satisfactorily with adults in both forensic (Morgan et al. 2008) and nonforensic settings (O'Reilly et al. 2007), its use in children requires the participation and satisfaction of both the child and the parent or care provider, and such studies are currently under way (Myers et al. 2008).

Liability Considerations

Once the provider–patient relationship is established, the provider has the responsibility to either be available to provide care or refer the patient to someone who is able to do so. In child and adolescent psychiatry, there will likely be an alternate decision maker and care provider who participates in treatment as well, making the situation somewhat more complex (Ash 2002). In the case of telepsychiatry, abandonment claims may arise when equipment failure prevents adequate access to the responsible provider or when treatment needs outstrip the ability of the remote psychiatrist to provide care (Miller et al. 2005). As has been noted previously, the involvement of a local care team utilized in the consultation model reduces the risk of intended or unintended patient abandonment and thus is preferable over the direct care model in remote service delivery when risk minimization is desirable.

Although documents such as "Telepsychiatry Via Videoconferencing" by the American Psychiatric Association (1998), "A Teleconsultation Practice Guideline" by the G8 Global Health Applications SP4 Group (Nerlich et al. 2002; see also Asbach and Nerlich 2003), and a practice parameter by the American Academy of Child and Adolescent Psychiatry (Myers and Cain 2008) all suggest best practices, there is no established standard of care in the United States specific to the practice of telepsychiatry (Hyler and Gangure 2004). The prevailing *reasonable care* standard, which dictates that the practitioner should exercise the skill and prudence that a reasonable practitioner would exercise in similar circumstances, would likely be applied to the telepsychiatry situation as questions about standard of care are raised (Miller et al. 2005). Negligence may be claimed when videoconferencing is deemed inferior to in-person services in conducting an adequate assessment or conveying a treatment plan (Miller et al. 2005). Although some data indicate that telepsychiatry encounters are not uniformly inferior to in-person services, very little, if any, data currently exist indicating that the two are equivalent.

Providers choosing to use telepsychiatry must verify with the carrier, preferably in writing, that malpractice coverage is in place for planned activities (Hyler and Gangure 2004). Providers should also utilize legal consultation to develop practice policies, documentation procedures, and contractual language that maximizes transparency with the site, facilitates clarity of communication with patients, and minimizes risk exposure.

Licensure

While the practice of telepsychiatry within a single state is relatively uncomplicated from the standpoint of licensure, the practice of telepsychiatry extending beyond state or national borders presents significant challenges regarding licensure (Hyler and Gangure 2004) since national medical licensure is not yet on the horizon in the United States. Telepsychiatrists (and their risk managers) must address the question of whether their activities trigger the requirement for licensure in the "remote" state (Gunter et al. 2003). A total of 30 states require some kind of licensure for the practice of telepsychiatry (24 require full licensure and 6 require a special purpose license for telehealth; www.telemed.org). The remaining 20 states do not specifically address the delivery of services via telemedicine in licensure law, regulation, or policy, so particular care should be undertaken in determining the definition or interpretation of the "practice of medicine" (www.telemed.org). Active consultation with all applicable medical boards is advisable to ensure that the telepsychiatrist is aware of practice issues that typically vary by state and impact licensure, including mandatory reporting and civil commitment procedures, required documentation of the process of care, and regulations related to the prescription of medications.

Credentialing

Regardless of the proximity of the sites, the telepsychiatrist will need to be credentialed at each practice site (Hyler and Gangure 2004). The credentialing process will ensure that telepsychiatrists are familiar with the services provided, equipment used, and policies and procedures at the provider site and all remote sites. Following initial credentialing at both sites, continuing education in telepsychiatry must occur at regular intervals. Staff development and periodic monitoring at both the provider and patient sites are essential to ensure that quality services are being provided. Issues of credentialing, standards, protocols, and quality will likely be queried in the courtroom. The telepsychiatrist should be well versed and articulate in these matters.

Site Issues

Regardless of the service undertaken by a remote consulting telepsychiatrist, strong local support is essential (Greenberg et al. 2006). In the consultation model, the local site will be invaluable in providing background information, assessing the quality of commu-

nication, conducting in-person evaluations (e.g., vital signs), and coordinating local care (Boydell et al. 2007). A technical consultant should be available to both sites to advise on major difficulties and downtime procedures established to guide staff at both sites in dealing with situations in which the network may not be available. In the direct care model, the telepsychiatrist must develop strategies to accomplish these tasks directly with the participant and pertinent decision makers.

For the forensic psychiatrist, the judicial system will be an important stakeholder to consider. Given that telepsychiatry is a relatively new tool in conducting court-ordered evaluations and delivering treatment, the forensic telepsychiatrist should make every attempt to determine that the retaining attorney has sought agreement from the judge and other parties involved concerning the likely acceptance of videoconferencing for conducting the requested evaluation, using the information obtained as the foundation for subsequent sworn testimony, and providing testimony during depositions, hearings, and/or trials (Miller et al. 2005).

Health Information

Both sites involved in the delivery of telepsychiatry services must provide appropriately equipped private interview rooms with secure communications lines. The patient and patient's decision maker must be educated about the nature and purpose of the session, any limitations in confidentiality, the use and operation of the equipment, and any security risks inherent in the particular technology implemented for the encounter. Prior to the first session, written informed consent should be obtained from the parent or guardian and assent obtained from the minor patient. A particular concern for all participants is the ease with which data exchanged by this technology can be recorded by either party, and this must be addressed in all discussions and written documents. All remote participants should be encouraged to raise any concerns about the service provided or technology used as they arise, and the patient or evaluee should be specifically queried about satisfaction with the service at its conclusion.

In order for the interaction to be most useful, the patient's complete medical record should be available to the telepsychiatrist. This is most easily accomplished if a longitudinal electronic medical record can be accessed by both sites, but more traditional forms of communication such as mailing or faxing portions of the paper record for review may produce a satisfactory exchange of information. The systems used and information exchanged in the provision of mental health services will likely be subject to federal security and privacy rules under the U.S. Health Insurance Portability and Accountability Act of 1996 (HIPAA), which were designed to protect identifiable health information by providing a uniformly minimum standard and may be subject to more stringent protections in some states (Hyler and Gangure 2004).

In the case of forensic evaluations, the issues regarding information handling are often even more complex. Even with a longitudinal electronic medical record, there will often be case-specific legal information in paper form for review prior to the telepsychiatry encounter. Therefore, the likely record generated will be an electronic-paper hybrid composed of both medical and legal information. Strategies for handling this scenario to ensure that a complete secure record is available at all times should be detailed in the agreement with the retaining attorney or agency. The additional issues of whether the evaluation will be recorded, who will have access to the recording, and how the recording would then be stored should also be discussed with the consulting party and evaluee (and decision maker if applicable) in advance.

Financial Considerations

One of the greatest challenges to creating a sustainable telepsychiatry program is securing a satisfactory financial platform for the service provider or party bearing the expense of the technology (Hilty et al. 2008; Kennedy 2005; Sulzbacher et al. 2006). Telepsychiatry programs have direct and indirect costs that occur in both the setup and maintenance phases of program development. Though programs offer cost savings in some situations (Hyler and Gangure 2003), often the expenditures and benefits are not direct, immediate, or experienced equally by the parties involved in the telepsychiatry service (Smith 2007a). For instance, if a university-based telepsychiatry clinic delivers a mental health intervention to a remote rural center that is successful in lowering hospital admission rates, then both the patient and the community experience time and cost savings. The patient has not been inconvenienced by an expensive inpatient stay, nor has the patient traveled outside of his or her home community to gain the benefits of an intervention that has also likely improved quality of life. Though the local center has experienced capital costs in setting up the equipment ini-

tially, it experiences decreases in costs associated with both local service provider time and contracted bed space for each patient served by the telepsychiatry intervention who was not hospitalized. So, having described the advantages gained by the patient and outlying site, let us now consider the service provider. For the remote telepsychiatry provider, the situation is somewhat more complex. If the remote provider has an obligation to provide a service to the distant site regardless of the presence of technology, then the technology does in fact offer both cost and time savings for the provider. However, if the telepsychiatry provider would not otherwise provide the service, then the service provider has incurred charges related to equipment, time spent in the service, and decreased availability for other tasks. In order for the situation to be tenable then, the provider requires compensation.

Contracts between telepsychiatry providers and remote sites (or individual patients) may stipulate specific reimbursement for services or service hours, while other agreements may stipulate that services will be paid by reimbursement from third-party payers. Currently, only 19 states offer Medicaid reimbursement for telemedicine (Naditz 2008), and only 5 states (California, Kentucky, Louisiana, Oklahoma, and Texas) mandate equivalent reimbursement for telemedicine and in-person service by commercial insurers operating within those states according to the Telemedicine Information Exchange (www.telemed. org). Although some have proposed that reimbursement for a service should be based on the service and relatively independent of the technology utilized (Perednia and Grigsby 1998), the reality is that reimbursement, when available, is lower when practicing telepsychiatry than when providing in-person services most of the time. Thus, in addition to maximizing compensation, one must also calculate the volume needed to generate sufficient income to cover the expenditures and examine ways to minimize costs in order to enhance viability. From a technical perspective, the use of dedicated Internet protocol networks for telepsychiatry, as opposed to dedicated line-based services, may serve to lower costs and facilitate sharing of costs but brings with it additional concerns about security (McGinty et al. 2006). Additionally, the use of the consultation model may be more cost-effective (Hilty et al. 2008) than the direct care model because the codes used for initial evaluation are often among the best compensated and professional time needed beyond the initial consultation is minimized. Other ways to minimize costs might include diversifying services delivered via telepsychiatry, sharing resources across programs, and involving trainees in telepsychiatry service delivery (Hilty et al. 2008).

In the case of a forensic evaluation conducted under retainer, payment arrangements will likely be detailed in the contract between the expert and the attorney or agency rather than the remote site directly. These payment arrangements must be explicit and should incorporate the areas discussed above.

Conclusion

Telepsychiatry is a rapidly evolving tool in the provision of mental health services to children and adolescents. In studies involving adults, and in demonstration projects involving rural care, telepsychiatry appears to be efficient for providers who are unable to travel to areas of need and acceptable to patients for whom there are few, if any, other options for accessing services (Grubaugh et al. 2008). Significant knowledge gaps remain in determining specific systems and services best suited to telepsychiatry, patient acceptance where other care options exist, and equality to in-person evidence-based psychiatric services (Myers and Cain 2008; O'Reilly et al. 2007). There are many programs, organizations, agencies, and researchers currently investigating these and many other questions about this emerging technology (Nguyen et al. 2007). While telepsychiatry in particular, and electronically mediated health care in general, offer great promise in equalizing access to quality care in an efficient and cost-effective manner, their place in the spectrum of mental health services provided to children and adolescents and impact on traditional services should be critically evaluated at each step in their evolution (Ratner 2002).

—Key Points

— Electronically mediated health care is changing the practice of medicine. The legal and regulatory environments are rapidly changing. Providers not only need to keep abreast of current legislation and regulation but also must advocate for reasoned policies appropriate to each of the emerging technologies. One area that providers should be particularly vigilant and vocal about is the outsourcing of care enabled by electronically mediated health care.

— Telepsychiatry is one of the most traditional and least controversial of these evolving electronic tools. Despite this, significant indeterminacies exist concerning technical standards, practice standards, licensure, liability, and reimbursement. Service providers and their risk managers should consider legal consultation before beginning service delivery, especially if they contemplate an interstate or international practice situation.

— Telepsychiatry is an effective and appropriate tool for delivering forensic subspecialty services to geographically isolated and underserved populations. A priori consultation with the court system regarding issues of acceptance and admissibility, however, is still advisable as telepsychiatry has not yet come into the mainstream.

— Clinical and technological standards for telepsychiatry remain works in progress. As an evolving field, telepsychiatry has a rapidly growing body of evidence outlining both its advantages and its limitations. Several separate groups of health care professionals, regulators, and other stakeholders are attempting to put forth practice guidelines for telepsychiatry. The recently published practice parameter by the American Academy of Child and Adolescent Psychiatry (Myers and Cain 2008) is an excellent resource for those working with children and adolescents.

— As telepsychiatry moves from demonstration projects and pilot studies to the mainstream, critical issues concerning utilization and cost-effectiveness must be addressed to facilitate the definition of the niche that it will occupy in the range of services offered to patients and evaluees. Models for assessing costs, cost savings, and outcomes need to be developed and rigorously applied in future studies so that incentives and facilitators can be used to overcome both real and perceived barriers for each stakeholder involved in this enterprise.

References

American Psychiatric Association: Telepsychiatry via Video-conferencing. July 1998. Available at: http://archive.psych.org/edu/other_res/lib_archives/archives/199821.pdf. Accessed March 31, 2008.

Asbach P, Nerlich M: A telemedicine guideline for the practice of teleconsultation. Stud Health Technol Inform 97:1–14, 2003

Ash P: Malpractice in child and adolescent psychiatry. Child Adolesc Psychiatr Clin N Am 11:869–885, 2002

Barton PL, Brega AG, Devore PA, et al: Specialist physicians' knowledge and beliefs about telemedicine: a comparison of users and nonusers of the technology. Telemed J E Health 13:487–499, 2007

Boydell KM, Volpe T, Kertes A, et al: A review of the outcomes of the recommendations made during paediatric telepsychiatry consultations. J Telemed Telecare 13:277–281, 2007

Bryant B: Telepsychiatry gets good reception with Texas high school students. Psychiatric News 42:22a, March 2, 2007

Dwyer TF: Telepsychiatry: psychiatric consultation by interactive television. Am J Psychiatry 130:865–869, 1973

Elford R, White H, Bowering R, et al: A randomized, controlled trial of child psychiatric assessments conducted using videoconferencing. J Telemed Telecare 6:73–82, 2000

Ferrante FE: Evolving telemedicine/ehealth technology. Telemed J E Health 11:370–383, 2005

Gibbons MC: A historical overview of health disparities and the potential of eHealth solutions. J Med Internet Res 7:e50, 2005

Graeff-Martins AS, Flament MF, Fayyad J, et al: Diffusion of efficacious interventions for children and adolescents with mental health problems. J Child Psychol Psychiatry 49:335–352, 2008

Greenberg N, Boydell KM, Volpe T: Pediatric telepsychiatry in Ontario: caregiver and service provider perspectives. J Behav Health Serv Res 33:105–111, 2006

Grigsby B, Brega AG, Bennett RE, et al: The slow pace of interactive video telemedicine adoption: the perspective of telemedicine program administrators on physician participation. Telemed J E Health 13:645–656, 2007

Grigsby J, Sanders JH: Telemedicine: where it is and where it's going. Ann Intern Med 129:123–127, 1998

Grubaugh AL, Cain GD, Elhai JD, et al: Attitudes toward medical and mental health care delivered via telehealth applications among rural and urban primary care patients. J Nerv Ment Dis 196:166–170, 2008

Gunter TD, Srinivasaraghavan J, Terry NP: Misinformed regulation of electronic medicine is unfair to responsible telepsychiatry. J Am Acad Psychiatry Law 31:10–14, 2003

Hilty DM, Alverson DC, Alpert JE, et al: Virtual reality, telemedicine, web and data processing innovations in medical and psychiatric education and clinical care. Acad Psychiatry 30:528–533, 2006

Hilty DM, Cobb HC, Neufeld JD, et al: Telepsychiatry reduces geographic physician disparity in rural settings, but is it financially feasible because of reimbursement? Psychiatr Clin North Am 31:85–94, 2008

Hyler SE, Gangure DP: A review of the costs of telepsychiatry. Psychiatr Serv 54:976–980, 2003

Hyler SE, Gangure DP: Legal and ethical challenges in telepsychiatry. J Psychiatr Pract 10:272–276, 2004

Keilman P: Telepsychiatry with child welfare families referred to a family service agency. Telemed J E Health 11:98–101, 2005

Kennedy CA: The challenges of economic evaluations of remote technical health interventions. Clin Invest Med 28:71–74, 2005

Khasanshina EV, Wolfe WL, Emerson EN, et al: Counseling center-based tele-mental health for students at a rural university. Telemed J E Health 14:35–41, 2008

Mack D, Brantley KM, Bell KG: Mitigating the health effects of disasters for medically underserved populations: electronic health records, telemedicine, research, screening, and surveillance. J Health Care Poor Underserved 18:432–442, 2007

Mackert M, Whitten P: Successful adoption of a school-based telemedicine system. J Sch Health 77:327–330, 2007

May C, Gask L, Atkinson T, et al: Resisting and promoting new technologies in clinical practice: the case of telepsychiatry. Soc Sci Med 52:1889–1901, 2001

McGinty KL, Saeed SA, Simmons SC, et al: Telepsychiatry and e-mental health services: potential for improving access to mental health care. Psychiatr Q 77:335–342, 2006

Miller TW, Burton DC, Hill K, et al: Telepsychiatry: critical dimensions for forensic services. J Am Acad Psychiatry Law 33:539–546, 2005

Morgan RD, Patrick AR, Magaletta PR: Does the use of tele-mental health alter the treatment experience? Inmates' perceptions of telemental health versus face-to-face treatment modalities. J Consult Clin Psychol 76:158–162, 2008

Myers K, Cain S: Practice parameter on telepsychiatry with children and adolescents. J Am Acad Child Adolesc Psychiatry 47:1468–1483, 2008

Myers K, Valentine J, Morganthaler R, et al: Telepsychiatry with incarcerated youth. J Adolesc Health 38:643–648, 2006

Myers KM, Valentine JM, Melzer SM: Child and adolescent telepsychiatry: utilization and satisfaction. Telemed J E Health 14:131–137, 2008

Naditz A: Medicare's and Medicaid's new reimbursement policies for telemedicine. Telemed J E Health 14:21–24, 2008

Nerlich M, Balas EA, Schall T, et al: Teleconsultation practice guidelines: report from G8 Global Health Applications Subproject 4. Telemed J E Health 8:411–418, 2002

Nguyen HQ, Cuenco D, Wolpin S, et al: Methodological considerations in evaluating eHealth interventions. Can J Nurs Res 39:116–134, 2007

Norman GJ, Zabinski MF, Adams MA, et al: A review of eHealth interventions for physical activity and dietary behavior change. Am J Prev Med 33:336–345, 2007

O'Reilly R, Bishop J, Maddox K, et al: Is telepsychiatry equivalent to face-to-face psychiatry? Results from a randomized controlled equivalence trial. Psychiatr Serv 58:836–843, 2007

Oh H, Rizo C, Enkin M, et al: What is eHealth (3): a systematic review of published definitions. J Med Internet Res 7:e1, 2005

Perednia DA, Grigsby J: Telephones, telemedicine, and a technologically neutral coverage policy. Telemed J 4:145–152, 1998

Pesamaa L, Ebeling H, Kuusimaki ML, et al: Videoconferencing in child and adolescent telepsychiatry: a systematic review of the literature. J Telemed Telecare 10:187–192, 2004

Ratner RA: Ethics in child and adolescent forensic psychiatry. Child Adolesc Psychiatr Clin N Am 11:887–904, 2002

Shore JH, Hilty DM, Yellowlees P: Emergency management guidelines for telepsychiatry. Gen Hosp Psychiatry 29:199–206, 2007a

Shore JH, Savin D, Orton H, et al: Diagnostic reliability of telepsychiatry in American Indian veterans. Am J Psychiatry 164:115–118, 2007b

Singh SN, Wachter RM: Perspectives on medical outsourcing and telemedicine—rough edges in a flat world? N Engl J Med 358:1622–1627, 2008

Singh SP, Arya D, Peters T: Accuracy of telepsychiatric assessment of new routine outpatient referrals. BMC Psychiatry 7:55, 2007

Smith AC: Telemedicine: challenges and opportunities. Expert Rev Med Devices 4:5–7, 2007a

Smith AC: Telepaediatrics. J Telemed Telecare 13:163–166, 2007b

Strecher V: Internet methods for delivering behavioral and health-related interventions (eHealth). Annu Rev Clin Psychol 3:53–76, 2007

Sulzbacher S, Vallin T, Waetzig EZ: Telepsychiatry improves paediatric behavioural health care in rural communities. J Telemed Telecare 12:285–288, 2006

Thomas CR, Miller G, Hartshorn JC, et al: Telepsychiatry program for rural victims of domestic violence. Telemed J E Health 11:567–573, 2005

Wachter RM: The "dis-location" of U.S. medicine—the implications of medical outsourcing. N Engl J Med 354:661–665, 2006

Wagnild G, Leenknecht C, Zauher J: Psychiatrists' satisfaction with telepsychiatry. Telemed J E Health 12:546–551, 2006

Whitten P, Zaylor C, Kingsley C: An analysis of telepsychiatry programs from an organizational perspective. Cyperpsychol Behav 3:911–916, 2000

Yellowlees PM, Hilty DM, Marks SL, et al: A retrospective analysis of a child and adolescent eMental Health program. J Am Acad Child Adolesc Psychiatry 47:103–107, 2008

Chapter 8

Cultural Competence in Child and Adolescent Forensic Mental Health

Todd S. Elwyn, J.D., M.D.
Wen Shing Tseng, M.D.
Daryl Matthews, M.D., Ph.D.

The United States is often likened to a melting pot because of the diverse mix of immigrant groups constituting its population since its birth as a nation. Foreign-born persons continue to compose a significant percentage of the population—estimated to be 12.4% in 2000 (Dumont and Lemaitre 2005). Approximately 4% of all children in the United States younger than 18 were born outside of the United States and its territories in 2005 (KewalRamani et al. 2007). Of the immigrant population, 53.3% come from Latin America, 25% from Asia, 13.7% from Europe, and 8% from other regions of the world (Larsen 2004). Foreign-born persons constitute a significant percentage of the population in several other English-speaking nations, such as Australia (23.0%), Canada (19.3%), and the United Kingdom (8.3%) (Dumont and Lemaitre 2005). In addition to immigrants, international tourists and their families regularly travel to the United States and other countries for short-term stays.

As the world has grown smaller, health care providers have increasingly recognized the importance of developing cultural competence. Cultural factors are known to influence the development, expression, and interpretation of symptoms, especially in the area of mental health. Understanding cultural factors allows

clinicians to perform better assessments that improve diagnostic accuracy and provide care in an appropriate manner to their diverse patient population. Similarly, forensic mental health examiners have recently begun to appreciate the value of developing cultural competence in order to conduct thorough forensic assessments and provide appropriate and relevant opinions (Tseng et al. 2004). The issues at stake for the forensic examinee potentially have significant ramifications for an individual's or family's liberty, finances, and happiness. Being able to recognize cultural issues and account for them appropriately helps improve the accuracy and responsiveness of forensic evaluations and may help minimize the chance of an unjust outcome resulting from expert opinion.

What Is Cultural Competence?

The word *culture* has been defined in various ways since it began to be used in this context in the late eighteenth century. A simple definition might be, "the customary beliefs, social forms, and material traits of a racial, religious, or social group" (Merriam-Webster Online Dictionary 2009). A culture typically is formed over many generations and changes slowly. Whether consciously or unconsciously, culture shapes one's beliefs about the world, one's behaviors, and one's attitudes about those behaviors, including notions of right and wrong and what constitutes appropriate punishment for transgressions. On a larger level, culture and religion influence the development of legal systems around the world. Accordingly, in some countries or regions, rules defining right and wrong are based on or influenced by religious law (such as Islamic law or Talmudic law); based on the common law (as in the United States and the United Kingdom); based on civil law (as in France and Germany); based on customary law (as in Cambodia); or based on a mixed system of one or more of the above. Immigrants and others coming from a different culture may find the rules and mores of the new country to differ widely from their own.

Although the terms *culture, ethnicity, race,* and *minority* are often used interchangeably, they differ in important ways. The terms *ethnicity* and *ethnic group* refer to a group of persons that shares a common identity based on historical lineage and behavioral norms that separates and distinguishes it from other groups. An ethnic group may share a common culture with other groups but have characteristics that identify them as a distinct group. *Race* refers to a group of people that are distinguishable by characteristic physical features such as the color of their skin and hair, their physical size, or their facial features. Race is a socially constructed category based on observed differences in phenotype rather than a biologically based distinction rooted in genotype. The term *minority* refers to any group within a society that differs from the larger group of which it is a part on the basis of politics, religion, or race. The status of a group as a minority is a social construct that may or may not be related to matters of culture or ethnicity (Tseng et al. 2004).

Cultural competence in forensic mental health consists of the ability to recognize that cultural factors may be contributory whenever an examiner is performing a forensic assessment of someone from another culture, to identify relevant cultural issues, and to determine the best way to appropriately address them. Cultural competence begins with the recognition that each evaluator carries into the examination room beliefs, attitudes, assumptions, and interpretations that have been shaped by his or her own cultural background. Examiners who lack cultural competence may believe that their own culturally conditioned ex-

perience serves as a reliable guide for understanding the actions and behaviors of others, regardless of their culture of origin. In contrast, the culturally competent examiner seeks to understand the actions and beliefs of the examinee from the perspective of the examinee. Thus, examiners must become aware that other cultures may view numerous things differently and then be open and receptive to learn about the beliefs, attitudes, perceptions, and ideas of the other culture. This quality is called *cultural sensitivity* and is one of the foundations of cultural competence.

Other key aspects of cultural competence include cultural knowledge, cultural empathy, culturally relevant interactions with examinees, and culturally informed presentations of the forensic results. *Cultural knowledge* refers to developing at least a basic knowledge of the culture of the examinee. *Cultural empathy* describes understanding the emotional valence attached to various cultural practices. For example, if mental illness is stigmatized in a culture, the examiner should understand this fact as well as consider how difficult admitting one has a mental illness may be for a person of that culture, such as when raising an insanity defense. Finally, the examiner should be aware that the interaction between examiner and examinee may have culturally influenced implications because of the power imbalance inherent in the evaluation or because of the race or sex of the examiner. Cultural consultants such as anthropologists or professionals belonging to the relevant cultural group may be necessary to fully understand the issues involved. The forensic examiner then must provide a report for the court or the retaining attorney that conveys the important cultural information in such a way that the receiving party can understand the significance of the information conveyed. That is, the report must be written with enough detailed description and in a manner appropriate to the forum so that the recipient judge or attorney can realize its import (Tseng 2003, pp. 219–225).

The process of forensic examination involves gathering the relevant data, correctly interpreting the data, and synthesizing the data to present it in a coherent and cohesive manner. Cultural competence in forensic examination recognizes that cultural factors can influence any aspect of this process. Accurate data gathering, such as may occur when observing the examinee's behavior or responses during an interview, requires that the examiner has eyes to see what is actually taking place rather than merely seeing an image produced by one's own cultural lens. If the examinee's behavior is not recorded correctly, then the error introduced will taint one's interpretation of the behavior and how it is synthesized with the other data. Important cultural issues may present in the form of subtle misunderstandings or misperceptions that have gone unnoticed, or they may involve more dramatic cultural issues, such as may be the case when culture-bound syndromes are present. A careful inquiry on a case-by-case basis will be needed to tease out the relevant issues.

Cultural competence has been recognized only recently as an important aspect of forensic practice. As such, many facets of cultural competence have yet to be rigorously studied in a systematic fashion. In this chapter, we highlight the current state of the literature and provide direction for those who confront in daily practice these important issues. We begin by describing some of the important cultural considerations attendant to performing a forensic examination. Next, we discuss how the law handles culture, including culture-bound syndromes. Finally, we describe the role of culture in the specific kinds of assessments the child and adolescent examiner typically performs.

Culturally Competent Forensic Examination

Initial Tasks

The culturally competent forensic evaluation begins with obtaining from the referral source as much relevant information as possible about the examinee. Private attorneys sometimes can provide a greater level of detail than can other sources of referral, such as courts, or government or private entities, such as schools, hospitals, or social service agencies. At a minimum, information about the examinee's country of origin, the language spoken, and the degree of fluency in English is necessary to make decisions about using an interpreter. Whenever possible, the examiner also should obtain information about the city, town, or village from which the person or family hails; whether the person or family belongs to an ethnic or religious minority within that country; the family's socioeconomic status within the country; the number of siblings; when the person and family left that country; any significant issues that arose with emigration from the country; and when the person and family arrived in the United States. Learning as much as possible about the examinee from the beginning will save time and facilitate understanding of the areas that require further inquiry.

Armed with this preliminary knowledge, a useful next step in the evaluation process is to take time to reflect on one's own biases, experiences, and beliefs about the culture of origin of the examinee. Our formative life experiences involving the culture of the examinee may influence and distort how we perceive the examinee. For example, if one's wallet was stolen by someone of a certain ethnic or racial background, one might harbor the suspicion that all persons of that ethnicity or race are thieves. Such biases will impede the forensic evaluator's ability to understand the experience of the examinee from the examinee's perspective, which is an important goal of forensic evaluation. Qualitative research theory suggests that developing an understanding of the biases and faulty assumptions one brings into the investigation of a topic improves the clarity of one's vision. McCracken (1988) recommends writing down and analyzing one's experiences in a detailed and systematic way, examining them, and examining the associations, incidents, and assumptions that surround the topic in one's own mind as a useful step to overcome personal biases and develop a more accurate understanding of the issues.

Maintaining an ongoing sensitivity to one's biases throughout the evaluation process is an important task for the culturally competent examiner. Fontes (2008) identified several specific types of bias that may influence an examiner. *Motivational bias* refers to the desire on the part of the evaluator to arrive at a particular outcome to please someone else, such as a retaining attorney. *Notational bias* refers to ways in which our categories or terms can bias the outcome, such as diagnosing a condition even though the person does not fit neatly into the category. *Cognitive biases*, including observational biases, are thinking errors that arise from using simplified information processing strategies. Cognitive biases include confirmatory bias (seeing what we expect to see), fundamental attribution error (attributing a person's actions to his or her personality rather than to situational factors such as fatigue or illness), halo effect (allowing one aspect of a person to influence the perception of other aspects), in-group bias (giving preferential treatment to others who are like us), and self-fulfilling prophecy (eliciting results that confirm one's preconceptions.) For example, cognitive bias may be present in child custody evaluations when an evaluator preferentially weighs the responses of the divorcing parent who is of the same ethnicity or race as the examiner when assessing what is best for the child.

Collateral Information

Obtaining collateral information for review may be more difficult when evaluating the foreign-born examinee. Sources of collateral information may include written documents that must be obtained from the examinee's country of origin, such as medical records or school records. Problems may arise in obtaining these documents when organizations in the home country have kept limited records or have limited technology available to copy and send them. Regardless, efforts should be made to obtain them because they may be helpful to understanding the case. The referral source may be able to provide assistance in arranging this, especially when the records are likely to be helpful in establishing an element of the case. The obtained records may require both translation into English and consultation with someone familiar with such records in order to be properly understood and applied to the case.

Collateral information will include interviews with family members, friends, teachers, and other persons who are important in the life of the examinee. Interviews also may be needed from individuals living outside the host country, especially those living in the country of origin. Setting up such interviews may require significant effort and expense. Collateral informants, including those living in the host country, may have little familiarity with the laws, customs, or procedures of the host country, which may invite misunderstandings, confusion, fear, or other problems. Some topics the examiner may wish to pursue may be considered off limits, and certain questions may be seen as unfriendly, inappropriate, or insensitive. Other questions that are considered a normal part of an evaluation may be confusing or of little importance to an informant. For example, questions about developmental milestones, such as when a child first spoke, may be difficult to answer if such information is not tracked by persons in a specific cultural group (Fontes 2008).

Preparing in advance of the interview will help to avoid cultural misunderstandings. The examiner should become familiar enough with the culture to understand issues such as how to convey respect appropriately, how to handle sensitive topics, the pacing of the interview, the appropriate and inappropriate use of body language and nonverbal communication, how to ask follow-up or clarifying questions appropriately, and the culturally appropriate ways to address the individual. Preparing the collateral informants in advance also may be necessary. Arrangements can be made for the interpreter to carefully explain the nature and purpose of the interview, its importance, and any culturally related issues likely to be a source of confusion to the interviewee. The interpreter also can describe for the family the logistical aspects of the interview, such as, for example, the order in which the examiner will meet with the parents and the child or adolescent. The goal of the interview is to obtain all relevant information. Devoting one's efforts to preventing cultural impediments to achieving this goal will be time well spent.

The Interview

By giving thought before the interview to the potential culturally related problems that might affect the relationship with the examinee or the examinee's family, the examiner may better make arrangements to overcome them. For example, the examinee and family are in a subordinate position to the forensic examiner, who is an authority figure. In some cultures, this difference in status may influence the quality and amount of information gained during an interview. The examiner will wish to consider how this can be addressed so that the examinee or family does not, for example, merely seek to please the examiner by providing answers he or she thinks will result in a favorable outcome. The examiner who knows how members of a culture view an issue will be better able to probe the examinee's attitudes and beliefs. For example, if a culture stigmatizes mental health problems, the examiner may be better able to probe for the presence of mental illness that might, for example, lead to successfully asserting an insanity defense.

The examiner will wish to consider potential transference reactions in the relationship, such as when a youth or family member has a history of negative dealings with authority figures or persons from the government in his or her home country. Persons from some cultures may react differently to being questioned by a female examiner than by a male examiner or by a white examiner rather than an examiner who is a person of color. Children may respond differently to a young male examiner than to an older female examiner. Finally, the examinee may react differently depending on whether the examiner is a member of his or her own culture or other cultures. Understanding how members of a culture behave and think will help to minimize emotional discomfort that might otherwise impair the relationship between examiner and examinee (Silva et al. 2003).

The examiner's approach to the interview may require modification to better elucidate the examinee's symptoms and clarify the diagnosis. Mental health assessment usually involves asking the examinee questions about symptoms. Examinees from other cultures may be unfamiliar with this approach and not provide the sought after information. For example, asking an adolescent if he or she feels depressed may work with those who understand what depression means. For those unfamiliar with the concept or unaccustomed to being asked directly, a more culturally appropriate approach will need to be followed. Questions designed to assess fund of knowledge or to assess understanding of proverbs also may need to be modified for the examinee with a different cultural background.

Before beginning the forensic evaluation of a child or an adolescent, examiners typically explain to the examinee and his or her parents or guardian the nature and purpose of the examination, the limits on confidentiality, how the information obtained will be used, and related information (American Academy of Psychiatry and the Law 2005). This approach may seem overly legalistic and off-putting to members of some cultures. Discussing such "business" details at the outset before getting to know one another would be considered impolite or improper in their culture. The forensic examiner may need to modify his or her approach to accommodate cultural differences. Initiating a conversation by making "small talk" about general matters such as the weather, the season, or some equally benign topic may prove a nonthreatening inroad to then raising the issue of informed consent.

During the interview, the forensic examiner's assessments of the behavior and words of the examinee will influence the direction of the interview and the examiner's findings and conclusions. Through possessing an understanding of normative behavior in the culture of origin, the examiner may more accurately interpret his or her observations and formulate clarifying follow-up questions. The examiner's knowledge of whether an examinee's behavior would be considered normal in his or her culture will help to distinguish behavior that is truly abnormal from that which is different because of culture. The examiner will need to assess the extent of the examinee's acculturation to be able to interpret the observed behavior.

Care must be exercised so as not to misattribute reasons for an attitude or a behavior observed in a child or an adolescent. Behaviors may be explained by several different factors, some of which are related to immigrating to a new country. For example, children who appear aloof and unsociable may simply speak English poorly and so may be reticent to engage in conversation. Such children may have trouble following the conversation, appearing distractible, or being inattentive, impulsive, or hyperactive. They may have difficulty registering or remembering what has been said and appear forgetful or may be slow to begin or complete tasks. Children who have undergone little formal schooling may have trouble staying organized. The child who appears unruly may have yet to internalize the norms of his or her new society. The child who has undergone trauma in the home country may appear oppositional, hyperactive, or detached (Fontes 2008). The stress of being involved in a forensic examination may result in regression by the child or adolescent such that English language skills and behavior worsen.

The ways in which cultural differences can confound interpretations about behavior and thereby complicate forensic assessments are too numerous to recount. However, caution must be exercised when attributing a behavior to cultural differences so as to avoid stereotyping or justifying misbehavior. For example, persons from certain Asian cultures may appear more distant or reserved, avoiding open displays of physical affection, but this does not necessarily mean that the coldness shown by a youth toward a parent is the result only of culture. Careful questioning is needed to elucidate other possible reasons, such as abuse. Adequately sorting out and addressing cultural and culture-related factors can be a difficult task for the forensic examiner. After the examiner has conducted the examination, collateral sources may be used as a way to check whether the examinee's thoughts and behaviors deviate from the norms of that culture (Tseng et al. 2004).

Psychological Testing

Forensic examiners use psychological and neuropsychological testing as a part of the assessment process. Such testing can be especially helpful with cases that are complicated or do not follow the usual pattern. Persons from other cultures may present in atypical ways such that examiners may seek psychological testing to clarify diagnosis or gain valuable supplemental information. Caution must be exercised, however, because the use of psychological or neuropsychological testing with persons from different cultures presents several challenges.

Cultural values, assumptions, and beliefs are embedded within psychological testing instruments. Tests are authored by persons from one culture and, as such, may reflect the cultural biases and constructs of the authors. The assessment of depression, for example, in one culture may involve asking questions different from those needed to assess depression adequately in individuals from another culture. Accordingly, an examiner cannot simply administer a test to a person from another culture using an interpreter or a translation of the test and assume that the test has adequately measured what it is supposed to measure.

Proper selection of a testing instrument requires confirming that the proposed instrument has been administered to a sufficient number of persons of the same culture and ethnicity that norms are available for use with that population. By using such norms, the performance of an individual can be compared with the performance of a group of individuals with similar characteristics. In some cases, the process of developing norms may have been inadequate. For example, a test with norms that have been developed on a Hispanic population may not have norms for all subgroups and cultures that make up the Spanish-speaking population. Certain beliefs held by Mexican people may differ from those held by persons in Spain or Puerto Rico.

Cultural issues may arise during the administration of the test. An examinee may communicate in such a way that competence on a test becomes confused with communication style (Gopaul-McNicol and Armour-Thomas 2002). The examinee may come from a culture in which psychological testing is rarely performed and may find it an unfamiliar experience. The examinee may be uncomfortable providing private or personal information to a stranger. The examinee who comes from a culture in which great deference is paid to authority may respond in ways he or she thinks the examiner would find pleasing (Tseng et al. 2004).

Interpreting the data obtained from the testing will require cultural competence. Many instruments have a subjective component that requires the examiner to make judgments regarding the meaning of the answers given. An examinee's answers may express cultural values or attitudes that the uninformed evaluator may be unable to grasp properly. For example, the teenager who answers "I don't know" in response to questions that are not overly difficult may simply be following a cultural tendency to avoid making mistakes and thinking independently. The response, however, may be incorrectly interpreted as making inadequate or invalid effort (Judd and Biggs 2005). The psychologist should assist with interpreting the data in a way that accounts for the effects of culture and integrates the results appropriately.

In no area has the use of psychological testing proven more controversial than in the assessment of intelligence and achievement in the public school setting. In the late 1960s, the overrepresentation of culturally, ethnically, and racially diverse children in special education programs began to be challenged in the courts. The first such case, *Hobson v. Hansen* (1967), found that the IQ tests used to track students were culturally biased as applied to lower-class and black students because they were standardized on a white, middle-class sample. In *Diana v. Board of Education* (1970), the placement of Mexican American and Chinese students in special education was challenged because the intelligence tests used for determining placement were administered in English. Many such challenges resulted in the current amalgamation of state and federal laws that today require, among other things, that the student be assessed in his or her own language, that the tests measure what they are supposed to measure, and that the test results accurately indicate the student's ability (Gopaul-McNicol and Armour-Thomas 2002).

The inappropriate use of psychological or neuropsychological testing invites challenges to one's opinion. We recommend working with a psychologist trained in and experienced with the kinds of cultural issues that may complicate assessment. Judd and Biggs (2005) opined that the psychologist should possess general knowledge about cross-cultural evaluation (e.g., how to work with an interpreter, acculturation principles, principles of test translation and adaptation), knowledge about the specific culture and language of the examinee, knowledge of the neuropsychological literature on the culture and language of the examinee, access to appropriate test materials and norms, knowledge of the forensic question, and knowledge of applicable professional ethics (Judd and Biggs 2005).

The validity of data collected in a multicultural or multilingual assessment is dependent on how well the methods and procedures used for evaluation and interpretation have minimized the potential biasing influences arising from linguistic and cultural differences (Rhodes et al. 2005). To avoid problems with admissibility of evidence, these issues need to be considered and addressed from the start of the forensic evaluation.

Presentation of Results

The culturally competent forensic examiner's final task is presenting the results and recommendations to the retaining party in a manner that is appropriate and that accurately conveys the relevant information. The better the examiner understands the legal issues bearing on the case, the better he or she can provide useful assistance to the retaining party. The legal system itself may be viewed as a separate culture, complete with its own language and rules. The forensic examiner is, in effect, already functioning as a bridge between cultures: making the mental and emotional world understandable to those in the legal system. The presence of cultural issues layers another dimension of complexity onto this process. To make the cultural issues clear in this forum, the examiner may need to provide basic education about the practices and attitudes of the culture of the examinee.

Work With Interpreters

When examining someone whose native language is not English, the use of a qualified interpreter may be required. Interpretation consists of the oral translation of one language into another. Simultaneous interpretation, which is typically used in courtroom proceedings, involves translating spoken words into another language as soon as they are spoken. Consecutive interpretation, which is more common in forensic evaluations, involves the speaker pausing after speaking so that the interpreter may translate what the speaker has said.

The decision of whether to use an interpreter should be made carefully. Failing to use an interpreter when an examination requires one may result in an inaccurate assessment that jeopardizes the foundation of one's opinion. The retaining attorney may express an opinion about whether an interpreter is needed. In practice, examinees with little or no fluency in English typically are provided interpreters, and examinees who appear proficient are interviewed without one. However, attorneys and examiners may be ill-equipped to assess an examinee's level of fluency in English.

One may simply decide to use interpretation services for all examinees whose native language is not English. This strategy may be useful when examining children and adolescents because although they may be able to speak with little trace of an accent and sound fluent, they may actually have only a limited vocabulary. Furthermore, some research suggests that using an interpreter may lead to greater accuracy because non-native English speakers may have greater psychopathology when speaking in English than when using their native tongue (Marcos et al. 1973). Finally, using an interpreter may prevent later claims that the examiner misunderstood the examinee or that the examinee could not express himself or herself adequately. Although an examinee may be asked whether he or she would like to have an interpreter present, in general the examiner should make this decision.

The use of an interpreter interjects into the evaluation process an additional barrier between examiner and examinee. The examiner's accuracy is influenced by limitations in the quality of the interpretation services. The examiner is subject to the interpreter's distortions, misunderstandings, and inaccuracies. Errors may occur as a result of the interpreter's lack of lan-guage competence and translation skills, the interpreter's lack of psychiatric knowledge, or the interpreter's attitudes (Marcos 1979). Key messages may be omitted or paraphrased by the interpreter, information may be added, concepts may be substituted, the form of the question may be altered (such as making an open question into a closed one), the interpreter may replace the examiner's questions with his or her own, or the information may be normalized (Farooq and Fear 2003). The interpreter may even seek to dissuade the examinee from disclosing information that would be stigmatizing within his or her culture or religion.

Accordingly, care in selecting a qualified interpreter must be exercised. The use of friends or family members of the examinee to function as interpreters should be avoided in the forensic setting. Having bilingual abilities does not guarantee skill in interpretation. Also, the examiner's questions may probe sensitive areas such as sex or financial matters about which the interpreter would be uncomfortable hearing and which the examinee would not want him or her to know. Using bilingual health care professionals is better than using family members, but their use still may result in significant distortions that could lead to misevaluation of the patient's mental status (Marcos 1979).

The danger of errors in translation may be especially pronounced in mental health examinations in which distortions or abnormalities in thought are sometimes subtle and require teasing out. For example, forensic examiners typically seek to hear the raw, uncensored answers given by the examinee without correction of syntax, relevance, or content to assess accurately the presence of psychopathology. Interpreters who lack training in mental health interpretation may feel the need to "make sense" of an examinee's nonsensical answers. Some interpreters may paraphrase rather than provide literal translations, which may result in the comic-appearing situation when an examinee provides a very long reply to a question but the interpreter gives only a very short interpretation.

So far as possible, forensic examiners should use interpreters who have undergone training in both mental health interpretation and legal interpretation. Although interpreters may be culturally competent about their culture and the host culture, the world of forensic mental health is a specialized subculture of medicine and law that requires specific knowledge. Certification by a professional organization helps ensure that this foundational knowledge is present. In California, for example, the State Personnel Board provides certification for medical interpreters who provide interpreting services at medical examinations conducted for the purpose of determining compensation or monetary award in civil or workers' compensation cases. Many court systems have their own certification process for interpreters.

When working with interpreters, some useful tips have been proposed (California Department of Education 2006; Farooq and Fear 2003). The examiner should meet with the interpreter before the interview to explain its purpose and content and to review any technical jargon that may be used. If technical words or phrases will be used during the examination, the examiner may wish to provide the interpreter with a list of them. The examiner should make certain the interpreter is familiar not only with the language of the examinee but also with the culture of the examinee.

When conducting the interview, the examiner should exercise care to make eye contact with and speak to the examinee rather than to the interpreter. Words should be spoken clearly, slowly, and loudly, using simple grammatical constructions. The examiner should avoid slang, idiomatic words or phrases, and long strings of sentences. The examiner should then allow adequate time for the interpreter to interpret the full message before proceeding with further questioning. While the interpreter is speaking, the examiner can observe nonverbal behavior and jot down notes. Unclear or confusing responses should be clarified. A verbatim interpretation of the examinee's words that is not "cleaned up" by the interpreter may be especially revealing of mental status. Finally, after the interview, the examiner should meet with and obtain feedback from the interpreter about the examinee's responses and behaviors and impressions of the conversation's normalcy.

Work With Cultural Consultants

No single forensic examiner is expected to have expertise regarding every culture and subculture. Even examiners who routinely work with a particular foreign population may benefit from consultation with a cultural consultant to understand better cultural nuances, confirm assumptions, and gain another opinion about the behavior of the examinee within the framework of the culture. The consultant should be able to provide general information about cultural issues as well as specific advice about topics such as whether the behavior of the examinee is common in the culture and how it might be viewed by other members in the culture. Even when the forensic examiner does not find the services of a cultural consultant to be necessary, the attor-

ney may still wish to consult with one when important cultural issues need to be explained to the jury.

As with using an interpreter, establishing a relationship with a cultural consultant can be especially helpful if an examiner evaluates many persons from that culture. The cultural consultant should possess excellent credentials and a thorough knowledge of the culture of the examinee. Well-qualified consultants often can be found working in academic university or college settings in anthropology departments. Interpreters or translators who are familiar with court proceedings can be used, although their qualifications must be scrutinized carefully.

Culture in the Law

Over the past 30 years, questions about how the law should deal with cultural differences have been hotly debated. In the arena of criminal law, courts have grappled with the question of how best to accommodate defendants from different cultural backgrounds. Should, for example, a foreign national be prosecuted just as a local defendant if he or she engages in behavior that might be accepted in the home country but is unlawful in the host country? Proponents of the use of "cultural defenses" argue that recognizing cultural factors promotes individualized justice because each person is judged according to the standards of his or her culture, which is appropriate given the culturally diverse and pluralistic society in which we live ("The cultural defense in the criminal law" 1986). Opponents argue that excusing a crime based on culture undermines the deterrent effect of the law by providing different standards of accountability to different groups in a society and discriminates against the victims of the crime, who are generally women or children from the same culture (Coleman 1996).

In practice, courts in the United States have been willing to consider the cultural and religious backgrounds of litigants in arriving at a result they deem just or appropriate. Although culture is most commonly raised in the context of criminal proceedings in adult criminal cases, courts have allowed cultural issues to play a role in civil litigation and in family law matters. For example, the state of New York was sued in a civil case by a 16-year-old Orthodox Jewish girl for negligent operation of a ski lift after the chairlift she was riding in with a male friend stopped halfway down the mountain. To avoid violating the prohibition against being alone with a man overnight, she jumped off of the ski lift and suffered physical injuries. The court awarded monetary damages to the girl after finding that she was, in fact, a member of that branch of Judaism that believed as she did and that the state had been negligent (Renteln 2004).

Cultural issues may be taken into consideration at any stage of criminal proceedings. Defense attorneys regularly raise cultural issues when serving immigrant clients in criminal cases to mitigate fault or lessen punishment (Renteln 2007). Culture defenses also may be raised with juvenile defendants in the context of adult criminal court or juvenile justice. Although courts have yet to adopt culture as one of the available formal legal defenses to a charge, cultural issues continue to be raised in a variety of cases and contexts resulting in various ad hoc dispositions.

Law enforcement personnel may take cultural issues into consideration in deciding whether to arrest or take into custody an alleged offender, although how often this happens is unclear. Prosecutorial agencies may consider cultural issues when deciding on the appropriate postarrest disposition, such as prosecution in family court or adult criminal court. In some cases, charges may be dropped. For example, charges against a South American woman for child abuse because she stroked her male toddler's genitals were dropped after investigation because the district attorney concluded that her culture had taught her that this was the proper way to put healthy young boys to sleep (Lacayo 1993). Charges may be modified or subject to plea bargaining, especially in cases in which the crime is of such severity that not punishing the defendant would offend the sensibility of American society but in which cultural factors clearly played a role. For example, an Iraqi father who followed the traditional custom of marrying his 13- and 14-year-old daughters to countrymen twice their ages was initially charged with child abuse, and his wife was charged with contributing to the delinquency of minors (Terry 1996). In return for pleading no contest to child neglect charges, they were sentenced to attend parenting and anger control classes (Talbot 1997).

If raising of cultural issues is unsuccessful at earlier stages, cultural issues may be reintroduced during the trial or during the sentencing phase of a case. During the trial, cultural issues may be raised by the defense to show that the defendant lacked the requisite *mens rea* for the crime and thus should be acquitted. This may occur in cases involving a specific intent crime (i.e., that the accused committed the crime with the specific intention of doing so). For example, an Inupiat Eskimo man was charged with molesting his son, his grandson, and their friend because he "swat-ted" their "crotch areas" over their pants and attempted to pull down their pants while wrestling with them at a party. He asserted that such behavior was part of a cultural tradition of "teasing behavior meant to teach young boys to laugh off adversity, protect themselves from attack and respond quickly." The court agreed and acquitted him based on the testimony of experts who affirmed that his behavior was "within the bounds of traditional Eskimo culture and had no erotic intent" (Sikora 2001, p. 1701).

In some cases, the judge will not allow the introduction of cultural evidence, ruling it "irrelevant" to the issues (Renteln 2004). However, in other cases, courts have allowed culture to be incorporated into traditional legal defenses such as self-defense, diminished capacity, and the insanity defense. With diminished capacity, for example, cultural issues may be raised to show that a defendant knew the act was illegal but was impaired in the ability to control his or her actions because of cultural factors. With the insanity defense, cultural factors may overlap with psychiatric ones such that questions are raised about the defendant's state of mind at the time of the crime. For example, in the case of *People v. Metallides* (1974), a Greek immigrant, after learning that his daughter had been raped by his best friend, killed the friend and claimed temporary insanity under the irresistible impulse test. The attorney reportedly constructed an argument based on the cultural idea that in traditional Greek culture you do not wait for the police if your daughter has been raped. The jury was charged with determining whether the accused had temporary insanity, and nine psychiatrists testified in the course of the trial. The man was found not guilty by reason of insanity in large measure because of Greek culture (Renteln 2004).

In assessing whether a litigant is eligible to raise culture as a defense, commentators have recommended that three considerations be met. First, the defendant must be a member of the ethnic group that claims the cultural tradition. Second, the group actually must have the cultural tradition the defendant claims. Because culture is fluid and dynamic, the defendant must show that the custom or practice has not changed over time. Third, the defendant must have been influenced by that tradition when he or she acted (Renteln 2004). To these requirements may be added two more: that the act, in its original setting, should advance social rather than personal goals; and that the defendants should not have known of the antisocial or criminal nature of the acts (Donovan and Garth 2007). These guidelines may be useful in assessing whether a defense based on culture is likely to be recognized by the court system.

Specific Culture-Related Psychiatric Syndromes

The expertise of a culturally competent forensic mental health examiner may be required in cases in which the litigant's mental health issues correspond to a recognized "culture-bound syndrome," as described in Appendix I of DSM-IV-TR (American Psychiatric Association 2000). Because these syndromes may not be limited to just one culture but may occur in many cultures, we prefer the term *culture-related specific (psychiatric) syndrome*. DSM-IV-TR sets forth 25 syndromes, although many more have been identified in the literature. These syndromes are defined as "recurrent, locality-specific patterns of aberrant behavior and troubling experience that may or may not be linked to a particular DSM-IV diagnostic category" (American Psychiatric Association 2000, p. 898). The syndromes described in DSM-IV-TR represent "some of the best-studied culture-bound syndromes and idioms of distress that may be encountered in clinical practice in North America" (American Psychiatric Association 2000, p. 899).

The brief descriptions of each culture-related specific syndrome in Appendix I provide little information about the age distribution for these conditions. Two culture-bound syndromes are explicitly recognized as occurring in children or adolescents. First, *mal de ojo*, or the "evil eye," is known to especially affect infants and children in Mediterranean cultures. The afflicted may experience fitful sleep, crying without apparent cause, diarrhea, vomiting, and fever (American Psychiatric Association 2000, p. 901). Second, brain fag is experienced by high school and university students from West Africa. In response to the pressures of school, students note symptoms of difficulties with concentration, remembering, and thinking (American Psychiatric Association 2000, p. 900). All other culture-bound syndromes appear to occur primarily in adults, although DSM-IV-TR does not exclude the possibility that they might occur in children or adolescents.

Several of the specific culture-related syndromes included in DSM-IV-TR could appear in a forensic context. Syndromes that may result in aggressive or violent behavior and that might form the basis for an insanity defense include amok, *ataque de nervios, boufée de-lirante, locura, pibloktoq,* and *zar* (Parzen 2003). In addition, lesser-known syndromes not included in DSM-IV-TR that are associated with violent or aggressive behavior could serve the same function. Forensic mental health examiners should develop some level of knowledge about these disorders so that they can be recognized in the event that they best describe the experience of a foreign individual accused of a crime.

Amok, of all the culture-bound syndromes, is the syndrome that perhaps best lends itself to an insanity defense. The term *amok* is derived from the Malay word *amuk*, meaning "mad with rage," and is described in DSM-IV-TR as a "dissociative episode characterized by a period of brooding followed by an outburst of violent, aggressive, or homicidal behavior directed at people and objects" (American Psychiatric Association 2000, p. 899). Amok is found in Southeast Asian countries such as Malaysia, Indonesia, Laos, Thailand, and the Philippines. In a typical case of running amok, a male who has shown no previous sign of anger or any inclination to violence will acquire a weapon and, in a sudden frenzy, will attempt to kill or seriously injure anyone he encounters. Amok episodes of this kind normally end with the attacker being killed by bystanders or committing suicide. Persons who carry out such attacks are often young males who have social isolation, anger, depression, loss, and delusions. This has led Hempel et al. (2000) to argue that the condition should not be considered a culture-bound syndrome. The age range of persons who have experienced amok has not been well defined, but in one study of Laotians who had perpetrated grenade amok, the ages ranged from 17 to 35 (Westermeyer 1972).

Culture-bound syndromes rarely appear in the forensic setting. A review of case law finds few examples in which a recognized culture-related specific syndrome has been raised. In a criminal prosecution for murder in Hawaii, an adult defendant unsuccessfully raised the defense of amok (*State v. Ganal* 1996). Another adult defendant, from Laos, also argued unsuccessfully that he was experiencing extreme emotional disturbance when he killed his wife, asserting a defense based on culture similar to amok (*State v. Aphaylath* 1986). *Oyako-shinju* is a culture-bound syndrome unique to Japan that is not found in DSM-IV-TR in which the parent kills the child before committing suicide. The parent kills the child because death is deemed preferable to making one's way in the world alone without a family. Although parent–child suicide is proscribed by law in Japan, it reportedly rarely results in harsh punishment (Matsumoto 1995). In *People v. Kimura* (1985), a Japanese woman living in California drowned her two children and attempted to kill herself after learning that her husband had been secretly keeping a mistress. In her defense, she relied on psychiatric expert testimony that she was mentally disturbed at the time, and thousands of people in the community signed a petition requesting leniency by asserting that her actions were rooted in Japanese culture. The court allowed her to plead guilty to manslaughter. She was sentenced to 1 year in county jail and was placed on 5 years' probation with psychiatric treatment. A review of the literature found no cases in the United States in which culture-bound syndromes have been raised by children or adolescents. Perhaps future cases will raise such issues.

Areas of Forensic Practice: Cultural Issues

Juvenile Justice

The forensic examiner working in the area of juvenile justice may encounter issues related to ethnicity and race more commonly than issues of culture. In 2006, the racial composition of juveniles in the United States was 78% white (including Hispanic), 17% black, 5% Asian or Pacific Islander, and 1% Native American. However, the juvenile arrest rate for violent crimes showed black youth to be overrepresented (51% of arrests) and Asian youth to be underrepresented (1% of arrests.) The findings were similar for property crimes: 31% involved black youth, and 2% involved Asian youth (Snyder 2008).

Racial and ethnic factors may affect the process of forensic evaluation through complicating diagnostic assessment. In one study, 4.5% of African American youth and 4.9% of Hispanic or Latino youth were diagnosed with psychosis compared with just 2.5% of white children and adolescents (Muroff et al. 2008). Black and Native Hawaiian youth were more likely than white youth to be given the diagnosis of disruptive behavior disorders. Hispanic and Native Hawaiian youth were less likely than white youth to be given the diagnosis of depression or dysthymia (Nguyen et al. 2007).

Cultural issues also may affect the process of forensic evaluation of youth. One role the forensic examiner may serve for the courts is to evaluate issues such as amenability to treatment and make recommendations that assist the court in deciding on an appropriate disposition. Factors relevant to the examination often include amenability to treatment, risk for future offend-

ing, and level of maturity. The criteria examiners use to make these determinations deserve careful attention to ensure they do not simply reflect the examiner's culturally influenced beliefs. Komen (2006) described the difficulties experienced by forensic psychiatrists in the Netherlands in evaluating juvenile offenders from culturally and ethnically diverse backgrounds when making recommendations to the courts regarding type and duration of legal sanction. The forensic psychiatrists reported more difficulty in performing assessments of these juveniles than in assessing ethnically Dutch offenders. For example, several psychiatrists viewed Moroccan youth as "excessively polite" and insincere in their efforts to present themselves in a socially desirable manner. In other words, the psychiatrists interpreted the behavior as merely trying to gain favor with the psychiatrist and obtain a lighter sentence. Other culturally related factors that complicated assessment included the presence of manipulative behavior, a lack of perceived empathy and emotional responsiveness, the way in which a youth behaved toward the examiner, differing concepts about the use of mendacity, and the difficulty in determining the level of intelligence (Komen 2006).

Forensic clinicians working in the correctional setting may find little accommodation made for youth from a foreign culture. The youth must experience the normal stress that comes from living in a foreign country and speaking a foreign language in an environment that is often harsh and unfriendly. The demands of uniformity will take precedence over individual cultural preferences in all areas of life. The youth will eat whatever is served by the facility during mealtime, will sleep in a cell or dorm, and may have limited ability to interact with persons from his or her culture speaking his or her language. Rehabilitative activities may be limited, uninteresting, or unsuitable for foreign-born youth. Because of language difficulties, youth may be less aware of what is going on in the facility, have more trouble meeting their needs, and be more vulnerable to exploitation.

Competency

Cultural factors may affect determinations regarding the competency of a child or an adolescent involved in the justice system. The issue of competency to stand trial in adult criminal court has perhaps received the most attention. The minimum competency standard for standing trial in adult criminal court was supplied by the Supreme Court of the United States in the *Dusky* case (*Dusky v. U.S.* 1960). Although many questions remain regarding competency standards for juveniles, in most states the definition of competency to stand trial in juvenile court is similar or identical to the *Dusky* test (Melton et al. 2007).

Commentators have divided the competency question into various component parts suggested by the language in the *Dusky* opinion. This division is useful when considering how culture plays a role. First, a factual understanding of legal proceedings must be present. Many immigrant youth may be even less familiar with the workings of the court and the justice system than are local youth because they may have had fewer opportunities to learn this kind of information. A thorough assessment is important because some youth may attempt to act as though they possess this information out of a desire not to appear stupid, uninformed, or foreign. Follow-up questions should probe the depth of knowledge possessed by the youth. A deficit of knowledge often can be remedied with instruction and enough time.

Second, the *Dusky* test requires a rational understanding of the court proceedings. This means that the defendant must be able to apply and use the information about the court proceedings in a rational manner. Because our cultural background and experience shape how we use the information we know, a defendant from a different culture may be able to memorize the factual information but either not know how to use it or use it inappropriately. Culturally conditioned expectations, experiences, and beliefs may undermine understanding of the relevant information. For example, a youth from a culture in which women traditionally do not function in professional roles may have trouble working with his female attorney, despite knowing the role of the attorney in the court. As Grisso (2005) has pointed out, developmental immaturity may be a reason for incompetence for youthful defendants. Gaining a rational understanding of court proceedings in the presence of some degree of immaturity may take substantially more time to remedy for the defendant from a different culture than for a local one.

Third, according to the *Dusky* test, the defendant must be able to consult with counsel with a reasonable degree of rational understanding. To prepare an adequate defense, the attorney requires the collaborative participation of the defendant. For a defendant whose cultural experience is to be wary of authorities or outsiders, participation may be impaired. Similarly, youth from a culture that prizes respect for authority may have trouble "speaking up" and challenging the attorney's misconceptions. A youth may believe that the truth will somehow "win out" without realizing that the model for seeking truth in the American system of justice is adversarial requiring debate and the clash of competing stories in which the youth must be an active participant.

Malingering

Feigning mental illness for the purpose of achieving a secondary gain, such as evading prosecution or obtaining financial compensation, is not uncommon in adult psychiatric patients. In children and adolescents, the practice is thought to be less common because of their comparatively low level of sophistication. Cultural factors may influence aspects of the malingering assessment, including interpreting the behavior as exaggerated or feigned when it is not. In some cultures, loudly complaining when experiencing symptoms may be appropriate but may be seen as exaggerating symptoms in another culture. The way in which symptoms present themselves may vary among cultures. The symptoms shown by an examinee from a different cultural background deserve careful investigation before a determination of malingering is made.

Child Abuse and Neglect

Parenting practices are influenced by culture and so vary greatly from country to country. Just as there is no unanimity regarding what constitutes ideal parenting, cultures do not always agree about what practices constitute child maltreatment. For example, American culture, with its emphasis on autonomy and individualism, fosters parenting practices that might be viewed as inappropriate or even abusive by other cultures. Even within the same society, we often find disagreement regarding parenting practices. Most people would agree that selling children into sexual slavery constitutes child maltreatment, but they might disagree about whether corporal punishment so qualifies.

The World Health Organization has defined the term *child maltreatment*, which encompasses child abuse and child neglect, as including "all forms of physical and emotional ill-treatment, sexual abuse, neglect, and exploitation that result in actual or potential harm to the child's health, development or dignity. Within this broad definition, five subtypes can be distinguished—physical abuse; sexual abuse; neglect and negligent treatment; emotional abuse; and exploitation" (World Health Organization 2008). In the United States, the federal Child Abuse Prevention and Treatment Act (2008) sets forth a minimum standard of what constitutes child abuse and neglect:

[T]he term "child abuse and neglect" means, at a minimum, any recent act or failure to act on the part of a parent or caretaker, which results in death, serious physical or emotional harm, sexual abuse or exploitation, or an act or failure to act which presents an imminent risk of serious harm.

Entrusting to the states the ability to craft their own laws regarding child abuse has invited different views and different standards as to what constitutes maltreatment.

Some states with substantial ethnic minority populations have acknowledged the role of culture in determining child abuse. California, for example, explicitly provides that "cultural and religious childrearing practices and beliefs shall not in themselves create a need for child welfare services unless the practices present a specific danger to the physical or emotional safety of the child" (California Welfare and Institutional Code 1996, § 16509). In the same vein, Colorado law requires those investigating reports of child abuse to take into consideration the accepted child-rearing practices of the parents' culture (Colorado Revised Statutes 1997, § 19-1-103(b)). Children of Native American heritage facing foster care placement, termination of parental rights, or preadoption or adoption placement will fall within the embrace of the Indian Child Welfare Act, which sets forth special rules for such cases.

We recommend that examiners routinely consider the parenting practices and attitudes of the culture of the parents. Seeman (2008) illustrated the perils associated with failing to consider cultural differences in her description of a Chinese woman with schizophrenia who had just given birth. The newborn was removed from the mother and placed in foster care because the mother behaved differently toward her child than hospital staff expected her to. The reasons for her behavior were fully explained by cultural differences surrounding childbirth (Seeman 2008). Similarly, children from Asian countries such as Cambodia, Vietnam, Laos, or China may develop bruises or skin irritation from the use of traditional Asian medical practices such as coining or cupping to treat mild maladies. These marks may be mistaken as evidence of child abuse, and referral may be made to Child Protective Services. Coining is thought to restore balance to the body and treat maladies such as the common cold. Coining is done by rubbing or scratching with a coin on the skin of the back, neck, upper chest, and arms. Water, lotion, medicine, or Tiger Balm may be applied to the skin before it is rubbed with a quarter or a similar-sized coining tool. Cupping involves burning a small candle or cotton ball to remove the air and create a vacuum inside the cups, which may be sucking cups, glass jars, or medicine bottles. The cups are then rapidly applied to the skin of the forehead, back, and upper chest, creating red circular lesions. Pinching involves using the first and second fingers to pull upward hard on the skin of the neck, back, chest, and between the eyebrows. Pinching may be done with enough force that it causes bruising (Graham and Chitnarong 1997).

Statistics on child maltreatment indicate a higher incidence among certain ethnic minorities. In 2006, the rates of victimization per 1,000 children were highest for African American (19.8), American Indian or Alaska Native (15.9), and children of more than one race (15.4). The rate for Asians was the lowest (2.5), followed by whites (10.7) and Hispanics (10.8) (U.S. Department of Health and Human Services 2008). Economic disparities are thought to account for much of this difference because low-income families are more likely to be the subject of scrutiny by social service organizations than are middle-class families (Campbell 2005).

Child Custody

In determining what parenting arrangement is in "the best interests of the child," forensic examiners must consider a variety of important factors such as parenting style, quality of attachment, and social support systems. For families with a cultural background different from the majority, such as immigrants or refugees, an examiner also must consider cultural issues. The American Academy of Child and Adolescent Psychiatry's "Practice Parameters for Child Custody Evaluation" (Herman 1997) recommends that the examiner "assess the availability of cultural and ethnic influences and their importance to the growth and development of the child."

Taking cultural issues into consideration in child custody disputes is important because a child of diverse heritage should have access to opportunities that maintain his or her cultural ties. Custody plans for parents who are from different ethnic or cultural backgrounds should afford opportunities for the child to share in the language, customs, and culture of both parents. A child is unlikely to be confused by partaking of two cultures because children are fully capable of integrating highly diverse and contradictory cultural and religious identity fragments (Roll 1998).

Culture may affect factors commonly considered by evaluators, such as parental fitness (Hicks 2004). How one determines what constitutes a healthy bond between parent and child is influenced by one's culturally conditioned beliefs. Reebye (2008) recommends evaluating one's own cultural background before engaging in a custody evaluation and then constructing a cultural profile of a family consisting of three axes. Axis 1 involves estimating how great a deviation exists between the family's values and the mainstream culture. Axis 2 involves determining the degree of acculturation and assimilation of the family. On Axis 3, the examiner determines the effects of culture on the problem-solving strategies of the family. The examiner then can perform an analysis of family functioning and the cultural issues that are relevant (Reebye 2008).

Summary

Cultural competence has emerged as an important component of forensic practice. Providing forensic opinions that accurately determine the cultural issues that are present enhances accuracy and, therefore, may enhance justice. Cultural issues may affect any evaluation performed by a child and adolescent forensic examiner. Developing cultural competence is a lifelong process that evolves, requiring flexibility and adaptability.

—Key Points

— To prepare for assessment of children and families from diverse backgrounds, the examiner should study other cultures and become aware of how culture has conditioned his or her own attitudes, practices, and beliefs.

— The examiner must obtain all relevant collateral information about all examinees and use translation and interpretation services as needed.

— The examiner should review his or her own beliefs, attitudes, and biases as they relate to the culture of the examinee.

— The examiner should prepare thoroughly in advance of the interview and pay close attention to cultural differences that might result in misunderstanding.

— The examiner should use interpreters trained in mental health and legal interpretation.

— The examiner should prepare in advance the examinee and his or her family as needed for the examination.

— The examiner should obtain cultural consultation with an expert in the culture of the examinee as needed to better understand the relevant issues.

References

American Academy of Psychiatry and the Law: Ethics guidelines for the practice of forensic psychiatry, adopted May 2005. Available at: https://www.aapl.org/pdf/ETHICS-GDLNS.pdf. Accessed June 16, 2008.

American Psychiatric Association: Diagnostic and Statistical Manual of Mental Disorders, 4th Edition, Text Revision. Washington, DC, American Psychiatric Association, 2000

California Welfare and Institutions Code § 16509, 1996

California Department of Education: Quality Indicators for Translation and Interpretation in Kindergarten Through Grade Twelve Educational Settings. Sacramento, California Department of Education, 2006. Available at: http://www.cde.ca.gov/re/pn/fd/documents/qualityindicators.pdf. Accessed April 7, 2008.

Campbell ET: Child abuse recognition, reporting and prevention: a culturally congruent approach. Journal of Multicultural Nursing and Health, Summer 2005. Available at: http://findarticles.com/p/articles/mi_qa3919/is_/ai_n14825657. Accessed December 17, 2008.

Child Abuse Prevention and Treatment Act of 1974, 42 USC § 5106g. Available at: http://www.acf.hhs.gov/programs/cb/laws_policies/cblaws/capta/capta1.htm#106. Accessed September 16, 2008.

Coleman DL: Individualizing justice through multiculturalism: the liberal's dilemma, 96 COLUMBIA L. REV. 1093–1167 (1996)

Colorado Revised Statutes 1997, § 19-1-103(b)

Diana v. State Board of Education, CA 70 RFT (N.D. Cal. 1970)

Donovan JM, Garth JS: Delimiting the culture defense. 26 QUINNIPIAC L. REV. 109–146 (2007)

Dumont J-C, Lemaitre G: Counting immigrants and expatriates in OECD countries: a new perspective (OECD Social, Employment and Migration Working Papers No. 25). OECD, Directorate for Employment Labour and Social Affairs, 2005. Available at: http://www.oecd.org/dataoecd/27/5/33868740.pdf. Accessed May 2, 2008.

Dusky v US, 362 US 402 (1960)

Farooq S, Fear C: Working through interpreters. Advances in Psychiatric Treatment 9:104–109, 2003

Fontes LA: Interviewing Clients Across Cultures: A Practitioner's Guide. New York, Guilford, 2008

Gopaul-McNicol SA, Armour-Thomas E: Assessment and Culture: Psychological Tests With Minority Populations. San Diego, CA, Academic Press, 2002

Graham EA, Chitnarong J: Ethnographic study among Seattle Cambodians: wind illness. 1997. Available at: http://ethnomed.org/ethnomed/clin_topics/cambodian/ethno_wind.html. Accessed March 4, 2008.

Grisso T: Evaluating Juvenile's Adjudicative Competence. Sarasota, FL, Professional Resource Press, 2005

Hempel AG, Levine RE, Meloy JR, et al: A cross-cultural review of sudden mass assault by a single individual in the oriental and occidental cultures. J Forensic Sci 45:582–588, 2000

Herman SP: Practice parameters for child custody evaluation. American Academy of Child and Adolescent Psychiatry. J Am Acad Child Adolesc Psychiatry 36 (10 suppl):57S–68S, 1997

Hicks JW: Ethnicity, race, and forensic psychiatry: are we color-blind? J Am Acad Psychiatry Law 32:21–33, 2004

Hobson v Hansen, 269 F Supp 401 (D DC 1967)

Indian Child Welfare Act of 1978, 25 USC 1901 et seq.

Judd T, Biggs B: Cross-cultural forensic neuropsychological assessment, in Race, Culture, Psychology and Law. Edited by Barrett KH, George WH. Thousand Oaks, CA, Sage, 2005, pp 141–162

KewalRamani A, Gilbertson L, Fox MA, et al: Status and Trends in the Education of Racial and Ethnic Minorities (NCES 2007-039). Washington, DC, National Center for Education Statistics, Institute of Education Sciences, U.S. Department of Education, 2007. Available at: http://nces.ed.gov/pubs2007/2007039.pdf. Accessed August 25, 2008.

Komen M: Difficulties of cultural diversity: an exploratory study into forensic psychiatric reporting on serious juvenile offenders in the Netherlands. Crime, Law and Social Change 45:55–69, 2006

Lacayo R: The "cultural" defense. Time, December 2, 1993. Available at: http://www.time.com/time/magazine/article/0,9171,979741,00.html. Accessed April 2, 2008.

Larsen LJ: The Foreign-Born Population in the United States: 2003. Current Population Reports, P20-551. Washington, DC, U.S. Census Bureau, 2004. Available at: http://www.census.gov/prod/2004pubs/p20-551.pdf. Accessed April 24, 2008.

Marcos LR: Effects of interpreters on the evaluation of psychopathology in non-English-speaking patients. Am J Psychiatry 136:171–174, 1979

Marcos LR, Alpert M, Urcuyo L, et al: The effect of interview language on the evaluation of psychopathology in Spanish-American schizophrenic patients. Am J Psychiatry 130:549–553, 1973

Matsumoto A: A place for consideration of culture in the American criminal justice system: Japanese law and the Kimura case. Detroit College of Law Journal of International Law and Practice 4:507–538, 1995

Melton GB, Petrila J, Poythress NG, et al: Psychological Evaluations for the Courts: A Handbook for Mental Health Professionals and Lawyers, 3rd Edition. New York, Guilford, 2007

Merriam-Webster Online Dictionary. 2009. Available at: http://www.merriam-webster.com/dictionary/culture. Accessed January 11, 2009.

McCracken G: The Long Interview. Newbury Park, CA, Sage, 1988

Muroff J, Edelsohn GA, Joe S, et al: The role of race in diagnostic and disposition decision making in a pediatric psychiatric emergency service. Gen Hosp Psychiatry 30:269–276, 2008

Nguyen L, Huang LN, Arganza GF, et al: The influence of race and ethnicity on psychiatric diagnoses and clinical characteristics of children and adolescents in children's services. Cultur Divers Ethnic Minor Psychol 13:18–25, 2007

Parzen MD: Toward a culture-bound syndrome-based insanity defense? Cult Med Psychiatry 27:131–155, 2003

People v. Kimura, No. A-091133 (Los Angeles Cty Super. Ct. filed April 24, 1985)

People v Metallides, Case No 73-5270 (1974)

Reebye P: Child custody-access evaluation: cultural perspectives. Available at: http://priory.com/psych/custody.htm. Accessed September 16, 2008.

Renteln AD: The Cultural Defense. New York, Oxford University Press, 2004

Renteln AD: Raising cultural defenses, in Cultural Issues in Criminal Defense, 2nd Edition. Edited by Ramirez LF. Huntington, NY, Juris Publishing, 2007, pp 423–466

Rhodes RL, Ochoa SH, Ortiz SO: Assessing Culturally and Linguistically Diverse Students: A Practical Guide. New York, Guilford, 2005

Roll S: Cross-cultural considerations in custody and parenting plans. Child Adolesc Psychiatr Clin N Am 7:445–454, 1998

Seeman MV: Cross-cultural evaluation of maternal competence in a culturally diverse society. Am J Psychiatry 165:565–568, 2008

Sikora DW: Note: Differing cultures, differing culpabilities? A sensible alternative: using cultural circumstances as a mitigating factor in sentencing. Ohio State Law Journal 62:1695, 2001

Silva JA, Leong GB, Weinstock R: Culture and ethnicity, in Principles and Practice of Forensic Psychiatry, 2nd Edition. Edited by Rosner R. London, Arnold, 2003, pp 631–637

Snyder HN: Juvenile arrests 2006. Juvenile Justice Bulletin, November 2008. Available at: http://www.ncjrs.gov/pdf files1/ojjdp/221338.pdf. Accessed November 25, 2008.

State v Aphaylath, 502 NE2d 998, 999 (NY 1986)

State v Ganal, 917 P2d 370 (Hawaii 1996)

Talbot M: Baghdad on the plains. The New Republic, August 11, 1997. Available at: http://members.tripod.com/jummahcrew/baghdad.htm. Accessed June 9, 2008.

Terry D: Cultural tradition and law collide in middle America. New York Times, December 2, 1996. Available at: http://query.nytimes.com/gst/fullpage.html?res=9D01E7D9 133CF931A35751C1A960958260andsec=andspon= andpagewanted=print. Accessed November 25, 2008.

The cultural defense in the criminal law. 99 HARV. L. REV. 1293–1311 (1986)

Tseng WS: Clinician's Guide to Cultural Psychiatry. San Diego, CA, Academic Press, 2003

Tseng WS, Matthews D, Elwyn TS: Cultural Competence in Forensic Mental Health. New York, Brunner-Routledge, 2004

U.S. Department of Health and Human Services, Administration on Children, Youth and Families: Child Maltreatment 2006. Washington, DC, U.S. Government Printing Office, 2008. Available at: http://www.acf.hhs.gov/programs/cb/stats_research/index.htm#can. Accessed April 24, 2008.

Westermeyer J: A comparison of amok and other homicide in Laos. Am J Psychiatry 129:703–709, 1972

World Health Organization: Child maltreatment (Health Topics). Available at: http://www.who.int/topics/child_abuse/en/. Accessed September 16, 2008.

Supplemental Reading

Barrett KH, George WH (eds): Race, Culture, Psychology and Law. Thousand Oaks, CA, Sage, 2005

Fontes LA: Child Abuse and Culture. New York, Guilford, 2008

Herndon E, Joyce L: Getting the most from language interpreters. Fam Pract Manag 11(6):37–40, 2004. Available at: http://www.aafp.org/fpm/20040600/37gett.html. Accessed April 21, 2008.

PART II

Legal Regulation of Practice

Peter Ash, M.D.

Chapter 9

Legal Issues in the Treatment of Minors

Vivek S. Sankaran, J.D.

JoAnn E. Macbeth, J.D.

Mental health professionals who treat minors—children and adolescents—face the same legal issues and challenges as those who treat adults. However, the resolution of these problems may require a different approach and additional steps because of two factors that distinguish a treatment relationship and legal situation when the patient is a minor from that when the patient is an adult. The first factor is that the patient, a minor, has limited, if any, legal capacity. The second factor is that the mutual relationship between clinician and patient must bend to accommodate a third party (or third and fourth parties)—the parent(s). This chapter reviews the legal issues and problems that derive from these differences, summarizes the situations in which they are most likely to occur, and offers a framework for their resolution.

Both the case and the statutory law in this area reflect a tension and a balance between 1) the presumptions that parents have a fundamental right to direct the upbringing of their children,[1] that their "natural bounds of affection" will lead them to act in the best interests of their children,[2] and that parents have the "maturity, experience, and capacity for judgment" that their child lacks to make difficult decisions[3] and 2) a recognition that children, particularly teenagers, possess independent liberty interests that must be considered regardless of their parents' wishes.[4] These tensions are complicated by the changing structure of the family unit as it is no longer uncommon for a minor to have parents who are separated or divorced and who may disagree about important medical decisions in the minor's life or for a minor to live with a nonparent, such as an extended family member.

An introductory word of caution: this is an area of the law that has been changing relatively rapidly and is governed primarily by state-specific statutes. Changes have tended to give minors—particularly adolescents—greater autonomy with regard to treatment and related decisions. Beyond this, generalizations about changes are not possible. It would be prudent for a practitioner to review periodically the basic statutes and regulations in this area. Legal resources can be found at a local law school library or on the Internet. For example, FindLaw (www.findlaw.org) is a free legal

---

[1] *Pierce v. Society of Sisters*, 268 U.S. 510 (1925).

[2] *Parham v. J.R.*, 442 U.S. 584, 602 (1979).

[3] Id., at 602.

[4] *Tinker v. Des Moines*, 393 U.S. 503, 511 (1969) ("Students in school as well as out of school are 'persons' under our Constitution").

resource that contains information about many areas of the law. Pay services such as WestLaw and Lexis-Nexis can also provide reference materials. Clinicians may also want to identify an attorney with expertise in these issues who can be consulted if a difficult case arises.

Consent to Treatment: Who Makes Medical Decisions for a Minor?

As is the case with treatment provided to adults, a mental health professional who provides treatment to a minor[1] without legally adequate consent risks suit and potential tort or malpractice liability. The practitioner will be responsible for any untoward consequences of, or damage caused by, such unauthorized treatment, even if the care was entirely appropriate and satisfied all applicable standards of care. As is also the case with adults, in order for the consent to treatment to be effective, it must be informed. In other words, the consent must be given after the decision maker has received a fair and reasonable explanation of the proposed treatment. The explanation must include an appropriate explanation of all the risks, as the decision maker cannot make a knowledgeable choice if he or she is not aware of all risks.[2] On the basis of this information, the decision maker can then make a knowing and willful decision (see also Chapter 1, "Introduction to the Legal System").

These basic principles apply whether the patient is a minor or an adult. However, in almost all circumstances involving adults, the person with the power to make decisions regarding treatment is the patient, that is, the person who can be expected to both enjoy the benefits of the treatment and suffer the side effects, risks, and other potential ill effects. The source of the challenges that this situation presents for those working with children is that in many situations the individual with decision-making authority is not the child patient but a third party—an adult—who has legal authority to make decisions for the patient. Ascertaining who has the authority to consent to treatment for the child patient can be complicated.

General Principles

The law has traditionally considered minors to be incompetent for most purposes, for example, entering into contracts, incurring debts, and retaining lawyers. This has included the making of decisions about medical treatment. This reflects the judgment that, as a general matter, individuals younger than age 18 cannot fully appreciate the potential consequences of receiving or forgoing treatment. As such decisions must be made, the law has provided that those persons legally responsible for minors—in most cases, their parents—will make these decisions on their behalf.

Thus, as a traditional matter, for a physician to be protected against charges of battery or unauthorized treatment, a minor's parents (or legal guardian) have to consent to the treatment in question.[3] To the extent this general rule applies, it means both that the clinician will be safe as a legal matter if he or she acts as directed by a minor's parents and that the clinician will be at risk to the extent he or she follows the directions of the minor and they diverge from those of the minor's parents.[4]

Two caveats are in order. First, as discussed, there are many exceptions, defined by both statutes and case law, to this rule. These exceptions vary significantly from one jurisdiction to another, and it would be prudent for a clinician to become familiar with the major relevant exceptions in his or her state or jurisdiction. However, although there are many potentially relevant exceptions, it would be inadvisable to assume in any given situation that it is safe to treat minors without obtaining parental consent. Particularly with a young minor, unless the practitioner is aware of an exception

---

[1] A psychiatrist should make certain as to the age of majority in the jurisdiction in which he or she practices. Although the age of majority is 18 in most states, it is higher (age 19 or 21) in a number of states.

[2] See, e.g., *Goodman v. United States*, 298 F.3d 1048, 1058 (9th Cir. 2002), describing the duty to explain and warn to require the physician to disclose "the nature of the proposed treatment, the probability of success of the contemplated therapy and its alternatives, and the risk of unfortunate consequences associated with such treatment."

[3] See, e.g., *Rishworth v. Moss*, 159 S.W.122 (Tex. Civ. App. 1913).

[4] The physician who provides services to a minor on the mistaken, though good-faith, belief that the minor is an adult is likely to be protected if that belief appears reasonable. A number of state statutes and regulations address this situation directly. For example, in the District of Columbia, "[i]f having acted in good faith, no physician...shall be liable on the basis of a minor's representation." D.C. Mun. Reg. tit. 22 § 602.3 (2008).

valid in the jurisdiction in which he or she has seen the patient, the practitioner would be well advised to obtain the consent of the minor's parent. As is the case with adults, this is not merely general consent to treatment but specific consent tailored to any particular intervention at issue, for example, medication, that provides sufficient information about potential risks, such as side effects, for the parent to make an informed decision.

Second, as stated, these principles reflect society as it used to be: most children lived with, and were cared for by, two parents. In these circumstances, the law was based on the presumption that parents were in accord as to decisions such as medical treatment or, at least, that there was agreement that one would make the decisions for both. As is discussed below, both society and the law have changed; a practitioner needs to stay alert to the possibility that he or she may be dealing with a parent but that the parent may not have the legal right to make decisions regarding the child's treatment. This does not mean that the practitioner needs to investigate to make certain that he or she is dealing with an adult with decision-making authority. Although only a parent with legal custody has authority to consent to a child's treatment, without some information that calls into question the authority of the parent, there is no duty to affirmatively inquire about custody when a parent first brings a child for evaluation and/or treatment.

A practitioner's duties in this regard may well change if, during the course of treatment, the practitioner develops a reason to believe that the parent who brought the child for treatment does not have legal custody. This could result from statements made by the child patient or the parent, from notification of changed living circumstances, from a subpoena attempting to secure the psychiatrist's testimony in connection with divorce or custody litigation, and so forth. Once the practitioner is put on notice that there may be some question as to the legal authority of the parent to consent to treatment on the child's behalf, the practitioner has the duty to clarify the situation. The practitioner will be required to take reasonable steps to determine which parent has legal custody and confirm the consent of this parent. If the practitioner receives conflicting information about this, he or she may even need to consider requiring some proof of custody, for example, a copy of the custody decree.

Treatment When Parents Are Divorced or Separated

A practitioner needs to be particularly careful about issues involving consent when a minor patient's parents are divorced or separated—or where there is reason to believe that they may be. In these circumstances, the practitioner should take reasonable steps to determine which parent has legal custody of the minor, and particularly whether the parent who consents to treatment has legal custody. Obtaining and reviewing a copy of the custody order are essential. If the clinician believes that involving the noncustodial parent is therapeutically appropriate, the clinician should get the custodial parent's consent prior to doing so. In the event that both parents share legal custody of the child and disagree about treatment, then the court may have to intervene to determine whether treatment is in the child's best interest.

The situation may be even more difficult when a minor's parents have both been involved in the minor's treatment but separate or divorce during the course of treatment. It is probably safe for a practitioner to continue treatment when this occurs unless the practitioner is told by one of the parents to stop treatment. If this occurs, the practitioner should consult the parent continuing to request treatment and ask for some confirmation of authority to consent to treatment, which will typically be contained in the custody order. The practitioner should also be careful before proceeding with treatment based solely on the consent of a stepparent or a relative without legal authority over the child, as in many states those individuals do not have the power to consent to treatment.[1]

Treatment Without Parental Consent: Exceptions

Although it would be prudent for a practitioner to assume that he or she should obtain the consent of a custodial parent before undertaking treatment of a minor, there are a number of exceptions to this general rule. As the nature and availability of such exceptions vary significantly from one jurisdiction to another, it would be advisable for a practitioner who treats minors to become familiar with relevant exceptions in the jurisdiction(s) in which he or she practices. The following exceptions may be available.

---

[1] See, e.g., *In re Care and Protection of Sharlene,* 445 Mass. 756 (2006).

Emergency Exception

In most jurisdictions, no consent is necessary if the situation is an emergency. The practitioner will not risk exposure if he or she proceeds to treat a child in such circumstances, regardless of who brought the child in for treatment. The exception reflects the assumption that if there were sufficient time to consult a parent, the parent would consent to the provision of emergency medical treatment.

Although this is a common exception, the foundation of the exception as well as its contours varies. In a number of states, the rule that protects a physician who provides services to an adult in an emergency extends to minors as well. Courts have struggled to define what constitutes a sufficient emergency to proceed without consent, recognizing that an overly broad definition could subsume the informed consent doctrine, whereas one that was too narrow could leave physicians who respond to life-threatening situations at risk and, thus, potentially unwilling to provide such care. The resulting case law does not always seem consistent.

The case law that specifically addresses the treatment of children in emergencies indicates that courts are especially willing to invoke this exception when obtaining or attempting to obtain consent would delay treatment and this delay would significantly increase the risk to the minor's life. In a number of jurisdictions, courts apply the exception more broadly, permitting treatment without parental consent when the delay would endanger the health of the minor.[1] There also seems to be a tendency to lower the gravity requirement and permit treatment in situations that are only semiemergent when the minor is older, is aware of the treatment, and cooperates with it.[2] As discussed below, this is particularly the case under some of the statutes that address emergency situations.

In addition to exceptions made by judges, many states have now enacted emergency statutes that are specifically applicable to minors. A few states will endorse proceeding without consent only in a "life-threatening situation."[3] Others permit emergency treatment without a parent's consent if the delay would endanger the health of the minor.[4]

Some states have also broadened the circumstances in which care can be provided without parental consent to situations that are not emergencies but in which the delay involved in securing parental consent would increase the risk of danger to the minor's health. For example, in the District of Columbia, there is a standard regulation authorizing the provision of emergency services to any person when the professional believes "that the giving of aid is the only alternative to probable death or serious physical or mental damage."[5] However, there is also a regulation that addresses only the provision of "health services" to minors of any age without parental consent. This requires only a judgment by the treating physician that the delay that would result from attempting to obtain consent would "substantially increase the risk to the minor's life, health, mental health, or welfare, or would unduly prolong suffering."[6] Of course, the clinician should look to state law to ascertain whether mental health services are included in the definition of "emergency services" or "health services."

Children in Foster Care

Mental health professionals may provide treatment for children placed in foster care. Studies show that children in foster care have significant mental health needs caused by myriad factors, including physical abuse, neglect, the trauma caused by removal, and the uncertainty of being in foster care. Foster children may be referred to the psychiatrist by a variety of people, including the parent, judge, case worker, foster parent, or child's attorney or guardian ad litem.

Determining which of the different actors holds the authority to consent to treatment can be challenging and varies from state to state. Obtaining a copy of the court order or seeking clarification from the court as to

---

[1] See generally Annotation, *Medical Practitioner's Liability for Treatment Given Child Without Parent's Consent*, 67 A.L.R. 4th 411 (1989) and supp. (2007).

[2] See, e.g., *Younts v. St. Francis Hospital & School of Nursing*, 469 P.2d 330 (Kan. 1970).

[3] See, e.g., N.D. Cent. Code § 14-10-17.1 (2008).

[4] For example, in Minnesota, such treatment can be rendered to minors without the consent of the parent or legal guardian when "in the professional's judgment, the risk to the minor's life or health is of such nature that treatment should be given without delay and the requirement of consent would result in delay or denial of treatment." Minn. Stat. § 144.322 (2007).

[5] D.C. Mun. Reg. tit. 22 § 600.5 (2008).

[6] Id. at § 600.4 (2008).

who possesses decision-making authority may be necessary. Generally, the parent will continue to retain the right to consent to medical treatment of their child until a finding is made that the parent abused or neglected the child, which then empowers the court to assume jurisdiction (or temporary custody) over the child. At that point, typically the court, the child's case worker, or the temporary custodian of the child may be granted medical decision-making authority.[1] In some states, however, parents will retain this authority until their parental rights have been terminated.[2] Again, practitioners should consult the specifics of their state statutes and review the court's order should this situation arise.

Emancipated Minors

In most jurisdictions, parental consent is not necessary for the provision of treatment to an emancipated minor, that is, a minor who is no longer under the control of his or her parents. In deciding whether a child should be (or has been) emancipated—which may occur in the context of litigation contesting the physician's treatment—courts may base their decisions on an agreement between the child and the parent or on the conduct of the child and the parent. Typically, the youth must be a minimum age, usually 16 years old, and must place himself or herself beyond the control, custody, and care of the parents.[3] Marriage, military service, and parenthood may support a finding of emancipation. Financial independence is also an important factor, although emancipation will not necessarily be defeated by some financial assistance from parents if the minor is living on his or her own and managing his or her own financial affairs.[4] Emancipated minors are considered adults for a variety of purposes, including the ability to rent an apartment, enter into contracts, and consent to medical care. These minors, however, relinquish the right to parental support.[5]

Most states have also adopted legislation that identifies specific criteria that will be adequate to guarantee minors who satisfy them the right to make decisions about medical or mental health treatment.

Mature Minor Exception

An additional exception may be available to a minor who is "mature," even if he or she would not meet the test for being legally emancipated. The test is whether the minor is capable of appreciating (and does appreciate) the nature, extent, and consequences of the medical treatment to which the minor is giving consent.[6] Again, there is significant variability in the circumstances in which this exception has been available to a minor. However, the case law that recognizes this exception frequently involves older minors, those whose parents were not available when the treatment decision was made, and/or treatments that were relatively low risk and clearly of benefit to the minor. Several states have also enacted statutes based on this doctrine.[7]

Cardwell v. Bechtol demonstrates the principle in operation.[8] The case involved a 17-year-old girl who had gone to a family osteopath on her own. The treatment resulted in a herniated disc, bladder and bowel problems, and decreased sensation in her legs. Finding the girl able to give effective consent to treatment, the Tennessee Supreme Court explained that whether a minor is sufficiently mature "depends upon the age, ability, experience, education, training and degree of maturity or judgment obtained by a minor, as well as upon the conduct and demeanor of the minor at the time of the incident involved."

---

[1] For example, in California, once a child is made a ward of the court, only the juvenile court judge can authorize the use of psychotropic medication for the child. Cal. Wel. & Inst. Code § 739.5 (2007).

[2] See, e.g., Mich. Comp. Law 722 § 124(a), which notes that until parental rights have been terminated, "[o]nly the minor child's parent or legal guardian shall consent to nonemergency, elective survey for a child in foster care."

[3] For example, in *Harris v. Rattini*, 855 S.W.2d 410 (Mo. Ct. App. 1993), the Missouri court determined that a child was emancipated because he dropped out of high school before his 18th birthday, took a part-time job, and had no mental or physical incapacity.

[4] In *Ireland v. Ireland*, 855 P.2d 40 (Idaho 1993), the court held that a 16-year-old child who was working full time while attending high school at night, who was able to pay for his own groceries, and owned his own truck was emancipated.

[5] See, e.g., *Carter v. Cangello*, 105 Cal. App. 3d 348 (Ct. App. Cal. 1980).

[6] See, e.g., *In re E.G.*, 133 Ill. 2d 98, 109 (Ill. 1989), observing that the "[r]ecognition that minors achieve varying degrees of maturity and responsibility (capacity) has been part of the common law for well over a century."

[7] For example, Arkansas and Nebraska permit unemancipated minors to authorize treatment when they understand and appreciate the nature of the proposed examination and voluntarily request it. See Ark. Code § 20-9-602(7) (2008); Nev. Rev. Stat. § 129.030(2) (2007).

[8] *Cardwell v. Bechtol*, 724 S.W.2d 739 (Tenn. 1987).

Although relatively few states have adopted mature minor exceptions, courts in recent years have seemed reluctant to hold a physician liable for treatment of an older minor who has consented to treatment. For a psychiatrist, the risks of providing treatment when only the minor patient consents are likely to be lower when only psychotherapy—as opposed to medication or electroconvulsive therapy—is involved. Even in jurisdictions that have explicitly recognized the exception, care should be taken in relying on it. The rule's subjective nature requires the practitioner to make judgments about the individual minor's capacity to comprehend the nature and purpose of the treatment in question. Those who are considering proceeding with treatment in reliance on this exception should familiarize themselves with the contours of the rule in their state. Practitioners should also document in their records the basis for their conclusions that the minor satisfies the requirements.

Specific Consent Statutes

Increasingly, state legislatures are addressing the question of when minors should be able to consent to medical treatment by identifying specific kinds of treatment decisions that minors may make, rather than the characteristics of minors who may make the decisions (which is the case involving emancipated or mature minors). These frequently involve treatment that is necessary, in circumstances in which requiring parental consent would discourage the minor from receiving care. For example, minors are likely not to tell their parents about drug problems, pregnancy, or sexually transmitted diseases. If their parents must consent to treatment for such conditions—which inevitably requires that they know of the problem—the minors will be much less likely to receive required treatment. To encourage minors to obtain treatment in these types of situations, the overwhelming majority of states have provided minors with the ability to seek specific types of treatment without the knowledge or consent of the parent or guardian.[1]

Who Pays?

As the discussion above indicates, there are an increasing number of circumstances in which a minor can validly consent to the medical treatment that he or she wishes to receive. This ability protects the physician against charges of assault and battery, unpermitted touching, malpractice, and so forth. However, it may create situations in which the physician is unlikely to be paid for his or her services. If services are provided pursuant to the emergency exception, it is likely that a physician would, as a legal matter, be able to look to the parent or guardian for payment. In other circumstances, however, it is likely that the minor's ability to consent to treatment means that when he or she does so, it is to the minor that the clinician must look for payment.

Some jurisdictions address this issue directly in their statutes or implementing regulations. For example, the District of Columbia regulations that authorize consent by minors in certain circumstances provide both that a minor who consents to the provision of health care services to himself or herself as permitted by the regulations will be liable for payment for the services and that the parents or legal guardians of a minor who consents to such services will not be liable for payment for those services unless they expressly agree to pay.[2]

Limits of Parental Authority: A Minor's Right to Refuse Treatment Arranged or Consented to by Parents

The converse of the question of whether a minor may consent to treatment without parental consent or involvement is whether a minor may effectively refuse treatment requested or arranged by a parent with legal custody of the minor. Again, this is a very difficult question to generalize. Some states have addressed this question through legislation or regulations that relate to specific situations, others have case law that provides some guidance, and still others have not yet addressed the issue.

Perhaps the only generalization that is possible is that states seem to be reluctant to permit a minor—even an older or "mature" minor—to refuse medical treatment requested by the parent or legal guardian if that treatment is necessary to save the minor's life. The

---

[1] For example, in Maryland, minors have the capacity to consent to treatment or advice about, among other issues, drug use, alcoholism, venereal disease, pregnancy, contraception, or injuries resulting from rape or sexual offense. Md. Health-General Code Ann. § 20-102. (2008).

[2] D.C. Mun. Reg. tit. 22 §§ 601.1 and 601.2 (2008).

result is asymmetrical. In other words, while the law may uphold or reflect the right of a minor to consent—without parental consent—to life-sustaining treatment, it is much less likely to permit the minor to refuse such treatment when the parent has requested it.

In re E.G.[1] involved a decision by a 17-year-old to refuse, on religious grounds, blood transfusions that were necessary to prevent her from dying of leukemia. Her mother acquiesced in this decision, also for religious reasons. When the case reached the Illinois Supreme Court, the court reached out to address an issue that was not before it: whether the minor's rejection of treatment would have been effective if the mother had wanted her to receive the treatment. In this situation, the court said, "If a parent or guardian opposes an unemancipated mature minor's refusal to consent to treatment for a life-threatening health problem, this opposition would weigh heavily against the minor's right to refuse."[2]

This asymmetry is reflected in statutory and regulatory provisions in a number of jurisdictions. For example, in Maryland, a minor has the same capacity as an adult to consent to a number of specific kinds of treatment, including treatment for drug abuse or alcoholism.[3] However, the Maryland code specifically provides that the capacity of a minor to consent to this treatment "does not include the capacity to refuse treatment for drug abuse or alcoholism in an inpatient alcohol or drug abuse treatment program…for which a parent or guardian has given consent."[4]

Commitment Proceedings

Issues involving consent often arise when a psychiatrist must determine whether to recommend that a child be placed in an inpatient mental health facility. This situation may arise based on a request made by a parent or an adolescent child or based on the medical necessity for a hospitalization when consents are lacking. Laws governing civil commitments vary depending on the state in which the request is being made,

and within each state, different procedures may apply based on who is requesting the hospitalization. Practitioners must familiarize themselves with the law governing commitments in their jurisdiction should the need arise. General observations about the process are discussed below.

Voluntary Admissions

Voluntary admissions of children refer to the inpatient hospitalization of children in which the facility has obtained the consent of the child's parent and/or of the child prior to the hospitalization. Most states permit a parent, for a child of any age, to request that the child be admitted to a mental health facility.[5] Additionally, many states permit an adolescent to make such a request as well. For example, a number of states permit children age 14 and older to make such requests.[6] Some states also require parental notification when a child requests the hospitalization. Again, the procedures vary significantly among jurisdictions, and broad generalizations are difficult to draw. One consistent principle emerges, however. Prior to voluntarily admitting a child, the clinician must make sure that the person requesting the commitment has the legal authority under state law to make such a request. If a parent or child bearing that legal authority makes a request for admission, then generally the request will be legally permissible if there is a clinical finding that the child has a mental illness or a disorder and that the inpatient treatment will benefit the minor.

Subsumed in the category of voluntary admissions are situations in which a child may object to a parent's decision to commit him or her. Such an admission against the child's wishes infringes upon the child's constitutional rights under the Fourteenth Amendment because it deprives the child of his or her liberty for a significant period of time. In *Parham v. J.R.*,[7] the U.S. Supreme Court determined the level of due process required when a parent seeks to admit a child against the child's wishes. When such a conflict arises, the Court held that an inquiry must be held by a neutral fact finder to determine whether statutory admis-

---

[1] *In re E.G.*, 549 N.E.2d 322 (Ill. 1989).

[2] Id. at 328.

[3] Md. Health-General Code Ann. § 20-102(c)(1) and (2) (2008).

[4] Id.

[5] See, e.g., Ind. Code Ann. § 12-26-3-2 (2008); 405 I.L.C.S. 5/3-503 (2008).

[6] See, e.g., Vt. Stat. Ann. tit. 18, § 7503(c) (2008); Conn. Gen. Stat. § 17a-79(a) (2008); Idaho Code § 66-318 (2008).

[7] *Parham v. J.R.*, 442 U.S. 584 (1979).

sions criteria to the facility have been met. This inquiry must examine the child's background and must include an interview of the child. The decision maker must also have the authority to refuse to admit any child who does not satisfy the medical standards for admission and the decision to admit must be reviewed periodically. Most notably, however, the Court refused to hold that the neutral decision maker must have any legal training, that a formal or quasi-formal hearing be held, that any adversarial process be required, or that the hearing be conducted by someone other than the admitting physician.

Parham established the minimum due process requirements that a state must provide to children when their parents decide to admit them. Many states have chosen to go beyond the minimum guarantees of due process and have afforded additional procedural protections for children, including judicial review, the right to legal representation, and the presentation of evidence at an adversarial hearing. For example, in Iowa, if a child objects to a parent's request for admission, even if the medical officer agrees, the parent must petition the juvenile court for admission.[1] Other states have determined that, when faced with a child's objection, a parent must petition for admission under the more stringent standards for an involuntary admission discussed below.[2]

Involuntary Admissions

A decision to admit a child to an inpatient facility against the wishes of both the parent and the child significantly infringes upon the constitutional rights of both. Supreme Court case law clearly holds that absent compelling circumstances, parents have a constitutional right to direct the upbringing of their children. Additionally, as noted above, since commitments deprive children of their liberty interests, their due process rights are implicated as well. The state's police powers and *parens patriae* interest in protecting children, however, have been used to trump the rights of both parents and children. The burden, however, on the state to justify such an involuntarily commitment is quite high.

As with voluntarily admissions, state laws vary considerably on the issue of involuntary admissions.

Generally, to justify an involuntary commitment, most states require that the child have a mental illness and that a serious likelihood of harm to the child exists that cannot be addressed by less restrictive means.[3] Although all state statutes permit emergency hospitalizations where a mental health professional certifies that immediate action is necessary to protect the child, a judicial hearing is afforded to the parents and the child soon thereafter to contest the commitment decision. At this hearing, evidence will be presented to determine whether the legal standard for the commitment has been met. Psychiatrists who testify without their client's consent at a commitment hearing do not violate their client's privilege.[4] If the court determines that the statutory criteria for the involuntary admission have been met, then commitment for a specific period of time will be authorized. After that period elapses, the burden typically rests on the treatment facility to bring another petition before the court requesting a longer commitment period. Details such as length of the initial commitment order, standards of proof justifying the entry of the order, and procedural safeguards such as the right to an attorney for the child and/or the parent are different in each jurisdiction.

Clinicians involved in commitment proceedings must ensure that they carefully document their observations and diagnoses regarding the children to ensure that only those children with behaviors and circumstances that meet the statutory criteria are actually committed. Clinicians must be able to convince themselves and the court that there is indeed a sufficient reason for infringing upon the significant liberty interests of both the parent and the child.

Confidentiality and Privilege

Mental health professionals are both legally and ethically bound not to disclose information learned from a patient or information about a patient learned through, or in connection with, a treatment relationship. That duty is reflected in two overlapping but distinct areas of law that are frequently confused: privilege

---

[1] Iowa Code § 229.2. (2008).

[2] See, e.g., Hawaii Rev. Stat. Ann. 334-60.1 (2008).

[3] See, e.g., Wash. Rev. Code § 71.34.710 (2008).

[4] See, e.g., *In re Dennis W*, 717 N.W.2d 488 (2006).

and confidentiality. Privilege rules are rules of evidence; they govern disclosure of information in judicial, quasi-judicial, or administrative proceedings. Information disclosed to a practitioner during treatment is "privileged"—that is, absent some applicable exception, the patient may prevent the practitioner from disclosing it in such a proceeding. Confidentiality rules are much broader, barring disclosure of any information learned from the patient to any person not directly involved in the current patient's care. Privilege and confidentiality rules apply to the oral or written disclosure of information learned from patients as well as to the release of written notes, records, and so forth.

Confidentiality

Confidentiality is essential to the therapeutic relationship and effective treatment. Its importance is reflected in the double duty—ethical and legal—to maintain patient confidences. Unfortunately, the legal status of minors complicates the rather clear-cut rules that apply in the treatment of adults and results in countervailing duties running to different interested parties. On one hand, it is clear both that a minor's parents generally are entitled to more information about the patient than family members of an adult patient would be and that they may make certain decisions about the release of information about the minor that would ordinarily only be made by the patient. On the other hand, it is also clear that minors possess certain independent, albeit relatively limited, rights of confidentiality, which must be considered and which will outweigh parental rights in certain situations. Thus, practitioners must proceed with care when parents seek information and minor patients resist disclosure.

Risks of Confidentiality Breach: General Principles

In all jurisdictions, what was solely an ethical obligation to keep patient information confidential is now also a legal duty. Suits for breach of confidentiality have been brought under various theories.[1] Patients have sued for invasion of privacy, tortuous breach of a duty of confidentiality, breach of an implied contract to maintain confidentiality, and breach of duties derived from state licensing statutes or testimonial privileges. Although not all such theories have been successful, the trend is clearly in the direction of recognizing a legal duty and concomitant right of recovery, regardless of the legal theory on which this duty is based. In addition, in recent years, the federal government and an increasing number of states have enacted statutes that provide for the confidentiality of information and records of mental health treatment and set out any exceptions to that rule.

It would be reasonable to assume that the rules governing who may authorize the release of confidential treatment information would derive from those governing who may authorize treatment and that where a parent controls consent to treatment, the parent also makes all decisions regarding waivers of confidentiality and the release of information. Although this is a good starting place for analyzing confidentiality questions and this approach has been explicitly adopted in a number of jurisdictions (and seems to be implicitly followed in others), it will not always yield the right result. Assuming that it is universally followed could create exposure for the clinician. This is an area in which there may not be an easy legal answer; there may not always be a statute or regulation that sets out in what circumstances and at what age a minor enjoys independent confidentiality rights. Nevertheless, there are generally ways in which a clinician can control and minimize risk.

Health Insurance Portability and Accountability Act of 1996

Any analysis of a clinician's legal obligation to preserve the confidentiality of a patient's medical information must begin with the Health Insurance Portability and Accountability Act of 1996 (HIPAA), which established a foundation of federally protected rights permitting individuals to control certain uses and disclosure of their protected health information. In August 2002, the U.S. Department of Health and Human Services published a comprehensive set of rules, known as the *privacy rule*, which implements the requirements of HIPAA.[2] The statute and rules create a complex set of standards to which clinicians must adhere, as evidenced by the array of guides and handbooks written to help practitioners. More detailed in-

---

[1] See Annotation, *Physicians' Tort Liability for Unauthorized Disclosure of Confidential Information About Patient*, 48 A.L.R. 4th 668 (1986) and supp. (2007).

[2] See 45 C.F.R § 160.101 et seq. (2008).

formation about HIPAA and the privacy rule can be found at http://www.hhs.gov/ocr/hipaa.

A clinician must first determine whether he or she is subject to the requirements of HIPAA. A "covered entity" under HIPAA includes any health care provider who electronically transmits health information in connection with certain transitions, including processing claims, benefit eligibility inquiries, referral authorization requests, or other transactions for which the Department of Health and Human Services has established standards under the HIPAA transactions rule.[1] Any provider of medical services should immediately determine whether compliance with HIPAA is legally required.

HIPAA imposes a number of requirements on covered entities. These obligations include providing privacy notices to patients, permitting patients to see their records with limited exceptions, and restricting third-party payer requests for information to the "minimum necessary" information. HIPAA and the subsequent privacy rule also prevent covered entities from disclosing a patient's protected health information (PHI) unless 1) the privacy rule permits or requires the disclosure or 2) the individual who is subject of the information (or the individual's personal representative) authorizes the disclosure in writing.[2] PHI includes information such as a patient's past, present, and future physical or mental health condition and the provision of health care to the individual.[3] The privacy rule permits the use and disclosure of PHI without the patient's authorization or permission for 12 national priority purposes including public health activities; protection of victims of abuse, neglect, or domestic violence; law enforcement purposes; serious threats to health and safety; and judicial and administrative proceedings.[4] These exceptions are specifically laid out in the privacy rule.

Unless the PHI falls under one of these exceptions, the covered entity must obtain the written consent of the patient prior to disclosing the information. For most minors, however, the privacy rule gives the right to consent to the disclosure of the PHI to the child's personal representative, who is the person legally authorized (under state or other applicable law) to make health care decisions for the child.[5] In most cases, parents are the personal representatives for their minor children. This, however, may not be the case in a number of situations. For example, a custody order may empower one parent with the sole authority to make these decisions for a child. A state may not require the consent of a parent or other person before the minor can consent to obtaining a particular health care service, or a parent may agree to a confidential relationship between the minor and the doctor, which may or may not be legally enforceable. These exceptions, in which the parent is not the personal representative, are all determined by state law. When a parent is not the child's personal representative, then HIPAA defers to state law to determine the rights of parents to access and control the PHI of their children. When state or other applicable laws are silent regarding a parent's access to a child's PHI, a covered entity has the discretion to provide or deny a parent's access to the records provided that the decision is made by a licensed health care professional in the exercise of professional judgment.

Once the personal representative of the child is identified, the privacy rule requires that he or she be treated the same as the adult patient with respect to uses and disclosures of the child's PHI. The privacy rule, however, does permit an exception when a covered entity has a reasonable belief that the personal representative may be abusing or neglecting the child, or that treating the individual as the personal representative could otherwise endanger the child. In such situations, the covered entity may choose not to treat the individual as the child's personal representative if, in the exercise of professional judgment, doing so would be contrary to the best interests of the child.

Clinicians who fall under the scope of HIPAA must carefully follow the requirements in the statute. In addition to general tort claims that may be filed against the clinician for breach of confidentiality, HIPAA permits individuals to file complaints with the Department of Health and Human Services alleging violations of the statute, which can result in substantial civil and criminal penalties.[6] Because the obligations imposed by HIPAA on clinicians treating children may vary depending on the specifics of state law, clinicians

---

[1] 45 C.F.R. §§ 160.102, 160.103 (2008).

[2] 45 C.F.R § 164.502(a) (2008).

[3] 45 C.F.R. § 160.103 (2008).

[4] 45 C.F.R. § 164.512 (2008).

[5] 45 C.F.R. § 164.502(g) (2008).

[6] 42 U.S.C. §§ 1320d-5, 1320d-6 (2008).

must familiarize themselves with state laws governing confidentiality. Although laws vary significantly from jurisdiction to jurisdiction, some general principles are discussed below.

Release of Information to Custodial Parents

Generally, the issue of what information about the minor and his or her treatment may be released to the minor's parents is a question that arises frequently and is one of the more difficult confidentiality questions a practitioner faces. The closeness of the parent–child relationship, the anxiety a parent is likely to feel about a child in treatment, and the fact that the parent is likely to be paying for treatment lead many parents to ask for and expect complete information about a child in treatment.

As a strictly legal matter, unless there is a statute to the contrary, it is fair to assume that if a parent is legally entitled to authorize treatment for a minor child, that parent has a legal right to full information disclosed by the minor, until the minor reaches the age of majority. This legal rule poses obvious clinical problems. Even when patients are young, many practitioners would feel uncomfortable if parents actually sought to exercise their right of full access to complete information about the treatment. The potential damage to the therapeutic relationship with the minor is the most obvious risk. In addition, certain disclosures may well exacerbate family problems.

To avoid such risks, when parents appear to have a legal right to full information—or to more information than practitioners may feel it is appropriate to give them—it is advisable to lay out ground rules regarding confidentiality and disclosure at the outset of treatment. Practitioners should explain what they will tell the parents, what they will withhold, and what their reasoning is. Most parents will understand. If the parents elect to go forward with treatment, practitioners may assume that they have agreed to those terms.[1]

The problem of disclosure to parents assumes even greater importance with adolescent patients. As discussed later, statutes frequently give adolescents greater authority regarding the release of information about them and their treatment. Even in the absence of such statutes, parents of adolescent children may well not be entitled to the same amount of information as are parents of very young minors. To begin with, as discussed earlier, in many circumstances and jurisdictions, it is likely that minors who are legally able to give effective consent to treatment will also be entitled to control the release of information about that treatment. The statutes of some states specifically link consent to treatment and disclosure authority. Even without such a statute, unless there is a statute or regulation specifically giving the parents control over disclosure, there is little risk in relying on an adolescent's consent to release confidential information when that adolescent was legally entitled to consent to the treatment in question.

When it is not clear that the adolescent controls consent to treatment, it is essential that the practitioner make disclosure rules clear to both the adolescent and his or her parents. The risks of not doing so are significant. If the matter is not discussed, the adolescent and parent(s) each may well assume that he or she controls confidentiality. Both the adolescent and the parents should be informed at the outset of treatment to what extent the adolescent will control the disclosure of the information—including disclosure to the parents—and to what extent or in what situations information will be shared with the parents regardless of the adolescent's wishes.

The decision of where this line will be drawn should be informed by both legal and ethical[2] considerations. As a legal matter, practitioners will be at risk if they withhold information that could enable parents to protect their adolescent from serious harm. When the interests involved are less vital, but practitioners feel that certain information would benefit the family, practitioners should attempt to arrange this disclosure without breaching confidentiality and, thus, endangering the therapeutic relationship with the adolescents. First, practitioners may be able to work with the adolescents, encouraging them to disclose the information to their parents themselves. If the adolescents are unwilling to do this, they may be willing to permit

---

[1] Whereas obtaining written agreement to such conditions offers the greatest degree of protection, many psychiatrists are unwilling to go beyond an oral explanation to their patients' parents. An intermediate approach would be to develop a standard statement regarding confidentiality to go over with, and provide to, the parents.

[2] The American Psychiatric Association's (APA) *Principles of Medical Ethics With Annotations Especially Applicable to Psychiatry*, section 4, annotation 7 (2008 Edition), addresses the countervailing ethical interests as follows: "Careful judgment must be exercised by the psychiatrist in order to include, when appropriate, the parents or guardian in the treatment of a minor. At the same time, the psychiatrist must assure the minor proper confidentiality."

the practitioners to do so. If the adolescents resist both options, practitioners may be able to accomplish this purpose by discussing with the parents a general problem without disclosing anything the adolescents may have said about themselves or any specific information about the adolescents.

State statutes and regulations. Much of the preceding discussion has been predicated on the assumption that there is no statute specifically addressing the confidentiality rights of minors, or at least no statute that speaks to the situation at issue. Increasingly, this is not the case. It would be advisable for practitioners whose work involves minor patients to become familiar with any statutory or regulatory provisions relevant to these issues in the jurisdictions in which they practice. Although there is still great variability in the legislative approaches of different jurisdictions, several approaches are common. As suggested earlier, a number of jurisdictions have adopted an approach under which, as a general matter, a minor's ability to control the release of information is coterminous with his or her ability to consent to treatment. For example, in Massachusetts, when a minor is able to consent to treatment, absent limited exceptions, all information is confidential between the minor and the physician.[1]

The District of Columbia's confidentiality rules reflect another common approach—one based on the age of the minor—and also have a consent to treatment overlay. The District of Columbia Mental Health Information Act provides that if a patient is between age 14 and 18, both patient and parent must authorize, in writing, the disclosure of confidential information. Disclosures about a patient younger than age 14 may be authorized by a parent or legal guardian alone; however, if the parent has not consented to the minor's receipt of services, the minor alone may authorize the release of information.[2]

In some jurisdictions, the parent or legal guardian is generally exempted from a requirement that the minor authorize the release of any mental health information. For example, New Mexico requires the minor to authorize the release of any information from which he or she could be identified and establishes clear rules as to who acts for the child if he or she is in-

capable of giving or withholding consent. (Parents may act for children younger than age 14; a treatment guardian must be appointed for older minors.) However, the statute provides that no authorization by the child is required if either 1) the disclosure is to the parent or legal guardian and is essential for the treatment of the child or 2) the disclosure is to the primary caregiver and is only of information necessary for the continuity of the child's treatment.[3]

Even when minors appear to have a clear legal right to control the release of information, practitioners should be alert to exceptions that may either permit or require them to provide certain information to parents. For example, in Massachusetts, even if the minor in question is able to give consent and, thus, controls disclosure, a practitioner must notify parents of a medical condition so serious that "life or limb is endangered."[4] In Maryland, a minor has the same capacity as an adult to consent to treatment for a variety of conditions (including drug abuse, alcoholism, venereal disease, and pregnancy). Nevertheless, a physician, without the consent of the minor, or even over the express objection of the minor, may, but is not required to, give information to a parent or guardian about treatment needed by or provided to the minor (other than abortion).[5] In the District of Columbia, rather broad provisions permitting a physician to give information to parents are trumped by the district's Mental Health Information Act, discussed earlier. However, the District of Columbia still requires providers to inform parents about treatment needed by a minor who is infected with a sexually transmitted disease and has refused treatment.[6]

Parental separation or divorce. The divorce or separation of the parents of a minor patient further complicates the situation. Traditionally, the principles discussed above applied: the parent(s) with legal custody enjoyed whatever legal rights existed to obtain information about the minor's treatment, including information disclosed by the minor in the course of therapy. Increasingly, however, the law protects the interests of the noncustodial parent to access such information. The provision of the Michigan code is typical: "Notwithstanding any other provision of law, a parent shall

---

[1] Mass. Gen. Laws ch. 112 § 12F (2008).

[2] D.C. Code § 7-1202.05 (2008).

[3] N.M. Stat. Ann. § 32A-6A-24 (2008).

[4] Mass. Gen. Laws ch. 112 § 12F (2008).

[5] Md. Gen. Code Ann. § 20-102 (2008).

[6] D.C. Mun. Reg. tit. 22 § 602.7 (2008).

not be denied access to records or information concerning his or her child because the parent is not the custodial parent, unless the parent is prohibited from having access to the records or information by a protective order."[1]

Note that this does not give the noncustodial parent any greater right to information than he or she would otherwise have—that is, such a provision must be interpreted through the overlay of other provisions of state law that may limit even a custodial parent's right to information regarding a child.

Even in the absence of such a statute, a practitioner would be ill advised to treat the parent who does not have legal custody as an ordinary third party. Particularly if the parent has actual custody, arrangements should be made to provide the noncustodial parent with any information the practitioner believes is essential, for example, information about medications, behavior that has signaled trouble in the past, and concerns about the minor's safety. If possible, consent should be obtained from the parent with legal custody. If the custodial parent is unwilling, the parent with the child can seek assistance from the court or guardian ad litem, if one has been appointed to represent the child's best interests, to resolve the issue. Practitioners may also want to condition the acceptance of the child patient on the custodial parent's willingness to permit the involvement of the other parent in the child's treatment.

Release of Information to Third Parties

The rules that govern the release of information about minors to unrelated third parties—schools, researchers, insurers—are somewhat less clear. The principles discussed earlier would suggest that at least in the absence of specific statutory provisions addressing the situation, custodial parents may consent to such releases unless the minor controls the right to consent to the underlying treatment. However, both ethical and legal concerns suggest that this general rule needs to be tempered somewhat when the information is to be released to someone other than the minor's parents.

In addition, in this area in which statutory and regulatory provisions are proliferating, it is critical to determine whether there is a statutory provision on this point. Most of the statutes discussed earlier in the context of the release of information to a minor patient's parents have provisions that address the release of information to third parties. For example, as indicated, the New Mexico code, which permits the disclosure of information to parents if it is essential to the minor's treatment or necessary for the continuity of treatment, provides that the minor controls the release of information in most other circumstances.

Even when the practitioner has authorization for the disclosure of information from the appropriate party, the practitioner has an ethical obligation to limit disclosures to those necessary in the particular situations.[2] Practitioners should be particularly sensitive to this obligation when the person authorizing the disclosure (the parent) is someone other than the person who may be harmed by the disclosures (the minor). Moreover, as the foregoing discussion indicates, increasingly, minors have some independent right of confidentiality. Although its contours are far from clear, courts may be more willing to protect this right when information is being withheld from third parties rather than from the minor's parents.

Particular caution should be exercised when the disclosures are to benefit someone other than the child. The practitioner who wants to write about the minor or use information about the patient in some other kind of research would be well advised to obtain the consent of both the parents and the minor before doing so. Additionally, federal law requires that the assent of children be obtained prior to being used as research subjects.[3]

Exceptions to Consent Requirement: Reporting Statutes and Other Public Safety Considerations

Both federal and state laws define important exceptions to the requirement that confidential information be disclosed to third parties only with consent. HIPAA and the privacy rule lay out 12 national priority purposes that permit the use and disclosure of protected

---

[1] Mich. Comp. Laws Ann. § 722.30 (2008). Florida has enacted a similar statute authorizing noncustodial parents to have access to records and information pertaining to a minor child. Fla. Stat. § 61.13 (2008).

[2] The APA's *Principles of Medical Ethics With Annotations Especially Applicable to Psychiatry*, section 4, annotation 5, provides that "[e]thically, the psychiatrist may disclose only that information which is relevant to a given situation. He/she should avoid offering speculation as fact. Sensitive information such as an individual's sexual orientation or fantasy material is usually unnecessary."

[3] 45 C.F.R. § 46.408 (2008).

health information without first obtaining consent.[1] The statute, however, relies extensively on state law to define the precise nature and scope of the exceptions. Some of the more common exceptions found under state law are detailed below.

Child abuse reporting.   Most clinicians, whether treating children or adults, are aware that they are obligated to report known or suspected abuse or neglect of children. In 2006, there were 3.3 million reports of child maltreatment involving 6 million children.[2] Of the 3.3 million reports referred to Child Protective Services, 60% of them were accepted for investigation and approximately 905,000 children were found to be victims of abuse or neglect.[3] More than 60% of those children were determined to be victims of neglect, more than 15% suffered physical abuse, and less than 10% endured sexual abuse.[4]

Federal law requires that states designate certain professionals as mandatory reporters of child abuse or neglect. However, the exact circumstances in which this duty arises are often unclear, as is the approach to be taken in analyzing the situation. Although child abuse statutes vary from one jurisdiction to another, there are some constants that underlie most: 1) practitioners' duty to report child abuse generally derives from their licensure in a state, which makes their duties less clear if the abuse has occurred or the victim lives in a different state; 2) as statutes give little or no discretion regarding reporting, patients may need to be warned before they make disclosures; 3) reports must generally be made very quickly, that is, within 24 to 48 hours; and 4) because all states also have statutes granting reporters immunity from civil liability for reports made in good faith, a practitioner who believes that abuse has occurred should not be dissuaded by the risk of a lawsuit by enraged parents or others reported. Beyond this, state legislative schemes vary, following one of several different approaches, and each practitioner should become familiar with the basic elements of the scheme in the state(s) in which he or she practices.

Regardless of the approach, the determination of whether to report child abuse or neglect generally should be made through a two-step process. First, the practitioner must determine whether the reported behavior constitutes abuse or neglect under the operative statute. Most statutes contain precise definitions of physical, emotional, and sexual abuse and of neglect. These should be reviewed in connection with any difficult questions, for example, whether corporal punishment would be considered abuse. Statutory definitions are also likely to control what abuse will have to be reported. In a number of states, for example, conduct that would otherwise qualify as abuse does not have to be reported as child abuse unless a parent, guardian, or caretaker inflicts the abuse or allows it to occur.[5]

If the practitioner determines that the alleged conduct would qualify as reportable child abuse, he or she must determine whether there is an actual duty to report. States take many different approaches to this issue. It is not unusual for a state to require reporting upon the receipt of any indication that there may have been abuse, even when the practitioner may have suspicions about the veracity of the reporter, for example, a young minor.[6] This approach reflects the belief that children are optimally protected when a state investigative process, rather than the variable responses of individual professionals, is used to screen out unsubstantiated reports.

Many other states take a different approach, requiring reporting only when the reporter has "reason to believe" or "reasonable cause to suspect" that abuse has occurred. For example, in Washington State, a practitioner needs to report only when he or she "has reasonable cause to believe that a child…has suffered abuse or neglect."[7] This would appear to permit the exercise of some discretion, for example, when the practitioner believes that the report is false. Care should be taken in deciding not to report, however, and

---

[1] 45 C.F.R. § 164.512 (2008).

[2] Children's Bureau, U.S. Department of Health and Human Services, Child Maltreatment 2006, at xiv (2008).

[3] Id.

[4] Id. at xv.

[5] See, e.g., N.Y. Fam. Ct. Act § 1012 (2008).

[6] For example, Texas has a relatively broad reporting requirement, extending the duty to cases in which the reporter has concern about the child's future welfare. It requires reporting by "[a] person having cause to believe that a child's physical or mental health or welfare has been adversely affected by any abuse or neglect by any person." Tex. Fam. Code Ann. § 261.101 (2007).

[7] Wash. Rev. Code § 26.44.030(I) (2008).

the reasoning for such a conclusion should be carefully documented. Failure to report child abuse or neglect could result in civil and criminal penalties.

Finally, although this may be less relevant for the practitioner who treats minors, some states make the decision to report contingent on whether the reporter has had professional contact with the alleged victim. In Wisconsin, for example, the duty to report arises only for "a physician...having reasonable cause to suspect that a child seen in the course of professional duties has been abused or neglected."[1]

Whether the decision is to report or not to report, once the question of possible child abuse has surfaced, the practitioner should carefully document the reasoning that led to his or her decision. State statutes can be useful in this effort, offering a framework for analysis and the decisions that need to be made to decide about reporting.

Other reporting statutes. In some states, other statutes require the practitioner to report infectious diseases and other conditions that may affect children. The requirements vary significantly from state to state; practitioners should familiarize themselves with the law of the jurisdictions in which they practice. Statutes adopted in a number of jurisdictions may have implications for those who treat adolescents. These require a physician to report to state motor vehicle authorities the identity of patients suffering from certain disorders that might impair their driving. At their broadest, these statutes require the reporting of identified conditions if the condition is likely to impair the ability to control a vehicle and drive safely. The conditions are likely to include mental or emotional disorders and chronic abuse of substances that may impair motor skills.

Duties imposed by permissive reporting statutes. State confidentiality statutes sometimes authorize psychiatrists to breach confidentiality in order to protect both the patient and others from harm. These statutes obviously apply to minors as well as to adults. Although these statutes are only permissive in nature, that is, they do not by their terms require reporting, practitioners should be extremely careful if they practice in a jurisdiction with such a statute. It is likely that in the presence of such a statute, the common, or judge-made, law of such a jurisdiction would be interpreted as imposing a duty to protect.

Duties in the absence of specific reporting statutes. Even in the absence of statutes that impose, or are likely to be interpreted as imposing, a duty to report, in most jurisdictions a practitioner will be at risk if he or she does not appropriately disclose information that suggests that another person is endangered by the patient, minor or adult. Most courts that have considered the issue have held not only that a physician may warn a third party of threatened harm but also that the physician can be held responsible for the consequences of not doing so. Similarly, as with adult patients, if a practitioner possesses information about a minor's suicidal intent, it must be disclosed as necessary and appropriate to prevent suicide. In both cases, the interests of the patient and the state in confidentiality are considered outweighed by the interest in preservation of life and safety.

Custody Disputes

The issues a clinician must consider when a minor's custody has been settled through a separation agreement or divorce decree have been addressed. When parents separate during the course of a minor's treatment, different problems may arise. It is not uncommon in such a situation for one or even both parents to seek the practitioner's assistance in the custody contest. As discussed below, the physician–patient privilege may permit one parent or the other to prevent this testimony. Even if it does not, and even if the practitioner has very clear opinions as to where the patient's custody interests lie, the practitioner should resist being drawn into the case.

The risks are many. If the minor is aware of the practitioner's appearance in court, particularly if it is "in support of" one parent and "against" the other, it may seriously undermine the treatment relationship. Nor are the risks confined to the minor patient's reactions. One or both parents may resent the practitioner's expressed views and may refuse to continue to work with the practitioner or to pay for treatment. The practitioner should explain to the parents that the child is best served by the practitioner remaining solely in a therapeutic role and that they can obtain an independent evaluation for purposes of the litigation. The following section on privilege will discuss how to proceed if the parent or counsel persists and seeks to compel the practitioner's involvement.

[1] Wis. Stat. Ann. § 49.981(2) (2007).

Authorization to Release Information: Formalities of Consent

Regardless of who—minor, parent, both parents, other persons, or a combination—has the authority to consent to the release of confidential information, the practitioner should make certain that the consent on which he or she relies is legally valid. A practitioner should make certain that the authorization actually extends to the information in question and that it satisfies federal and state confidentiality law requirements. Both HIPAA and a number of state laws have provisions that specify the form and content of effective authorization.[1] Practitioners should familiarize themselves with the specifics, because there may be elements that they would not otherwise include, for example, a statement that the consenting party has the right to revoke consent at any time, a description of the use that may be made of the information released, and a statement that the consenting party has the right to examine any information disclosed.

As a general rule, these statutes require written authorization to release information. Even when there is no such statutory requirement, it is advisable to obtain written consent. The use of a consent form both encourages a patient to focus on the process and the rights being waived and serves as documentation of consent. This is particularly useful when children and adolescents are involved and consent may become a contentious issue between them and their parents.

Before releasing the information in question, practitioners should satisfy themselves that the patient's and/or parents' consent is informed.[2] Those authorizing disclosure should be aware of the nature of the information sought as well as what will be included in the information released. If release of the patient's medical record is at issue, the patient should be informed of the types and sources of information in the record. This is particularly important when the consent of a minor is involved, because the record is likely to include significant information from parents and other sources of which the patient is unaware.

Authorization for the release of information frequently comes indirectly from third parties—such as insurance carriers or schools—who have obtained written authorization from the patient or parent. If the practitioner believes that the patient or parent would not have consented if fully aware of the nature of the information involved or was not aware that the authorization would be used to obtain mental health information, the practitioner should contact the patient to discuss authorization and disclosure. The most effective consent is that made with knowledge of exactly what the practitioner will be disclosing. This would require the practitioner to make all disclosures in writing and to provide the patient a copy to review and approve prior to release.

Privilege

Privilege rules govern the disclosure of confidential information in judicial, quasi-judicial, or administrative proceedings. Privileges were created by statute in recognition that certain social values—the protection of certain kinds of relationships—were more important than the need for full disclosure. Privileges encourage full and frank communication in these relationships. The rationale for the physician–patient privilege is that without full communication between doctors and patients, effective treatment cannot take place.

Scope of the Privilege

The law of virtually every state includes a psychotherapist–patient or physician–patient privilege that applies to communications between mental health professionals and their patients, including minor patients. Whether or not particular information from or about the patient will be found privileged—and therefore subject to exclusion by the patient (or the person legally authorized to exercise the privilege on the patient's behalf)—depends on a variety of factors that vary considerably from jurisdiction to jurisdiction. These state law rules will apply in proceedings in state courts or administrative bodies. Federal courts apply both state and federal laws, depending on the nature of the claim at issue. When entertaining a federal claim, federal courts will apply federal privilege law. In *Jaffe v. Redmond* (1996), the U.S. Supreme Court recognized a federal psychotherapist–patient privilege. Reasoning that "[e]ffective psychotherapy...depends upon an atmosphere of confidence and trust in which

---

[1] 45 C.F.R. § 164.508 (2008).

[2] Ethical considerations also warrant such an action. Section 4, annotation 2, of the APA's *Principles of Medical Ethics With Annotations Especially Applicable to Psychiatry* provides that "[t]he continuing duty of the psychiatrist to protect the patient includes fully apprising him/her of the connotations of waiving the privilege of privacy."

the patient is willing to make a frank and complete disclosure of facts, emotions, memories, and fears," the Supreme Court held that "confidential communications between a licensed psychotherapist and her patients in the course of diagnosis or treatment are protected from compelled disclosure under [the federal rules of evidence]."[1]

In most jurisdictions, the privilege protects not only appropriate communications from the patient to the psychotherapist but also any information learned in the course of examination and the diagnosis and other conclusions about the patient and diagnosis.[2] The privilege is usually held to apply only to communications between the clinician and patient that relate to the patient's treatment. This should cover virtually all information learned by a clinician from a patient.[3] On the other hand, information such as billing records and the fact that a certain individual is a patient may not be privileged.

An important issue in the treatment of children and adolescents is whether information disclosed in the presence of another person is privileged. The traditional rule was that such communications were not privileged—that there could be no expectation of privacy when a third person, including a parent, was present. However, this rule is under modification as courts examine and acknowledge the reality of child and adolescent therapy and other family treatment situations.

Another issue of importance in the treatment of children and adolescents is whether information received from a minor patient's parents, family members, and other third parties is protected by the privilege. Important interests are served by including this information within the privilege. Some of the most sensitive information about both the patient and the family—and the information most critical to successful treatment of the minor—may come from the family. If the confidentiality of such information is not assured,

family members may not be willing to provide it. To date, although some courts have understood the importance of extending the privilege to such third-party communications, there is no uniformity on this point.[4]

Exceptions to the Privilege

Virtually every privilege statute contains significant exceptions—circumstances in which the privilege does not apply and the clinician may have to testify regardless of the confidential treatment relationship. Courts have developed other "exceptions," reasoning that the patient has waived the privilege by various means. Commitment proceedings, will contests, and criminal matters are frequently excepted from the privilege, as are cases in which the patient seeks to prove a particular mental health condition in court, such as posttraumatic stress disorder. Particularly important to the practitioner who treats minors is the common abrogation of the privilege in proceedings relating to child abuse or neglect.[5] The scope of this exception varies from state to state, depending on the language of the state's statute and subsequent judicial interpretations. In some states, such as Alaska, the privilege is abrogated only in proceedings brought under the state's child abuse acts.[6] In other states, the exception is broader, and courts have held that the privilege does not apply in a range of civil proceedings.[7]

Some state statutes have created a possible exception in child custody cases. In these jurisdictions, a minor's treating psychiatrist can be compelled to provide testimony and disclose confidential information learned through treatment even over the objection of the minor patient and the minor's parents. However, some courts have recognized that there are countervailing interests and that the evidence can be obtained in other ways. These courts have upheld the privilege, requiring an independent examination instead. For example, in Massachusetts a clinician's testimony will

---

[1] *Jaffe v. Redmond*, 518 U.S. 1 (1996).

[2] This is the case even in most jurisdictions that have statutes that only refer to patient communications. See, e.g., *State v. Henneberry*, 558 N.W.2d 708, 709–710 (Iowa 1997).

[3] Communications made during the course of examinations undertaken for purposes other than treatment usually will not be protected. This exception would likely include court-ordered or school-requested forensic evaluations.

[4] See, e.g., *Grosslight v. Superior Court*, 72 Cal. App. 3d 502 (Ct. App. Ca. 1977).

[5] For example, in Michigan, "[a]ny legally recognized privilege communication except that between attorney and client or that made to a member of the clergy... is abrogated and shall not constitute grounds for excusing a report otherwise required to be made or for excluding evidence in a civil child protective proceeding." Mich. Comp. Laws Ann. 722.631 (2008).

[6] See, e.g., Alaska Stat. § 47.17.060 (2007); Colo. Rev. Stat. 19-3-311 (2007).

[7] See, e.g., *State ex rel D.M. v. Hoester*, 681 S.W.2d 449 (Missouri 1984).

be permitted only if the judge determines after a hearing not only that the witness has significant evidence regarding the parent's ability to provide custody but also that the disclosure of the evidence is more important to the child's welfare than is the protection of the therapeutic relationship.[1]

Waiver of the Privilege

Explicit waiver. The physician–patient and the psychotherapist–patient privileges may be waived. If the patient or the person authorized to act on the patient's behalf waives the privilege (does not choose to exercise it), the confidential information that would otherwise be privileged may be introduced into the judicial proceeding. Practitioners who treat children and adolescents face the uncertainty of whether a minor patient may decline to exercise (and therefore waive) the privilege. Although this depends on state statutes and case law, which differ from state to state, if the patient is a minor, the parent or legal guardian will ordinarily have the power to waive the privilege on behalf of the child. If the parents are divorced or separated, the parent with legal custody traditionally has controlled the exercise of the privilege.

Although it is generally safe for a practitioner to rely on the waiver of one parent, he or she should be cautious if the minor's parents are separated or divorced or custody seems unclear. The most difficult questions arise in the context of custody disputes, in which the practitioner's testimony is likely to be central to the dispute and the parents frequently disagree about whether the privilege should be exercised or waived. The law in this area varies dramatically from state to state. In *Nagle v. Hooks*,[2] Maryland's highest court held that when a child was too young to make decisions about the privilege himself, the decision in a custody dispute could not be made by either parent or even by both together. The court explained that a custodial parent has an inherent conflict of interest in acting on the child's behalf in asserting or waiving the privilege in the context of a continuing custody dispute. The court required that a neutral party be appointed to serve as guardian for the limited purpose of deciding whether or not to assert the privilege. The guardian was to be guided by what was in the child's best interests.

Implied waiver. Courts have also recognized implied waiver of the privilege in a variety of circumstances. These include cases in which the patient has testified about his or her treatment, in which the patient has testified about his or her condition at the time of the communications in question or has called another physician to testify about his or her condition at that time, and in which there has been a waiver in another case or disclosure of the confidential information outside the courtroom.

The extent to which the privilege is held to be waived in these or other circumstances varies from one jurisdiction to another. Because the applicability of the privilege is often unclear, a practitioner should never disclose information in reliance on a litigant's or lawyer's representation that the patient has waived the privilege or waived confidentiality. Unless the practitioner is provided with a signed release from the patient (or person authorized to act on the patient's behalf), the practitioner should explain that the information will not be turned over without a subpoena, and the procedures outlined in the next section for responding to a subpoena should be followed.

Response to a Subpoena

Responding to a subpoena may be one of the most common legal problems or issues a practitioner faces. This is certainly the case with child mental health professionals, who have information that most divorce and custody lawyers are likely to believe is relevant, even critical, to their client's case. Although subpoenas frequently look quite formal and can be difficult to interpret, the rules for responding to them are straightforward. As a general matter, information sought by a subpoena can be provided if the patient—or the individual who controls the privilege on the patient's behalf—waives the physician–patient or psychotherapist–patient privilege, that is, consents to the information's release, or if there has been a judicial determination that the privilege does not apply or has been waived by some conduct of the patient's.

As discussed earlier, privilege statutes and interpretive case law can be confusing, contradictory, and unclear. Nevertheless, a practitioner's obligation on receipt of a subpoena is simple: the practitioner should

---

[1] Mass. Law ch. 233, § 20B(e) (2008).
[2] *Nagle v. Hooks*, 296 Md. 123, 460 A.2d 49 (Md. 1983).

attempt to determine whether there has been a waiver by the patient and, unless it is completely clear that there has been such a waiver, should take necessary steps to protect the information within the context of responding to the subpoena and, as appropriate, securing judicial direction as to his or her obligations. These steps will depend to a certain extent on whether the subpoena is for trial or for deposition and/or document production.

Deposition and Document Subpoena

A subpoena for a deposition should first be reviewed to determine whether written authorization or consent from the patient—or whoever controls the privilege— is included. Such authorization is not unusual. If the patient must waive the privilege in order to pursue the litigation, opposing counsel will generally have requested a release from the patient for this purpose. The subpoena should include the name, address, and telephone number of the attorney who has issued it. If an authorization is not included, a call or brief letter to the attorney may yield one. If not, the practitioner can contact the patient's attorney to determine if the patient consents to the deposition or document production.[1] If consent is not forthcoming from one source or another, the practitioner must contact the attorney who issued the subpoena to notify him or her that it will not be possible to provide any substantive information about the patient—including confirmation of treatment—without authorization by the patient or a court order. The attorney should then take steps to secure one or the other.

If the practitioner receives neither—or the issuing attorney makes it clear that he or she will not take steps to secure one or the other—the practitioner should make it clear that without a court order, the practitioner will appear as the subpoena requires, will provide information about him- or herself and his or her practice, but will provide no information about the patient. To avoid a useless deposition session and the attendant waste of time and money, attorneys who are notified of this position are likely to take steps to secure consent or a court order before the deposition—or to cancel the deposition.

If the attorney insists on going forward with the deposition, the practitioner is obligated to appear unless he or she has taken steps to quash the subpoena.[2] At such a deposition, the practitioner should remember not to provide any information about a patient. If asked questions that seek such information, the practitioner should respond that the information is confidential and privileged. It is possible that another deposition will be scheduled after the issuing attorney has obtained a court order or consent.

Trial Subpoena

As with a subpoena for a deposition, when a practitioner receives a trial subpoena, the practitioner should attempt to determine whether the patient has authorized his or her testimony. Although subpoenas usually come from someone other than the patient, that is not always the case, particularly at trial.[3] If the subpoena has been issued by the attorney for the patient, a practitioner can assume that the patient has consented to the testimony sought. The situation when the patient is a minor is somewhat more complicated and is discussed later.

If the situation has not been resolved before the date on which the practitioner has been ordered to appear for trial, the practitioner should appear as directed. As at deposition, at trial, the practitioner can testify about matters that do not involve the patient or confidential information, for example, his or her name, address, and credentials. When asked the first question the answer to which would entail confidential information, the patient's attorney or opposing counsel may object on terms of the physician–patient or psychotherapist–patient privilege. If this occurs, the practitioner may follow the judge's subsequent decision and direction. To the extent a judge has considered a claim of privilege and ordered the testimony in question, the physician is protected. If there is no objection

---

[1] Although oral consent may be effective in some circumstances, it is preferable to obtain written consent. Unless there has been a judicial determination that the privilege has been waived or does not apply, written consent that conforms to statutory or regulatory specifications may be necessary in jurisdictions with such provisions.

[2] Absent special circumstances, for example, an impending trial date or a deposition conducted by out-of-town counsel, deposition scheduling is generally flexible. Although the subpoena may specify a date and time, it is usually possible to negotiate a more convenient time. Opposing counsel may be helpful in this effort.

[3] Trial counsel frequently issue subpoenas for witnesses they have worked with and who will be supporting their case. This permits the rescheduling of testimony should the witness not appear for some reason.

but the practitioner does not feel that there has been adequate consent or that the issue of privilege has been considered and resolved, the practitioner may raise the issue. It would be appropriate for the practitioner to state the concern (that it is the practitioner's understanding that the information is privileged and confidential) and to ask whether he or she should testify.

Minor Patient

This discussion has focused on the issues all practitioners face when they receive a subpoena. As is the case with other issues discussed in this chapter, although the analytical framework remains the same, minor patients are likely to pose special challenges. The practitioner should not assume, as is the case with an adult patient, that the minor patient may authorize deposition and trial testimony. Instead, the rules discussed in the context of privilege will prevail. As there remains uncertainty in this area, the practitioner should be cautious about assuming that an authorization is valid.

As with other issues, the greatest uncertainty is in the custody area. To begin with, it is common in a custody case for one parent to consent to disclosure and testimony and for the other parent to oppose it adamantly. As discussed previously, a practitioner is generally safe in relying on the consent of one parent, but it would be risky to do so in the custody context unless the practitioner has confirmation that the consenting parent has sole legal custody of the minor patient. In any other case, if parental consent is to be the basis of the practitioner's disclosure, it must be the consent of both parents. The situation may be even more complicated when adolescents are involved. Because there is an increasing tendency to accord adolescents greater control over the release of information about themselves and their treatment, in contentious situations, the practitioner may need to consider proceeding as if there were no consent, even when the parent with legal custody or both parents have authorized the practitioner's testimony.

For clinical reasons, even when there appears to be effective consent or waiver of the privilege, practitioners should attempt to negotiate a solution that would allow them to restrict their role to treatment. The practitioner may be able to convince a minor's parents of the importance of protecting the treatment relationship with the child. Offering assistance in locating another professional to evaluate the child may encourage the parents in this regard. It may also help to discuss these matters with the attorney(s) for the parent(s). To the extent the attorneys are looking for inexpensive expert testimony, they may be convinced to turn elsewhere for assistance if they understand that the practitioner will testify only to issues of fact, not opinion, and that any testimony will be given reluctantly. Most attorneys will not want to call experts who are reluctant to testify. If parents and their attorneys cannot be convinced, the practitioner may want to consider contacting the judge to urge the appointment of an independent expert to conduct an evaluation and testify in the custody proceedings.

Conclusion

Practitioners who work with children face many challenges. Issues involving consent to treatment, commitment of children, and confidentiality of information are complex, and practitioners may incur liability by making decisions that violate statutes and case law. Those working in this area are urged to familiarize themselves with relevant federal and state laws and to obtain written copies of court orders detailing the legal rights of the parties. Additionally, where uncertainties exist, seeking the advice of legal experts is highly recommended.

—Key Points

- Clinicians should familiarize themselves with relevant state and federal statutes and case law and should consult legal experts when they are uncertain about what actions to take.

- The main differences in the regulation of child and adolescent mental health treatment derive from the fact that minors are presumed incompetent and third parties (parents) are involved in the treatment.

— As is the case with treatment provided to adults, a mental health professional who provides treatment to a minor without legally adequate consent risks suit and potential tort or malpractice liability.

— When treating children following parental separation or divorce, clinicians must be sure to identify which parent is able to provide legal consent for treatment and should obtain a written copy of the custody order for their records.

— When treating a child in foster care, the clinician should obtain a copy of the court order or seek clarification from the court as to who possesses the authority to make medical decisions for the child.

— Prior to voluntarily admitting a child into a mental health facility, the clinician must make sure that the person requesting the commitment has the legal authority under state law to make such a request.

— The involuntary commitment of children involves heightened procedural protections for children and their parents.

— Federal law and state law require certain professionals to mandatorily report suspicions of child abuse and neglect. Clinicians who are mandatory reporters should educate themselves on their legal responsibilities.

— Although federal law and the law of most states recognize a psychotherapist–patient privilege, that privilege may be waived by the patient or be deemed waived by the type of legal proceeding initiated, the presence of third parties during a therapy session, or other factors.

References

American Psychiatric Association: Principles of Medical Ethics With Annotations Especially Applicable to Psychiatry. Arlington, VA, American Psychiatric Association, 2008

Annotation, Medical Practitioner's Liability for Treatment Given Child Without Parent's Consent, 67 ALR 4th 411 (1989) and supp (2007)

Annotation, Physicians' Tort Liability for Unauthorized Disclosure of Confidential Information About Patient, 48 ALR 4th 668 (1986) and supp (2007)

Cardwell v Bechtol, 724 SW2d 739 (Tenn 1987)

Carter v Cangello, 105 Cal App 3d 348 (Ct App Cal 1980)

District of Columbia Mental Health Information Act, DC Code § 7-1202.05 (2008)

Goodman v United States, 298 F3d 1048, 1058 (9th Cir 2002)

Grosslight v Superior Court, 72 Cal App 3d 502 (Ct App Ca 1977)

Harris v Rattini, 855 SW2d 410 (Mo Ct App 1993)

Health Insurance Portability and Accountability Act of 1996 (HIPAA), 45 CFR § 160.101 et seq (2008)

In re Care and Protection of Sharlene, 445 Mass 756 (2006)

In re Dennis W, 717 NW2d 488 (2006)

In re EG, 133 Ill 2d 98, 109 (Ill 1989)

In re EG, 549 NE2d 322 (Ill 1989)

Ireland v Ireland, 855 P2d 40 (Idaho 1993)

Jaffe v Redmond, 518 US 1 (1996)

Nagle v Hooks, 296 Md 123, 460 A2d 49 (Md 1983)

Parham v JR, 442 US 584 (1979)

Pierce v Society of Sisters, 268 US 510 (1925)

Rishworth v Moss, 159 SW122 (Tex Civ App 1913)

State ex rel DM v Hoester, 681 SW2d 449 (Missouri 1984)

State v Henneberry, 558 NW2d 708, 709–710 (Iowa 1997)

Tinker v Des Moines, 393 US 503, 511 (1969)

Younts v St Francis Hospital & School of Nursing, 469 P2d 330 (Kan 1970)

Chapter 10

Legal Aspects of Intellectual Disability

James C. Harris, M.D.

The mental health professional may be requested to evaluate persons with intellectual disability in a variety of situations that have legal implications. Most people with intellectual disability are law-abiding citizens, but a small minority do have legal difficulties. It has long been recognized that the law should deal with them differently than those in the general population (Jones 2007). Moreover, behaviors that might be considered criminal by the courts might be seen as reflecting behavior problems by clinicians.

Because intellectual and development disabilities have multiple etiologies, forensic assessment of individuals with these disabilities requires an understanding of the nature and etiology of the specific cognitive developmental disorder and associated symptoms. Ethical issues related to care, the individual's legal rights, his or her vulnerability to being a victim of abuse (Horner-Johnson and Drum 2006; Reiter et al. 2007) and a victim or perpetrator of criminal acts, and the risk for mental disorders must all be taken into account.

There is a long history of stigmatization of persons with intellectual disability and an ongoing effort to define their condition in terms that are not stigmatizing. This effort has resulted in the diagnostic label being changed nine times over the past 100 years. Currently, *mental retardation* is the designation used in the World Health Organization and DSM-IV-TR (American Psychiatric Association 2000) definitions; however, this designation is no longer current. In 2008, the American Association on Mental Retardation (AAMR)

changed its name to the American Association on Intellectual and Developmental Disabilities (AAIDD). In the federal government, the President's Committee on Mental Retardation is now known as the President's Committee for People With Intellectual Disabilities. These changing concepts and legal issues related to intellectual disability have been reviewed recently (Harris 2006).

The mental health professional must appreciate that intellectual disability is a vulnerability factor in mental illness and be aware of how developmental progression is affected by cognitive deficits. Developmental milestones involving infant attachment, sexuality, aggression, moral development, attention processes, and memory formation all may be affected. Brain dysfunction in persons with intellectual disability increases the risk of aggressive behavior and social disinhibition. Psychotropic drugs must be used with caution and their complications (e.g., tardive dyskinesia) (Gualtieri and Hawk 1980) fully understood. Intellectual disability is heterogeneous and has multiple causes. Thus, knowledge of intellectual disability syndromes such as Down syndrome, fragile X syndrome, and XYY syndrome; their natural histories and behavioral features; and their vulnerabilities must be considered.

In this chapter, I provide an overview of intellectual disability and discuss legal rights and legal issues, including culpability, legal competency (to stand trial, to testify, to make confessions) and how it is evaluated, sterilization, and guardianship. I also address clinical assessment and discuss psychiatric diagnosis and human rights issues.

Overview of Intellectual Disability

Definition

Intellectual disability refers to significantly subaverage intellectual functioning along with concurrent deficits or impairments in current adaptive functioning (i.e., the person's effectiveness in meeting the standards expected for his or her age by his or her cultural group in at least two of the following skill areas: communication, self-care, home living, social and interpersonal skills, use of community resources, self-direction, functional academic skills, work, leisure, health, and safety). The onset is before age 18 years (American Association on Mental Retardation 2002; American Psychiatric Association 2000). DSM-IV-TR and AAMR classifications should be consulted for further details regarding definition. Table 10–1 provides guidelines to consider in the assessment process.

General intellectual functioning refers to the ability to learn and is measured by the intelligence quotient (IQ). Subaverage intellectual functioning is defined as an IQ of lower than 70 with a variation in measurement error of approximately 5 IQ points. However, the intelligence test alone is not an adequate assessment because an individual may come from deprived circumstances, and the test itself could be culturally biased. More specifically, IQ tests are not accurately measuring how an individual may function in society, although they may predict educational progress. The deficits in adaptive behavior are critical because IQ tests alone are not an accurate measure of an intellectually disabled person's overall functioning. *Adaptive behavior* has been defined as "the effectiveness or the degree with which the individual meets the standards of personal independence and social responsibility expected of his age and cultural group" (Grossman 1983, p. 11). This includes areas of social skills and responsibility.

Intellectual disability is not a disease or an illness in itself. In intellectual disability, thinking is not characteristically disordered and perception is not distorted unless a concurrent mental disorder or brain damage is present. It is made up of a heterogeneous group of conditions that range from genetic and metabolic disorders to functional changes that follow trauma to the nervous system at birth or later in the developmental period. Because of this heterogeneity, each case must be considered independently according to whether an associated syndrome (e.g., Down syndrome) or an associated etiology (e.g., head trauma) is present.

Although the intellectually disabled person also may have a diagnosis of a major psychiatric condition, his or her day-to-day problems ordinarily relate to difficulties in developmental functioning. Depending on the degree of cognitive ability, the person may have deficits in abstract thinking, in social judgment, and in his or her fund of general information. Difficulties in these areas, if appropriate to the person's cognitive level, are not evidence of a mental disorder. (At the time of examination, it should be ascertained whether the individual was previously functioning at a higher level and has lost skills and regressed.) The intellectually disabled person will develop over time and pass through the same developmental stages as a non–intellectually disabled person does but not reach the higher levels of cognitive functioning. Abilities are re-

---

TABLE 10–1. Assessment of intellectual disability

Be familiar with the definitions of intellectual disability (American Association on Intellectual and Developmental Disabilities, DSM-IV-TR).

Remember that assessment of adaptive function is a crucial element in the definition.

Consider variability in cognitive profile on IQ tests, level of language functioning, and presence of neurological conditions.

Keep in mind that intellectual disability includes a heterogeneous group of individuals who range from mildly to profoundly intellectually disabled and includes specific syndromes as well as intellectual disability secondary to traumatic head injury occurring during the developmental period.

Be cognizant of developmental level and IQ test data.

Record data in a multiaxial classification format.

duced in all areas of functioning, including language, language communication, memory, attention, self-concept, suggestibility, knowledge base, control of impulsivity, moral development, and overall motivation. From a legal perspective, difficulty in logical thinking, planning strategies for action, and foresight are among the most important deficits. Furthermore, those with intellectual disability have an intellectual rigidity, which is established by impaired ability to learn from mistakes and difficulty in mentally generating a range of options to choose from in a new situation, particularly when stressed. An intellectually disabled adult with a mental age of 6 years will be less flexible in thinking than will a non–intellectually disabled 6-year-old. However, the adult intellectually disabled person will have more life experience than will a child of equivalent mental age on which to base his or her options in decision making.

Levels of Severity

Intellectual disability is divided into four degrees of severity reflecting the amount of intellectual impairment: mild, moderate, severe, and profound. Although intelligence tests are not the sole basis for determining intellectual disability, these tests are the accepted standard to measure the degrees of severity of intellectual disability. *Profound* intellectual disability is an IQ of 20 or lower (adult mental age younger than 3 years), *severe* is an IQ of 20–34 (adult mental age 3 to younger than 6 years), *moderate* is an IQ of 35–49 (adult mental age 6 to younger than 9 years), and *mild* is an IQ of 50–69 (adult mental age 8–11 years) (World Health Organization 1992). Intelligence scores are based on the assessment of a variety of relatively specific skills. Although these skills generally develop together, there may be wide discrepancies between subtest scores (Jones et al. 1988) (e.g., language functioning may be low and performance on tests of visuospatial skills higher). Because of this scattering of skills, the test profile must be considered in regard to adaptive functioning. Moreover, if large discrepancies are seen between verbal and performance scores, the full-scale IQ may not adequately reflect true ability level. In these cases, neuropsychological testing may be needed to clarify specific cognitive functions. Tests of adaptive behavior that are used together with intelligence tests include the AAMR Adaptive Behavior Scale (Lambert et al. 1993) and the Vineland Adaptive Behavior Scales (Sparrow et al. 1984). In addition, the AAIDD focuses on the extent of supports needed for each person in addition to their level of functioning. The AAIDD has de-

veloped a Supports Intensity Scale (SIS) to measure support requirements in 57 life activities and 28 behavioral and medical areas. The assessment is done through an interview with the individual, staff, family, and others who know the person well (see also Chapter 5, "Special Education: Screening Tools, Rating Scales, and Self-Report Instruments," and Chapter 6, "Psychological Testing in Child and Adolescent Forensic Evaluations").

Prevalence

The overall prevalence rate of intellectual disability (Harris 2006) is estimated to be approximately 3% of the school-age population. In the adult population, the prevalence of intellectual disability is about 1% because many mildly intellectually disabled people may adapt in society following an appropriate education and no longer meet the adaptive function criteria, and the more severely intellectually disabled people with medical complications may not survive into adulthood. Eighty-five percent of the intellectually disabled population fall into the mildly intellectually disabled range, and the remaining 15% are moderately, severely, or profoundly intellectually disabled. It is those who function in the mildly intellectually disabled range who are most likely to be involved in criminal proceedings and may be found to be legally competent.

Multiaxial Classification

DSM-IV-TR includes mental retardation on Axis II, the designated developmental axis. Mental disorders occurring in mentally retarded persons are coded on Axis I, and multiple psychiatric diagnoses may be listed. Medical conditions that relate to mental retardation are classified on Axis III. Psychosocial complications that commonly occur in the lives of persons with mental retardation are coded on Axis IV, and global adaptive functioning is coded on Axis V. This multiaxial approach allows for the diagnosis of mental retardation, mental disorders that may be associated with mental retardation, and physical conditions that may be etiologically important in regard to mental retardation. The designation of the nature of psychosocial complications that impinge on the mentally retarded person and an overall global adaptive function rating complete this system. This diagnostic approach is descriptive in nature rather than etiologically based. Concurrent physical disorders or conditions can be indicated without necessarily suggesting that these conditions are etiologically related to a mental disorder in the person with mental retardation. Medical conditions, particularly those involving the brain, may be additional vulnerability factors that increase the risk for a mental disorder. *In program planning, the multiaxial classification is of particular importance* because it designates each of the areas that are important in treatment planning and highlights those areas that are of most importance in evaluating the overall function of the mentally retarded person. The AAMR (Luckasson et al. 2002) uses a multidimensional approach.

Normalization—The Developmental Model

Intellectual disability is a permanent condition and is not curable, although the degree of habilitation that can be accomplished for the intellectually disabled person can be substantial (Wolfensberger 1972). Deficits in current adaptive functioning are major targets for intervention. During the past 20 years, a focus on a developmental model that acknowledges the capability for growth, of developing independence in social skills, and of new learning has been emphasized. The developmental model specifically addresses the fact that the intellectually disabled person's level of functioning is not static and that an individual's adaptive behavior may be improved through habilitation. Because an intellectually disabled person is capable of learning and adapting, legal approaches need to take into account that the intellectually disabled person may require additional education and instructional effort but can learn new information.

The focus on normalization (Wolfensberger 1972) for persons with intellectual disability emphasizes the importance of intellectually disabled persons being entitled to services that are as culturally normative as possible to help them establish and maintain more appropriate personal behavior. Normalization emphasizes that intellectually disabled persons should live in the community, go to regular schools, seek competitive employment, and behave as closely as possible to the standards of the non–intellectually disabled persons at a comparable developmental age. Furthermore, they should be responsible for their own behavior, and others should not assume that because they are intellectually disabled, they are not capable of doing so. Still, their differences and their need for individual assessment must be recognized to guarantee that services are provided (Simpson 1998). For normalization, it is proposed that not only is a focus on social competence critical in treatment programs but also an ethical approach is needed that recognizes interests, desires, and preferences of the individual (Simpson 1998). One risk is excessive programming for an individual with a lack of allowance for leisure time and for personal choices of activities.

Special features of persons with intellectual disability that need to be taken into account in normalization are their communication skills, their previous life experiences, and any associated physical disorders. Many intellectually disabled people have concurrent difficulties in language expression and articulation. Consequently, a special effort may be required to communicate with them, and in some instances, "signing" may be necessary to communicate. In other instances, the nonverbal intellectually disabled person with a physical handicap, such as cerebral palsy, may require a speech synthesizer or other language devices to assist in communication. The intellectually disabled person may have lacked certain life experiences because of poor programming, which may then influence his or her ability to respond to new situations. Finally, physical disorders involving the brain and other organ systems that are quite commonly found in intellectual disability syndromes must be considered in normalization.

Sexuality in Intellectual Disability

Intellectually disabled persons may be stereotyped in regard to the expression of sexuality (Abram et al. 1988; Harris 2006); considered to be sexually uninhibited, eternal children, or asexual; or believed even to have no sexual interest and needs. Because of concerns about sexuality and disinhibited social behavior and fears that the intellectually disabled individuals would indiscriminately procreate, leading to an increase in the incidence of intellectual disability, involuntary sterilization (Appelbaum 1982; Denekens et al. 1999) has been practiced in the past, and marriages between intellectually disabled persons often were prohibited. In some circumstances, an intellectually disabled person was even denied the opportunity to socialize and develop an intimate relationship with someone of the opposite sex. Fortunately, involuntary sterilization is no longer practiced, but residual fears remain in some communities.

The onset of sexual interest is variable, and ordinarily it is after puberty that sexual interest becomes apparent. Puberty may be delayed in some intellectually disabled persons secondary to the disorder that underlies their intellectual disability. Regardless of the age at pubertal onset, most severely intellectually disabled individuals show little interest in sexual behavior toward others. However, mildly intellectually disabled people and many moderately intellectually disabled people may have normal pubertal development, show appropriate sexual interests, and establish sexual identities.

When expressions of their sexual interests are denied, sexual activity may be a response used to indicate a sense of self-importance and be aimed at gaining acceptance from others. Sexual status may be important for their peer group just as it is for those who are not intellectually disabled. The encouragement of a relationship with others of the same developmental level and the learning of social skills are essential and must precede specific instruction about sexual activity.

Intellectually disabled persons, particularly women, may be exploited sexually. Their knowledge of sexuality is often not fully developed because the usual sources of information may not be available to them. Peer relationships, printed reading material, and sex education in school are often limited or unavailable for intellectually disabled persons. Furthermore, family members may be reluctant to review sexual matters with them. Mildly and moderately intellectually disabled adolescents frequently lack basic information on sexual anatomy, contraceptive issues, and venereal disease. Their knowledge of sexuality often is related more to life experience and opportunity than to intelligence level.

Legal Issues

Scope of Involvement of the Mental Health Professional

Mental health professionals may evaluate intellectually disabled persons in a variety of settings, such as emergency departments, where aggression toward self or others may present or where abuse of the intellectually disabled person is questioned; the court, where there may be questions of competency to stand trial or to act as a witness; the clinic, where a diagnostic evaluation may be requested; and the school, where questions are raised about the least restrictive environment for education. Questions of legal rights are common—for example, access to education, participation in decisions about medical treatment, use of a guardian to guarantee the rights of an incompetent intellectually disabled person, and participation in research. To adequately conduct these evaluations, the mental health professional must be aware of legal rights legislation that relates to intellectually disabled individuals as well as the more traditional forensic concerns that re-

late to competence. Table 10–2 outlines considerations for the forensic evaluation.

Insanity Defense/Culpability

Formulations of the insanity defense traditionally base the defense on "mental disease or defect" (Giorgi-Guarnieri et al. 2002), the latter referring to intellectual disability. Intellectual disability can be used as a basis for the insanity defense (Menninger 1986). Ordinarily, the culpability of persons with intellectual disability can be considered to be reduced, so intellectual disability can be considered to be a mitigating circumstance in criminal proceedings. Mental disorder and intellectual disability both must be considered in decisions regarding the insanity defense. This distinction between them is clearly made in international classifications of disorders and diseases. However, this distinction is sometimes blurred in the court. This blurring may occur because cases brought for criminal action may involve intellectual disability and a mental disorder, both of which then must be taken into account in the assessment process.

When applied to intellectually disabled individuals, the insanity defense is most frequently considered in murder cases when the question of the culpability of an intellectually disabled person is raised. This issue may arise if an adolescent with an intellectual disability is referred to adult court. Culpability involves the capacity of the accused to distinguish right from wrong. The legal standard that is applied most often is the M'Naghten Rule, which requires that there be a lack of knowledge of the nature and wrongfulness of the committed act for the person to be found not responsible. The American Law Institute (1962) modi-

---

TABLE 10–2. Forensic assessment

Find and make careful use of multiple informants for data collection.

Be aware of issues of stigma in intellectual disability.

Consider the cognitive and adaptive limitations of the intellectually disabled person.

Remember that there may be considerable variability in cognitive profile.

Use specific measures of adaptive functioning such as American Association on Mental Retardation Adaptive Behavior Scale and the Vineland Adaptive Behavior Scales because adaptive skills deficits are required for diagnosis.

fication of this rule is commonly used: "A person is not responsible for criminal conduct if at the time of such conduct as a result of mental disease or defect, he lacks substantial capacity either to *appreciate* the criminality (wrongfulness) of his conduct or to conform his conduct to the requirements of the law." The difference in wording focuses on substituting the word "appreciate," which suggests both emotional and cognitive awareness, for the word "know." Knowing that an act is wrong may indicate only surface knowledge of its wrongfulness without a full appreciation of why it is wrong (Menninger 1986). Furthermore, although knowing an act is wrong, because of excessive impulsiveness or enhanced suggestibility or acquiescence to authority, he or she may have difficulty in conforming his or her conduct to the law (Luckasson 1988).

Competency

Issues related to competency of minors in criminal context include the basic legal competency to stand trial in those jurisdictions or venues (adult court) that require it and the ability to be a competent witness (Buescher and Dinerstein 1999; President's Committee on Mental Retardation 1991; Smith and Kunjukrishnan 1986). Assessment in civil contexts, such as competency to manage one's own affairs, seldom arises for intellectually disabled minors. Table 10–3 summarizes issues to be considered in competency evaluations.

Competency to Stand Trial

Competency to stand trial refers to the ability to comprehend the nature and quality of the legal proceedings and advise counsel in preparation and implementation of one's own defense (*Dusky v. U.S.* 1960; see also Chapter 26, "Juvenile Waiver and State-of-Mind Assessments"). Some states require competence to stand trial in juvenile court, and all states require competence in minors waived to adult criminal court. An intellectually disabled person may have difficulties because of limited ability to understand the charges or their consequences as a result of reduced intelligence, lack of life experience, inadequate education, tendency to overcompliance to please others, or fear of the authorities.

Competency to Testify

In certain circumstances, intellectually disabled persons may be asked to testify for the prosecution in a criminal case (Gudjonsson and Gunn 1982). The defense may argue that they are not competent to be witnesses and raise questions about their reliability. A witness is not specifically disqualified by law because he or she is intellectually disabled, but an individual assessment of his or her competency to testify may be required. To do so, the prospective witness must understand that he or she may be punished for not telling the truth. He or she must be able to show the ability to recall and to report past events accurately. The assessment of the intellectually disabled person to testify will require an evaluation of his or her language and memory capabilities, his or her personal understanding of the meaning of the alleged crime, the pressures exerted by others on him or her, and his or her capacity to differentiate reality from fantasy. The final determination of credibility of the intellectually disabled witness will be up to the court and jury. The evaluation of a potentially intellectually disabled child or adolescent witness should include whether he or she has a history of compulsive reporting of fantasy stories regarding the issue in question. The effect on him or her of testifying on the witness stand also should be considered, particularly if testimony is directed toward a family member or guardian who has a supervisory role for the intellectually disabled person (Harris 1998).

Competency and Confessions

Intellectually disabled persons are at risk for giving a nonvoluntary confession (Praiss 1989). In confessions, it is important to measure understanding and suggestibility in defendants (Everington and Fulero 1999). A criminal confession in response to questioning while in custody cannot be used in evidence unless the defendant voluntarily, knowingly, and intelligently waived Miranda rights. These rights ensure that when a person is taken into custody, he or she is informed of the Fifth Amendment right to remain silent and have counsel retained or appointed before an admissible confession can be obtained. An intellectually disabled person requires a thorough explanation of these rights. Because of adaptive problems and intellectual limitations, care is needed in determining whether the waiver of rights is valid. Because of the special needs of intellectually disabled persons, counsel should be sought as early as the precustodial stage. With early access to an attorney as well as a familiar person, the intellectually disabled person's waiver is best protected and more likely to be voluntary.

Parental Competency

The ability to care for a child on a day-to-day basis, to make future plans for his or her child, and to consistently set limits on behavior must be evaluated in the

TABLE 10–3. Considerations in the evaluation of competency

Review the accuracy of the assessment that determined the level of intellectual disability.

Be familiar with definitions of competency and culpability as they relate to criminal responsibility.

Consider the stresses that may be involved when an intellectually disabled person is asked to testify.

Carefully review the circumstances in the elicitation of confessions.

Use all means to facilitate communication (e.g., communication boards, speech synthesizer, drawings) at the appropriate cognitive level.

Be aware of the legal rights for the incompetent intellectually disabled person.

Consider the following factors in assessment:

- Lack of life experience
- Inadequate education
- Problems with over- or undercompliance
- Fear of authority
- Associated deficits such as seizure disorder

intellectually disabled parent who is a minor (Feldman 1986; Keltner et al. 1999). Intellectual disability per se is not automatically considered evidence for lack of competency in child care, although it is increasingly evident that successful parenting by an intellectually disabled person is fraught with difficulty, particularly in the care of children beyond infancy (Whitman and Accardo 1989). Children of intellectually disabled parents are at risk for intellectual disability, but a substantial number, 60%–70% in one study (Accardo and Whitman 1990; Whitman and Accardo 1989), were not intellectually disabled. Factual evidence of competence is necessary for mildly and moderately intellectually disabled parents; however, if a parent is severely and profoundly intellectually disabled, then the child will ordinarily require placement. In some settings, both the parent and his or her child may be placed in a foster home. Here, the foster parents can assume overall responsibility for the child's care, and the natural parent can assist them as he or she learns new skills. Issues of parenting by an intellectually disabled person are of particular importance when multiple children are in the home and when the intellectually disabled person has a normally intelligent child.

Rights of Incompetent Persons

Some intellectually disabled individuals will be mentally incompetent from birth, and the protection of their constitutional rights is an ongoing consideration throughout their lifetime. The issues that come up most often relate to procreation, the issue of steriliza-

tion (Denekens et al. 1999), rights in regard to involuntary institutionalization, the consent to sexual activity (Stavis and Walker-Hirsch 1999), and the right of others to initiate medical intervention (Sundram 1988) or to terminate life-sustaining treatment. A mentally incompetent, developmentally disabled individual is generally unable to exercise these rights. The procedural safeguards necessary to guarantee his or her rights even though he or she is incompetent are important to consider. How best to preserve the developmentally disabled person's autonomy despite his or her incompetence has been considered in several ways. Legislation focusing on the best interest test is one recent standard. This standard is contrasted with the substituted judgment test.

An incompetent intellectually disabled person cannot function normally in society or voluntarily consent in regard to decisions about his or her well-being. Others must make decisions for him or her, including the choice to undergo or terminate life-sustaining treatment; the right to reproduce or procreate; and the right to remain in the community and not be institutionalized. These rights have been considered constitutionally protected (Roesch and Golding 1979). However, the right of self-determination is exercised not by the intellectually disabled person but by another person—a parent or guardian appointed by the state through the courts.

The approach to the right of self-determination for incompetent individuals includes 1) the best interest test and 2) the substituted judgment test. In the best interest test, the focus is primarily on the needs of an incompetent person. His or her expressed desires or intentions are considered but may be disregarded depending on the circumstances. In the substituted judgment test, the court renders the decision for the developmentally disabled person that it believes the person would render for himself or herself if he or she were competent. The substituted judgment test has been questioned because it may lead to excessive involvement of the courts in matters that can be handled more personally and expeditiously by a guardian or family member. The best interest procedure may lead to better accountability and avoids the abstractions inherent in the court's assumptions of how a person who has never been competent would make a decision.

Procedural safeguards that are available to protect the rights of the incompetent individual include 1) the appointment of a guardian ad litem, 2) an adversarial hearing, and 3) limits on the control by the court. This last precaution considers whether the judge has the expertise to resolve the issues that arise.

Guardian Ad Litem

A guardian ad litem is appointed to represent an incompetent person. This guardian may be appointed by the court either on a motion to the court or following a statute. The guardian's responsibility is to defend the rights of an incompetent person and represent his or her best interests. He or she also may help resolve differences between medical and legal issues (Martyn 1994).

Adversarial Hearing

A mandatory due process hearing may be required for specific issues regarding the intellectually disabled person (e.g., sterilization). In the due process hearing, several issues must be addressed. These include 1) the opportunity to be heard, 2) the opportunity to question and cross-examine witnesses, and 3) the right to offer evidence. Such hearings may be necessary when there is a question as to whether a family is acting in the best interest of their intellectually disabled family member and whether that intellectually disabled person's constitutional rights are not being protected.

However, in other instances, adversarial hearings have not been mandated; for example, in *Parham v. J.R.* (1979), the Supreme Court upheld a Georgia law that permitted the parents of a mentally ill child to commit their child on their petition along with the recommendation of a mental health professional but without a formal hearing. The Court indicated that the commitment was purely medical and suggested that a hearing "could exacerbate whatever tensions already exist between child and parent."

Role of the Court

The judge must weigh the overall circumstances in regard to determining the rights of an incompetent litigant and those of family members. Family stability must be considered in reviewing the constitutional rights of the intellectually disabled person. For example, a family might not be able to control a very aggressive child or may not be able to provide for the basic physical needs, such as dressing, toileting, and transporting their intellectually disabled adolescent or young adult family member. The court would need to balance the constitutional interests of the child and the reasonable interests of the family who cannot properly care for the child at home.

Sterilization and Intellectual Disability

Because of past abuses, the use of sterilization in intellectual disability has been an area of continuing concern (Webster 1985). The Mental Health Law Project (Rousso 1984) has recommended standards. These require representation by a disinterested guardian ad litem, independent evaluation of the individual, and findings that the individual is not capable of making and not able to develop the capacity to make an informed judgment. The individual also must be physically capable of procreation and likely to engage in sexual activity but permanently incapable of taking care of a child. Furthermore, there must be no alternatives to sterilization. The major concerns are to protect the individual's rights and to follow due process.

Clinical Issues

Considerations in Forensic Assessment

It is a basic right of an intellectually disabled person to be responsible for himself or herself and to be held accountable for his or her own behavior (Harris 2006). Suggesting incompetence based on intelligence alone without considering adaptive ability diminishes the mentally intellectually disabled person as an individual. In criminal cases, the opportunity to stand trial offers the chance for probation, whereas being found incompetent may lead to an indeterminate sentence.

When brought in for a forensic assessment, an intellectually disabled person may be overwhelmed, particularly if there are legal proceedings that he or she does not understand. Time and patience will be needed to establish a sense of trust and rapport and to gain his or her assent to continue with the assessment. An intellectually disabled person may not understand the officer's recitation when his or her rights are read to him or her, may not understand the nature of the offense that he or she is accused of, may not appreciate the consequences of the accusation, and may not know how to defend himself or herself. A more gradual and considered approach that acknowledges his or her disability may render the individual competent. If one makes the necessary initial efforts at gaining the intellectually disabled person's confidence, the assessment can be direct and detailed. The focus is on his or her self-care skills, his or her comprehension of the meaning of others' social behavior, and his or her facility in interpersonal communication. The psychiatric examination is comprehensive and deals with all these issues: co-occurring psychiatric diagnosis, the specific legal questions of competency to stand trial, and the kind of service programs needed by the individual. Detailed information about therapeutic programming can be used by the court in making the final disposition.

Intellectually disabled minors are ordinarily taken by their caregivers for psychiatric assessment rather than self-referred. Because an intellectually disabled person often has difficulty in verbal expression, either in articulation or in expressive language; may have problems in memory; and is generally dependent on the caregiver, the caregiver's history is of paramount importance. A variety of special approaches may be needed in interviewing the intellectually disabled person, which include devices to augment communication (communication boards, computers, signing) and interviewing methods used for establishing therapeutic contact with younger, normally intelligent children (drawings, stories, structured settings). In assessing the intellectually disabled child or adolescent, one must consider, for example, his or her capacity to understand basic explanations for medical procedures, his or her degree of credibility, the ability to advocate for his or her own rights, and his or her ability to postpone immediate gratification for subsequent benefits. A history of ability to carry out these activities is central and should be confirmed in the examination.

In obtaining the history, several sources are needed in addition to the family and the intellectually disabled person himself or herself (e.g., schools, community programs, sheltered workshop staff, job coaches). When eliciting historical information, one must consider not only the specific behaviors of concern but also the circumstances under which the behaviors were said to have occurred and how they were responded to by others. The caregiver's relationship with the intellectually disabled person also must be taken into account. The extent of parental recognition of the handicap and its meaning to the parents must be considered in the assessment. Their ability to see the referred person's strengths as well as his or her weaknesses should be investigated.

Criminal Liability

Most individuals with intellectual disability are not prone to criminal or violent behavior. Those who are prone to such behavior frequently have multiple risk factors, as pointed out by Lewis et al. (1988). They reported on 14 juveniles condemned to death in four states and found that 1 had an IQ score in the 60s and that 5 had scores in the 70s. All had a history of head trauma in childhood, with 9 of 14 requiring hospitalization. Twelve of the group had a history of abuse in childhood. Most had severe deficiencies in abstract reasoning.

In the past, it has been suggested that the XYY chromosomal abnormality may be associated with antisocial behavior (Telfer et al. 1968); however, this has not proven to be the case. Because of these misconceptions, when individuals with intellectual disability become involved with the criminal justice system through misunderstanding of this kind, they are at risk for being treated unfairly (Biklen 1977; McAfee and Gural 1988).

The current evidence is that intellectually disabled persons may have a higher likelihood of being arrested for criminal behavior, especially for minor delinquent behavior (President's Committee on Mental Retardation 1991). Crimes involving impulsive acts may be increased among intellectually disabled individuals. One study found no increase in fantasies of aggression among intellectually disabled offenders but suggested possible difficulties in inhibiting impulses (Silber and Courtless 1968), a finding that bears replication. Fire setting also has been associated with intellectual disability (Foust 1979; Kearns and O'Connor 1988; Yesavage et al. 1983). Rather than a specific cause of criminal behavior, intellectual disability and its associated features are risk factors for legal difficulty. It is not intellectual disability per se but rather the higher rate of associated behavior and emotional problems in intellectually disabled people that is of particular concern (Feinstein and Reiss 1996). The likelihood of emotional and behavior problems is enhanced by frequent psychosocial adversity and central nervous system dysfunction. This increased prevalence of mental disorder further increases their vulnerability to acting antisocially. The issue of stigma also must be considered because "being different" and "being intellectually disabled" are factors that influence attitudes in the community. Often, intellectually disabled persons are the first suspected of delinquency in their neighborhoods because of these attitudes in the community. Yet in criminal proceedings, intellectual disability may be a mitigating circumstance that may lead to a reduction of the offender's personal culpability and moral blameworthiness for the act committed.

Confessions

Clinically, intellectually disabled persons should be considered to be individuals with limited learning capacity and problems in social adaptation. Still, characteristics of intellectual disability may impede voluntary and intelligent constitutional waiver of rights by an intellectually disabled person. Competency also must be considered in regard to the reliability of a confession to a crime made by an intellectually disabled person (Praiss 1989). An intellectually disabled defendant who has pleaded guilty may be referred to a mental health professional to determine whether he or she was competent to plead guilty. In some instances, intellectually disabled persons have insisted that they were guilty and should be in prison. Here, individuals may be responding to the attention accorded them at the time of the examination with the hope that this recognition might elevate their standing in the community because they may feel that their self-esteem as individuals is enhanced by the proceedings. Thus, it is important to carefully assess the degree of understanding and extent of suggestibility found in intellectually disabled persons (Everington and Fulero 1999).

Initially, there may be confusion in the setting where the intellectually disabled person is interviewed, such as a police station or courthouse. An intellectually disabled person may be compliant, seek approval, and have a desire to be accepted as well as show easy suggestibility. In this way, a compliant intellectually disabled person is not a major problem for the police, but the police in the process of interrogation may be a major problem for the intellectually disabled person. Although no specific correlation exists between intellectual disability and criminal behavior, many intellectually disabled persons have been incarcerated. Despite the 1%–3% of the general population who are intellectually disabled, 10%–25% of the prison population have tested in the intellectually disabled range. In some instances, intellectually disabled people may be easily apprehended and less often paroled. When they are apprehended, they may assume blame to "please their accuser." Intellectually disabled persons also may be implicated and used by others who have encouraged them to assist in antisocial behavior.

Nevertheless, intellectual disability does not necessarily exclude the ability to understand constitutional rights to remain silent or to obtain legal counsel (Buescher and Dinerstein 1999). To reach the appropriate level of comprehension, rights must be slowly and carefully explained in terms that can be understood at the appropriate cognitive and developmental level. Moreover, adaptive impairments can cause intellectually disabled persons to become confused and more dependent in stressful circumstances. This may further inhibit their ability to understand new concepts and make independent decisions. Consequently, a police officer's recitation of the standard Miranda warning may not be understood, and the person may not appreciate or have a requisite understanding of his or her rights and the consequences of waiving them, nor will the person necessarily be able to make a voluntary decision to waive those rights. A further complication is that even if police officers are trained to identify intellectually disabled persons and to provide an appropriate setting and explanation of their constitutional rights and the consequences of abandoning them, the creation of a favorable environment of warmth and friendliness may, in itself, result in the intellectually disabled suspect making a voluntary confession or being induced to make an involuntary confession after waiving his or her rights. Consideration also must be given to the family in regard to confession (Cockram et al. 1998).

Psychiatric Diagnosis in Intellectual Disability

Vulnerability to Mental Disorder

An intellectually disabled and mentally ill defendant raises concerns in regard to the relation between the legal and the mental health systems (Kearns and O'Connor 1988; Williams and Spruill 1987). The prevalence of psychiatric disorders in the intellectually disabled population is three to five times that found in the general population (Bregman and Harris 1995).

The more severely intellectually disabled the child, the greater the likelihood of disturbed behavior and impaired interpersonal relationships (Harris 2006). The term *dual diagnosis* has been used in describing psychiatric disorders in intellectually disabled individuals. Mildly intellectually disabled individuals are prone to the same range of psychiatric disorders as seen in the general population, but their vulnerability is increased as a result of cognitive deficits and their difficulty in social adaptation. More severely and profoundly intellectually disabled children are more likely to be vulnerable because of brain disorders that are often associated with genetic syndromes, metabolic diseases, and trauma. Seizure disorders are the most common neurological problem seen in the intellectually disabled population. Brain dysfunction is a vulnerability factor that increases the likelihood of behavioral and interpersonal difficulties; however, all behavior problems cannot be ascribed to brain dysfunction. Table 10–4 summarizes issues to consider in the assessment of co-occurring mental disorders.

Intellectually disabled persons are just as likely as others in the population to be given diagnoses of major mental illnesses, such as depression and schizophrenia (Feinstein and Reiss 1996). Pervasive developmental disorders, which include autism and other forms of pervasive developmental disturbances in language and social behavior, are particularly important to recognize. Services for the latter group must include intensive training in social skills. The American Academy of Child and Adolescent Psychiatry has published practice parameters for the treatment of mental illness in intellectually disabled persons (Szymanski and King 1999) as a guide to more effective practice.

TABLE 10–4. Intellectual disability and mental disorder

Consider all DSM-IV-TR diagnoses that may be pertinent on Axis I.

Appreciate how diagnostic criteria may require modification for the intellectually disabled person.

Use all five DSM-IV-TR axes to facilitate treatment planning.

Remember to consider how cognitive deficits affect diagnoses such as mood disorder and schizophrenia. Use caution in diagnosing psychosis.

Issues in Treatment

Following multiaxial diagnosis (DSM-IV-TR) or multidimensional assessment (AAIDD), treatment is specified for the disorder or disorders that are identified, and a disposition may be recommended (American Association on Mental Retardation 2002; Quinsey and Maguire 1983; Roesch and Golding 1979). Issues commonly addressed in an interdisciplinary assessment include psychosocial stressors, disruptive behaviors, appropriate use of psychopharmacological agents (Fielding et al. 1980; Nisonger Center for Intellectual Disability and Developmental Disabilities 1998), and concerns that relate to the use of aversive conditioning procedures (National Institutes of Health 1990; Nolley et al. 1980).

Sexual Misconduct and Intellectual Disability

A minority of intellectually disabled individuals may show socially unacceptable sexual behavior that brings them into conflict with the legal system. Early studies of criminology reported an increase in sexual offenses by intellectually disabled persons. These studies, however, are questionable on methodological grounds. The prevalence of intellectual disability among male sexual offenders may be similar to the prevalence in the general population. Still, intellectually disabled persons may be involved in initiating sexual offenses, and if so, special considerations are necessary for their treatment (Lindsay 2002; Lindsay et al. 1999).

Legal issues in regard to the use of antilibidinal agents (Clarke 1989) may come to the attention of the court in relation to legal rights and when sexual deviancy is at issue and when an intellectually disabled adolescent is sexually aggressive. Pharmacological agents, particularly medroxyprogesterone acetate, have been used to reduce libido in intellectually disabled individuals—for example, when excessive masturbation has prevented participation in programming and in cases of sexually deviant behavior. Authors working in this area have suggested that a small reduction in sexual drive may be sufficient to enable a patient to avoid acting on an impulse that would lead to unacceptable behavior. Treatment with antilibidinal drugs in combination with psychotherapy is more effective than treatment with antilibidinal agents alone. The drug treatment will reduce the intensity of the drive but will not alter the direction of the drive.

Rights of Intellectually Disabled Persons

Legislation providing for the rights of intellectually disabled persons to self-determination has substantially increased. The Education of All Handicapped Children Act (Public Law 94-142), Individuals With Disabilities Education Act, Americans With Disabilities Act, reimbursement provisions under Title XIX, and amendments to the Vocational Rehabilitation Act have addressed restrictive treatment plans and focused on elimination of discrimination and provision of protections similar to those for other citizens.

—Key Points

The mental health profession should consider the following key points when undertaking a forensic assessment:

— *Attitude toward intellectual disability.* Self-assessment of one's attitudes and beliefs about intellectual disability is critical. Intellectually disabled persons may be stigmatized because of their appearance, social habits, and history of behavior with others in the community. Reminders are continually needed to clarify that, with adequate social supports, normalization is, to a considerable extent, possible.

— *Adequacy of the assessment of cognitive functioning.* The determination of intellectual disability requires both individual testing and interpretation of results on tests, such as the Wechsler Intelligence Scale for Children—III, and assessment of adaptive functioning. It is absolutely critical to understand that a diagnosis of intellectual disability is *not* based on the IQ test alone. A mildly intellectually disabled person may acquire sufficient adaptive skills and no longer be eligible for this diagnosis. Pitfalls in testing include reliance on the group administration of tests rather than one-to-one testing and general descriptions of adaptive functioning when more formal measures, such as the AAMR Adaptive Behavior Scale (Lambert et al. 1993) or Vineland Social Maturity Scale, are indicated.

— *Failure to understand the law by the intellectually disabled person.* Understanding of the law by the intellectually disabled person is a major concern. The professional must make certain that the parent or guardian was notified immediately after arrest and that legal counsel was made available at an early stage to ensure that the intellectually disabled person was provided a requisite understanding of his or her constitutional rights to remain silent and to retain counsel. Effective safeguards for these constitutional rights are needed so that an intellectually disabled citizen will not be vulnerable to mistreatment by the justice system.

— *Understanding the law in regard to intellectual disability by the professional.* It is essential for mental health professionals to understand how intellectual disability affects a person's legal rights. A common misunderstanding is the confusion of legal and psychiatric issues in case assessment.

— *Increased risk for mental disorders.* Intellectual disability is a major risk factor for psychiatric disorders. Particularly when those with mild intellectual disability have legal difficulty, it must be borne in mind that they are susceptible to the same disorders as people without intellectual disability and for the most part respond to the same treatments.

References

Abram PR, Parker T, Weisberg SR: Sexual expression of mentally retarded people: educational and legal implications. Am J Ment Retard 93:328–334, 1988

Accardo PJ, Whitman BY: Children of mentally retarded parents. Am J Dis Child 144:69–70, 1990

American Association on Mental Retardation: Mental Retardation: Definition, Classification, and Systems of Support, 10th Edition. Washington, DC, American Association on Intellectual and Developmental Disabilities, 2002

American Law Institute Model Penal Code, sec. 401. Philadelphia, PA, American Law Institute, 1962

American Psychiatric Association: Diagnostic and Statistical Manual of Mental Disorders, 4th Edition, Text Revision. Washington, DC, American Psychiatric Association, 2000

Appelbaum PS: The issue of sterilization and the mentally retarded. Hosp Community Psychiatry 33:523–524, 1982

Biklen D: Myths, mistreatment, and pitfalls: mental retardation and criminal justice. Ment Retard 15:51–57, 1977

Bregman JD, Harris J: Intellectual disability, in Comprehensive Textbook of Psychiatry, 6th Edition. Edited by Kaplan E, Sadock BJ. Baltimore, MD, Williams & Wilkins, 1995, pp 2207–2241

Buescher M, Dinerstein RD: Capacity and the courts, in A Guide to Consent. Edited by Dinerstein RD, Herr SS, O'Sullivan JL. Washington, DC, American Association on Intellectual and Developmental Disabilities, 1999, pp 95–107

Clarke DJ: Antilibidinal drugs and mental retardation: a review. Med Sci Law 29:136–146, 1989

Cockram J, Jackson R, Underwood R: People with an intellectual disability and the criminal justice system: the family perspective. J Intellect Dev Disabil 23:41–56, 1998

Denekens JP, Nys H, Stuer H: Sterilisation of incompetent mentally handicapped persons: a model for decision making. J Med Ethics 25:237–241, 1999

Dusky v US, 362 US 401 (1960)

Everington C, Fulero SM: Competence to confess: measuring understanding and suggestibility of defendants with mental retardation. Ment Retard 37:212–220, 1999

Feinstein C, Reiss AL: Psychiatric disorder in mentally retarded children and adolescents: the challenges of meaningful diagnosis. Child Adolesc Psychiatr Clin N Am 5:827–852, 1996

Feldman MA: Research on parenting by mentally retarded persons. Psychiatr Clin North Am 9:777–796, 1986

Fielding LT, Murphy RJ, Reagan MW, et al: An assessment program to reduce drug use with the mentally retarded. Hosp Community Psychiatry 31:771–773, 1980

Foust JD: The legal significance of clinical formulations of firesetting behavior. International Journal of Law and Psychiatry 2:371–387, 1979

Giorgi-Guarnieri D, Janofsky J, Keram E, et al: AAPL practice guideline for forensic psychiatric evaluation of defendants raising the insanity defense. American Academy of Psychiatry and the Law. J Am Acad Psychiatry Law 30 (2 suppl):S3–S40, 2002

Grossman HJ: Manual on Terminology and Classification in Mental Retardation, Revised Edition. Washington, DC, American Association on Mental Deficiency, 1983

Gualtieri CT, Hawk B: Tardive dyskinesia and other drug-induced movement disorders among handicapped children and youth. Appl Res Ment Retard 1:55–69, 1980

Gudjonsson GH, Gunn J: The competence and reliability of a witness in a criminal court: a case report. Br J Psychiatry 141:624–627, 1982

Harris J: Intellectual disability, in Developmental Neuropsychiatry. Edited by Harris J. New York, Oxford University Press, 1998, pp 91–126

Harris J: Intellectual Disability: Understanding Its Development, Causes, Classification, Evaluation, and Treatment. New York, Oxford University Press, 2006, pp 11–41

Horner-Johnson W, Drum CE: Prevalence of maltreatment of people with intellectual disabilities: a review of recently published research. Ment Retard Dev Disabil Res Rev 12:57–69, 2006

Jones J: Persons with intellectual disabilities in the criminal justice system: review of issues. Int J Offender Ther Comp Criminol 51:723–733, 2007

Jones JM, Barnett RW, McCormack JK: Verbal/Performance splits in inmates assessed with the multidimensional aptitude battery. J Clin Psychol 44:995–1000, 1988

Kearns A, O'Connor A: The mentally handicapped criminal offender. a 10-year study of two hospitals. Br J Psychiatry 152:848–851, 1988

Keltner BR, Wise LA, Taylor G: Mothers with intellectual limitations and their 2-year-old children's developmental outcomes. J Intellect Dev Disabil 24:45–57, 1999

Lambert N, Kazuo N, Leland H: AAMR Adaptive Behavior Scale—School, 2nd Edition. Austin, TX, Pro-Ed, 1993

Lewis DO, Pincus JH, Bard B, et al: Neuropsychiatric, psychoeducational, and family characteristics of 14 juveniles condemned to death in the United States. Am J Psychiatry 145:584–589, 1988

Lindsay WR: Research and literature on sex offenders with intellectual and developmental disabilities. J Intellect Disabil Res 46 (suppl 1):74–85, 2002

Lindsay WR, Olley S, Baillie N, et al: Treatment of adolescent sex offenders with intellectual disabilities. Intellectual Disability 37:201–211, 1999

Luckasson R: The dually diagnosed in criminal justice, in Intellectual Disability and Mental Health: Classification, Diagnosis, Treatment, Services. Edited by Stark JA, Menolascino FJ, Albarelli MH, et al. New York, Springer-Verlag, 1988, pp 354–361

Luckasson R, Borthwick-Duffy S, Buntinx WHE, et al: Mental Retardation: Definition, Classification, and Systems of Supports, 10th Edition. Washington, DC, American Association on Mental Retardation, 2002

Martyn SR: Substituted judgment, best interests, and the need for best respect. Camb Q Healthc Ethics 3:195–208, 1994

McAfee JK, Gural M: Individuals with mental retardation and the criminal justice system: the view from states' attorneys general. Ment Retard 26:5–12, 1988

Menninger K: Mental retardation and criminal responsibility: some thoughts on the idiocy defense. Int J Law Psychiatry 8:343–357, 1986

National Institutes of Health: Consensus Conference on Treatment of Destructive Behaviors in Persons With Developmental Disabilities. Washington, DC, U.S. Government Printing Office, 1990

Nolley D, Butterfield B, Fleming A, et al: Non-aversive treatment of severe self-injurious behavior: multiple replications with DRO and DRI, in Life-Threatening Behavior. Edited by Hollis JH, Meyers CE. Washington, DC, American Association on Mental Deficiency, 1982

Nisonger Center for Intellectual Disability and Developmental Disabilities: The International Consensus Handbook: Psychotropic Medications and Developmental Disabilities. Edited by Reiss S, Aman MG. Columbus, Ohio State University, 1998

Parham v JR, 442 US 584 (1979)

Praiss DM: Constitutional protection of confessions made by mentally retarded defendants. Am J Law Med 14:431–465, 1989

President's Committee on Mental Retardation: Citizens With Intellectual Disability and the Criminal Justice System. Washington, DC, U.S. Department of Health and Human Services, 1991

Quinsey VL, Maguire A: Offenders remanded for a psychiatric examination: perceived treatability and disposition. Int J Law Psychiatry 6:193–205, 1983

Reiter S, Bryen DN, Shachar I: Adolescents with intellectual disabilities as victims of abuse. J Intellect Disabil 11:371–387, 2007

Roesch R, Golding SL: Treatment and disposition of defendants found incompetent to stand trial: a review and a proposal. Int J Law Psychiatry 2:349–370, 1979

Rousso A: Sterilization of the mentally retarded. Med Law 3:353–362, 1984

Silber DE, Courtless TF: Measures of fantasy aggression among mentally retarded offenders. Am J Ment Defic 72:918–923, 1968

Simpson MK: The roots of normalization: a reappraisal. J Intellect Disabil Res 42 (pt 1):1–7, 1998

Smith SM, Kunjukrishnan R: Medicolegal aspects of mental retardation. Psychiatr Clin North Am 9:699–712, 1986

Sparrow SS, Balla DA, Cicchetti DV: Vineland Adaptive Behavior Scales: Interview Edition, Survey Form Manual. Circle Pines, MN, American Guidance Service, 1984

Stavis PF, Walker-Hirsch LW: Consent to sexual activity, in A Guide to Consent. Edited by Dinerstein RD, Herr SS, O'Sullivan JL. Washington, DC, American Association on Intellectual Disability, 1999, pp 57–65

Sundram CJ: Informed consent for major medical treatment of mentally disabled people: a new approach. N Engl J Med 318:1368–1373, 1988

Szymanski LS, King BH: Practice parameters for the assessment and treatment of children, adolescents, and adults with mental retardation and comorbid mental disorders. J Am Acad Child Adolesc Psychiatry 38 (suppl), December 1999

Telfer MA, Baker D, Clark GR, et al: Incidence of gross chromosomal errors among tall criminal American males. Science 159:1249–1250, 1968

Webster F: A report on voluntary sterilization with special reference to minors and women who are intellectually disabled. Clin Reprod Fertil 3:99–106, 1985

Whitman BY, Accardo PJ: When a Parent Is Intellectually Disabled. Baltimore, MD, Paul H Brookes, 1989

Williams W, Spruill J: The criminal justice/mental health system and the mentally retarded, mentally ill defendant. Soc Sci Med 25:1027–1032, 1987

Wolfensberger W: The Principle of Normalization in Human Service. Toronto, Ontario, National Institute on Intellectual Disability, 1972

World Health Organization: International Statistical Classification of Diseases and Related Health Problems, 10th Revision. Geneva, World Health Organization, 1992

Yesavage JA, Benezech M, Ceccaldi P, et al: Arson in mentally ill and criminal populations. J Clin Psychiatry 44:128–130, 1983

PART III

Child Custody

Elissa P. Benedek, M.D.

Chapter 11

Child Custody Evaluation

Pamela S. Ludolph, Ph.D.

The law has long made provision for the custody of children whose parents do not live together. Before the early nineteenth century, English common law, on which U.S. law is generally based, gave absolute power to the father over his children (Gould and Martindale 2007). During the nineteenth century, this standard began to be replaced by the *tender years doctrine*, which increasingly advocated that children be raised by their mothers, especially when they were young. By the twentieth century, mothers had replaced fathers as the primary custodial choice for children of divorce. Only in the last two decades has empirical support emerged for the importance of fathers in the lives of children (Kelly and Lamb 2000), such that there is now serious question in many courts about maternal preference (Gould and Martindale 2007).

The standard that has replaced maternal preference is "the best interest of the child," which was enacted in the U.S. Congress in 1979 and has now been adopted as law throughout the United States. It is also the standard underlying the *Guidelines for Child Custody Evaluations in Family Law Proceedings* of the American Psychological Association (2009). Nonetheless, the best interest standard is problematic, primarily because its definition remains vague in most jurisdictions, though some states have enacted legislation specifying the factors that define "best interests." For instance, Michigan's Child Custody Act (1993) specifies 11 factors that the court must consider in determining a child's best interest. Recent commentary considers the advisability of moving beyond a simple best interests standard in evaluations to one which can more individually consider family dynamics and other factors, as indicated specifically by the court (Gould and Martindale 2007).

Evolving child custody evaluation practice involves the examination of various kinds of data for the purpose of giving information to the court about families in which parents or other legally defined caregivers are unable to derive their own parenting plans. The usual context of such evaluations is divorce. Child custody evaluations assess parenting and other factors requested by the court and, in some cases, give opinions as to custody.

Legal Issues in Child Custody Evaluations

Custody evaluators must be reasonably familiar with the law that applies to their endeavor. Most generally, they should know the controlling law with regard to the admissibility of evidence from expert witnesses in their state. Some states have law that derives from the *Frye* standard (*Frye v. United States* 1923), a standard that requires that the court permit expert scientific testimony if it is "generally accepted" in its field. Gould (2006) stated that most courts consider that the *Frye* standard is met if the data presented derive from peer-reviewed journals. Other states have adopted the more recent *Daubert* standard (*Daubert v. Merrell Dow Pharmaceuticals* 1993), which is similar to the *Frye* standard but emphasizes the role of the judge as gatekeeper as to whether the expert testimony is scientifically valid and has relevance to the issue before the court. The *Daubert* standard looks for expert testimony to be "helpful" to the court. Gould (2006) pointed out that the intent of the court in *Daubert* seems to have been to modify *Frye* to allow the presentation of "new, unconventional, or unpublished scientific principles and methods" (p. 52).

In addition, custody evaluators should know the law that applies to divorce and child custody in their state, including relevant case law. Evaluators should understand and respect the legal rights of those who participate in child custody evaluations. They should be aware of the hearsay rules in their state, particularly as they apply to the admission of information obtained from collateral sources. Evaluators should know the child protection law and the workings of the local Child Protection Department, as should all clinicians, both to interpret past Child Protective Services referrals and because issues of maltreatment sometimes make it necessary to report individuals to Child Protective Services in conjunction with the child custody evaluation.

Ethical Issues in Child Custody Evaluations

Child custody work is ethically complex. The ethical evaluator is often confronted with thorny dilemmas and is greatly assisted by the several ethical models that have been put forth by professional organizations in the last several years. Notably, these include the *Guidelines for Child Custody Evaluations in Family Law Proceedings* of the American Psychological Association (2009); the *Practice Parameters for Child Custody Evaluation* of the American Academy of Child and Adolescent Psychiatry (1997); and the *Model Standards of Practice for Child Custody Evaluation* of the Association of Family and Conciliation Courts (AFCC 2007). These documents amplify the general ethical standards of mental health professionals and the general forensic guidelines for psychologists and psychiatrists. Clearly, the ethics of child custody evaluation must be understood within these wider frames. There are differences in these documents and controversies in the field about these differences, particularly from supporters of the newer and more stringent AFCC Model Standards. Nonetheless, they share many core principles. Among the key ethical principles for child custody evaluators are the following:

1. The child custody evaluation is a forensic enterprise. A custody evaluator is not a therapist. As

Greenberg and Shuman (1997) outlined in the title of their article, there is an "irreconcilable conflict between therapeutic and forensic roles." The therapist is helpful and supportive and, for the most part, works confidentially. The forensic evaluator is objective and detached, and works to benefit the court. The evaluator has only as much privilege as the specific forensic role and the particular judge allow.

2. The evaluator is in an impartial role. If the evaluator has any conflict that might even appear to compromise his or her neutrality, it should be disclosed at the outset. If the conflict is significant, the evaluator should consider withdrawing from the case.

3. Evaluators should generally only give opinions about those whom they have directly evaluated. The common mistake here is acting on the sometimes desperate pleas of the noncustodial parent to evaluate a child who has allegedly been subject to maltreatment at the hands of the custodial parent, and then informing the court of recommendations as to parenting. There are, of course, appropriate roles for evaluators who are retained by only one party in child custody disputes. These roles are circumscribed, for instance, testifying about the empirical literature as to some relevant issue, or testifying as to the flaws in another expert's report, after thorough investigation (Gould et al. 2004). Such evaluators should still remain objective in their investigation and presentation of their comments to the court.

4. The evaluator's work is guided by current scientific and legal knowledge. Gould and Martindale (2007) made the point, however, that emphasizing the science of child custody evaluation does not eliminate reasonable clinical judgment; both are essential to forensic decision making.

5. The evaluator should avoid multiple relationships. Thus, the evaluator declines appointment if he or she has a personal relationship with any family members or has served in some other professional capacity for the family.

6. The evaluator is aware of his or her own personal and societal biases and seeks to eliminate their impact on his or her work.

7. The evaluator uses multiple methods of data gathering. This chapter will outline a widely accepted approach to child custody evaluation that includes interviews with family members, observations of parenting, psychological testing, and the examination of collateral documents and sources. Although there are reasonable arguments as to the

necessity of some of these approaches, there is no argument that child custody is too important a matter to be decided by cursory interviews and investigations.

The Empirically Grounded Child Custody Evaluation

Beginning the Evaluation

The evaluation will often begin with contact from one or both attorneys for the parties. From the outset, the evaluator should be cognizant of his or her neutral role and provide information symmetrically to both attorneys. After the initial telephone calls, information can often be shared by copied letters or e-mails or conference calls. Ex parte communication with the court should be avoided.

Although child custody evaluation can take place by consent of both parents, without an order, this has become an increasingly rare practice. An order of the court provides the evaluator with a measure of authority and information about the scope of the evaluation requested. In many jurisdictions, the court order allows the evaluator some degree of quasi-judicial immunity against malpractice allegations. In a practice in which one or both parties can be unhappy with the result of the evaluation, quasi-judicial immunity may be the only way an evaluator can work comfortably. Sometimes, the order comes from the court in a terse, unelaborated form. At that point, the evaluator may wish to contact the attorneys in the case and request a more detailed and comprehensive order, specifying matters such as the nonconfidentiality of the report as to the participants in the evaluation, their counsel, and the court; the need for the parties' full cooperation in the evaluation; the nature of contact with the expert by attorneys for the parties; fee arrangements, often including a clear statement that the report will not be released until the expert is paid; and arrangements for testimony, if the case proceeds to trial (Erard and Kirkendall 2003). The order may also include preferences of the evaluator, such as stating that the treating mental health professionals of family members should have access to the report and that the children and others not party to the case should not have access to it. Of course, such an order is subject to the strictures of relevant state law and local practice, and individual attorneys may wish to alter parts of it. In this event, the evaluator should decide whether the changes that the attorney wishes are acceptable or whether they require that the evaluator withdraw the offer of services.

Alternatively, the jurisdictional practice may be such that the evaluator must work with a brief order of the court in which all that is specified is the name of the expert. In this case, the kinds of information listed above can be made part of a "Statement of Understanding," which is discussed with the parties by their counsel before the first session and signed at or before that session (Gould 2006). In any case, the evaluator should go over the key points of the order or agreement with each parent in the first session and answer any questions. The goal in the first sessions and throughout the evaluation should be transparency with the parties about the process.

Interviewing Parents

Interviews with parents should emphasize parenting and issues that affect parenting. Parents should be asked to talk about each of their children and their parenting practices with regard to that child. The evaluator should carefully note the depth of the description of the child and assess its accuracy after comparison with other data. Children should emerge from these discussions as distinct individuals, with separate life histories, needs, talents, and weaknesses. Parents should be able to describe the temperamental idiosyncrasies of their infants and toddlers and to comment on their likes and dislikes. Mothers and fathers should describe their capacities to provide appropriate comfort and nurturance, yet promote independence as well. Evaluators should look into a parent's level of involvement in the child's life, for instance at school and extracurricular activities. In the course of the interviews, parents should present clear evidence of love and concern for the child, and an inclination to place the child's needs above their own. Parents should describe an approach to discipline that is age appropriate and neither overly harsh nor permissive. They should be able to outline how they comfort and encourage their child when he or she is having trouble and encourage and praise the child when he or she is doing well. In divorce, a parent should be able to communicate reasonably openly with the other parent, should portray the other parent in positive terms to the child, and should encourage the child to visit the other parent.

Parents should also have the opportunity to tell the story of what brings them to the evaluation, the history of their relationship with each other, and their concerns about each other's parenting of their children. These data can then be used to suggest appropriate collateral sources to address each parent's allegations and to promote discussion with the other parent. Toward the end of the evaluation, both parents should also be asked to respond to significant allegations against them made by the other parent or collateral sources.

Parts of the interview should inquire into signs and symptoms of mental illness. Some evaluators use questionnaires for screening; some conduct a formal mental status exam; most talk to the parent's mental health providers, with appropriate consents. If there are indications that significant mental health problems exist, the evaluator should inquire further. Substance abuse should also be assessed (Schleuderer and Campagna 2004). The possibility of domestic violence, child maltreatment, and alienation dynamics should be considered in the interview. The focus here, however, is not necessarily to provide the court with a firm diagnosis of the parent but to determine whether the parent's difficulties compromise parenting. I evaluated a family in which a parent had lost parenting time with his children because of an uncontrolled and severe bipolar illness; with medication, therapy, and a solid plan for the children in case there was a recurrence, this man proved a much more effective parent than the mother and was awarded primary physical custody of the children.

Interviewing Children and Observing the Family

Child forensic interviewing is among the most difficult tasks a mental health professional can take on. In the often incendiary context of high-conflict divorce, such interviews can present issues of extraordinary complexity. Suffice to list some of the necessary skills for the endeavor and, consequently, the areas in which the child custody evaluator must become expert. Especially with young children, evaluators must know the principles of child forensic interviewing, including accepted techniques for interviewing about allegations of maltreatment (Poole and Lamb 1998). Evaluators must be able to explain their role to the child so that the child will be inclined to cooperate with them. Evaluators must know how to use play to make the child comfortable and establish an alliance, but they must be aware that conclusions based solely on play therapy techniques have no place in a forensic evaluation (Gould 2006). The evaluator must make decisions about whether to inquire directly about the child's opinion with regard to custody, and if so, how to proceed without making the child feel too guilty or responsible. There should be assessment of the developmental aspects of children's cognition, language (Walker 1999), emotion, and general understanding of the divorce process (Garrity and Baris 1994). The competent evaluator must know about suggestibility in children (Ceci and Bruck 1995) and the effects of parental coaching in children of divorce. Knowledge of childhood psychopathology, disability, developmental delay, and learning problems is key, because many high-conflict divorces are fought out around disagreements in how to raise children with special needs (Saposnek et al. 2005). Psychological testing can be helpful in exploring problem areas in children who seem unusually troubled.

Many have talked about the importance of the child's voice being heard in the divorce process, whether in interviews with the court, increasingly in mediation, or in representation by a guardian ad litem or an attorney for the child. Most recently, the child specialist role in collaborative law provides a neutral mental health professional to interview and assess children of divorcing parents, bringing the children's wishes and needs to the forefront in the negotiations among parents and their attorneys (Gutterman 2004). Sensitive child interviewing by the child custody evaluator can also yield data that bring the voice of the child into play in the divorce proceedings. Children can, of course, advocate positions that are clearly not in their best interests. In my experience, however, most of them have valuable thoughts to contribute to the process. I remember a little girl, the youngest of her family, telling me simply that she was afraid of her mommy and she did not know why; after talking longer, the child slowly revealed a history of significant physical abuse. An older child told me that he feared that his father would kill all of the children in an accident after he had been drinking. I asked a 4-year-old how he would feel if he and his mommy moved to another state. He told me that he would be very, very sad, that he loved his mommy and his daddy and wanted his daddy close, so his daddy could read their favorite book to him at night. In all of these cases, a clear presentation of the children's statements was very important to the outcome of the litigation.

Observations of parent and child together are also a key part of child custody evaluation. In a nutshell, it is hard to evaluate parenting if you have not seen it. In general, an observation should be held with all members of the father's household, and then with all members of the mother's household. Thus, stepparents, live-in partners, and live-in stepsiblings should be included. Observations are most often conducted in the office. Sometimes they are held in the parties' homes for a variety of reasons, ranging from a wish to compare the physical living situations of both parents to an attempt to accommodate a fearful toddler who adapts slowly and painfully to new places and experiences. Some evaluators do a pure observation, just noting down what family members do and say for an hour or so, saying as little as possible themselves. Other evaluators have a number of tasks for the family to do together, each for some specific purposes. The majority of evaluators probably use a combination of unstructured and semistructured activities. It is astonishing how revealing these brief glimpses of family life can be. In my office, one mother threatened to send her mildly oppositional children to an orphanage, clearly terrifying them. Another mother was so undone by her toddler's tantrum that she burst into tears and needed assistance getting the child to her car.

Psychological Testing

Carefully chosen psychological tests are a valuable tool in child custody evaluation (Flens and Drozd 2005). Psychological testing often generates hypotheses that careful evaluators can then confirm or disconfirm with interview or collateral data. Gould (2006) suggested that evaluators who do not use psychological testing do well to remember that tests add normative information with regard to issues such as personality functioning, parenting, and attitudes about family violence. He also suggested that an evaluator can often compensate for the loss of testing by adding additional collateral and interview data.

The Minnesota Multiphasic Personality Inventory—Second Edition (MMPI-2; Butcher et al. 1989) and the Millon Clinical Multiaxial Inventory—Third Edition (MCMI-III; Millon 1997) are the most frequently used tests in the current child custody evaluation practice of psychologists (Quinnell and Bow 2001). The MMPI-2 assesses psychopathology in many areas; the MCMI-III focuses on psychopathology and personality disorder. Both have scales that assess the examinee's candor. Both have been subjected to normative study using groups of child custody litigants (Bathurst et al. 1997; McCann et al. 2001) and are often the centerpieces of the child custody evaluator's test battery. Both can be scored with the assistance of computer-generated reports, although such reports should be used carefully, if at all. The task of test analysis must be the province of a skilled psychologist, not a computer program with unknown specifications. It must be remembered, however, that although the

MMPI-2 and the MCMI-III provide useful information, they do not specifically address parenting.

Of course, many other tests are used in evaluations, and should be. It is very important to choose tests that are appropriate to the context of the specific evaluation. For instance, there are tests that are particularly constructed to assess issues such as an adult's propensity to abuse children, the ability to co-parent, or a parent's assessment of his of her children's behavior and symptoms. In selecting tests, evaluators should choose instruments with the kind of demonstrated reliability and validity likely to survive a *Daubert* challenge. Tests such as Incomplete Sentences or the House-Tree-Person test do not meet these psychometric standards and should not be used in a forensic context. Projective tests, and particularly the Rorschach test, are controversial at this time, with some authors arguing that the Rorschach, scored by the Exner Comprehensive System (Exner 1991), meets any psychometric standard in the family court (Erard 2007) and some arguing the contrary (Erickson et al. 2007) (see also Chapter 6, "Psychological Testing in Child and Adolescent Forensic Evaluations").

Corroboration and Collateral Sources

Corroboration of the statements of parents and children to the evaluator is essential. Greenberg and Schuman (1997) stated that the forensic role requires the verification of the litigant's statements with "historical truth." Collateral sources can be solicited from parents or specifically requested by the evaluator after interviewing the family. Careful consideration should be given to the credibility of different collateral sources (Austin 2002). Teachers, child care providers, and physicians of family members are examples of professionals who are frequently called upon. Psychotherapists are particularly key in the child custody evaluation process. Questioning them, however, can present ethical challenges. Therapists of vulnerable parents in the throes of high-conflict divorce may lose their effectiveness with a client if they speak candidly to the evaluator about the client's psychopathology. Therapists of children also risk damaging the child's trust and sense that the therapy can be a safe haven from the tribulations of parental divorce. Particularly with child therapists, I often suggest that the therapist speak with the child to discuss what the child is comfortable having shared with me. Sometimes, I have the same conversation with the child. In the end, I am generally able to secure helpful information without damaging the therapeutic alliance.

All collateral sources should be informed that the evaluation is not confidential and that the collateral's statements may be included in a report that will be shared with the parents and the court. After releases are signed by the parents, information from collateral sources can be collected in various ways. Some evaluators insist on written consents from collateral sources (Gould 2006), and some explain the collateral's role in a telephone call and obtain and note verbal consent (Austin 2002). Telephone interviews are frequently and effectively used. Some evaluators collect information in writing; occasionally, an important collateral source is best interviewed in the office. A new spouse or live-in partner of a child custody litigant is both a collateral source and an important and continuing presence in the life of the child. As such, the stepparent is usually subject to some level of assessment as well as questioning to provide collateral information, albeit likely biased information.

Document review also provides important collateral information. Police reports, Child Protective Services reports, records of psychiatric hospitalizations, report cards, and other school records provide important information to confirm or disconfirm interview data.

The Advisory Report and the Controversy About Recommendations

The advisory report should present the data objectively and comprehensively, bearing in mind its importance to the child and the family. Comprehensive reports do require some reading, but they give the court the necessary opportunity to understand why the evaluator reached whatever conclusions were reached. The report is usually the only place the data are fully presented, given that child custody evaluators rarely testify (Bow and Quinnell 2001). Detail and clarity are of the utmost importance if the report is not to be subject to cross-examination (Bow and Quinnell 2002).

Bow and Quinnell (2001) surveyed 52 child custody reports written by doctoral-level psychologists. The most frequent component of the reports were recommendations, present 96.2% of the time. Nonetheless, there is great controversy about whether child custody evaluators should offer recommendations to the court. A small group of attorneys and psycholo-

gists have argued that custody evaluators should not be permitted to offer opinions that speak to the ultimate issue of child custody (Melton et al. 1997; Tippins and Wittmann 2005). Their position is that mental health professionals do not have a solid enough scientific basis for their opinions to offer them to the court. Others have argued that custody opinions are based on growing scientific knowledge and are important to the judiciary in guiding its thinking about psychological issues in which mental health professionals can be expected to know more than judges (Kelly and Johnston 2005). Gould and Martindale (2005) pointed out the demand of attorneys and the courts for such recommendations and advocate recommendations only to the "psychological best interests of the child," leaving the "legal" best interests to the courts. Virtually all authors on child custody agree that if recommendations are made, they should be based on a thorough knowledge of the current literature and with humility and clear statements about their limitations. In the relatively rare event that the data and recommendations are presented to the court in testimony, the expert should be particularly careful to present evidence carefully and neutrally, noting the scientific evidence in support of and opposed to the expert's conclusions.

Parenting Plans

If recommendations are made, they will often involve a specific plan for the parenting of the children. In devising parenting plans, evaluators will usually be considering the best interests of children whose parents are involved with much conflict and chronic litigation. There is much empirical support for the association of exposure to high conflict and poorer child outcome, so effective parenting plans do well to minimize transitions between households that expose the children to significant acrimony between their parents (Kelly and Lamb 2000). Thus, transitions at school or day care often work well. Garrity and Baris (1994) offered numerous other suggestions for parenting plans for children of high-conflict divorce.

Parenting plans must also be suited to the developmental needs of the child. Older children, for instance, should be provided a schedule that allows for their increasing need to spend time with their peers. Parenting plans are particularly complex for infants and very young children. Gould and Stahl (2001) presented a number of factors that evaluators should bear in mind when they make plans for such children. Evaluators should take into account the parenting history of the child; if the child has been comfortable with a parent during the marriage, the child probably will be after the divorce. The authors also mentioned issues such as the strengths and weaknesses of the parent in parenting and the fit with the child, the temperament of the child, and the ability and inclination of both parents to discuss the needs of their young child.

Attachment issues and the importance of the primary parent to the later mental health of the child have often been cited as reasons that very young children should spend the bulk of their time with their mothers and avoid overnights with their fathers. Recent research, however, has called into question some of the tenets of traditional attachment theory, pointing out that other variables beside the relationship with the primary caregiver are important to the development of the young child and that early attachment status is not necessarily stable over time (Ludolph 2009). There has also recently been significant comment and research on the issue of overnights for young children with the noncustodial parent (Pruett 2005), something that had often been precluded on attachment grounds. Kelly and Lamb (2000) described the importance to the development of young children of substantial contact with both parents and have made the point that overnights with the noncustodial parent promote many aspects of healthy emotional development in the child.

Complex Evaluations

Allegations of Child Physical and Sexual Abuse

Allegations of abuse are common in child custody work. Johnston et al. (2005) surveyed 120 families referred for custody evaluation or specialized counseling for high-conflict divorce and found that 34% had allegations of child neglect or physical, emotional, or sexual abuse. Allegations were more often brought against fathers than mothers, though the allegations were substantiated about equally. These data make it clear that child abuse in divorce is much more than a matter of the false allegations of an angry parent and needs careful attention by any custody evaluator.

Sexual abuse in which one parent accuses the other has proved a particularly difficult area for child custody evaluators. At the outset of the evaluation, one parent has often been deprived of parenting time with the child based on very little substantial evidence, pending the evaluation. The issues involved are a breeding ground for bias: the allegations are often so heinous that there is an inclination to substantiate "just to be sure." There is also danger, however, in the child's spending all her time with a parent who is falsely accusing the other of a heinous crime and in the child's perhaps coming to believe that she was incestuously abused when she was not. The child custody evaluator needs to be well acquainted with forensic protocols for interviewing the child about abuse and follow them with skill and sensitivity (Kuehnle 1996; Kuehnle and Kirkpatrick 2005; Poole and Lamb 1998).

Allegations of Domestic Violence

Johnston et al. (2005) studied high-conflict, divorcing families and found that domestic violence allegations were brought against mothers in 30% of the families and substantiated in 15%; such allegations were brought against fathers in 55% of the families, with substantiation 41% of the time. There is no argument that domestic violence is a significant problem in general, and in high-conflict divorce in particular. There has been much argument in the field, however, about definitions of domestic violence. Increasingly, there has been a press to derive typologies that recognize a range of family violence that involves different levels of risk to the child and the abused parent, as well as different interventions and plans for the child's access to the perpetrator.

Kelly and Johnson (2008) derived a sophisticated typology that describes four types of violence. *Coercive controlling violence* generally describes the posture of the traditional batterer: intimidating, emotionally abusive, and physically very violent and dangerous. *Violent resistance* is the stance of the victim of coercive controlling physical violence who strikes back violently. *Situational couple violence* identifies partner violence that is generally less dangerous and not motivated by power and control. Finally, *separation-instigated violence* occurs in a couple only at the time of separation. The authors noted that it is now clear that both men and women can be violent in intimate partner relationships, although the most serious subtype of violence, coercive controlling violence, is perpetrated primarily by men. There is also abundant evidence that exposure to domestic violence is predictive of maladjustment in children. Kelly and Johnson recommended that child custody evaluators make distinctions among types of domestic violence, entertain multiple hypotheses, and avoid gendered biases. Skilled evaluators should make recommendations that take into account the type and level of violence and the likelihood that it will recur. There are useful models available for the assessment of risk in families where domestic violence is alleged, for instance those of Austin (2001) and Jaffe et al. (2008).

Allegations of Child Alienation

Gardner (1992) initially described the parental alienation syndrome, by which one parent, usually the mother, actively campaigned against the other to alienate the child. This model has come under widespread criticism and has largely been replaced by more complex thinking concerning why a child might align himself or herself with one parent and seek to minimize or eliminate contact with the other. The dominant model in the field is that of Kelly and Johnston (2001), who have moved the focus from the parent to the child. The model first distinguishes "estranged" children, those who resist spending time with a parent for understandable reasons, including the parent's history of significant psychopathology, family violence, and maltreatment. The responses of the estranged child should be assessed largely as healthy and protective.

In the case of the alienated child, however, the child's negative feelings about the parent are unreasonable and disproportionate to the actions of the parent. Kelly and Johnston (2001) outlined a number of reasons why this might be so, including problems in the aligned parent, such as deep hurt at the separation or false beliefs that the other parent is dangerous, and problems in the rejected parent, such as unavailability or harsh and unempathic parenting. The child, usually age 9 to 15 years, is often anxious and fearful, with a history of unsatisfactory contact with the rejected parent. The evaluator has only to see a few of these children to become familiar with the hollowness of their accounts of the rejected parent and their echo of the story of the aligned parent, very often including the use of that parent's exact words. Experts in the management of these cases advise timely custody evaluations, to determine the reasonableness and origin of the child's concerns, with contact and family therapy con-

tinuing during the evaluations (Sullivan and Kelly 2001). These authors also provided suggestions for the highly structured parenting plans that these and other high-conflict families generally require.

Issues of Relocation

There is much disagreement in legal and psychological thinking at this time concerning the approach the court should take when a custodial parent wishes to move away with the child, thus restricting access to the noncustodial parent. Some mental health professionals have argued that the move should be allowed, in that benefit to the primary parent from the move should constitute benefit to the child. Others have argued the contrary. Austin (2008a) presented a compelling review of the relevant research indicating the deleterious effects of relocation on children, and particularly on children of divorce. Such children are at significant risk of adjustment problems, including lower academic achievement, behavioral problems, and teen pregnancy. Nonetheless, of course, child custody evaluators evaluate specific children for whom a move might make sense, for instance, by significantly increasing the child's socioeconomic opportunities or improving educational options. Austin (2000, 2008b) proposed a model of relocation risk assessment by which evaluators can more scientifically estimate the risk of relocation. The risk factors described include the following: 1) age of the child, with younger children being more vulnerable; 2) geographical distance and travel time; 3) psychological stability of the relocating parent and parenting effectiveness of both parents; 4) individual resources and individual differences in the child, including temperament and special needs; 5) involvement by the nonresidential parent; 6) parental support of the other parent's relationship with the child; 7) interparental conflict and domestic violence; and 8) recentness of the marital separation, given that conflict tends to be highest early in the divorce (Austin 2008b). This model shows promise in assisting evaluators to come to empirically based and nonbiased conclusions about relocation.

—Key Points

— Child custody evaluation is conducted in the best interest of the child.

— Child custody evaluators must know the rules of admissibility of expert evidence in their jurisdiction and other laws applicable to child custody work.

— Ethical issues are paramount in child custody evaluation. Evaluators should be clear that they are functioning in an impartial role, guided by current scientific and legal knowledge. Evaluators should work to minimize bias. They should use multiple methods of data gathering to increase the accuracy of their findings.

— The focus of the interviews with parents is parenting, not psychopathology.

— Child interviews are key and require sophisticated knowledge of child development, high-conflict divorce dynamics, and child forensic interviewing techniques.

— Psychological testing can inject important normative data about many issues relevant to child custody evaluation. If psychological testing is not used, additional interviews and collateral information can be substituted.

— Collateral documents and sources are indispensable to the process of confirming and disconfirming information received from family members.

— Recommendations, if presented at all, should be made based on a thorough knowledge of the literature and with clear statements about their limitations.

— Certain issues present special concerns for child custody evaluators. Cases involving these issues should be accepted only if the evaluator gains special competency in the area designated for evaluation. Among these issues are allegations of child physical and sexual abuse, domestic violence, child alienation, and disputes involving relocation or parenting plans for very young children.

References

American Academy of Child and Adolescent Psychiatry: Practice parameters for child custody evaluation. J Am Acad Child Adolesc Psychiatry 36:57s–68s, 1997

American Psychological Association: Guidelines for Child Custody Evaluations in Family Law Proceedings. Washington, DC, American Psychological Association, February 2009. Available at: http://www.apa.org/practice/childcustody.pdf. Accessed June 9, 2009.

Association of Family and Conciliation Courts: Model standards of practice for child custody evaluation. Family Court Review 45:70–91, 2007

Austin WG: A forensic psychology model of risk assessment for child custody relocation law. Family and Conciliation Courts Review 38:192–207, 2000

Austin WG: Partner violence and risk assessment in child custody evaluations. Family Court Review 39:483–496, 2001

Austin WG: Guidelines for utilizing collateral sources of information in child custody evaluations. Family Court Review 40:177–184, 2002

Austin WG: Relocation, research, and forensic evaluation, Part I: Effects of residential mobility on children of divorce. Family Court Review 46:137–150, 2008a

Austin WG: Relocation, research, and forensic evaluation, Part II: Research in support of the relocation risk assessment model. Family Court Review 46:347–365, 2008b

Bathurst K, Gottfried AW, Gottfried AE: Normative data for the MMPI-2 in child custody litigation. Psychol Assess 9:205–211, 1997

Bow JN, Quinnell FA: Psychologists' current practices and procedures in child custody evaluations: five years after American Psychological Association guidelines. Prof Psychol Res Pract 32:261–268, 2001

Bow JN, Quinnell FA: A critical review of child custody evaluation reports. Family Court Review 40:164–176, 2002

Butcher JN, Dahlstrom WG, Graham JR, et al: Minnesota Multiphasic Personality Inventory–2 (MMPI-2): Manual for Administration and Scoring. Minneapolis, University of Minnesota Press, 1989

Ceci SJ, Bruck M: Jeopardy in the Courtroom. Washington, DC, American Psychological Association, 1995

Daubert v Merrell Dow Pharmaceuticals, 113 S Ct 2786 (1993)

Erard RE: Picking cherries with blinders on: a comment on Erickson et al. (2007) regarding the use of tests in family court. Family Court Review 45:175–184, 2007

Erard RE, Kirkendall JN: A judge's guide to the testimony of mental health professionals. Presented at the Second Annual Family Law Institute, Institute of Continuing Legal Education, Ypsilanti, MI, November 2003

Erickson SK, Lilienfeld SO, Vitacco MJ: A critical examination of the suitability and limitations of psychological tests in family court. Family Court Review 45:157–174, 2007

Exner JE Jr: The Rorschach: A Comprehensive System, Vol 2: Interpretation, 2nd Edition. New York, Wiley, 1991

Flens JR, Drozd L (eds): Psychological Testing in Child Custody Evaluations. New York, Haworth Press, 2005

Frye v United States, 293 F 1013 (DC Cir 1923)

Gardner RA: The Parental Alienation Syndrome. Cresskill, NJ, Creative Therapeutics, 1992

Garrity C, Baris M: Caught in the Middle: Protecting the Children of High-Conflict Divorce. New York, Lexington Books, 1994

Gould JW: Conducting Scientifically Crafted Child Custody Evaluations, 2nd Edition. Sarasota, FL, Professional Resource Press, 2006

Gould JW, Martindale DA: A second call for clinical humility and judicial vigilance: comments on Tippins and Wittmann (2005). Family Court Review 43:253–259, 2005

Gould JW, Martindale DA: The Art and Science of Child Custody Evaluations. New York, Guilford, 2007

Gould JW, Stahl PM: Never paint by the numbers: a response to Kelly and Lamb (2000), Solomon and Biringen (2001), and Lamb and Kelly (2001). Family Court Review 39:372–376, 2001

Gould JW, Kirkpatrick HD, Austin W, et al: A protocol for offering a critique of a colleague's forensic work product. J Child Custody 1:37–64, 2004

Greenberg SA, Shuman DW: Irreconcilable conflict between therapeutic and forensic roles. Prof Psychol Res Pract 28:50–57, 1997

Gutterman SM: Collaborative Law: A New Model for Dispute Resolution. Denver, CO, Bradford Publishing, 2004

Jaffe PG, Johnston JR, Crooks CV, et al: Custody disputes involving allegations of domestic violence: toward a differentiated approach to parenting plans. Family Court Review 46:500–522, 2008

Johnston JR, Lee S, Olesen NW, et al: Allegations and substantiations of abuse in custody-disputing families. Family Court Review 43:283–294, 2005

Kelly JB, Johnson MP: Differentiation among types of intimate partner violence: research update and implications for interventions. Family Court Review 46:476–499, 2008

Kelly JB, Johnston JR: The alienated child: a reformulation of parental alienation syndrome. Family Court Review 39:249–266, 2001

Kelly JB, Johnston JR: Commentary on Tippins and Wittmann's "Empirical and ethical problems with custody recommendations: a call for clinical humility and judicial vigilance." Family Court Review 43:233–241, 2005

Kelly JB, Lamb ME: Using child development research to make appropriate custody and access decisions for young children. Family and Conciliation Courts Review 38:297–311, 2000

Kuehnle K: Assessing Allegations of Child Sexual Abuse. Sarasota, FL, Professional Resource Press, 1996

Kuehnle K, Kirkpatrick HD: Evaluating allegations of child sexual abuse within complex child custody cases, in Child Custody Litigation: Allegations of Child Sexual Abuse. Edited by Kuehnle K, Drozd L. New York, Hayworth Press, 2005, pp 3–39

Ludolph PS: Answered and unanswered questions in attachment theory with implications for children of divorce. J Child Custody 6:8–24, 2009

McCann JT, Flens JR, Campagna V, et al: The MCMI-III in child custody evaluations: a normative study. J Forensic Psychol Pract 1:27–44, 2001

Melton GB, Petrila J, Poythress MG, et al: Psychological Evaluations for the Courts: A Handbook for Mental Health Professionals and Lawyers, 2nd Edition. New York, Guilford, 1997

Michigan Child Custody Act of 1970, MCL 722.23 (amended 1993)

Millon T, Davis RD, Millon C: Manual for the Millon Clinical Multiaxial Inventory—III, 2nd Edition (MCMI-III). Minneapolis, MN, National Computer Systems, 1997

Poole DA, Lamb ME: Investigative Interviews of Children: A Guide for Helping Professionals. Washington, DC, American Psychological Association, 1998

Pruett MK: Overnights and Young Children: Essays From the Family Court Review. Madison, WI, Association of Family and Conciliation Courts, 2005

Quinnell FA, Bow JN: Psychological tests used in child custody evaluations. Behav Sci Law 19:491–501, 2001

Saposnek DT, Perryman H, Berkow J, et al: Special needs children in family court cases. Family Court Review 43:566–581, 2005

Schleuderer C, Campagna V: Assessing substance abuse questions in child custody evaluations. Family Court Review 42:375–383, 2004

Sullivan MJ, Kelly JB: Legal and psychological management of cases with an alienated child. Family Court Review 39:299–315, 2001

Tippins TM, Wittmann JP: Empirical and ethical problems with custody recommendations: a call for clinical humility and judicial vigilance. Family Court Review 43:193–222, 2005

Walker AG: Handbook on Questioning Children: A Linguistic Perspective, 2nd Edition. Washington, DC, American Bar Association Center for Children and the Law, 1999

Chapter 12

Parenting Assessment in Abuse, Neglect, and Permanent Wardship Cases

Jack P. Haynes, Ph.D.

Forensic Assessment and Parenting Assessment

Forensic assessment takes place at the interface of mental health disciplines and the legal process. It most often results from directives from the legal system for the purposes of the legal system, distinct from most traditional assessments that are based on the request of and on behalf of a patient. Melton et al. (2007) discussed extensively the differences of scope, autonomy, pace, and context between forensic assessment and therapeutic assessment.

Parenting assessment is a type of forensic assessment. Most parenting assessments take place post-adjudication and follow a determination by a court, although some assessments involve whether physical, sexual, or emotional abuse or physical neglect has taken place. Some assessments include evaluation in the context of termination of parental rights to determine if a parent is unable or unfit to care for the child.

Parenting assessment often includes recommendations about whether a child should be under the care and custody of the parent or parents versus another family member or a social agency, either temporarily or permanently. Parenting assessments assist the court by providing judges and other finders of fact with reasoned and scientifically related analyses upon which to make decisions about child welfare.

Child Abuse and Neglect

Etiology

According to the U.S. Department of Health and Human Services, more than 900,000 children annually are victims of abuse or neglect. Annually about 12 of every 1,000 children are abused or neglected, a rate consistent for more than 10 years (U.S. Department of Health and Human Services 2006). Child Protective Service agencies report a 30% substantiation rate for allegations. More than 60% of the children were involved for neglect, 16% for physical abuse, 8% for sexual abuse, 6% for psychological maltreatment, and 2% for medical neglect. Youngest children are at the highest risk, with 75% of the deaths being children age 4 years and younger (Tishelman et al. 2006).

Physical abuse can range from bruises and abrasions to fractures, internal trauma, and death. In recent years, there has also been focus on Munchausen by proxy, the creation of an actual or apparent illness in a child or the false reporting of illness by a parent

(Levin and Sheridan 1995). Neglect can be conceptualized primarily as involving physical, medical, educational, or emotional maltreatment or physical abandonment.

Social, economic, and psychological factors are associated with child abuse. Social isolation and lack of social support often are identified with child maltreatment (Coohey 1996; Gelles and Straus 1979). Lack of access to material resources and lack of involvement with relatives and friends can be significantly contributory. Social isolation and lack of social support may interact with economic factors (Garbarino and Crouter 1978; Garbarino and Sherman 1980; Melton 1992). Child maltreatment often occurs in the context of families with other significant problems such as substance abuse or unemployment (National Research Council 1993).

As for psychological factors associated with child abuse and neglect, severe mental illness is not typical among abusive or neglectful parents (National Research Council 1993). Gaudin et al. (1995) found specific clusters of family dynamics among low-income neglectful families to be more associated with maltreatment than mental illness of parents. Research has found stronger association between maltreatment and low parental empathy and low sense of competence more than with mental illness (Milner et al. 1995). Research to date does not appear to support the concept of a child abuser syndrome.

Prognosis

Relatively little published research exists on treatment of abused and neglected children or their parents (Melton and Flood 1994). Much of the existing research suggests apparent underutilization of resources regarding children and parents involved with maltreatment. There often is a lack of compliance by parents of abused and neglected children, even with court-ordered psychological treatment, parent education, and other treatment components.

Legal, Philosophical, and Policy Parameters

All states require identified professionals to report suspected abuse or neglect of children. However, the context of child abuse and neglect often includes competing interests. One perspective emphasizes active protection and broad authority for intervention regarding abuse and neglect and also emphasizes ex-

pending state resources and programs for rehabilitation. This viewpoint favors withdrawal of the child or children from the family of origin for the purposes of protection (Platt 1977).

A competing perspective emphasizes awareness of possible harm and disruption to a child resulting from dramatic intervention and withdrawal, except in severe cases. This viewpoint highlights that state agencies have limited resources and that there are dangers consequent to easy intervention. As an example, Goldstein et al. (1973, 1979), who articulated the concept of the best interests of the child, view the state or its surrogate as an unlikely satisfactory substitute for a family but recommend state intervention in situations of clear harm, situations most likely to end up in permanent wardship.

The jurisdiction of abuse and neglect cases resides within a variety of courts—family, juvenile, probate, or trial courts. Although legal definitions of abuse and neglect vary, all states sanction state intervention regarding allegedly physically abused, sexually abused, and neglected children. The Child Abuse Prevention and Treatment Act of 1974 (CAPTA) linked federal funding of state child abuse programs with certain requirements and fostered similarity of state laws. CAPTA has been amended, reauthorized as the Keeping Children and Families Safe Act of 2003.

Physical Abuse and Neglect

As for physical abuse, states vary regarding the extent of injury necessary to be relevant. This relates also to the issue of variability among investigators as well as triers of fact of what constitutes appropriate versus inappropriate discipline. There also is a variety of possible definitions of neglect, from physical care and supervision issues to failure to protect. Mental health clinicians who assess abuse and neglect should be familiar with the relevant statutes in their particular legal jurisdiction.

Sexual Abuse

Most states reference sexual abuse in both criminal and civil statutes. Sexual abuse allegations can emerge in various legal contexts, not only in juvenile or probate court but also through family or divorce courts and adult criminal proceedings.

The specific nature and extent of the abuse are important variables in sexual abuse cases. In sexual abuse, the psychological significance of the abuse to the child may be as important—or more important—than in physical abuse. There is a wide range of possible behaviors. The impact on the child may be related to the nature and frequency of the abuse. Sexual abuse, physical abuse, and neglect are broad concepts and may overlap. Clinicians need to focus on the specifics of each case.

Allegations of sexual abuse during or postdivorce, as well as during custody and parenting time disputes, have increased during the past 25 years. Allegations of sexual abuse in divorce, custody, and parenting time contexts may be controversial and intense because typically in traditional juvenile court contexts, no one could stand to "benefit" from such allegations, whereas in divorce, custody, and parenting time dispute contexts, often the person reporting abuse or neglect is the estranged spouse or partner of the person accused, either by direct report or through report to a mandatory reporting professional. Sexual abuse allegations can severely affect the process of divorce, custody, and parenting time, with a near universal cessation of contact between the accused and the child, and the interruption may extend for months or years, even when allegations are not substantiated.

Emotional Abuse

This chapter emphasizes neglect and physical and sexual abuse more than emotional abuse because some states cover this topic by statute and some do not. Some states allow for prosecution regarding emotional abuse and neglect, but clear and specific definition is difficult, and consequently the adjudication of it often is challenging.

Definitions regarding what constitutes emotional abuse lack consensus. In contrast to physical abuse, sexual abuse, and neglect, which have tangible aspects to them, emotional abuse as an allegation to be proved in court may be less tangible and also more challenging in terms of demonstration of cause and effect. Typically, psychological problems for a child must be demonstrated to have been caused by the behavior of the parent.

Termination of Parental Rights

In the most serious or repeated cases of child maltreatment, the state attempts to terminate the rights of the parents. Few states define standards of minimal parenting competence or describe specific behaviors.

The legal standard for permanent wardship established by the U.S. Supreme Court requires clear and convincing evidence (*Santosky v. Kramer* 1982). All states have statutes providing for court termination of parental rights. Approximately 15% of adjudicated abuse and neglect cases end in permanent wardship of the child, with the rights of the parents terminated (Herring 1992).

The legal standard considers the child's best interests to be most significant (National Clearinghouse on Child Abuse and Neglect Information 2001). The most common bases for termination of parental rights are severe or chronic abuse or neglect of a child or his or her siblings, abandonment, significant mental illness, long-term substance abuse problems, felony conviction regarding violence against the child or another family member, or involuntary termination of the rights of the parent to another of their children.

Parenting Assessment Content and Process

Legal Process

Other than as a mandated reporter of suspected child abuse, most often clinicians are not involved in the early, preadjudicative phase involving abuse and neglect. In some child custody and parenting time cases, clinicians are called upon by courts to review the findings of Child Protective Services and opine from their own contact with the child, though that clinician may be late in the sequence of professionals who have interviewed the child. Hence, a question may be raised if what a child reports has become contaminated. A question also may be raised regarding the role of the mental health clinician who is functioning as an investigator and who may not have access to all the facts.

Guidelines

The American Psychological Association (1998) and the American Academy of Child and Adolescent Psychiatry (1997) have produced guidelines regarding evaluations in child protection matters. The underlying principles recommend a systematic approach utilizing multiple methods of data gathering. Evaluators should be familiar with the guidelines for their profession. Table 12–1 provides a summary guideline of the structure and content of parenting evaluation.

Little empirical examination has been made of the extent to which parenting evaluations in child protec-

TABLE 12–1. Structure and content of parenting evaluation

1. Be familiar with guidelines of your profession for assessment in child protection cases.

2. Understand the specific referral question, what the court expects, the legal context, and the legal status of the case.

3. Oral and written informed consent should also include explanations of confidentiality and who the client is in the evaluation.

4. Review collateral information, including legal, social, educational, therapeutic, and medical, for parents and child.

5. Interview style and structure should focus on rapport building and should involve multiple interviews, both conjoint and individual for parents.

6. History components for parents should include interviews regarding the following:

    a. Family-of-origin experiences, including how the parent was parented as well as family-of-origin values, discipline experiences, rewards, punishment, rules, communication, expectations

    b. Educational, occupational, health, and legal history; traumas; disabilities

    c. Mental health treatment (inpatient and outpatient), substance use and abuse, psychotropic medication history

    d. Marital history/relationship of each parent, including violence

    e. Family and nonfamily relationships, support systems

7. Parenting capacity interview components should include the following:

    a. Capacity to care

        i.   Value system

        ii. Nurturance, attachment, emotional support, affection, sensitivities, empathy, responsiveness, communication abilities, awareness of child's needs

        iii. Involvement of parent with physician, dentist, psychotherapist, teachers, day care provider

        iv. Involvement of parent with homework, hygiene, school, clothing, child's friends

    b. Capacity to protect

        i.   Supervision, limit setting, discipline, guidance, safety

        ii. Parental tolerance for frustration and management of anxiety

        iii. Parental risk taking, parental advocacy

    c. Capacity to change

        i.   Assess parental intelligence

        ii. Parental reactions to mental health or substance abuse treatment, casework directives, parent education classes

        iii. Ability of parent to manage personal problems and to differentiate themselves from child

        iv. Mental status exam if needed

8. Parenting instruments

9. Parent psychological testing:

    a. Intelligence testing

    b. Objective and projective personality testing

10. Child interview should include the following:

    a. Developmental issues and developmental level of child; explore broad experiences and resilience of child

    b. Attachment, parent emotional availability, separation issues, suggestibility

TABLE 12–1. Structure and content of parenting evaluation *(continued)*

11. Child psychological testing:

    a. Intelligence

    b. Personality

    c. Academic achievement

12. Parent–child observations:

    a. Multiple occasions and locations desirable

    b. Parents observed separately with child

13. Court reports should be structured in the following manner:

    a. Documentation organized

    b. Legal issues, history and context

    c. Data logically connected to conclusions

    d. Test and instrument data connected to interview and collateral data, inconsistencies discussed

    e. Discussion of subspecialty consultations, if any

    f. Functioning level of child and of each parent

    g. Overview of parent capacity to care, protect, change

    h. Impact of child's maltreatment history, options, and prognosis

    i. Risks and benefits of reunification

tion matters conform to such guidelines. Two studies that investigated the topic found limited compliance (Budd et al. 2001; Morietti et al. 2003). It would seem likely that the emphasis on evidence-based practice will lead to further investigation.

Doing specialty work such as evaluation in matters of abuse and neglect assumes proper and adequate training and knowledge. Consultative work with colleagues is advised, especially in a matter such as termination of parental rights.

Parent Assessment

Referral Question

The most important part of the initiation of parent assessment (or any forensic evaluation) is to clearly understand the referral question. Clinicians must respond to the questions the court is posing to them. If needed, clarification should be obtained before proceeding, if possible in writing.

Legal Context

Understand the legal context. For example, the concept of "best interests" may have different applicability in a family court proceeding such as custody or parenting time than in a juvenile court proceeding involving abuse or neglect allegations in which best interests of

the child may be counterbalanced by consideration of the best interests of the parents.

Additionally, the current legal status of the case is important. Do the parents have contact with the child, and if so, what is the nature of the contact, what has been the timeline of legal decisions in the matter, and is there a legal guardian for the child?

Who Is the Client?

If the court has ordered the evaluation, the court is the client. Evaluation materials including reports are the work product of the court, releasable only with court permission. Any evaluations not directed by order of the court must proceed very carefully, especially in the area of recommendations. The only basis for recommendation is if all relevant parties have been evaluated directly. For example, the current American Psychological Association (2003) Ethical Principles and Code of Conduct states that assessment opinion contained in statements, recommendations, and conclusions must have adequate support and substantiation.

Ex Parte Communications

Avoid ex parte communications, such as communicating with one party or his or her attorney but not the other party or his or her attorney or the prosecutor. Best practice dictates that evaluator communication be conjoint. Written and electronic communications by the evaluator should be shared with each attorney (and prosecutor), and received communications from any of the attorneys should be shared with the other attorneys. Phone calls should be conjoint with all the attorneys. Stating this policy clearly at the outset simplifies matters and minimizes conflicts and issues.

Informed Consent

The evaluation typically begins with an explanation of informed consent and confidentiality. Informed consent needs to be clear, systematic, organized, operational, spoken, and written, signed at the outset of the evaluation.

The informed consent process should express in writing the basis of the evaluation, such as which court has ordered the evaluation and for what purpose. Informed consent should explain that the court is the client and the evaluee may or may not personally benefit from the evaluation. The distinction between forensic evaluation and psychotherapy should be stated, and the limits of confidentiality should be discussed. The assessment components should be described. The evaluator should explain that a report will be generated, that recommendations will be made, and that the examiner may testify in court and offer opinions and recommendations. The options of the evaluee to consult an attorney if he or she has any questions should be stated, and that the evaluator will answer questions about the evaluation.

I use a forensic informed consent form that delineates these elements and others. Adult evaluees are asked to read along as I slowly read aloud the informed consent form and are encouraged to ask any questions. They are asked to sign the form if they have understood and agree to the content.

Confidentiality

The limits to confidentiality in court-ordered evaluations should be discussed separately. The court as well as the defense, prosecuting, and child guardian attorneys, and sometimes Child Protective Services and other relevant individuals identified on the release of confidentiality form, will have knowledge of the content of the evaluation and will receive a copy of the evaluation report including conclusions and recommendations.

A parent in such situations may not have legal custody of the child at the time of the evaluation. If parents have custody, releases to obtain confidential information about the child or children from community sources should be obtained after the basis has been explained.

Review of Case History and Current Issues

One of the underlying issues to remember is that the majority of clinical literature is based on research and group data. The opinion of the professional in a particular case must be based on a particular child in a particular family in the context of the specific findings and what is known about the dynamics of abuse and neglect circumstances as indicated in the professional literature.

Interview Style and Structure

As in any clinical evaluation, establishing rapport in a parenting evaluation is important. Several interviews are preferable to a single extended interview. Multiple interviews repeatedly sample behavior and increase the likelihood of collecting reliable information. Parents should be seen individually as well as conjointly, if feasible. Questions should include both general and very specific inquiry. Care must be taken to ask questions in ways that do not suggest or imply any expected or desirable response in this highly motivationally distorted context.

Basic History Components of Interview

Obtain a detailed personal history of each parent. It is important to ascertain the experience of how the parent in question was him- or herself parented as a child and what implications this may have had for his or her behavior as a parent. Inquire about similarities and differences between the life of the parent as a child and the life of their child regarding values, discipline, punishment, rewards, rules, communication, and expectations.

Educational, occupational, health, and legal histories (civil and criminal, including Personal Protection Orders against them) should be taken. Are disabilities present? Has the parent experienced any significant traumas? Explore relevant cultural or subcultural issues.

Explore substance use and abuse as well as mental health treatment, both inpatient and outpatient treatment and participation in self-help groups. Have psychotropic drugs been prescribed, and is the parent currently being prescribed any?

Explore the marital/relationship history of each parent. Has there been violence, and if so, what kind, how often, and has the child witnessed violence? What has been the emotional climate of their relationship, and what has the child experienced?

What are the family and nonfamily relationships? What is the support system of the parent, and to what extent are they socially isolated or integrated? What are their most significant relationships? How does each parent choose to spend free time?

Parenting Capacity Components of Interview

Grisso (1986) presented several constructs regarding parenting capacity, a key aspect of parenting assessment in abuse and neglect evaluations. His constructs included recommended inquiry regarding nurturing and physical care, training and management of the psychological needs of the child, teaching and skill training regarding care and safety, orienting the child to the social aspects of his or her world, transmission of cultural and subcultural goals and values, promoting interpersonal skills and behaviors, and guidance regarding the child formulating his or her own goals.

Barnum (2001) focused on parenting capacities involving protection and care. Protection encompasses the extent to which a parent prevents a child from harm, including discipline and conflict resolution. Care refers to nurturance, growth-promoting activities, skill building, and related behaviors.

Budd's (2005) parenting capacity evaluation model proposed that the evaluation should center on parenting, should use a functional approach emphasizing behaviors and skills in daily performance, and should employ a minimal parenting standard rather than comparing parental behavior to optimal functioning.

My view regarding assessing parenting capacity in abuse and neglect cases focuses on parental capacities for protection and care but additionally emphasizes the capacity of a parent to change his or her own behavior, a central, disposition-related issue in cases of abuse and neglect. Assessing capacity is inferential, but the solidity of inference increases with the number of tangible behavioral anchors that are identified. Because statutes focus on levels of minimal acceptable care, the focus should be on minimal standards rather than optimal standards.

Interview Structure Regarding Parent Capacity to Care

Parents' information and perceptions about the matters before the court can provide useful information about their value system and the extent of their valuation of the child. Not only can questions about the nature of their relationship and their involvement with the child provide data that can be compared with reports by third parties of the actual behavior of the parents toward the

children, but what a parent says or omits can also be helpful in assessing parenting capacity to care.

Inquire about behaviors related to nurturance, attachment, emotional support, and affection. Inquiry about each parent's history of protecting the child can provide information about their sensitivities and capacities. Questions about the physical care of the child in actual or hypothetical situations in which the child has been or could be injured can reveal the degree of parental attachment and empathy. Explore parental responsiveness and communication abilities. How aware is the parent of the needs of the child, and is the parent capable of subordinating his or her own needs to the needs of the child? Inquire about the history of the parent's practical involvement with the child. Contact the child's physician, dentist, psychotherapist, counselor, teachers, day care provider. Ask questions about homework, hygiene, school activities, clothing, shopping, and the child's friends.

Interview Structure Regarding Parent Capacity to Protect

Inquiries about supervision, limit setting, discipline, guidance, safeguards, potentially dangerous behavior, and neighborhood problems are relevant in assessing a parent's capacity to protect. The content of inquiry can vary depending on the age of the child, with infants and other preschool children having different needs and being more dependent and more vulnerable.

Inquiries about parental response to challenging situations in child rearing, real or hypothetical, will provide information about the parents' tolerance for frustration and identification of and management of their own anxiety. Questions about child or parental risk taking as well as parental advocacy elicit information regarding the capacity to protect.

Interview Structure Regarding Parent Capacity for Change

Although controversies exist whether mental health clinicians in evaluation situations involving abuse and neglect should express an opinion regarding dispositional issues, including permanent wardship, many courts specifically direct clinicians to opine in those areas. The issue of capacity for change is central to disposition and important to assess. By definition, a parent against whom charges have been found to be true will be required to demonstrate change or capacity for change of behaviors from those that led to the abuse or neglect finding.

Parental intelligence level is a constant and can be relevant. Intellectual assessment is discussed in the psychological testing section below. A low level of measured intelligence can limit the ability of a parent to demonstrate insight into and basic understanding of his or her behavior and the behavior of the child. It also may influence the ability of the parent to understand and change his or her own problematic behavior.

Capacity for change can be reflected in parental behavior regarding psychological or substance abuse treatment, if any, or response to casework directives, and the extent of participation and compliance with parent education or other programs.

Inquiry about behaviors and experiences involving parental depression, anxiety, anger, impulse control, ruminations, and obsessions can reveal the extent to which the parents are focused on their own issues, how they differentiate themselves from their children, and how they respond to child-rearing demands. Do a mental status exam if indicated. The way a parent has handled treatment regarding substance abuse or mental illness also is germane to a parent's insight and capacity for change. Sattler (1998) suggested specific parenting assessment questions.

Parenting Instruments

Otto and Edens (2003) have comprehensively examined parenting instruments. As they pointed out, parenting instruments do not provide an empirical indication of present or future functional parenting ability; they do assess current characteristics of parents. The following instruments—all self-report measures—are used for assessing parenting characteristics and parenting orientation but do not focus directly on parenting issues as related to abuse or neglect.

The Child Abuse Potential Inventory (CAPI; Milner 1986) was developed to identify the risk of a parent physically abusing a child but not other forms of abuse or neglect. The 10 scales include a Child Abuse Scale and three validity scales. Fifty percent of the validation samples consisted of known physical child abusers. Cutting scores are used rather than normative tables. Scores do not represent the odds that an individual has abused a child nor the likelihood that an individual may abuse a child in the future. Some reviewers (e.g., Melton 1989) suggest that the CAPI shows more promise as a screening instrument than as a clinical tool.

The Parenting Stress Index (PSI; Abidin 1995) has been widely researched to measure parenting stress and has also been used as a measure of intervention effects. It has been used to measure dysfunctional parenting and predicts the potential for problematic parental behavior. Three areas of stress are measured. It can be used as a measure of parental effectiveness. The PSI is focused especially on preschool-age children but can be used with parents whose children are up to 12 years old.

The Parent–Child Relationship Inventory (PCRI; Gerard 1994) assesses parental attitudes toward parenting and toward their children. There are seven content scales and two validity scales. Among other things, the scales measure the perceived level of support a parent receives, parental experiences in disciplining a child, the ability of a parent to promote a child's independence, and the level of parental interaction with and knowledge of his or her child.

The Parenting Satisfaction Scale (PSS; Guidubaldi and Cleminshaw 1994) assesses parenting satisfaction along three dimensions: satisfaction with the parenting of the child's other parent, satisfaction with their own relationship with the child, and satisfaction with their own parenting performance. Like the PSI and PCRI, the PSS is not designed specifically for use with parents of reportedly abused or neglected children but may provide useful information about parenting dynamics.

Parenting instruments can provide related information in the context of clinical assessment regarding abuse and neglect, but the information is more general than specific and relates more to parental orientation than matching specific parental attributes of parenting with specific characteristics of the child or children in question in a specific case. There is a lack of necessary connection between specific parenting abilities and specific needs of a specific child.

Parental Psychological Testing

Psychological testing makes a strong contribution to assessment of parents in abuse and neglect situations. Testing provides independent, norm-based sources of data to understand the parents.

Psychological testing in parent assessment in abuse and neglect situations primarily involves personality testing of two types—standardized testing and projective testing—and may involve cognitive assessment, most often the Wechsler Adult Intelligence Scale, Third Edition (WAIS-III; Wechsler 1997). The WAIS-III is an individually administered instrument that assesses cognitive components, can determine suspected low intellectual functioning, and may help differentiate cognitive from personality dysfunction.

Standardized personality tests are norm-based, self-report instruments that produce scores on scales that have been shown to be valid and reliable. The two tests most commonly administered to parents in this context are the Minnesota Multiphasic Personality Inventory–2 (MMPI-2; Butcher et al. 2001) and Millon Clinical Multiaxial Inventory–III (MCMI-III; Millon 1997). Both are tests of psychopathology, have validity scales, are in a true/false format, are scored by computer, and produce norm-based scores on many scales.

Pathological personality functioning can be assessed and examined regarding the functioning of the child in question. These tests have not been constructed for specific use in assessing parents involved with abuse and neglect, but they measure coping style, adjustment, affective functioning, and perceptions. Tests such as the Beck Depression Inventory–II (Beck et al. 1996) or Psychopathy Checklist—Revised (Hare 2003) can be used when depression or psychopathy is suspected. If alcohol abuse is relevant, the Michigan Alcohol Screening Test (Selzer 1971) can be useful. If significant brain injury is suspected, referral for neurological examination or neuropsychological assessment may be indicated.

The Rorschach is a projective, unstructured measure of personality in which ambiguous stimuli are presented and interpreted according to principles to provide information about personality functioning. Typically, an empirically based system of scoring is used (Exner 2002).

Collateral Information Review

Primary sources are important and can provide a rich source of direct information about parent and child functioning. Collateral information includes court documents, Child Protective Services reports, police reports, and information about the parents from diverse but direct service provider sources to parents and children, such as psychotherapists, other types of therapists, physicians, schools, teachers, tutors, sports coaches, child care providers, probation officers, parent educators, substance abuse treatment or mental health facilities, and others. Hard copy of inpatient mental health or substance abuse treatment records should be obtained because of frequent situational motivational distortion as well as inaccurate or sketchy recall by evaluees.

Child Assessment

Assessment of the child in a parenting assessment is essential, though less an extended focus than the parents. Developmental issues, emotional functioning, school functioning, peer relations, and family relationships including sibling relationships need to be explored. Review of records and direct interview and contact with diverse sources of professionals who have been involved with the child are important. Information about the functioning of the child should be obtained separately from each parent. Information should also be obtained about such functioning from current caregivers and, if appropriate, from close relatives of the child and from potential caregivers of the child. The length of time the child has been separated from the parents and the nature of the specific abuse or neglect need to be considered during interview with the child.

It is important to explore the nature of attachment of the child to each parent as part of understanding the orientation of the child to the parents and to understand the likely experience by the child of each parent. From the perspective of the parent, attachment is part of parenting capacity to be caring, but it also is important from the perspective of the child's experience. It also is an important part of the parent–child relationship to be examined by inquiry of parents and child separately but also observed in the parent–child observations. Many of the areas of inquiry about parenting capacity to care and to protect can be reframed for interview of the child.

Interview of children can focus on aspects of attachment, such as the perceived emotional availability of each parent and the perceived capacity of each parent to focus on the child and be responsive and sensitive. Questions about resilience and about feelings of separation from the parents will be illuminating regarding the attachment by the child to each parent. Although measurement instruments have been constructed, they are at the research level and are not suitable for forensic clinical use in parenting assessment cases (Schmidt et al. 2007).

Interview Caveats and Developmental Issues

A thorough and detailed explication of interview considerations and specific techniques regarding interviewing children in forensic settings is available in Gudas and Sattler (2006), and more specifically regarding sexual abuse evaluation settings in Ceci and Bruck (1995). The focus of this chapter is parenting assessment, so child interviewing is referenced mostly in terms of caveats regarding structural issues on children that may affect the outcome of parenting assessment.

The memory of preschool children, relatively speaking, is immature, and their vocabulary is limited. As for suggestibility, preschool children can be highly suggestible, school-age children less so. Developmentally, with preschool children, wishful thinking may be mixed with factual events, and children of this age proceed in a highly egocentric manner. School-age children are highly variable in developmental level, think more factually than logically, typically understand cause–effect relationships, and may be vulnerable to negative feedback. Adolescents have a much greater capacity for abstract thought but may be impulsive, resistant, and negative. They may be very focused on confidentiality.

Psychological Testing of Children Ages 6 Years and Older

Psychological testing is often undertaken for abused and neglected children age 6 years or older. Children age 6 typically attend school, and achievement testing becomes feasible. Academic achievement is important to measure because school functioning is often a bellwether of problematic functioning for children with problematic home situations. Stresses from home are evident at school, and academic achievement often is one measure. A frequently administered individual achievement test in juvenile court circumstances is the Wide Range Achievement Test, the WRAT-4 being its current version (Haynes and Peltier 1983b; Pinkerman et al. 1993).

Individual intelligence testing by the current Wechsler test, currently the Wechsler Intelligence Scale for Children, Fourth Edition (Wechsler 2003), can give a current measure of a child's cognitive functioning and also may show or suggest possible personality dysfunction through the child's specific functioning and specific responses to test items. The specific issues of abuse or neglect may increase the value of information provided by testing a particular child with this instrument.

Personality testing of older children can be accomplished with some paper-and-pencil instruments, whereas projective instruments (e.g., Rorschach or Thematic Apperception Test/Children's Apperception Test) are much of what is available for younger children (Haynes and Peltier 1983a).

Psychological testing also can be useful for generating hypotheses about a child's functioning to be further explored by interview or examination of collateral materials or through making collateral professional contacts.

Collateral Information Review

It is important to determine the extent of involvement of the child with resources such as psychotherapy, medical care, social casework, school, church, tutoring, sports activities, and other community resources as connected with the actions of each parent and the needs of the child. These are relevant to the parent's ability regarding care, protection, and capacity for change.

Third-Party Information

The clinician should focus also on inquiry from direct service providers of their observations of the parent–child interaction. Open-ended inquiry works best initially, with follow-up questions framed in terms of apparent display of parent care, protection, and commitment to the child, exploring issues such as parental interest, responsiveness, perseverance, and advocacy.

Parent–Child Interaction: Format and Location

The format for evaluating parent–child interaction may be determined by the court. In some circumstances direct parent–child observation is not permitted because of the status of the case, as in permanent wardship. If possible, observation in the home or in community settings that are less controlled than the examiner's office is desirable. If the parents do not live together, each parent should be seen separately with the child. Multiple observations are desirable.

The working assumption is each parent will attempt to demonstrate his or her best behavior. Parameters to observe include nature of apparent attachment between parent and child; parental notice of and focus on the child's emotional or physical needs as demonstrated; parent understanding of developmental level of the child; parental response to handling of oppositional, aggressive, or frustrating behavior, if any, by the child; and an impression of the orientation of the parent to care and protect.

Report for the Court
Format and Structure

It is important to keep clear and organized documentation for the court or for others to review. The report should be clear, concise, issue focused, and data connected. The legal issue, legal context, and legal history should be stated. The procedures used and length of interviews should be specified so that what transpired is clear to the trier of fact and others involved in the legal process. Collateral material review and collateral contacts made should be documented in the beginning of the report and should be referenced in the body of the report. Data should be connected to conclusions. Psychological test results and any qualifications of results or inconsistencies should be stated. Any deviations from standard practice should be stated and explained.

If there are subspecialty areas involved, the evaluator should state the results of the consultations with experts in those subspecialty areas, including unusual injuries (such as shaken baby), unusual psychological trauma (such as Munchausen by proxy), a child's unusual traumatic experience (such as sexual assault or physical abandonment), or a child's special physical or cognitive needs. Koocher (2006) enumerated numerous issues to be considered in constructing a forensic psychological report involving children and adolescents.

Functioning Level of Child

The nature and extent of impact on the child from the maltreatment that has taken place should be discussed. The options for the child should be discussed in light of the data.

Functioning Level of Each Parent

Both parents (if there are two parents involved) should have their own conclusions and their own assessments regarding their capacity to care, to protect, and to change their behavior. Intellectual level, parenting history, assessment of parenting capacity, and likelihood of change all must be assessed in terms of the best interests of the child.

Recommendations

Some courts direct that recommendations be made in clinical evaluations; some do not want recommendations. This is particularly significant for termination of rights evaluations. Conclusions and recommendations should be clearly linked to the referral question and also to the data gathered. Uncertainties, ambiguities, and inconsistencies of results or viewpoints should be stated and explained, if possible.

Conclusions and recommendations should discuss risk–benefit issues to the child whose best interests are the focal issue. This is particularly the case regarding termination of rights and the risk–benefit to the child of not terminating rights.

—Key Points

— Understand the legal context of the case, including referral question and relevant statutes.

— Avoid the pitfalls of ex parte communications.

— Proceed with clear spoken and written informed consent, including explanation of confidentiality.

— History and information gathering should be shaped by consideration of parent capacity to care, to protect, and to change.

— Psychological testing and administration of parenting measures can broaden sources of data to consider.

— The report for the court should be concise, issue focused, and data connected. The nature and extent of impact of maltreatment on the child should be discussed.

References

Abidin RR: Parenting Stress Index Manual, 3rd Edition. Odessa, FL, Psychological Assessment Resources, 1995

American Academy of Child and Adolescent Psychiatry: Practice parameters for the forensic evaluation of children and adolescents who may have been physically or sexually abused. J Am Acad Child Adolesc Psychiatry 36:423–442, 1997

American Psychological Association, Committee on Professional Practice and Standards: Guidelines for Psychological Evaluations in Child Protection Matters. Washington, DC, American Psychological Association, 1998

American Psychological Association: Ethical Principles of Psychologists and Code of Conduct. Washington, DC, American Psychological Association, 2003

Barnum R: Parenting assessment in cases of neglect and abuse, in Comprehensive Textbook of Child and Adolescent Forensic Psychiatry. Edited by Shetky D, Benedek E. Washington, DC, American Psychiatric Press, 2001, pp 81–96

Beck AT, Steer RA, Brown GK: Beck Depression Inventory–II. San Antonio, TX, Psychological Corporation, 1996

Budd KS: Assessing parenting capacity in a child welfare context. Child Youth Serv Rev 27:429–444, 2005

Budd KS, Poindexter LM, Felix E, et al: Clinical assessment of parents in child protection cases: an empirical analysis. Law Hum Behav 25:93–108, 2001

Butcher J, Graham JR, Ben Porath YS, et al: Minnesota Multiphasic Personality Inventory—Revised Edition (MMPI-2): Manual for Administration, Scoring and Interpretation. Minneapolis, University of Minnesota Press, 2001

Ceci SJ, Bruck M: Jeopardy in the Courtroom. Washington, DC, American Psychological Association, 1995

Coohey C: Child maltreatment: testing the social isolation hypothesis. Child Abuse Negl 20:241–254, 1996

Exner J: The Rorschach, Basic Foundations and Principles of Interpretation. New York, Wiley, 2002

Garbarino J, Crouter A: Defining the community context of parent-child relations: the correlates of child maltreatment. Child Dev 49:604–616, 1978

Garbarino J, Sherman D: High-risk neighborhoods and high-risk families: the human ecology of child maltreatment. Child Dev 51:188–198, 1980

Gaudin JM, Polansky NA, Kilpatrick AC, et al: Family functioning in neglectful families. Child Abuse Negl 20:363–377, 1995

Gelles RJ, Straus MA: Determinants of violence in the family: toward a theoretical integration, in Contemporary Theories About Family, Vol 1: Research-Based Theories. Edited by Burr WR, Hill R, Nye FI, et al. New York, Free Press, 1979, pp 549–581

Gerard AB: Parent–Child Relationship Inventory Manual. Los Angeles, CA, Western Psychological Services, 1994

Goldstein J, Freud A, Solnit A: Beyond the Best Interests of the Child. New York, Free Press, 1973

Goldstein J, Freud A, Solnit A: Before the Best Interests of the Child. New York, Free Press, 1979

Grisso T: Evaluating Competencies. New York, Plenum, 1986

Gudas LS, Sattler JM: Forensic interviewing of children and adolescents, in Forensic Mental Health Assessment of Children and Adolescents. Edited by Sparta SN, Koocher GP. New York, Oxford University Press, 2006, pp 115–128

Guidubaldi J, Cleminshaw HK: The Parenting Satisfaction Scale. San Antonio, TX, Psychological Corporation, 1994

Hare RM: Manual for the Revised Psychopathy Checklist, 2nd Edition. Toronto, ON, Canada, Multi-Health Systems, 2003

Haynes J, Peltier J: Patterns of practice with the TAT in juvenile forensic settings. J Pers Assess 49:26–29, 1983a

Haynes J, Peltier J: Psychological assessment practices in juvenile forensic settings. Psychol Rep 52:759–762, 1983b

Herring DJ: Inclusion of the reasonable efforts requirement in termination of parental rights statutes: punishing the child for the failures of the state child welfare system. Univ Pittsburgh Law Review 54:139–209, 1992

Koocher GP: Ethical issues in assessment of children and adolescents, in Forensic Mental Health Assessment of Children and Adolescents. Edited by Sparta SN, Koocher GP. New York, Oxford University Press, 2006, pp 46–63

Levin AV, Sheridan MS: Munchausen Syndrome by Proxy: Issues in Diagnosis and Treatment. New York, Lexington Books, 1995

Melton GB: Review of the Child Abuse Potential Inventory, Form VI, in The Tenth Mental Measurements Yearbook. Edited by Conoley JC, Kramer JJ. Lincoln, NB, The Buros Institute of Mental Measurements, 1989, pp 153–155

Melton GB: It's time for neighborhood research and action. Child Abuse Negl 16:909–913, 1992

Melton GB, Flood MF: Research policy and child maltreatment: developing the scientific foundation for effective protection of children. Child Abuse Negl 18 (suppl 1):1–28, 1994

Melton GB, Petrila J, Poythress NG, et al: Psychological Evaluations for the Courts: A Handbook for Mental Health Professionals and Lawyers, 3rd Edition. New York, Guilford, 2007

Millon T: The Millon Inventories: Clinical and Personality Assessment. New York, Guilford, 1997

Milner JS: The Child Abuse Potential Inventory Manual. Webster, NC, Psytec Inc, 1986

Milner JS, Halsey LB, Fultz J: Empathic responsiveness and affective reactivity to infant stimuli in high- and low-risk for physical abuse mothers. Child Abuse Negl 19:767–780, 1995

Morietti MM, Campbell J, Samra J, et al: Final Report: An Empirical Evaluation of Parenting Capacity Assessments in British Columbia: Toward Quality Assurance and Evidence Based Practice. British Columbia, Canada: Family Court Centre, Provincial Services, Ministry for Children and Family Development, 2003

National Clearinghouse on Child Abuse and Neglect Information: Statutes at a Glance: Grounds for Termination of Parenting Rights. Washington, DC, 2001

National Research Council: Understanding Child Abuse and Neglect. Washington, DC, National Academy Press, 1993

Otto RK, Edens JF: Parenting capacity, in Evaluating Competencies, 2nd Edition. Edited by Grisso T. New York, Kluwer Academic/Plenum, 2003, pp 229–307

Pinkerman J, Haynes JP, Keiser T: Characteristics of psychological practice in North American juvenile court clinics. Am J Forensic Psychol 11:3–12, 1993

Platt AM: The Child Savers, 2nd Edition. Chicago, University of Chicago Press, 1977

Santosky v Kramer, 455 US 745 (1982)

Sattler J: Clinical and Forensic Interviewing of Children and Families. San Diego, CA, Jerome M. Sattler Publisher, 1998

Schmidt F, Cuttress LJ, Lang J, et al: Assessing the parent-child relationship in parenting capacity evaluations: clinical applications of attachment research. Fam Court Rev 45:247–259, 2007

Selzer ML: The Michigan Alcoholism Screening Test (MAST): the quest for a new diagnostic instrument. Am J Psychiatry 127:1653–1658, 1971

Tishelman AC, Newton AW, Denton JE, et al: Child physical abuse and neglect: medical and other considerations in forensic psychological assessment, in Forensic Mental Health Assessment of Children and Adolescents. Edited by Sparta SN, Koocher GP. New York, Oxford University Press, 2006, pp 175–189

U.S. Department of Health and Human Services: Child Maltreatment. Washington, DC, U.S. Government Printing Office, 2006

Wechsler D: Wechsler Adult Intelligence Scale—3rd Edition. San Antonio, TX, Harcourt Assessment, 1997

Wechsler D: Wechsler Intelligence Scale for Children, 4th Edition. San Antonio, TX, Harcourt Assessment, 2003

Chapter 13

Children in Foster Care

Thomas M. Horner, Ph.D.
James B. Gale, M.S.

Foster care is a major force and factor in the fabric of social services in the United States. *Fostering* has both generic and specific meanings, the former encompassing the broadly distributed motives of caring and promoting of growth and the latter entailing the practices of raising and rearing children who are not one's own. Human fostering is a special case of the larger biological activity of *alloparenting.* Many species, as well as humans, engage in fostering. In humans, the specific fostering of children (and adults who are of a determinably limited mental capacity) occurs both inside and outside of the legal (or custom-driven) frameworks of societies, many of which have meticulous laws concerning foster placement.

In recent years, in the United States, about a half million children are in legally determined and directed foster care at any one time (U.S. Department of Health and Human Services 2008a; Table 13–1). This does not include the number of children who are in de facto but not de jure foster care—that is, the number of children abiding for an extended period of care, sometimes for extenuating reasons, sometimes to avoid an anticipated state intrusion on the basis of inadequate parenting, with someone who is not their birth parent or close relative by birth. An estimated 34% of the children in legal foster care are younger than 6 years, 28% are between ages 6 and 12 years, and the remainder are teenagers (U.S. Department of Health and Human Services 2008b, pp. 1–2).

Of the children placed in foster care in 2006, 46% lived with a nonrelative, whereas about 24% lived with a relative. The remainder lived in group homes and institutions. About 2% were at runaway status at any given time (U.S. Department of Health and Human Services 2008b, p. 2). Children's individual lengths of stay in foster care vary immensely and range from days and weeks in many instances to years in other instances (U.S. Department of Health and Human Services 2008b; Table 13–2). The average length of stay in foster care in 2006 was 28 months, and the median length of stay was somewhat shorter but still sizable: 15.5 months (U.S. Department of Health and Human Services 2008b, p. 2).

Two other parameters of foster care pertain: 1) its frequency—that is, how many separate times a child enters into foster care following re-placement with a birth parent or relative, and 2) its multiplicity—that is, how many different foster placements occur within the scope of any single period of removal from parental (or birth relative) care. In the United States, many children come into foster care, are then returned to the care of a birth parent or close relative, but later re-enter the foster care system because of recurring parental inadequacies or endangerments, thus affecting the frequency of foster care. In other situations, a child may be placed in foster care only to be shifted across several other foster care venues before settling into a more extended stay. In 2006, about 50% of the children returned to the care of their parent(s) or principal caregiver(s), whereas 23% were adopted after permanent terminations of parental rights were enacted (U.S. Department of Health and Human Services 2008b, p. 3). Once permanent termination of parental rights occurred, the average wait for adoptive placement was

TABLE 13–1. Estimated numbers of children in foster care: October 2001 to September 2007

Fiscal year	Children in care	Entries	Exits
10/01/01–09/30/02	523,000	295,000	278,000
10/01/02–09/30/03	510,000	289,000	278,000
10/01/03–09/30/04	507,000	298,000	280,000
10/01/04–09/30/05	511,000	307,000	287,000
10/01/05–09/30/06	509,000	303,000	290,000
10/01/06–09/30/07	496,000	293,000	287,000

Note.   All figures are estimates and entail roundings.
Source.   Adapted from U.S. Department of Health and Human Services 2008a, p. 2.

14.5 months of additional foster care. Fifty-nine percent of adoptions out of foster care are by the foster parent(s) themselves, whereas 26% and 15% are by relatives and nonrelatives, respectively (U.S. Department of Health and Human Services 2008b, pp. 10–11).

The public images of child foster care are dominated at times by the circumstances that lead to it and by the fact that children seem, at least to many incidental observers, to remain so long in foster care. Added to these images are perceptions of foster care as a generically inferior alternative to so-called ordinary or "normal" parenting. The fact is, however, that children in foster care rarely come out of ordinary or normal circumstances and situations, burdened as those circumstances and situations are by parental problems in adjustment, by parental behavioral and relationship

TABLE 13–2. Estimated lengths of stay in foster care: fiscal year 2006

Durations of stay in foster care	Percentage of foster care population
<1 month	5
1–5 months	19
6–11 months	18
12–17 months	13
18–23 months	9
24–29 months	7
30–35 months	5
3–4 years	11
≥5 years	13

Note.   All figures are estimates and entail roundings.
Source.   Adapted from U.S. Department of Health and Human Services 2008b, p. 2.

dysfunctionality, by frank material poverty, or by combinations of these factors. None of these factors alone is sufficient for removal of children from their legal caregivers. The underlying (and unifying) force of removal, apart from these factors, is the determinably neglectful or abusive behavior of one or more adults in the child's immediate environment. Threading itself between these two traditional poles of maltreatment is the force of what is widely termed *failure to protect*, which entails a caregiver's failure to keep the child out of the thrusting distance of violent acts.

Sometimes, of course, determined acts of abuse or neglect are willful on the part of the adult who commits them. Other times, they are not so much willful as they are operative by dint of aforementioned stressors. Thus, they may occur as outcroppings of parental immaturity, misjudgment, ignorance, or altered states of mental capacity. Therefore, even though the language of abuse or neglect may permeate the documents that emerge from investigations and fact finding, frank inadequacy and endangerment are the ultimate criteria for removal.

The Legal Basis of Foster Care

The subject of child abuse and neglect, as well as its legal foundations and practices, is covered elsewhere in this volume (see Chapters 12 ["Parenting Assessment in Abuse, Neglect, and Permanent Wardship Cases"] and 17 ["Interviewing Children for Suspected Sexual Abuse"]). In this section, we focus on the foster care dimensions of interrupted parenting; we do not discuss the processes and criteria for determining abuse and neglect or the legal processes and criteria for terminations of parental contact and rights.

The foster care of children and adults is regulated by a broad network of federal and state statutes.[1] (This chapter deals only with children.) Federal laws are generally aimed at achieving uniformity of procedure and conditions of care across states, whereas state laws are specifically aimed along the same lines as well as defining jurisdictions, including empowering agents of children's protective services and the formulations of mandatory reporting duties (and protections from retaliations in relation to bona fide reporting) of various delineated groups of professionals.

Procedures leading to legal foster care are generally initiated after someone formally or anonymously notifies an established office of Child Protective Services that a child or group of children are being neglected or abused. The terms *abuse* and *neglect* are highly generic, and each encompasses a nearly innumerable set of conditions, situations, actions, and effects, which, singly or in combination with other variables, constitute neglectful or abusive circumstances and activity. Ultimately, determinations of abuse or neglect emerge from presentations of facts by designated authorities to judicial fact finders. It is the Child Protective Services agent's duty, notified of possible neglect or abuse, to investigate the initial allegations so as to make a determination of their validity, which then constitutes a basis for intervention. The latter itself may entail nonremoval of the child(ren) but with referrals to agencies that may assist the parent(s) with ongoing stressors that are creating an atmosphere of potential neglect or abuse Or, the child(ren) may be removed.

In many cases, a more elaborated set of clinically shaped interviews may be undertaken that will be used by the Child Protective Services agent and the court for further (or later) considerations of removal. Assistance to parents (and to the continuing investigation) may include provisions of parenting classes, anger management classes, substance abuse treatment, assessments of parental competence, assessments of child adjustment, and, in general, detailed descriptions of the general and specific qualities of family life that surround the child(ren). In either case—assistance or continuing investigations in conjunction with the Child Protective Services agent—the Child Protective Services agent is not likely to close an investigation until he or she is satisfied that the threshold for interventive removal has not been reached. (A closed record does not mean that the record is expunged, and Child Protective Services offices often have in their files documents relating multiple reports and investigations of children alleged to be neglected and/or abused.) Child protective agencies are burdened by the same decision-making dilemmas that burden all decision makers—namely, the error of deciding in favor of removal when the facts and circumstances of removal are later determined to have not warranted it (causing the public perception of their being overzealous and overriding of fundamental rights of parents), and the error of leaving intact a set of caregiving circumstances when a later event or tragedy makes one realize that the removal should have occurred (causing public outcries as to the neglect of children by the social services agencies that were established to prevent such occurrences).

Under the auspices of the state, child protective agents are authorized and empowered to remove children immediately from alleged (or observed) neglectful or abusive circumstances, and such removals generally will last until a court of jurisdiction, within an established length of time, affirms by order the placement into emergency—and therefore temporary—foster care. In any county or jurisdiction, a set of individuals exists who are willing and licensed to take such children into their care, for which they are remunerated at existing schedules, and who may have more than one such child in their care at any given time. As an alternative to placement in a foster care home as such, the child may be removed to the home of a determinably safe or appropriate relative, preference being given to relatives with whom the child is familiar.

Once a child is removed and placed into temporary alternative care (relative or specific foster care home), the Child Protective Services office assigns a caseworker whose duty it is

- To monitor the adjustment of the child in the foster care placement, engaging further medical, psychological, and/or social services for the child if they are warranted—services that are typically provided by individuals who receive contractually arranged compensation from the Child Protective Services office and whose duties are aligned with the mission and authority of that office.
- To monitor steps taken by the parent(s) of the child to meet criteria for recovering the care and custody of the child at issue.

---

[1] See, for example, the Adoption and Safe Families Act of 1997 (Pub. L. No. 105-89). See also the Adoption Assistance and Child Welfare Act of 1980 (Pub. L. No. 96-272).

Meanwhile, the court schedules a series of hearings concerning the child's and parent's status in relation to the original allegations and petitions. Children may not be maintained in foster care without such periodic hearings. At these points, progress reports generated by state caseworkers, usually augmented by reports of contracted medical and behavioral specialists, are presented along with recommendations. Actions by the court may either continue the status quo until a subsequent hearing or restore the parent's right to care for and possess the child (quite likely with continuing support, guidance, or monitoring services). Absent a qualified parent, a determinable relative may be designated as the recipient of the child, if such a relative can be found. Also, states are increasingly turning to the principle of geographic proximity to assign priority of placement to relatives or foster homes that are at least within the child's school district. (Other means of determining placement venue have included ZIP codes.) Even so, limitations in the availability of qualified relatives or foster homes often lead to a child being placed in a city, county, or even region (still within the state) *other* than the one in which the child was residing at the time of removal from the home. Although counties may assist and collaborate with one another in this regard, the county of origin remains the jurisdiction of ongoing decision making.

It is a ubiquitous principle of immediate postplacement hearings that it will not be at such hearings that parental rights termination proceedings will be initiated. This is because public policy is generally one that emphasizes rehabilitation and restoration over permanent removal and certainly over precipitous or premature termination. Thus, a court may seem at times to some observers to be (too) slow in deciding and in acting in relation to terminations of parental rights, when from the point of view of the court itself, its pace is determined by deliberation, appropriate cautiousness, and, ultimately, compassionateness. Certainly, some observers believe that courts are too hurried in terminating parents' rights.

Following are some of the factors affecting the pace of subsequent judicial decision making:

- The child's adjustment post foster placement, which may include not only the dynamics of actual adjustment reactions but also the continuing and complicating vicissitudes of preexisting psychological and behavioral conditions
- The dynamics of parental conduct both during the foster care placement of the child and prior to the foster care placement (as reconstructed from interviews with the parents themselves, neighbors, relatives, and, of course, the child himself or herself)

These points encompass not only the behavioral and relationship qualities and circumstances in the home but also its material and social qualities. Not only are the physical features and quality of the home of interest to the state but also the social network of the family—who comes and goes from the home, and what is the nature of their movements within the home and, thereby, the emotional zones of the child. (To give but one of the more familiar examples, children who have been removed from their mother may be returned to her care only *after* another relative or associate of hers [e.g., a violent boyfriend, a drug-abusing sister—aunt to the child] has vacated the home and has been determined to be staying away from the premises and the mother.)

During foster care, the parent's rights are not terminated but are placed in abeyance and therefore variously restricted. Thus, parents may be (and usually are, absent specific reasons) allowed to see their children under supervised conditions; meetings usually occur at the Child Protective Services office (or at the offices of one or more of its surrogates, including the offices of therapists and social workers who have made themselves available), and the frequency and duration may be weekly and for an hour or more at a time. The parent also may be (and usually is) allowed to send things to the child and to be informed of medical or other services that are being provided. The most common exceptions to this are the unavailability of the parent (e.g., because of incarceration; because of having absconded) or the determined or suspected dangerousness of the parent.

Restoration of parental rights following periods of temporary restrictions may occur with or without conditions (such as continuing counseling, attending parenting or anger management classes, enrolling in substance abuse rehabilitation, being available for visits by Child Protective Services agents) depending on the court's findings and determinations. In some states, the state reserves the right to remove children at birth from parents who have been previously determined to be unfit for parenting.

The Child in Foster Care

Entry Into Foster Care

Entry into foster care is nearly always abrupt. A child is removed from the home premises, or from day care or school premises, or perhaps even in a public place, and taken to a center. Usually, at least some of the child's belongings are removed with the child. Sometimes this cannot be immediately arranged. Contacts with established foster care providers are made by the Child Protective Services agent or an assigned caseworker. In large metropolitan areas, these providers may be arranged within specific agencies that are publicly funded but independently operated by licensees with various degrees of organization, executive administration, and elaborated services (including case management, clinical services, and consultative services). In such areas, the state itself may operate an agency for foster placement. In smaller communities, the state itself and alone may operate the foster care services agency. States structure and set the rules and requirements of independently operated foster care agencies. Foster care providers work and are remunerated on a per diem basis, the actual amount being determined by any special needs the placed child may present (e.g., in-home medical care such as monitoring ventilator support, giving injections, feeding via nasogastric or gastric tubing, and providing assistance in other such procedures).

At the point of child removal, a documentary record is launched, clothing and food may be provided at the agency, and then the child is transported to the home of the designated foster care provider. The child is introduced to the care provider, to any spouse or live-in partner of the provider if that person is present, and to any other occupants of the home including other children who are in foster care or who live there as part of the family. Meanwhile, a petition of removal is prepared for the court and is presented to the court with a time fixed by the particular jurisdiction but typically spanning between 24 and 48 hours. After a court order for temporary placement and assumption of control by the state has been issued, the child is then maintained in the home in which initially placed or transported to another foster home that will, events going as required, become the extended placement until future hearings determine otherwise (e.g., a return to the parental status quo ante, an extension of foster care, or a transfer of foster care venue as a result of extenuating occurrences or circumstances; see the following subsection, "Adjustments to Foster Care Placement").

During the initial period of foster care, the assigned caseworker is required to prepare a detailed report of the reasons for and circumstances underlying the decision to remove the child from the home and to initiate a series of steps toward a complete assessment of the child and of the caregiving circumstances from which the child has been removed. Within this period, a plan for restoration of parental rights must be initi-

ated as well, which, functionally, entails defining the conditions under which the child may be returned to the care and custody of the parent(s). Routine and expectable as this may seem, circumstances may delay or derail this part of the process. Sometimes the parents of the child abscond, or they are not permitted, for reasons relating to the child's removal, to have contact with the child.

Adjustments to Foster Care Placement

Initial Foster Care Placement

The adjustment dynamics of the child once placed in foster care are, of course, influenced by several factors, including 1) the child's age and correlative developmental status, 2) the conditions and dynamics leading up to removal, 3) the conditions and dynamics of the removal itself, and 4) the conditions and dynamics of the receiving foster care provider.

With regard to the child's age and correlative developmental status, established principles of child development and adjustment are instructive as to the normative issues most likely to be faced by helping authorities. Yet even as normative understandings of children's development and age-related coping capacities are used as guidelines for structuring and supporting their transitions into foster care, it is important to recognize that the home and developmental context from which a particular child has been removed may not be one that closely conforms to the kinds of normative rearing contexts that are broadly viewed to produce and promote normative coping capacities.

Thus, some children who are brought into foster care use coping behaviors that seem to reflect the aberrancies of their upbringing. Also, some children who are brought into foster care have surprisingly positive coping capacities. One can therefore never truly predict the course of a child's adjustment to foster care only on the basis of circumstances existing at the time of removal. One can, however, on the basis of professional knowledge and experience be prepared for a variety of adjustment dynamics.

The breadth of the array of the last of the factors listed earlier—the conditions of the receiving foster care provider—is beyond the scope of this chapter. It is nonetheless important to recognize its importance in considering children's adjustments to and in foster care, because foster care milieus are increasingly the targets of complaint on behalf of children by independent sponsors who report or otherwise present evidence of mistreatment in the foster care venues into which children have been placed. Adults in these venues serve as targets of such complaints, but other (usually other foster) children are targets as well, because they may behave aggressively toward or sexually provoke another child placed into that milieu as a result of their own problems in adjustment. It is also important to note that when such complaints arise, they increase the number of specific foster care placements in the child's life.

The challenges of initial child placement divide into two categories:

1. Meeting the needs of the child, many of which are unique to age and developmental status and some of which may be unique to an existing medical (e.g., chronic conditions such as asthma and epilepsy; acute medical conditions such as fractures or burns, which have been treated on an outpatient basis) or psychobehavioral (e.g., autism, attention-deficit/hyperactivity disorder) condition
2. Meeting the specific adjustment dynamics of the child

The enduring temperamental dynamics of the child, which may or may not be reliably evident during periods of acute crisis, are of central relevance to managing the child's adjustment. Issues of self-esteem, emotional regulation, and adaptive capacity, which have long been the bases of normative understanding of children's development and adjustment, are also centrally relevant.

From a psychiatric perspective, the dynamics of anxiety and depression, both of a preexisting kind and of an immediate kind, are at the forefront of assessments during the removal and immediate placement phases of foster care. The same is true of the kinds of preexisting and immediate conduct and adjustment conditions. The forces of preexisting and immediate reactive conditions are never easy to disentangle, particularly during the removal and placement phase, but also during the establishment of a stable fostering circumstance. Classifications of the immediate kind are generally assigned to Axis I of any DSM-IV-TR (American Psychiatric Association 2000) formulation that is made during the immediate placement phase—for example, acute stress disorder, 308.3 (which encompasses both anxious and depressed presentations), and physical or sexual abuse of child, V61.21. Adjustment disorders assigned at this point are usually premature unless the diagnostician is confident that the cur-

rently observed emotional tone and behavioral adjustment of the child are part of a response to the immediate removal and placement rather than to aspects of preexisting conditions. In either case, adjustment disorder is likely to be the principal diagnosis aside from any coexisting diagnoses (e.g., attention-deficit/hyperactivity disorder, oppositional defiant disorder) that are determined as observations and reports accumulate. Separation anxiety disorder (309.21), which, codewise, is on the adjustment disorder (with anxiety) spectrum, and reactive attachment disorder of infancy or early childhood (313.89) also may be applicable.

No child is immune to the potentially traumatic effect of abrupt removal from familiar and, safe to say in many or most instances, beloved caregivers—even when those caregivers have been definably abusive or neglectful. With respect to the larger subphases of development, issues unique to those subphases may, in fact, pose unique challenges and adjustment dynamics. Thus, infants and preschool children encounter unique sets of problems, for they lack what the much older child possesses in the way of capacities for verbalized cognitive mediation of the events. The emotional expressive and regulatory dynamics of infants and young children are also problematic not only for the children themselves but also for those who are now placed in the external regulatory roles foster parents occupy. Infancy and early childhood are phases in which emotional and behavioral regulation are exquisitely partnership-based, and if the partnership basis in the home from which the child has been removed has been deficient or defective (and very likely it has), then the grafted partnership of the infant and foster care parent may well pose great difficulties of adjustment.

Related to this, of course, is the difficulty infants and young children typically (but not universally) have in coping with the sudden novelties of Child Protective Services workers and, subsequent to removal, foster care figures into whose home the child arrives. The foster home itself inherently poses many features of disorganizing novelty, including its sights, sounds, and scents and also its interactive tones and dynamics. Sleeping arrangements may well be disturbingly new, and food availabilities and presentations and tastes may be disturbingly new as well. The voices are new, and the manners of communication and interaction are new—all of which challenge but hopefully soon augment the child's existing coping capabilities.

Many jurisdictions have on hand foster care homes into which only infants and young children are placed because of specialized talents or training or experience the foster care figures have in that respect. As a result of training and education in infant mental health concepts and practices, many jurisdictions have worked out, as far as expenses and logistics allow, procedures and parameters that are unique to developmental phases of infancy and very young children and that address in subphase-unique ways the issues just described.

School-age children and adolescents present different challenges. Verbally more competent and accessible than their infant and preschool counterparts, it may be "easier" to explain to them what is happening and to invoke hypotheticals and simple abstractions (possibilities) as cognitive organizing forces—for example, making explicit references to time and place and explaining contingencies. The cast of individuals who are impinging on the child's life at this time—the social workers, the foster care figures themselves, the counselors, the court—are more easily defined and delineated the older a child is, although during the removal and initial placement phases, these forces are likely to be as confusing and forgotten once introduced as such forces are even to adults who are undergoing rapidly unfolding events and/or abrupt transitions in their lives. It is almost universal that trauma temporarily functionally impairs the cognitive apparatus while it is ongoing.

School-age children and adolescents are often psychologically equipped to be politic during these times, and, according to their own perceptions of situations and events, they may be either cooperative or obstructive, particularly as they see their or their parents' interests, shared or independent, threatened or attacked. They may immediately campaign or act out against the placement, including running away. Just as likely, they may become somewhat inhibited or stunned by the events of removal and placement such that they are passive and acquiescent. They may withdraw. Finally, some may simply be able to comprehend the situation for what it basically is, and, with some feelings of guilt attached, they may feel relieved at removal and placement.

Collateral with these factors are how events proceed with (and for) the parent(s) during any period of foster care placement. There is, of course, no uniform unfolding or course of events when children are removed from their parents' care. It is a shock to most parents that Child Protective Services agents have even appeared at their door, and although schools are increasingly experienced in such matters, it is nevertheless sometimes unsettling when a Child Protective Services worker removes a child from their premises. When children are removed from the household, any number of events may occur, ranging from peaceful,

uncontested removals to desperate protests and attempts to block the removal, at which point police action is invoked, to part or all of which the child may be witness. The child herself or himself may be old enough to at least register a protest, and so her or his departure from the home may be agonized as well.

The child's entry into the foster home is likely, then, to be fraught with anxieties that are slow to remit even under the most supportive and receptive of conditions. Sometimes, between removal and entry into foster care, the child will have spent several or more hours in the office of the Child Protective Services worker or even an office in the police station as suitable placement is established. Not all removals occur during daylight hours, and not all removals occur in orderly sequence. Siblings may be involved, and the task of deciding whether they can (or should) be in the same placement immediately arises; also, caseworkers often must determine which foster placement, if any, can accommodate more than one, or many, children. Logistics are only sometimes straightforward or absent impasses.

Thus, the immediate placement phase of foster care placement may be very stormy and discombobulating for the child, when the immediate task is to provide physical safety and comfort.

Extended Foster Care

Within days or a few weeks of placement, inklings occur as to the likelihood that the placement period will be extended. When foster care placement becomes extended, the overriding administrative and monitoring principles and activities remain as they were at the outset of removal and placement—ongoing investigations, reports, recommendations, and plans (i.e., criteria setting and monitoring) for restoring the child's parents' rights of care, custody, and decision making.

By the time that a child's placement in foster care is undergoing transition to a more extended (and likely, therefore, indefinite) period of placement, that child usually has begun to show what will be the abiding adjustment dynamic. Stability of placement during this period is crucial to that dynamic's being manageable and uninhibiting of positive adaptation. Again, age and developmental status are factors that affect adjustment to the placement, just as the conditions and relationship dynamics of the foster care provider are contributing factors. (Again, though, the breadth of the array of the latter set of factors lies outside the scope of this chapter.)

Thus, infants and young children, once accustomed to the ambience and daily living cycles of the placement, generally settle and accommodate themselves. The inherent forces of attachment, although not commencing anew, lead to emotional connections with foster parents. Resilience is a more widely recognized quality of infant and early childhood adjustment than was once the case, and capacities for attachment to foster care figures are acknowledged more widely to rely on polytropic rather than sheer monotropic predispositions. Thus, within days to weeks, infants and children generally—with key and not infrequent exceptions—become attached to members of the foster care household, and, not surprisingly, they may concentrate their affections and approaches on the principal figure of the household. Foster parents also are likely to have bonded with the child, and for that reason, the point at which the child is returned to the care and custody of the original parent(s) may be emotionally distressing.

Nevertheless, we do not mean to declare that the birth parent(s) (and thus the presumptive principal attachment figures) are not missed or that the disruption of the primary attachment bond that has been caused by removal of the parent has no effect on the child's sense of continuity and security. But we do assert that young children's endowed normative capacities for extending or broadening the domain of beneficial attachment figures are (just as they are in stable day care settings and preschool settings) available and part of general positive adaptations made by infants and young children whose placements in foster care become extended. Separation anxiety—now centered on the foster care parent—may be heightened, just as it would be in relation to the birth parent himself or herself. Approaches for soothing also may now include the foster parent, just as they may have centered on the birth parent.[1]

With the emergence of attachment-related feelings and behaviors, the infant's and young child's vegetative and emotion-regulatory dynamics also generally stabilize. Sleep generally improves (although possibly remains prone to intermittent waking and waking-related anxiety), eating becomes more robust (although possibly excessive, sometimes diminished),

and expressions of sadness or worry become less predominating (although quite possibly persisting in sensitivity or reactivity thresholds) than was the case at the time of entry into foster care. These improvements notwithstanding, care and attentiveness must remain focused on the particular difficulties wrought by the nascent ego capacities of infants and young children in general.

Older children's and teenagers' adjustments to extended foster care placements are also generally positive, but preexisting behavior and emotional problems certainly influence the nature and vicissitudes of those adjustments. The older and more cognitively capable the child is, the more she or he is likely not only to understand the situation but also to play something of a calculating role in the course of events leading to continued placement, restoration of parental rights, or terminations of parental rights. The child in foster care remains an object of observation and query insofar as these issues and outcomes are concerned, and although the court and its agencies of determination strive to make decisions based on the facts in such instances, an underlying attention to the child's preference is often latently active in the communications occurring between and among the parties of foster care—that is, parents, foster parents, caseworkers, professional attachés, and children themselves.

Children who are relieved to be apart from their parents may develop strong opinions against returning to their care. Children who are angry at having been removed may lobby to be removed from the foster care placement, possibly by acting out their grievances or by making negative insinuations about the care they are receiving in the foster care home. Although most children and teenagers in most foster care circumstances, within most jurisdictions, adjust, survive, thrive (i.e., they go to school, participate in foster family activity, pursue interests in leisure or recreational activities and involvements, commence new recreational activities, comply generally with caseworkers' and foster parents' requests or instructions, eat, sleep, dress, carry out small but regular chores, and may even come to like the people with whom they are placed), and therefore

---

[1] In this regard, one cannot presume that the attachment dynamics of infants and young children placed in foster care will necessarily or neatly fit the categories and stages of normative development. Children removed from abusive or neglectful situations often do show attachment behaviors (albeit of an anxious, avoidant, or conflicted type) toward their parents, and they certainly have anxieties at points of separation from them. But in many, perhaps most, instances, because of existing relationship dysfunctionalities that are already embedded in the attachment relationship between the infant or young child and parent, the secure-base and haven-of-safety dynamics of the relationship may in fact be quite aberrant on entry into foster care. Thus, the attachment dynamics of the infant and young child in foster care may not always reflect a history of continuous positive attachment and attachment-related capacities for coping.

adapt to the necessity or inevitability of foster care placement—temporary or permanent—significant numbers of them try to influence their circumstances according to their perceptions or understandings of their situations in relation to their (self-constructed) self-interests. Teenagers especially, *as* teenagers, can be expected to make significant attempts to influence outcomes, sometimes benignly, but also sometimes emphatically even to the point of being disruptive if they believe it will further their preferences.

Of course, we are not implying that there are not many children who have trouble adapting, or who fail to adapt, which then may lead to changes of placement and, by extension, a series of changes in placement. All mental health officials, all agencies of jurisdiction, and all public policy analysts know and agree that multiple foster placements are both an index of something very wrong with a child's adjustment and a correlate of negative outcomes.

Terminations of Parental Rights

Most children who are in foster care eventually return to either their parent(s) from whom they were removed or a close relative. In some cases, guardianship by a relative of the parent is worked out with the parent's input and, once he or she submits emotionally to the inevitable impossibility of retaining possession of the child, ratification. Again, as stated at the outset, the prevailing policy and intent of the courts are to preserve and, when possible, restore parental possessions and care of their children, even if such restorations are not augmented or bulwarked by adjunct care providers in the form of guardians.

Legal procedures are used to permanently terminate the rights of the parents to care for the child. After all that has happened in the life of the child leading up to the original removal, all that has happened during the period of foster placement(s), and all that may in fact be conjectured by the child herself or himself in relation to failed visits and prolonged periods of parental absence and noncontact, most children are "ready for" the announcement that they will not be returning to the care of their parents. Infants and young children again are a special case of this realm of outcomes because permanent termination of their parents' rights, which leads to the community's seeking of a permanent placement for them, raises the specter of further interrupted attachments. When foster parents are in a

position, and want, to adopt infants and young children, the second interruption of the child's attachment (to the foster parent[s]) can be avoided. The same is true of older children as well, who also may have formed a positive attachment to the foster parent(s).

Role of the Forensic Mental Health Professional

Mental health practitioners are to be found during all phases of the foster care process. Most state caseworkers, both investigatory and case managing, are social workers of various levels of training and education and of certification. Additional mental health practitioners, including clinical social workers, psychologists, and psychiatrists, serve as consultants, adjunct investigators, and direct service providers. Any or all of the latter may function as part of the network of testimonies affecting the outcome of child removal and placement in foster care. The fact that they are active within and throughout the foster care system, combined with the fact that they therefore provide evaluative and consultative reports along with recommendations and associated commentary, certainly offers a patina of forensic function and purpose to many of their activities, including, of course, their direct testimonies in courts of law.

Almost any clinician with appropriate training and licensing credentials may, under the guidelines of federal and respective state rules of evidence, and with stipulation by contesting parties, be declared by a court of jurisdiction to be an expert in the case *at hand*. Apart from their giving testimony as to *fact* based on direct contact with one or several parties in a case, they are often granted by the court, at the conclusion of *voir dire*, a delimited field of *opinion* reporting, that is, the privilege of testifying as to meaning beyond the specific facts. The legal definitions and technicalities of forensic testimony are spelled out in detail in the Federal Rules of Evidence, as well as elsewhere in this volume (see Chapter 1, "Introduction to the Legal System").

However, other individuals—forensic specialists—have formal training, experience, and breadth of knowledge, and they provide specialized input and commentary not only about individual children's circumstances, dynamics, and considerable outlooks but also about the general and patterned issues that underlie such circumstances and outlooks. Forensic specialists are generally experts not only in interviewing and reporting but also in the specialized structures and dynamics of interviewing and reporting. They provide important information and clarifications to courts as to the quality and meaning of evidence adduced from interviews, testing, and observation. They are, then, in essence, experts on the multiple facets—cognate and technical—of clinical expertise.

As participants in the realms of determining abuse and neglect, as well as determining adjustment and outcome in foster care, forensic experts also provide practicing clinicians with useful guidelines for structured query that reduce or mitigate its more tainting aspects (e.g., leading and shaping responses, reliabilities and predictive limitations of children's communications). As participants in the realms of providing courts with useful testimony, forensic specialists help investigators and clinicians align their processes of inquiry with those of legal inquiry such that the logistics of clinical and legal inquiry are more congruent than not.

The standard of proof needed for terminations of parental rights is clear and convincing, or beyond reasonable doubt, depending on the state in which termination proceedings occur. Courts thus may rely on forensic specialists for a variety of tasks, including the submissions of amicus curiae communications, testimony concerning instant cases but from the perspectives of larger fields (e.g., adjustment patterns of [different-age] children *in general* in foster care, behavioral dynamics of children *in general* who have been abused, standards of care governing foster care settings, outcomes associated with defined conditions), and testimony concerning already gathered evidence (which typically includes reviewing and then testifying about clinical and investigative reports of record, depositions and transcripts of record, and other related documents).

As with all expertise, forensic expertise with respect to children in foster care divides into two domains, one that is cognate in its nature and scope and one that is technical. Cognate expertise is defined by the multiple areas of refined knowledge of child development and maturation, including their age-unique behavioral and emotional dynamics; family organizational and relationship dynamics, including those affected by economic stress; and categories of normative as well as clinically relevant adjustment.

Forensic specialists must be critical and discerning consumers of facts and theories—facts not as they are often constructed by theorists to fit the prevailing prejudices concerning children who are in foster care, but facts as they are encountered in the light of direct observation and cross-examination. Forensic expertise understands, and adheres to, the legal definitions of fact, which are often at variance with the kinds of fact that nonforensic clinicians adduce in their everyday work.

Technical expertise encompasses the expert's specialized skill not only in actual (i.e., case-centered) eliciting of information through observation, interviewing, and testing but also in clarifying (interpreting) information that is relevant to any of the several cognate categories just listed.

Conclusion

Children in foster care pose several challenges not only as objects of public policy but also to the specific individuals and agencies serving them. Children in foster care are not only children in foster care; they are also children whose parents are under close public scrutiny, who also find their practices and conceptions of parenting being confronted. Thus, the stresses of foster care placement are not only the stresses (or reliefs) of being placed outside their homes of origin but also the stresses of being separated from families. Foster caregivers also confront and bear the stresses of caring for these children, which entails not only providing shelter and certain material comforts but also acting as true and genuine surrogates of the emotional needs such children have. Finally, it is not easy at all for agents of the public's interests and intentions to act with universal approval from communities as a whole because sometimes conflicted communities are concerned about the rights and duties of children and their parents or caregivers. Thus, forensic specialists in child foster care placement practice within a complex world of competing values, motives, interests, and intentions. The chronic problem of shortages of available foster parents relative to community need compounds the challenges that all face when foster care is the necessary immediate option for those communities.

—*Key Points*

— About 500,000 children are in foster care in any given year.

— Lengths of stay in foster care vary greatly, the median length of stay being about 15.5 months, with lengths of care greater than 3 years being the case in about 24% of children.

— Foster care entails multiple adjustment challenges that occur in addition to stressors associated with being removed from parental care and placed into foster care.

References

Adoption and Safe Families Act of 1997 (Pub. L. No. 105-89)

Adoption Assistance and Child Welfare Act of 1980 (Pub. L. No. 96-272)

American Psychiatric Association: Diagnostic and Statistical Manual of Mental Disorders, 4th Edition, Text Revision. Washington, DC, American Psychiatric Association, 2000

U.S. Department of Health and Human Services: The Adoption and Foster Care Analysis and Reporting System Report for the Fiscal Year October 1, 2005–September 30, 2006. Washington, DC, Administration for Children and Families, 2008a

U.S. Department of Heath and Human Services: Trends in Foster Care and Adoption—Fiscal Years 2002–2007. Washington, DC, Administration for Children and Families, 2008b

Chapter 14

Adoption

Thomas M. Horner, Ph.D.
James B. Gale, M.S.

It has been estimated that about 1.5 million children in the United States today are adopted; this is about 2% of all children (Fields 2001). About one-third of these children live with one of their birth parents and have been adopted by a stepparent, leaving about 1 million who have been adopted by non–birth parents (Fields 2001). The precise number of adoptions occurring annually is not known because there is no overarching data-collecting authority that might provide such a number. Children are adopted through a number of channels, the most prominent of which are established state foster care agencies, licensed private adoption agencies, private independent adoption agents (facilitators), and the U.S. Department of State (which in April 2008 became the controlling representative of the United States to the 1993 Hague Convention on the Protection of Children and Cooperation in Respect of Intercountry Adoption, thereby activating the U.S. Intercountry Adoption Act of 2000 [Public Law 106-279]). By far, the largest number of adoptions in the United States occur through foster care agencies, and their figures lag (predictably) in their publication.

Adoption and Foster Care Analysis and Reporting System data provided to the U.S. Department of Health and Human Services Administration for Children and Families (2008) showed that 51,000 children had been adopted out of the foster systems of the 50 states in fiscal year 2007. This figure was quite stable from the previous year (also 51,000) and from 2002 (53,000) onward. From 2002 to 2007, between 129,000 and 134,000 children remained awaiting adoption on the last day of each reporting year. The median age of children adopted in 2006 was 5.4 years, while the median age of children waiting was 7.7 years. About 60% of the parents who adopted foster care children had been their child's foster parent.

Between 1989 and 2005, more than 234,000 children are said to have been adopted from countries other than the United States (National Data Analysis System 2007). Since 2004, the annual number of children legally adopted from other nations has been about 20,000 per year (Table 14–1).

The Thirteenth Amendment of the U.S. Constitution and the aforementioned Hague Convention on the Protection of Children and Cooperation in Respect of Intercountry Adoption expressly prohibit the selling and buying of human beings—hence the elaborate and often very technical itemizations of services and related costs associated with private, particularly international, adoption. The costs in fees and expenses of bringing forth these adoptions—typically in instances of adopting non-U.S.-born children—often far exceed the costs incurred by ordinary prenatal and obstetric care when parents conceive and give birth to children on their own. So, too, do they exceed the costs and fees associated with various in vivo and in vitro procedures that are used alternatively to create pregnancy. These domains—personal conception, legal adoption, and medically assisted pregnancy—constitute the pathways to primary child-rearing in the United States.

Certain contemporary celebrities and other high-profile individuals and their adoptions have cast particular hues in the spectra of public spotlights on adoption that, apart from the utter forms of publicity they

TABLE 14–1. Immigrant visas issued to adopted children: 2004–2008

	2004	2005	2006	2007	2008
China (mainland)	7,044 (1)	7,906 (1)	6,493 (1)	5,453 (1)	3,909 (2)
Russia	5,865 (2)	4,639 (2)	3,706 (3)	2,310 (3)	1,861 (3)
Guatemala	3,264 (3)	3,783 (3)	4,135 (2)	4,728 (2)	4,123 (1)
Ethiopia	289 (9)	441 (7)	732 (5)	1,255 (4)	1,725 (4)
South Korea	1,716 (4)	1,630 (4)	1,376 (4)	939 (5)	1,065 (5)
Subtotals[a]	18,178 (83%)	18,399 (84%)	16,442 (83%)	14,685 (78%)	12,683 (73%)
Tenth-ranked country	287	271	320	314	306
Fifteenth-ranked country	89	73	70	89	148
Twentieth-ranked country	57	62	56	54	59
Grand totals[b]	**22,884 (79%)**	**22,739 (81%)**	**20,679 (80%)**	**19,613 (75%)**	**17,438 (73%)**

Note. The countries listed are the top 5 for the years 2006 and 2007, 4 of which have consistently occupied the top 4 rankings across the 5 years that are listed. Ethiopia is listed across the 5-year period as it has became in 2007 and 2008 the source of the fourth highest number of internationally adopted children. Figures in parentheses beside the yearly totals by country refer to the rank of the listed countries. The tenth-, fifteenth-, and twentieth-ranked countries of origin are given for numerical referencing.
[a]Subtotals given are for the five countries listed. The figures in parentheses are the percentages of these adoptions in relation to the total number of adoptions for the top 20 countries.
[b]Grand totals are for all countries per year, the figures in parenthesis being the percentage of adoptions accounted for by the top 20 countries.
Source. Adapted from U.S. Department of State 2008.

engender, demonstrate a significant rotation from the cultural status of adoption that was at one time secretive and patently hidden or denied with falsifications and other confabulations. Such publicity has made the public more aware of the variants of adoption, though it cannot be correlatively argued that it has led to a greater public understanding of the mainstream issues of adoption.[1]

Because of the enduring primacy of so-called natural birth in large segments of the population, parents seeking adoption often feel that they are cast or relegated to an alternative class of parenting and childrearing.[2] Because adoption is usually considered and approached by parents following unsuccessful attempts at conceiving their "own," there are considerable internal emotional forces that reinforce this feeling. In other words, long before adoption is considered as a route toward child rearing, the values and habitviews of the dominant cultures of parenting have been absorbed by the individuals who now approach adoption. The counterpart of these values and habitviews is that many adoptive children grow to feel at some point that they have been deprived of their "real" parents. Another counterpart of these values and habitviews, this time in the professional community, is found in the common practice of referring to birth parents in a person's background as either the real or natural parents.

Most of the psychological challenges of adoption center on ancient and persisting notions of lineage, origins, identity in life, and fate-laden outcomes. Adoption is archetypal—Oedipus, Moses, Caesar Augustus, Jesus, Muhammad, Luke and Leia Skywalker, and Superman were, for various reasons and under widely differing circumstances, adopted children. Many individuals who thought (or fancied with longing implications) they had been adopted but never told of it (e.g., A. Freud 1942/1973; S. Freud 1909/1959; Rosenberg and Horner 1991) have been disappointed to find out that they were not; while many individuals in whom the thought of having been adopted never crossed their minds have discovered, with sudden implications, that they were.

Adoption has permeated human history and culture. Its practices and meanings are at the core of every society's kinship structures. Adoption has of course taken many forms and followed many practices, depending on the particular culture (or set of similar cultures) in which it has been carried out (Boswell 1988; Horner and Rosenberg 1991). Adoption, both de facto and de jure, has always and ubiquitously occurred.

Historical Perspectives

Contemporary Western laws concerning adoption have been shaped to a great extent by ancient Roman practices, which conferred legitimacy, permanence, and equality of status to the adopted child. Adoptions of many kinds were a conspicuous part of the ancient societies that became subsumed under Roman laws (Boswell 1988; Goody 1983; Howe 1983). Adoptions of children, and adoptions of adults as adults, permeate the written histories of Rome and since. Adoptions of children of non-Western countries have been less documented in writing.

For many centuries in Christianized Europe, adoption occurred mostly outside of the purview of established and formal law. Thus, Goody (1983) noted that children would frequently be given up by their parents at birth to be raised by others, sometimes giving token payments to the adopting parents for doing so. Sales, indenturements, oblatory commissions, and protection (rescue) of children have all constituted pathways toward adoption (Boswell 1988).

Adoption has served more than just personal or familial interests. Between 1874 and 1929, the New York Children's Aid Society, following the inspiration of certain reformers who viewed such practices as child improving, sent thousands of children to Midwestern and western farm communities to be adopted by farming families in need of workers to work beside their own children (Mintz 2004). Removals of children from Native American tribes were also once thought

---

[1] To be sure, adoption as a path toward raising a child "of one's own" differs from adoption that results from fostering; that is, for example, adopting that occurs because one's sister has died and her children are now taken in and therefrom raised. Thus, one can distinguish between adoptions that are pursued for purposes of creating a family and adoptions that are pursued in order to preserve a family.

[2] In this chapter, the use of either the word *parent* (or *parents*) will almost always carry with it both grammatically singular and plural meanings. In the United States, only individual people and legally married people may legally adopt children. In order to avoid the awkward forms of *parent(s)* and the various combinations of articles (*a/the*) and pronouns (*her/his/their*), the context of the statements that follow in this article will be allowed to determine the word usage. Similarly, the words *child* and *children* will be used individually with an expectation that the reader will aptly discern when either might apply.

to be "improving" of the children so removed (and adopted) (Anderson 2000; Jacobs 2004, 2005). Said Barbara Landis, biographer of the Carlisle Indian School: "There were kids who were Lakota, and there were kids who were Wampanoag. At Carlisle they became Indian" (Anderson 2000, p. 20).[1]

Adoption laws as such did not begin to reappear in Western Europe and the United States until recently. For example, in 1846 and 1850, respectively, Mississippi and Texas began to require registrations of private adoption agreements (Mintz 2004). In 1851 Massachusetts began to require judges to determine adoptive parental adequacy and to require birth parents to certify in writing their consent to the adoption (Mintz 2004). France (in 1892) and England (in 1926) later adopted similar principles (Sorosky et al. 1975). Since then, adoption has evolved to its present-day forms and regulations. The greatest proportions of contemporary adoption in the United States entail individuals and couples earnestly wishing to parent and individuals wishing to formalize de facto parent–child relationships (e.g., stepparents who legally adopt a spouse's children, guardians or foster parents who wish to complete a relationship through legal formalization).

Biological Perspectives

In everyday discourse, but also in professional parlance and discourse, adopted children are typically referred to as *nonbiological* children of the parents who adopt them. Coordinately, parents of adopted children are typically referred to as their nonbiological parents. A variant of the aforesaid terms often occurs in obtaining developmental histories of individuals who have been adopted; both the clinical interviewer and the interviewed adoptee slip into references to the "real" parents—that is, birth parents—rather than "the parents who raised me/you." These terminological distinctions again reflect the aforementioned implicit societal-cultural primacy of the birth parent over the adoptive parent.[2] Whereas the distinction between biological parent and adoptive parent is often encountered in the literature on adoption and in coverage of legal perspectives on adoption, and whereas this distinction in terms is common in clinical and everyday parlance concerning adoption, it is a terminological distinction that in the so-called natural order of things is more misleading than not with regard to the larger realms and distributions of child care and child rearing.

From a biological—that is, phylogenetic—perspective, (auto-)parenting by those who gave birth to the child from the womb and (allo-)parenting by those who have taken over the care of another's offspring in infancy following the loss of the birth parent are both part of the "natural" order of things insofar as child (offspring) survival and care are concerned. The fostering/adoption of abandoned young is practiced within and across species on a broad scale (Riedman 1982).

Ontogenetically, the individual offspring of parents is in search of a protective and nurturing environment from the point of its conception (Horner 1992). The first week or so of life is spent in intrafallopian and intrauterine space, the conceptus operating in a biologically framed search for an endometrium at which to implant itself toward pursuit of its genetically coded purposes, including, of course, the preservation of its own life. In the modern era, that endometrium may or may not (as in the case of in vitro impregnation) be that of the mother who dispensed half the genetic material it is carrying.[3] Although the physiological (i.e., placental) processes that eventually bind the embryo and the mother are most certainly physiologically reciprocal, it is important to retain the knowledge that the origin of the placenta is within the cell matrices of the future embryo; that is, the child itself. Thus, early placental implantation is as much a function of embryonic reaching for as it is a function of endometrial readiness for. From a biological perspective, adoptive parenting is *a* form of parenting rather than a *substitute* or *alternative* or *less normal* form of parenting. Culture, of course, may (and typically does) define things otherwise.

None of the foregoing discussion is stated to discount or otherwise dismiss the relevance and importance of certain genetic continuities between progenitive parents and their genetic children. But it is stated

---

[1] The Indian Child Welfare Act of 1978 was intended to rectify past practices of Indian removal (see Jones 1995, 1996; Thoma 2006).

[2] For an incisive treatment of the semantic and conceptual faults within the realms of so-called biological and adoptive parenting, including their implications for kinship definition, identity formation, and cultural attitudes, see Leon (2002).

[3] It is not at all inconsistent with or contradictory of established biological principles to view, when they entail embryos donated by nongenetic parents, in vitro pregnancies as adoptions of a kind. In point of biological fact, that is precisely what they are.

in order to assist the framing of any discussion concerning how it is, and with what meanings, children come to be loved and reared by the parents, whether through adoption or physical birth.

Legal Perspectives

Adoptions come about from the commingling of forces emanating from two sources: an abandoned, rescued, but otherwise dislocated child in search (need) of continuing care and the individual who either 1) is in search of a child to raise and to love or 2) may be obligated by the customs and rules of the community to take the child in. In all societies, various forms of custom and rule or law create a framework for transferring the care of children, and it is a framework that establishes status, right, and duty for each of the figures involved in transfers of care and custody. This framework is maintained by a system of brokers, arbiters, and decision makers within or attached to the legal (or decision-making) system that governs the community, who then enact procedures that lead toward a solemn consecration of such transfers.

As previously stated, adoption in the United States descends from Roman models of law as filtered through and annealed by English law and modern legislation.[1] Adoption is, for the most part, regulated by (and in all cases consummated through) each of the states, though federal governing statutes are applicable as well (e.g., the Adoption Assistance and Child Welfare Act of 1980 [Public Law 96-272], which among other policies established permanency planning as a standard of child welfare practice and preservation of reunification of children and parents where possible; the Adoption and Safe Families Act of 1997 [Public Law 105-89]).

Adoption is a shared process initiated by and affecting several parties. At the center of the process, of course, is the child, whose interests and ultimate disposition are closely regulated by the state. The state declares the eligibility of a child for adoption, and it determines the suitability for adoption. Eligibility for adoption is established by the child's loss of a parent through death or disappearance, by the parents' voluntary giving over of a child for adoption through either private or public channels, or by the state's determina-

tion of parental unfitness, which in turn leads to a termination of that parent's rights (see Chapters 11 ["Child Custody Evaluation"] and 13 ["Children in Foster Care"] in this volume). In each of these scenarios, the child's coming into the state's purview triggers a series of placements and transitions, which may include foster care, forms of temporary guardianship, and eventual availability of the child for adoption. When adoptions occur privately, the state is still superordinately involved and consecrating of the process, though the transfer of the child typically omits the transitional stages of fostering and guardianship.

Converging on these processes are members of a pool of parent-candidates who have come into that pool by self-presentation and who remain in the pool through processes of observation, investigation, and evaluation by the courts in conjunction with a number of state-sponsored agents and functionaries whose roles and qualifications are to determine their fitness to parent, that is, to adopt. (In private adoptions, these processes of assessment and determination may be abbreviated and handled more subtly, and they are therefore less conspicuous.) Depending on the state in which an adoption takes place, some quantity of interviews, observations in the prospective parent's home, collateral interviews with people who know and can vouch for the prospective parent, and consultations by known local experts in child development, family adjustment, and adoption itself may be undertaken. It is fashionable to refer to an *adoption triangle* or *triad* when defining the major sets of psychoemotional forces that converge on adoption. That triangle consists of the birth parent, the child, and the adoptive parent. But the power and ubiquitousness of the state is such that a tetrahedron may more accurately illustrate the interplay of forces that are active up to, at, and even following (for at least several months to a year, when a final assessment may be made) an adoption.

To be sure, there is quite a bit of variation in how eligible children and prospective parents gain access to each other. States typically license certain individuals who may serve the adoption process as intermediaries (often specializing attorneys) and facilitators of adoption, and who, by dint of contacts and knowledge they have established, may in fact bring eligible children and prospective parents into contact with each other. Such intermediaries have increasingly tapped populations of eligible children who live overseas, whose na-

---

[1] For much more detailed descriptions of the legal processes governing adoption, including comparisons of processes that vary from state to state, see Adamec (2004), Barr and Carlisle (2003), and Hicks (1993).

tions of origin are prepared to facilitate adoptions in the United States. The signatory nations of the Hague Convention on the Protection of Children and Cooperation in Respect of Intercountry Adoption (including the United States) have agreed to procedures and standards by which international adoptions may occur.

Legal adoption in the United States and most other nations establishes two overarching principles: to the adopting parent are conferred the full spectrum of parental rights and duties, and to the child are given the full spectrum of privileges and benefits of childhood. In the United States, adoption makes the resultant parent–child status equal with all other parent–child relationships whatever their physical or social biological origins. Once an adoption occurs and is consecrated as such, the law ceases to make distinctions.

Psychological Perspectives

A fundamental feature of forensic consultations concerning adoption is the set of principles and prescriptions consultants carry into the consultative arena, these principles ultimately applying to the question of whether (and if so, how much) it makes a difference— in experience, in life trajectory, in outcome—to have been adopted. Most authorities agree easily that it does make a difference, though they often disagree— sometimes slightly, sometimes significantly—as to how much the difference makes and of what kind it is. Certainly, all of the parameters and features of adoption—its timing, its permanence, who should and should not adopt, what to do about adoption searches, and more—have been sharply debated at one time or another (see, for example, Harnack 1995).

All children—adopted and not—have basic needs that may be met with varying but adequate degrees of efficacy by the caregiving persons in their lives. At the same time, all children, to varying degrees, express inherent interests and self-constructing and world-constructing dynamics that are designed (within their biology) to engage others (and things) occurring in their lives. Central to these dynamics are what are conventionally termed *attachment needs and interests*. They entail, following John Bowlby's original precepts, finding and fastening to a figure or set of figures who are consistent in their facilitating and growth-enhancing dynamics and who can thereby function as secure bases of exploration and emotional regulation as well as safe havens of emotional restoration and rebalancing when stresses (or threats of distress) arise. Such figures, apart from their biological functions, become objects of affection and affiliation.[1] These attachment figures center on the child's parents, though the realm of such figures expands once the child is exposed to day care and/or to preschool settings and, later, elementary school settings.

Correlatively, parents develop, seemingly instinctively—but also as a function of strong cultural forces, prescriptions and preparations, and the frank inherent characteristics and attractions of children—emotional attachments toward their children. In the developmental literature these attachments have generally been treated under the rubric of parental "bonding." Authorities in the past have theorized as to how parental bonds with children arise (or fail to arise), become (or fail to become) sustained, and flourish (or fail to flourish). It was once a strongly held view within the adoption literature that birth parents were more likely to establish positive bonding with their children than adoptive parents were with children "not their own." This view was anchored to the assumption, only partially supported by evidence from *some* animal species, that if one had not given physical birth to the child one was to be rearing, the ability to form the necessary parental bond was likely to be correlatively weaker by some margin. This view is not as broad or influential today as it once was, particularly as the processes of attachment and parent–child bond formation have been more widely and intricately studied.

This is not to say, of course, that processes of bonding and relationship formation following adoption are not affected by, even complicated by, adoption, particularly when children are adopted beyond infancy or very early childhood. The life history of the child up to the point of adoption is likely to have created continuing reverberating effects in terms of, say, learned (and perhaps maladaptive) coping dynamics and emotional predispositions involving sadness, anger, guilt, self-doubt, and so forth. For all children, but for some children in seemingly intractable ways, being adopted entails as much (and maybe more in some instances) a sense of change–loss as it does a sense of being found, or restored, or desired. All of these issues percolate, usually out of view, sometimes only dimly in view, and

---

[1] For thorough coverage of attachment in children, but also across the life span, see Cassidy and Shaver (1999) and Grossmann et al. (2005).

sometimes blaringly in view of those adopting the child (Eldridge 1999; McCreight 2002; Rosenberg 1992). There are certainly older children who have just been adopted who are ready to make the issues open and challenging. Most are not so immediately inclined, and many are inhibited for obvious reasons about doing so. Issues that relate to evident racial or ethnic incongruities, identity formation, and related processes of development and adaptation, circulate around everyday events and circumstances. Other issues are equally important: birth siblings and other relatives whose existence and whereabouts are not known, or if they are known, they are inaccessible. For discussions of the many others issues, see Eldridge (1999), McCreight (2002), and Rosenberg (1992).

All children ask about their origins, and in their conversations with each other and with adults they talk about them. (Many children are quite direct and even blunt with these subjects—sometimes with patent misconceptions underlying their assertions—but are typically also receptive to conversations of this nature.) Their assertions often put parents or other adults on guard or at unease, especially when the former sense or worry lest too much be known too soon in the child's development about "those kinds of matters." In some quarters, adoption bears the same kinds of weights of family taboo that sexuality and family finances carry in the lives of families. It is there to be addressed, but it is not always or easily addressed. Adopted children are therefore normative when they make such assertions, or make inquiries, or begin to explore the hidden regions of their backgrounds.

Adoptive parents (like all parents), when it concerns their children, want as much as possible to control the flow of information about the family business, so to speak; and whereas many are open about such flows, many are not.[1] Many adoptive parents are, of course, ready and willing to address these matters if they can feel that the information being sought fits with their (the parents') sense of proper timing. That timing in turn relates to the child's age, the parent's perception of the child's cognitive and emotional

readiness for information, and the perceived impacts conversations of this nature might have on their own or other family members' feelings and understandings. There is, of course, no undebatably correct way of communicating in these areas of potential sensitivity (Harnack 1995). Counselors specializing in adoption issues and challenges seek to facilitate children's and adults' finding the ways that fit for them.

At the core, then, of considering not whether but how adoption makes a difference are on the one hand, the appraisals one makes of a particular child's capacities and inclinations to form attachment bonds—that is, to target and to fasten emotionally to caregiving presences—at the point of adoption and to sustain them once made; and on the other hand, the appraisals one makes of particular prospective parents' abilities to reciprocate those attachments and to form specific bonds of their own with the adopted child. Although the afore-cited and oft-made presumption of a primacy of birth parenting over adoptive parenting still exists in many forensic consultants' minds, it is increasingly being recognized that this presumed primacy is more an expression of sociocultural construction than biological necessity (Leon 2002). If Leon is correct, then the "difference" adoption makes is rooted more in the attitudes (powerful, to be sure) people carry into the adoption process and its aftermath and in the child-rearing process than in the fact, as such, of adoption itself.

Another general axiom of child development is that children develop best in positive emotional contexts. Starting with safety and continuity, such contexts provide opportunities for optimal cognitive maturation, the broadening of social experiences and abilities, and the development of effective emotional regulatory capacities and social productivity. Extending out of these sectors are the formations of particular interests, ambitions, and standards of conduct. Uniting the sectors subjectively are such abstractions as the developing individual's feelings of identity, autonomy, and worth. Therefore, also at the core of considerations of the differences adoption makes are the

---

[1] It has been just short of a century since Jean Piaget first reported his investigations of the predictable queries of children during conversations with each other and with interested adults (e.g., Piaget 1923, 1936). Of importance in the present context are the questions children seem universally to ask (and answer!) concerning where things and, more apropos, where people themselves come from. Studies of children have consistently reiterated the importance of kinship belonging (Parkin and Stone 2004; Strathern 2005). It is thus quite predictable that the subject will come up soon in the developing child's life, that it will come up often, and that it will be introduced not only by the child's agemates but by adults themselves. Kinship knowledge, organization, and hierarchies are a basic element of social life, and conversations about kinship are a constant occurrence throughout a child's development. It is fashionable in U.S. early education venues to assign children to carry out classroom projects by which they report and delineate who their family members are.

opinions experts form of the competence of prospective parents to provide and maintain such contexts.

The literature on mental health expertise and its limitations is extensive and does not need to be summarized here. Forensic expertise from the mental health community, as it relates to cases of adoption, will be found clustered at points of adoption, at which experts may be recruited for either assessments of parental fitness or for opinions concerning future pathways and outcomes of children deemed, either physically or on the basis of past experiences, at risk for troubled or troubling outcomes. Expertise as such divides into two basic realms: *cognate expertise,* consisting of experts' refined knowledge of child development and correlative outcomes, particularly as they affect or are affected by adoption, and *technical expertise,* consisting of experts' specialized skills (e.g., interviewing, testing) at eliciting, organizing, and interpreting information that is relevant to any of several cognate areas.

Special Issues Related to Adoption

Availability

There are two large pools of individuals in search or need of adoption: parents wanting to adopt and children awaiting adoption, nearly all of which are living in foster care of some kind. This chapter cannot cover all of the permutations of factors affecting availability and selection, but it will be of no surprise that they revolve around (prospective) parental desires and definitions of child acceptability, on the one hand, and child characteristics and potential liabilities, on the other hand. Issues of community "standards" and "custom" play a large, often latent, role in how easy or difficult it is for cross-racial adoptions to occur or how easy or difficult it is for gay and lesbian individuals to adopt. It has been estimated that a half-million prospective parents in the United States are awaiting a child to adopt, while one-third of that number of children are awaiting adoption. It is obvious that some elements of preference and selectivity exist in relation to the child's origins and other characteristics.

On the child's side of things, whether or not the child is defined as having special needs or physical or psychological handicaps plays a role in determining eligibility for public subsidy of at least some of the care costs that may be entailed. Such children may also be

less acceptable to prospective parents who want what they deem to be a "normal" child with "normal" potentials. So, too, may the age, background (many prospective parents try to learn as much about the genetic and experiential background of the child as they can), or other characteristics of the child be blocks to adoption for some parents.

Adoptions occur, then, as stated earlier, both through public agencies, who harbor large numbers of children in foster care that are available for adoption, and through a large number of networks that have been developed to channel available children to available parents. Prospective parents not wanting to draw from the pool of such kids seek private arrangements either in the United States, or, increasingly, overseas. This undertaking requires the prospective parent to connect with an agency or organization that specializes in the legal transfer of children from birth parents to adoptive parents. The undertaking usually begins with a published guide or handbook of procedures and accesses (e.g., Ademec 2004; Barr and Carlisle 2003; Beauvais-Godwin and Godwin 2005; Sember 2007) or an Internet search.

Closed and Open Adoptions

A relatively recent development in adoption is the open adoption. The previous system of adoption in the United States emphasized the closing (sealing) of adoption records so as to keep adopted children (and the adoptive parents) from ever knowing the identities of birth parents and, likewise, to keep birth parents from ever finding their children. That system is still in effect in most locales. In the 1970s, based on principles postulated by Sorosky et al. (1978, 1989), experimentations in open adoptions (i.e., adoptions in which birth parents and adoptive parents were allowed and encouraged contact during the preadoption phase) began to occur. Open adoptions were followed by a worked-out plan of postadoption contacts between the child and the birth parents for information and photograph exchanges that would allow the birth parents to receive updated reports as to how the child was doing, and in many instances at least an annual physical contact between the child and the birth parents for conversation and interaction. Such contacts provided, then, a long-range platform for more openly and realistically coping with the child's developmentally emerging issues surrounding her or his birth and related matters. Some states provide for and support open adoptions, though none, of course, require it.

Searches for Birth Parents and for Children Placed Into Adoption

Two of the more compelling subjects associated with adoption are adopted children's searches for their birth parents and/or siblings, and birth parents' searches for children they placed into adoption long ago. Several organizations have been established to assist individuals from both groups in finding each other (see Adamec 2004; Barr and Carlisle 2003; Beauvais-Godwin and Godwin 2007). They may assist one party in a search for the other even though the other may be unaware of that search or perhaps not open (at least without a period of contemplation of it) to being located. Many states have constructed registries that are intended to facilitate searches, and there are some specialists who can assist, with added confidentiality, as honest intermediaries in setting up contacts between children and their birth parents. It has been estimated, however tenuously, that over one-half of the individuals who have been adopted would want to reunite with a birth parent if that were possible (e.g., Pertman 2000).

Controversy, some of it very sharp, exists as to whether or not such searches are appropriate or even legal, since at the time (and in many places) that adoptions occurred, the records were sealed in order to conceal the identities of children that were given over to adoption and the identities of parents who released them for adoption. Many children who are adopted only slowly or inadvertently learn that their names are not the names they bore as infants. Thus, the search process is often obstructed by legal barriers as well as barriers created by time, changes of names, locales, and so forth. Many of these barriers can be circumvented with the assistance of these organizations or intermediary specialists.

Perhaps the easiest reunions to enact are those in which the birth parent and released child are each in search of the other, and in which the only barriers really are those of tracing records and then locating the subject of the search. Where each is desiring and consenting of contact, and where the child is now of age to be able to decide for her- or himself as to the search, it is usually only a matter of time and the cooperation of those who might know what happened to one or the other of these individuals along life's paths. Some are pleased—overjoyed would not overstate the reactions in many of those instances—to have made the reunion and then go on to establish relationships of varying depths and extents, while others either are frankly disappointed or find that the search did not result in what was desired in the way of information, explanations, or outcomes encountered. Psychotherapists of varying theoretical orientations can certainly describe plausible, and in some cases seemingly applicable, motives (both conscious and not conscious) for these searches, and most of these descriptions will feature terms such as *loss, guilt, incompleteness,* and the like, to frame the motive constellations of searchers (and blockers of searches). Most will also feature explanations of why the successful search was pleasing or disappointing to the searcher and the found.

Each of the members of the aforementioned adoption triangle may be affected, or even deeply impacted, by adoption searches, particularly, for example, when either the child or the adoptive parents feel the adoption has not gone well by one or another criterion or when birth parents feel that events they thought they left behind are once again in the fore of their lives. As in the case of a mother, for example, who never told her present husband, or children, that there is another child out there, who is the blood sibling of their marital children. The father, for example, who never knew or had been informed that he had such a child, or who, knowing, had intended for that to remain a part of the past.

Adoptive parents sometimes divorce, and it is often the case that their child will ascribe the divorce to her- or himself as an adopted child. Generally, children of divorce often ascribe blame to themselves in this regard, though children who have been adopted may, perhaps even with subtle reinforcements from parental statements or allusions, confound the feeling of blame with her or his adoptive status. Certainly there are specialists in the field of adoption who would assert that adoption itself is a stressor on many levels and that both personal and family issues of a troubling nature are to be expected. Because of inherent behavioral and adjustment problems posed by the adopted child, his or her adoption status can become a focus of attention and ascription of "cause" in how things feel to people in the family. In each of these cases, an adoptee may feel impelled to search out her or his birth parents as a path or means of coping with feelings wrought by life within the adoptive family. The popular literature that is concerned with searches and reunions is an expanding one, and any browsing of the Internet on those subjects will encounter an abundance of individual case stories (see, for example, Schein and Bernstein 2007).

Adjustments to Adoption

The issues and dynamics of adjusting to adoption are in many respects similar to the adjustment issues and dynamics of children entering foster care—except, of course, that the child just adopted, not yet aware, convinced, or confident of any permanency to ensue, will now in fact remain where she or he has been placed. Her or his average age at the time of placement is about 5 or 6 years, perhaps younger if she or he has come through an international route. (The younger the child [e.g., infancy], the fewer background, experiential, and permanent conditions are likely to apply and therefore affect transition to adoption.) Several factors converge at the point of adoptive placement: on each side of the relationship are the child's and parents' respective objective and experiential histories and their respective natural temperamental and coping capacities. Each member of the adoption dyad—considering in this particular regard the older child more than, say, the infant as such—possesses hopes and expectations about the relationship, including its intrinsic qualities, its desired outcomes and fulfillments, and meanings. For the adopting parent there are adjustment challenges during adoption and the period following that resemble, in their own ways, the adjustment dynamics of any new parenting situation, including postadoption blues and postadoption adjustments to ordinary child care demands, scheduling, and turmoils. Of course, the routes toward birth and adoptive parenting are different, but it is not at all facetious when adoptive parents talk about their own gestational feelings, postpartum-like blues (Foli and Thompson 2004), and exhilarations at the arrival of their child (Rosenberg 1992). With or without adoption, child rearing *is* child rearing, and falling in love *is* falling in love.

The adjustment dynamics of the child, then, once adopted, are influenced by the usual factors of age and correlative developmental status, conditions, and dynamics leading to the adoption, including the conditions and dynamics of the child's having departed the birth parents (as well as foster parents) in the first place (which included any residual or permanent physical [e.g., handicapping] and mental/behavioral [e.g., attention-deficit/hyperactivity disorder, autism] conditions) and the child's perceptions of his or her new living circumstances, the home of the adoptive parent.

In these respects, what can be said by any expert at this point is the same that was said of transitions made by children to foster care (see Chapter 13, "Children in Foster Care," in this volume): whereas the child's age and correlative developmental status, along with established principles of child development and adjustment, may be instructive as to the normative issues most likely to be encountered and traversed, the light beams of normative pathways may fade as guideposts as the realities of actual adoption come into play.

Thus, as with regard to the situation of being placed into foster care, some children who are now placed into an adopted home will employ coping behaviors that seem to reflect the aberrancies of earlier care (though, as has been observed in relation to children living in foster care [see Chapter 13, "Children in Foster Care," in this volume], many children coming to adoption exhibit surprisingly positive coping capacities). As an expert, one can therefore never truly predict for a court or for an interested party to an adoption the course of a child's specific adjustment to adoption based only on the circumstances existing at the time of removal, nor can one ever truly predict that course from the time of adoption. One can, though, on the basis of professional knowledge and experience, be prepared for a variety of adjustment situations and dynamics, which in turn alert one to possible preventive measures or solutions once difficulties arise.

There is, on the adoptive parent's side, a set of adjustment factors to be considered as well; this is why legal adoptions are preceded by parent and home studies. The underlying assumption of such studies is that through them at least a basic degree and capacity for positive and appropriate parenting can be secured (or ruled out), the further assumption being that when at least a basic degree and capacity have been secured, there can be a reasonable expectation that things will generally work out positively if the adoption being considered goes forward. It is also reasonably posed and expected that as situations unique to being adopted (and to adopting) are encountered, positive resolutions can (and therefore will) be achieved.

From a psychiatric perspective, the dynamics of anxiety and depression, both of a preexisting kind and of an immediate kind, are at the forefront of assessments that may be solicited during the phases preceding and following adoption. Most children coming into adoption have had at least one period of living in foster care or (in international populations) an orphanage. They thus have a greater likelihood of cumulative experiences of multiple placements and large group living than of individualized and concentrated parenting. As such, they have often been regulated by schedules of eating, sleeping, and recreation that are now significantly different in an adoptive home—which may itself have multiple other children living within who have varying backgrounds and adjustment characteristics. Some children come to adoption having been patently sexually or physically abused at one (or successive) time(s) in their lives, or having been starved or left alone for long periods of time, prior to being removed from those conditions. When the child has been cared for effectively in foster care, where the foster parent is not the adoptive parent, elements of grief may come to the fore once adoption has occurred. Issues of race, culture, and gender will also be faced—by child and adoptive parent alike—as the adopted child now moves into a community of children and families.

Infants and preschool children pose unique sets of problems, for they lack what the much older child possesses in the way of capacities for verbalized cognitive mediation of the events. The emotional expressive and regulatory dynamics of infants and young children are also problematic, not only for the children themselves but also those who now occupy the external regulatory roles that parents occupy. Infancy and early childhood are phases in which emotional and behavioral regulation are exquisitely partnership based, and both members of the adoptive dyad are drawn to make adjustments to and within this context. In this, except for the details and the separated courses of events, adoptive and birth parents face the same challenges and prospects in regard to their infant children.

The Role of the Forensic Specialist

The two principal roles of the forensic specialist—that of cognate expert, entailing refined knowledge of child development and correlative outcomes, and technical expert, entailing specialized skills of observation and interviewing—have been alluded to above. Courts may thus rely on forensic specialists for a variety of tasks at points of adoption, including the submissions of *amicus curiae* communications or the provision of direct testimony concerning instant cases. Such testimony may be from the point of view of the child who is available to be adopted (e.g., defining special needs, offering opinions concerning potential outcomes or risks) or from the point of view of the parent who seeks to adopt (e.g., fitness to parent).

Sometimes adoptions are contested by competing parties, and forensic specialists may be recruited to assist in the process of determination when legal doctrines and standards are not directive. Each disputant may secure the services of such specialists, and of course, the court may appoint its own.

Finally, many cases of wrongful adoption include numbers of forensic specialists typically recruited by competing parties, but also sometimes appointed by the court, who may debate the principles and provisions for the putative "best interests" of the children involved.[1] Apart from these expert opinions, the judiciary typically decides in these matters, as ultimately it is tasked to do, on the basis of law.

Conclusion

Adoption poses many challenges that are framed by legal, cultural, and personal circumstances. There can be no overlooking the unique features and events of adoption and its course in the lives of those affected by it. But adoption in the twenty-first century and in the United States is more visible, more broadly accepted, and more widely supported than it once was. Forensic specialists have important consultative roles to play as courts encounter particular issues of psychological and developmental natures relating to a child's adoption status.

---

[1] The best interests standard, according to Rodham (1973), is not so much a standard as it is a set of rationalizations used by decision makers to justify judgments about children's futures, thereby to act in relation to a present disposition. According to Rodham, then, the child in judicial circumstances is "an empty vessel into which adult perceptions and prejudices are poured" (p. 513). Everyone knows what the best interests of the child are, but they often cannot agree on how to get to them.

—*Key Points*

— About 51,000 children are adopted each year in the United States out of the foster care system, while about 20,000 children are adopted each year through international channels. Private and independent adoptions account for a comparatively smaller number of adoptions per year.

— Special issues in adoption include availability of children, open adoptions, searches, and adjustment challenges.

References

Adamec C: Adoption. New York, Penguin Group, 2004

Adoption and Safe Families Act of 1997 (Pub. L. No. 105-89)

Adoption Assistance and Child Welfare Act of 1980 (Pub. L. No. 96-272)

Anderson S: On sacred ground: commemorating survival and loss at the Carlisle Indian School. Central PA Magazine, May 2000

Barr T, Carlisle K: Adoption. New York, Wiley, 2003

Beauvais-Godwin L, Godwin R: The Complete Adoption Book: Everything You Need to Know to Adopt a Child, 3rd Edition. Avon, MA, Adams Media, 2005

Boswell J: The Kindness of Strangers: The Abandonment of Children in Western Europe From Late Antiquity to the Renaissance. New York, Pantheon Books, 1988

Cassidy J, Shaver PR (eds): Handbook of Attachment: Theory, Research, and Clinical Applications. New York, Guilford, 1999

Eldridge S: Twenty Things Adopted Kids Wish Their Adoptive Parents Knew. New York, Bantam Dell, 1999

Fields J: Living arrangements of children. Washington, DC, U.S. Census Bureau Current Population Reports April:70–74, 2001

Freud A: Annual report (1942), in The Writings of Anna Freud, Vol 3. New York, International Universities Press, 1973, pp 142–211

Freud S: Family romances (1909), in The Standard Edition of the Complete Psychological Works of Sigmund Freud, Vol 9. Translated and edited by Strachey J. London, Hogarth, 1959, pp 237–241

Foli KJ, Thompson JR: The Post-Adoption Blues: Overcoming the Unforeseen Challenges of Adoption. New York, St. Martin's Press, 2004

Goody J: The Development of the Family and Marriage in Europe. New York, Cambridge University Press, 1983

Grossmann KE, Grossmann K, Waters E: Attachment From Infancy to Adulthood: The Major Longitudinal Studies. New York, Guilford, 2005

Harnack A (ed): Adoption: Opposing Viewpoints. San Diego, CA, Greenhaven, 1995

Hicks RB: Adopting in America. Sun City, CA, Wordslinger, 1993

Horner TM: The development of the symbiotic wish. Psychoanalytic Psychology 9:25–48, 1992

Horner TM, Rosenberg EB: The family romance: a developmental-historical perspective. Psychoanalytic Psychology 8:131–148, 1991

Howe RL: Adoption practice, issues and laws. Fam Law Q 17:173–197, 1983

Jacobs MD: A Battle for the Children: American Indian Child Removal in Arizona in the Era of Assimilation. Lincoln, University of Nebraska, 2004

Jacobs MD: Maternal colonialism: white women and indigenous child removal in the American west and Australia, 1880–1940. West Hist Q 36:453–476, 2005

Jones BJ: The Indian Child Welfare Act Handbook. Chicago, IL, American Bar Association, 1995

Jones BJ: The Indian Child Welfare Act: The Need for a New Law. Chicago, IL, American Bar Association, 1996

Leon I: Adoption losses: naturally occurring or socially constructed? Child Dev 73:652–663, 2002

McCreight B: Parenting Your Adopted Older Child. Oakland, CA, New Harbinger, 2002

Mintz S: Huck's Raft. Cambridge, MA, Harvard University Press, 2004

National Data Analysis System: International Adoption: Trends and Issues. Arlington, VA, Child Welfare League of America, November 2007

Parkin R, Stone L (eds): Kinship and Family: An Anthropological Reader. New York, Wiley-Blackwell, 2004

Pertman A: Adoption Nation. New York, Basic Books, 2000

Piaget J: The Child's Conception of the World. New York, Harcourt Brace, 1923

Piaget J: The Origins of Intelligence. New York, International Universities Press, 1936

Riedman ML: The evolution of alloparental care and adoption in mammals and birds. Q Rev Biol 57:405–537, 1982

Rodham H: Children under the law. Harv Educ Rev 43:487–514, 1973

Rosenberg EB: The Adoption Life Cycle: The Children and Their Families Through the Years. New York, Simon & Schuster, 1992

Rosenberg EB, Horner TM: Birth parent romances and identity formation in adopted children. Am J Orthopsychiatry 61:70–77, 1991

Schein E, Bernstein P: Identical Strangers: A Memoir of Twins Separated and Reunited. New York, Random House, 2007

Sember BM: Adoption Answer Book. Naperville, IL, Sphinx, 2007

Sorosky AD, Baran A, Pannor R: Identity conflicts in adolescence. Am J Orthopsychiatry 45:18–27, 1975

Sorosky AD, Baran A, Pannor R: The Adoption Triangle. New York, Anchor, 1978

Sorosky AD, Baran A, Pannor R: The Adoption Triangle: Sealed or Opened Records: How They Affect Adoptees, Birth Parents and Adoptive Parents. San Antonio, TX, Corona, 1989

Strathern M (ed): Kinship, Law and the Unexpected: Relatives Are Always a Surprise. New York, Cambridge University Press, 2005

Thoma R: Under seize: the Indian Child Welfare Act of 1978. 2006. Available at: http://www.liftingtheveil.org/icwa.htm. Accessed December 4, 2008.

U.S. Department of Heath and Human Services Administration for Children and Families: Trends in Foster Care and Adoption—Fiscal Years 2002–2007 (Adoption and Foster Care Analysis and Reporting System data). Washington, DC, U.S. Children's Bureau, Administration on Children, Youth and Families, 2008

U.S. Department of State: Total Adoptions to the United States. Washington, DC, Office of Children's Issues, 2008

U.S. Intercountry Adoption Act of 2000 (Public Law 106-279)

Chapter 15

Special Issues in Transcultural, Transracial, and Gay and Lesbian Parenting and Adoption

Frank E. Vandervort, J.D.
Robert B. Sanoshy, LCSW

The adoption of children whose natural parents are unable to or incapable of caring for them by adults who are able to provide for them has existed throughout human history in one form or another (*In re Smith Estate* 1955; Miller et al. 2007). Before the mid-1800s, however, there was no formal mechanism for a person interested in adopting a child in the United States to do so (Bartholet 1999). In 1851, the Massachusetts legislature enacted the Massachusetts Adoption of Children Act (General Court of Massachusetts 1851). Though enacted more than 150 years ago, the act's basic structure is clearly recognizable in many states' present adoption laws. The Massachusetts act permitted any person to petition a probate court to adopt a child; required the child's parents, if one or both were alive, to consent to the child's adoption; required that if an adoption petitioner was married, his or her spouse was required to join a petition to adopt a child; provided that children age 14 years or older also must consent to their adoption; provided for the court to make a determinate judgment that the proposed adoption would serve the child's welfare; and extinguished all rights of the natural parent while granting to the adoptive parents all the rights and responsibilities that would inure to a natural parent. The Massachusetts statute served as a model for other states' adoption

laws (*In re Smith Estate* 1955). Many of the requirements of that earliest American adoption law are still present in twenty-first-century adoption statutes.

Courts have consistently held that there is no constitutionally protected right for a person to adopt a child (*In re Adams* 1991; *In re Opinion of the Justices* 1987; *Webb v. Wiley* 1979). Rather, the adoption of children is a "legal creation governed by statute" (*In re Opinion of the Justices* 1987, p. 1098). Indeed, courts consistently hold that adoption law is entirely or exclusively statutory (*Adoption of Tammy* 1993; *In re Adams* 1991; *Lindley for Lindley v. Sullivan* 1989). As such, courts have generally held that a person will be prohibited from seeking to adopt only when the jurisdiction's adoption statute expressly forbids the individual from doing so (e.g., *Adoption of B.L.V.B. and E.L.V.B.* 1993; *Adoption of Tammy* 1993). In *Adoption of Tammy*, for example, the Massachusetts Supreme Judicial Court, the state's highest court, held that a lesbian woman's partner was not prohibited from seeking to adopt the woman's child where the statute required that if two persons were married the adoption petitioner's spouse was required to join in the petition to adopt. In part the court reached this conclusion because the statute did not expressly prohibit two unmarried persons from adopting a child together.

In all adoption proceedings, the overarching issue to be addressed is the best interests and welfare of the child (*In re C.D.M.* 2001; *Lindley for Lindley v. Sullivan* 1989; S.D. Codified Laws § 25-6-2, 2008). South Dakota's adoption statute is typical in this regard. It provides that "[i]n an adoption proceeding or in any proceeding that challenges an order of adoption or order terminating parental rights, the court shall give due consideration to the interests of the parties to the proceedings, but shall give paramount consideration to the best interests of the child" (S.D. Codified Laws § 25-6-2, 2008). Courts and legislatures generally define the phrase "best interests of the child" broadly so as to encompass virtually any factor that may affect a child. For example, the Supreme Court of Arkansas has noted that "The phrase 'best interest of the child' means more than station in life and material things. 'Best interest of the child' includes moral, spiritual, material and cultural values, matter of convenience and friends and family relationships" (*Bush v. Dietz* 1984, p. 707). Michigan's adoption statute (Mich. Comp. Laws Ann. § 710.22[g], 2008) contains a detailed definition of what the legislature intends for courts handling adoption proceedings to consider when addressing the child's best interests. The definition sets out 10 specific and one general consideration that the court must address in each adoption proceeding by making specific findings. For example, the court must make findings regarding "The capacity and disposition of the adopting individual or individuals…to provide the adoptee with food, clothing, education, permanence, medical care or other remedial care" and "The ability and willingness of the adopting individual or individuals to adopt the adoptee's siblings." Because of the prominence of the child's best interests and welfare, mental health professionals are frequently called upon to assess the child's needs and the prospective adoptive parents' capacities to meet those needs and to render an opinion to the court as to whether the adults are able to meet the child's needs. Where there are competing adoption petitioners, evaluators may be asked to opine as to which of two prospective petitioners is best equipped to meet the child's needs.

As with other areas of family life, adoption practices have evolved over time, and they continue to evolve (Groza et al. 2005). Today more than at any time in U.S. history, adoption law recognizes the changing structure of the American family, although the law in various jurisdictions is far from recognizing the true complexity of family structures. So, for example, single individuals may adopt children, and some states permit a lesbian woman's partner to adopt her children (*Adoption of B.L.V.B. and E.L.V.B.* 1993; *Adoption of Tammy* 1993) or gay couples to adopt (Vt. Stat. Ann. 15A § 1-102, 2008).

While historically, agreements for postadoption contact between the child and natural parent were unenforceable and contrary to public policy (*In the Matter of the Adoption of Moore-Tillay* 2006), today some states' laws provide for open adoption, that is, adoption with postadoption contact between the biological parent and the child (Ann. Laws Mass. GL Ch. 210 § 3, 2008; Ore. Rev. Stat. § 109.305, 2007). Oregon is a leader in open adoption; its adoption statute provides that "[a]n adoptive parent and a birth parent may enter into a written agreement, approved by the court, to permit continuing contact between the birth relatives and the child…." Under that state's law, the agreement for postadoption contact must be agreed to by the adopting parent, who cannot be forced into such an agreement, and then must be approved by the court in which the adoption takes place. Where the agreement for postadoption contact is not approved by the court, it cannot be enforced (*In the Matter of the Adoption of Moore-Tillay* 2006). Additionally, while most states address postadoption contact by way of a statute, some states permit courts, in exercise of their equitable powers to act in the child's best interests, to order contact with an adopted child and his or her biological parent (e.g., *Adoption of Vito* 2000). Even where a court has authority to order postadoption contact between a child and his or her biological parent, that decision must be made on the basis of the needs and best interests of the child and not the parents' needs or desire for continuing contact with the child (*In re Melanie S.* 1998). So, while the law has changed over time, it still seeks to ensure the rights of the child and the adoptive parents to control the child's upbringing and makes these determinations based on the child's best interests. These are just a few of the ways in which adoption law has changed over the past 20 years.

After addressing some general issues relating to adoption—definitions, forms of adoption, and the basic adoption process—this chapter will look in more depth at three areas of adoption law: transcultural (i.e., intercountry) adoption, transracial adoption, and adoption by gay and lesbian individuals and couples. In considering each topic, we address the implications for forensic mental health practice. Before doing so, a few words about limitations: the adoption of children is generally governed by state law, and every state's law is different. This chapter does not attempt to address the tremendous complexity in adoption law generally, or in any of the three specific areas subsequently considered. Rather, this chapter seeks to highlight a number of practices that are fairly uniform and to address the potential clinical issues of which mental health professionals working in the forensic arena should be aware.

Definitions

For purposes of this chapter, we refer to adoption as the process by which the parental rights of a child's biological parents are legally extinguished and the child is provided new legal parents. Transcultural adoption refers to adoption of a child into a family in the United States from another country. This form of adoption may be referred to as intercountry adoption; for example, when an American couple adopts a child from China or Vietnam. We use the term *transracial adoption* to refer to the adoption of a child by parents of a different race or ethnicity. An example of transracial adoption would be when a white mother adopts an African American or Native American child who had been initially placed with her for foster care. Finally, this chapter considers adoption by gays and lesbians, whether individually, as second parents, or as couples. Such adoptions may involve a woman adopting her partner's biological child, a gay couple adopting a foster child for whom they have provided care for years, or a single gay man seeking to start a family through adoption.

The parties to an adoption process are typically the natural parents, the prospective adoptive parents, an adoption agency, and, depending on the child's age, the child. If the child is an "Indian child" as defined by the Indian Child Welfare Act of 1978 (i.e., an unmarried person younger than 18 years who is a member of a federally recognized tribe or is the biological child of a member of a tribe and is eligible for membership), the child's tribe will also be a party to the proceeding whose interests may differ from those of both the child and the parents, and failure to involve the tribe in adoption planning may result in disruption of the adoption (e.g., *Mississippi Band of Choctaw Indians v. Holyfield* 1989).

Forms of Adoption

Adoption of a child may come about in any one of several forms or processes. This section briefly describes the basic forms adoption may take.

Release to Agency

The law of every state permits a parent wishing to relinquish a child for adoption to release his or her parental rights to an agency (Gregory et al. 2001). A parent may release his or her rights to either a public agency, such as the state's Department of Human Services, or to a private adoption agency licensed by state authorities to provide adoption services. Private adoption agencies may serve the general population in need of adoption services, or they may serve a niche constituency. For example, some adoption agencies serve a particular religious sect (e.g., *Scott v. Family Ministries* 1976), while others serve the adoption needs of the black community (e.g., "Homes for Black Children," n.d.). If the parent releases the child to the agency, the agency will typically select the adoptive parent.

Direct Placement

Most states permit a child's natural parents to select the adoptive parents for their child (Gregory et al. 2001). In a direct placement adoption, parents wishing to place a child for adoption may select an individual or couple to adopt their child with or without the assistance of a child placing agency. Michigan's law is typical and provides that "A parent or guardian...having legal and physical custody of a child may make a direct placement of a child for adoption....A parent or guardian shall personally select a prospective adoptive parent in a direct placement. The selection shall not be delegated" (Mich. Comp. Laws Ann. § 710.23a[1] and [2], 2008). When the parents have not identified a person or couple to adopt their child, they may turn to a child placing agency and seek its assistance in identifying adoptive parents. From among the possible adoptive families, the parent will then select one. Biological relatives of a child other than the parents have neither the authority to consent to a child's adoption nor any right to be notified when a biological parent releases a child for adoption (*Farnsworth v. Goebel* 1921).

Stepparent Adoption

Historically, before a stepparent could adopt a child, the child's natural parent had to release his or her parental rights to make the child available for adoption, then the couple could adopt the child jointly. However, with the increasing divorce and remarriage rates in the latter half of the twentieth century, a number of states amended their adoption laws to permit a child's stepparent to adopt without the rights of the biological parent having to be released (e.g., *Delgado v. Fawcett* 1973; Mich. Comp. Laws Ann. § 170.5, 2008). In a stepparent adoption, the child's parent consents to the child's adoption by the parent's spouse (Kan. Stat. Ann. § 59-2112, 2006).

Second-Parent Adoption

Second-parent adoption is the analogue in gay and lesbian adoption of stepparent in the heterosexual context. In a second-parent adoption, a gay or lesbian parent—whether biological or adoptive—consents to the adoption of his or her child by his or her life partner without having to first release his or her parental rights. Vermont's Supreme Court was one of the first courts in the country to interpret its adoption statutes to permit second-parent adoption by a lesbian couple (*Adoption of B.L.V.B. and E.L.V.B.* 1993). The legislature subsequently amended the state's Adoption Act to explicitly provide for second-parent adoption (Vt. Stat. Ann. 15A § 1-102, 2008). That statute now provides that "[i]f a family unit consists of a parent and the parent's partner, and adoption is in the best interest of the child, the partner of a parent may adopt a child of the parent. Termination of the parent's parental rights is unnecessary in an adoption under this subsection."

Involuntary Termination of Parental Rights

Every state's law provides a mechanism for state authorities or, in most instances, private actors to involuntarily terminate the parental rights of an abusive or neglectful parent or one who has abandoned or failed to support his or her child. In many instances, the parental rights to these children are terminated only after the child has suffered significant trauma and has spent some considerable period of time in the foster care system. Where the parents' rights have been involuntarily terminated, the state or private agency typically has the authority to consent to the child's adoption. Because the trauma—often multiple traumas—these children have experienced often leads to emotional or behavioral problems, they can be difficult to place and are at increased risk of adoption disruption. It is clear, however, that many children who have suffered multiple traumas do very well in adoptive homes (Bartholet 1999).

In an effort to move these children from temporary placements in the foster care system into permanent adoptive homes, since 1980 the federal government has provided funding for adoption incentive payments to offset some of the additional burdens these children experience as a result of their abusive and neglectful histories (42 U.S.C. § 670 et seq.). These payments may be in the form of either monthly cash assistance payments or the provision of Medicaid to address the child's medical and emotional needs. Additionally, adoptive parents may receive tax credits for adopting a child from the foster care system (Bartholet 1999). Despite the existence of these subsidy programs, large numbers of children in the foster care system remain in need of adoptive placements (Gregory et al. 2001; Pew Commission on Children in Foster Care, n.d.).

Children who have experienced involuntary termination of parental rights may be at heightened risk. They will have typically spent time, in some cases years, in temporary foster care. They may have experienced instability in placement, and their capacity to attach with an adoptive family may be impaired. This group of children may be at increased risk of adoption disruption because of emotional, behavioral, and physical challenges (Festinger 2005; Roberts 2002).

Standby Adoption

In the mid-1990s, largely in response to the AIDS epidemic, a number of state legislatures adopted standby guardianship statutes, which permit parents to name a guardian for their child in the event of their becoming debilitated or dying (McConnell 1995/1996; e.g., Fla. Stat. § 744.304; N.J. Stat. Ann. § 3B:12-68). One state, Illinois, took this concept one step further and permits a terminally ill parent to nominate a standby to adopt his or her child (Ill. Comp. Stat., 750 ILCS 50/1, 1950). Illinois law defines a standby adoption as "an adoption in which a parent consents to custody and termination of parental rights to become effective upon the occurrence of a future event, which is either the death of the parent or the request of the parent for the entry of a final judgment of adoption" (750 ILCS 50/1). In general, the process for putting in place a standby adoption is the same as establishing a typical adoption.

Basic Adoption Process

While there are variations in every jurisdiction, in general adoption follows a standard process. First, before a child may be adopted, he or she must be legally available for adoption. Availability for adoption in circumstances other than stepparent or second-parent adoptions requires that the parental rights of the child's biological parent be terminated. Termination of the natural parents' rights typically comes about by way of either release of parental rights directly to an adoptive parent or parents or release to an agency and then entry of a court order terminating rights (e.g., Kan. Stat. Ann. § 59-2136, 2006; Minn. Stat. § 259.24, 2007) or through involuntary termination of parental rights (Gregory et al. 2001). Some states' laws permit a public or private agency to seek adoption even without parental consent and over a parent's objection (Ann. Laws Mass. GL Ch. 210 § 3, 2008; Petition of New England Home for Little Wanderers 1975). (See also Chapter 14, "Adoption," in this volume.)

Once a child is available for adoption, the next step in the process is an evaluation of the child's needs and readiness for adoption. In this child assessment, the agency facilitating the adoption or a court social worker assesses the child's needs, details the child's attitude toward adoption if the child is old enough to express a preference, and makes a recommendation about whether a proposed adoptive plan will meet the child's needs.

Next, a home study of the prospective adoptive parent(s) is conducted to determine whether they are able to meet the child's needs. Most state laws contain very few disqualifiers for persons wishing to adopt a child but rely on the adoption study process to screen inappropriate candidates and to match a child with an appropriate individual or family (Gregory et al. 2001). The precise content of the home study varies from jurisdiction to jurisdiction and from agency to agency (Crea et al. 2007). Generally, a home study will include information about the home, community, work history, family life and history, health information, relationships between the adults seeking to adopt, information about other children who may reside in the home, and what categories of children the parties would be interested in adopting or not adopting (e.g., age, race, physically or mentally disabled; Ark. Code Ann. § 9-9-212, 2008; Crea et al. 2007). There is a criminal background check and a check of Child Protective Services records to determine whether there has ever been a referral concerning a child from the family home. Finally, the home study contains a recommendation regarding whether the investigating adoption worker approves the home (Crea et al. 2007). Home studies are also utilized as an opportunity to convey to an adoptive family information about the adoption process and the child the family may be interested in adopting. Because there is a subjective element to adoption home studies, some commentators are con-

cerned about the impact of bias or prejudice in decision making (Mallon 2007; McRoy et al. 2007). A number of jurisdictions have moved to establish more uniform measures to reduce the subjectivity and to facilitate adoption across jurisdictional lines (Crea et al. 2007).

When a child has been matched with an adoptive family, the next step is to initiate a petition seeking court authorization to complete the adoption. While specific state practices vary widely, there is typically a temporary order for adoption issued that permits the court and agencies to monitor a child's placement for a period of time before a final order of adoption is issued. Once the final order is issued, the court case is closed and the adoptive parent has the full rights of a natural parent.

Clinical Issues

A forensic mental health specialist may be called on to provide an opinion as to a child who is in need of adoption services or may be asked to render an opinion as to an adult's or couple's fitness to parent, either generally or in relation to a specific child. Careful, objective assessment of both the strengths and weaknesses of the child's adoptability and each prospective parent's ability and willingness to parent the child is crucial. As noted earlier, the primary guidepost for courts when making determinations about proposed adoptive placements is the "best interests of the child." Some jurisdictions define the meaning of this amorphous phrase in their statutes, whereas others leave it to courts to make determinations in individual cases. Before undertaking an evaluation for adoption purposes, a forensic expert should take the time to familiarize him- or herself with the jurisdiction's definition of best interest and the factors that courts may use in considering what is best for a child.

Forensic specialists should obtain as much documentary information as possible before undertaking such an evaluation. Reports from social workers, medical providers, schools, and similar agencies may contain crucial information about the child—including special needs he or she may have—and the prospective adoptive parents. Similarly, information regarding criminal histories and histories of contacts with Child Protective Services would be essential to understanding the needs of the child and the capacities of the adoption petitioners.

With this background information, the evaluator should meet with the child and each prospective parent individually to conduct a careful interview to gain additional information and to further assess the needs and capacities of the parties. Next, if the proposed adoption is with two parents, the evaluator should meet jointly with the prospective parents to assess their interactions with one another as well as their interaction with the child by observing them together. Finally, while adults wishing to adopt children typically must provide letters of reference, the evaluator may need to make contact with collateral sources of information, such as extended family members, friends of the family, or members of the clergy, to fully understand the family's circumstances.

Any chapter about adoption would be missing something if it failed to discuss attachment theory. Developed by John Bowlby (1973), attachment theory explains how human beings attach to one another. For adopted children and families, the challenge of attachment can be quite significant as children sometimes come from multiple attachments prior to placement, making attachment to their adoptive parents more difficult. Bowlby suggested that one of the primary goals of any infant is to establish a secure attachment to a parental figure. If a parent or caregiver does not attach to a child in a healthy and safe way, there is little a child can do to change this. When children come from multiple placements and have had a number of caregivers, especially early on in their life, the challenge of attaching to new caregivers can result in difficulties forming a healthy attachment with the adoptive parent and may result in behavioral problems.

Mary Ainsworth's work, in conjunction with Bowlby's research, identified three types of major attachments in her "Strange Situation" experiment (Ainsworth and Bowlby 1965): secure attachments, anxious–ambivalent insecure attachment, and anxious–avoidant insecure attachment. In anxious–ambivalent insecure attachment, the child is anxious about strangers even in the presence of an attachment figure, becomes quite distressed when the attachment figure leaves, and is ambivalent toward him or her upon return. In an anxious–avoidant insecure attachment, the child is avoidant of the attachment figure whether he or she is in the room or not, and strangers are treated similarly to the attachment figure.

Preplacement meetings and postadoption family and individual therapy can assist in the healthy attachment between adoptive parents and adopted children and teens. In a case in which attachment is or may be a problem, forensic evaluators should consider making a recommendation for the number of preplacement meetings and possibly therapy that they be-

lieve will help facilitate relationships that are rooted in safety and connection.

On occasion, there may be individuals or couples competing to adopt a single child. This sometimes happens when, for example, a child is in foster care and both the foster parents and a relative, say, an aunt or biological grandparents, are seeking to adopt. In such a circumstance, the forensic evaluator would want to meet with the child and each of the possible parents, conducting evaluations of each individually as well as their workings as a family unit. In circumstances in which there is a contest regarding an adoption, it is tempting for the forensic expert to be pulled in one direction or the other. It is essential, both to the proper working of the legal system and for the expert's own credibility, that she or he remain as objective as possible. In such circumstances an evaluator may be tempted to make comments about or provide opinions regarding an individual the evaluator has not assessed. It is crucial that the evaluator resist this urge. If the forensic evaluator has seen documentary information that suggests concern about one of the parties whom the evaluator has not personally evaluated, it is best to suggest that this information raises concerns that should be evaluated further rather than to take a position or articulate an opinion based on such information.

Transcultural Adoption

The international adoption of children is a fairly recent phenomenon. Before World War II, there were few international adoptions (Barthelot 1999). After the war, the adoption of children internationally into the United States, largely as a result of American soldiers fathering children in European and Asian countries, as well as the visibility of refugees of war and famine in Asia and Africa (Adoption History Project 2007), grew steadily until 2004 when there were 22,884 such adoptions (Navarro 2008). Between 2004 and 2007, international adoptions declined, mainly due to concerns about the ethical practices of some agencies facilitating international adoption. Several of these agencies apparently paid poor birth parents in countries such as Vietnam to release their rights to their children to be adopted or deceived birth parents as to their ability to have ongoing contact with their child (Navarro 2008; Olson 2008). As a result, some countries have stopped sending children to the United States for adoption, whereas other countries, such as Guatemala, have recently slowed the process of international adoption to ensure that birth parents were not deceived into giving up their children for adoption (Navarro 2008).

Hague Convention

On May 29, 1993, the Hague Conference on Private International Law concluded the Hague Convention on Protection of Children and Cooperation in Respect of Intercountry Adoption ("The Convention"), which entered into force internationally on May 1, 1995. The Convention was ratified by the United States on December 12, 2007, and took effect on April 1, 2008. The Convention is implemented in the United States through the federal Intercountry Adoption Act (P.L. 106-279), which establishes procedures to be used when American citizens adopt children from other countries that are parties to The Convention. When the country from which a child is being adopted is not a party to The Convention, the adoption is governed by the Immigration and Nationality Act and the Child Citizenship Act, which provides for an automatic grant of U.S. citizenship for a child who is adopted abroad.

The Convention establishes procedures to ensure that international adoptions are conducted in an ethically sound manner. Basically, an American citizen wishing to adopt from another Hague Convention state must apply to the U.S. State Department, which must make a determination that the prospective adoptive parent(s) is suitable to adopt a child. If the State Department is satisfied that the parent is suitable, it must prepare a report detailing information about the applicant's identity, suitability to adopt, family and medical history, background including reasons for wishing to adopt, and the characteristics of the children for whom the person would be qualified to care. The State Department must then forward this report to the comparable authority in the child's country of origin. If the designated officials in the child's country of origin are satisfied that the child is suitable for adoption, they must prepare a report regarding the child detailing the child's identity, adoptability, social, familial, and medical histories, as well as any special needs the child may have. In preparing the report, the authorities must take into consideration the child's upbringing and his or her ethnic, religious, and cultural background. The child's state of origin must, consistent with its laws, determine that the appropriate parental consents to adopt have been obtained. Finally, the authorities in the child's country of origin must determine that the adoptive placement would serve the child's best interests. If the authorities in the child's state of origin are satisfied that these requirements have been fulfilled, they must transmit the report detailing these matters as well as the consent of each parent to the U.S. State Department.

The Convention does not specify in which of the two countries the adoption will actually occur. Rather, this issue is to be determined by the laws of the respective countries. If the laws of the child's country of origin require that the child be adopted in that country, The Convention requires that the adoption actually take place there.

Recognition of Adoptions From Other Countries

When a child is adopted in another country, one question becomes whether a state in the United States will provide full recognition to that adoption. Generally, American states provide comity—that is, legal recognition and enforceability—to the decrees of foreign courts so long as the parties to a proceeding in that other country benefited from fair procedures unless that order or decree is repugnant to the law of the receiving state (Seymore 2004). The Convention addresses this issue (United Nations 1995). It allows a country to refuse to recognize an adoption if that adoption is "manifestly contrary to its public policy, taking into account the best interests of the child" (United Nations 1995, Ch. V, Art. 24). Additionally, some states have adopted statutes that specifically provide for recognition of adoption decrees issued by other countries (Seymore 2004; e.g., Fla. Stat. § 63.192, 2008; Mich. Comp. Laws Ann. § 710.21b, 2008). Michigan's law provides:

> A court order or decree establishing the relationship of parent and child by adoption and issued by a court in another country is presumed to be issued in accordance with the laws of that country and shall be recognized in this state. The rights and obligations of the parties as to matters within the jurisdiction of this state shall be determined as though the order or decree were issued by a court of this state. (Mich. Comp. Laws § 710.21b, 2008)

But this leaves open a question as to whether a properly issued court order of adoption issued in another country is enforceable in a particular state within the United States. A short example may help to illustrate these principles and the issues that may arise as a result. Imagine that a gay couple from Michigan adopts a child in Ontario, Canada, where gay couples can legally adopt children jointly. They then return with their child to Michigan. As noted, Michigan generally recognizes adoption decrees granted by other countries. However, Michigan's Attorney General has interpreted Michigan law to decline to permit homosexual couples, even those who are legally married in a state which permits same-sex marriage, to adopt within the state (Opinion of Michigan Attorney General 2004). This opinion is binding on state agencies unless a court arrives at a different conclusion (Mich. Comp. Laws Ann. § 14.32, 2008). That is, marriages performed in states that permit same-sex marriage are not entitled to comity in Michigan. While Michigan's legislature has adopted a statute that generally requires the recognition of foreign orders of adoption, it has also provided that the rights and obligations of the parties are as they would be under Michigan law, which would not grant the adoption. So, it is unclear whether the gay couple's Canadian adoption order would be valid in Michigan.

Clinical Concerns

This section looks at potential clinical vulnerabilities and resiliencies when exploring the effects of transcultural adoption. Two of the potential problematic areas for the transculturally adopted child are the possibility of an ambiguous history and a stressed connection to culture of origin and loss of family.

In some cases, Americans who adopt transculturally may not have accurate or complete information on their adopted child's biological background or social history that precluded their adoption. Poverty is a leading reason that children in foreign countries are in need of adoption services (Groza et al. 2005). This may help to explain why most children who are adopted internationally experience one or more prenatal risk factors such as low birth weight, prematurity, and a lack of prenatal medical care (Miller et al. 2007). Moreover, while most children who are awaiting adoption in the United States are placed in foster family homes, many children adopted from abroad are cared for in congregate care settings such as orphanages or other institutional settings (Groza et al. 2005). As a result, these children may have experienced early deprivation of nurturance and attentive care necessary for optimal development, and specifically may experience problems forming healthy attachments (Groza et al. 2005). These children may have difficulty adjusting to the emotional intensity of family life in their adoptive placements, and they may prove challenging for adoptive parents either immediately or later in adolescence when behavioral

problems may manifest. These factors may combine to place internationally adopted children at higher risk of maltreatment and may help to explain why some researchers and clinicians have expressed concern that internationally adopted children may be disproportionately represented among child maltreatment deaths (Miller et al. 2007). While not all children adopted internationally have experienced traumatic events, some of these children may have, and there remains the possibility that an adoptive parent will not be privy to this information. Additionally, for children who have experienced time in the streets, in abusive homes, or in overcrowded orphanages, their issues around attachment may be heightened.

Second, while many adoptive parents do their best to create an environment that is culturally familiar to their adopted child, there are only so many ways an adoptive parent can create lasting and meaningful connections to a child's culture of origin. More often than not, this connection to culture comes later in life, when the child seeks it out. While there are many cities and communities in which children may feel as though they see other individuals who look like them physically, the disconnection from a country of origin can be palpable when trying to form an identity. In transcultural adoptions, issues tend to be more about differences in race as opposed to culture, and although the two may seem similar, they are separate. When children are brought into the United States from countries whose culture differs drastically from American culture, parents may have a difficult time finding those connections for their children. This may be especially true of children from distinct subcultures. As adopted children grow up, their interest in their culture of origin may increase, and if they have a difficult time seeking out information and experiences that are directly relatable to their culture of origin, they may begin to develop an ambiguous feeling toward their adoption.

Transracial Adoption

Few issues in the field of adoption have proved as controversial as transracial adoption. Scholars from various disciplines have hotly debated the propriety and impact of this practice on minority communities and individual children (e.g., Bartholet 1999; Kennedy 2003; Roberts 2002). For instance, the National Association of Black Social Workers has long opposed the adoption of African American children by white parents (Bartholet 1999; Kennedy 2003). Harvard Law School Professor Randall Kennedy (2003) pointed out that during the time of slavery in the United States, children were assigned one race in part to prevent interracial child rearing, a practice which continued well into the twentieth century. He observed that before 1950 the question of transracial adoption "was hardly ever posed, simply because the very idea of interracial adoption was inconceivable" (Kennedy 2003, p. 387). In the decades between the enactment of the first modern adoption law by an American state in 1851 and the civil rights movement, interracial adoption was so stigmatized that it was not a serious issue, although two states' statutory law prohibited the adoption of children by parents of a different race (Bartholet 1999; Kennedy 2003). Louisiana's statute, for instance, provided that "A single person over the age of twenty-one years, or a married couple jointly, may petition to adopt any child of his or their race" (*Compos v. McKeithen* 1972). Similarly, Texas law provided that "No white child can be adopted by a negro person, nor can a negro child be adopted by a white person" (*In re Gomez* 1967). These statutes were challenged by persons wishing to adopt children across racial lines, and courts struck them down as violating the federal and state constitutions (e.g., *Compos v. McKeithen* 1972; *In re Gomez* 1967).

Even though the Federal District Court for the Eastern District of Louisiana struck down Louisiana's statute prohibiting all interracial adoption, the nation's last such law, it made clear that race could be legitimately considered as one factor in assessing a child's best interests in an adoption process. The court said:

> Cognizant of the realities of American society, this Court would agree that an interracial home in Louisiana presents difficulties for a child, including the possible refusal by a community to accept the child, and other community pressures, born of racial prejudice, on the interracial family. A determination of reasonableness of racial classification in this statute would seem to follow recognition of such difficulties, but we regard the difficulties inherent in interracial adoption as justifying consideration of race as a relevant factor in adoption, and not as justifying race as the determinative factor. (*Compos v. McKeithen* 1972, p. 266)

Such consideration of race as a factor in assessing an adoptive placement was commonplace and persisted until the 1990s (e.g., *Drummond v. Fulton County Department of Family and Children's Services* 1977; Groza et al. 2005; *In re Adoption of Minor* 1955; *In re Moorhead* 1991; Kennedy 2003).

In 1994, Congress enacted the Multiethnic Placement Act (MEPA; P.L. 103-382), which sought to pro-

hibit the routine consideration of race, color, or national origin in adoption planning for children from the public foster care system. This statute, which provides a private right of legal action against officials who violate its provisions, sought to speed the exit of children from the foster care system, to increase the number of foster and adoptive homes to meet the needs of children in the child welfare system awaiting adoption, and to eliminate discriminatory actions in relation to placement in foster or adoptive homes (Groza et al. 2005). Congress amended the law to make the prohibitions against the consideration of race stronger, in part by eliminating the use of the word *routine*, which seems to imply that race can never be considered in making adoption placement decisions for children in the foster care system (Roberts 2002). This amendment, referred to as the Interethnic Adoption Provisions (IEP; P.L. 104-188), was enacted in 1996. As Groza et al. (2005) pointed out, "This is contrary to what is known about the needs of some children for support in the development of racial or ethnic identity" (p. 436). In interpreting the statute as amended, the Children's Bureau, the agency within the federal Department of Health and Human Services responsible for administering the nation's child welfare system, has made clear that while any consideration of race, color, or national origin will be subjected to strict scrutiny, it is permissible to consider these factors if doing so is necessary to meet the needs of an individual child for whom placement decision making is being made (Herring 2007; Hollinger 1998).

Most advocates who have argued that race should be considered in adoption decision making have done so based on a belief that children, particularly African American children, benefit psychologically and culturally from being raised by parents of the same race (Bartholet 1999; Kennedy 2003; Roberts 2002). They assert that for these reasons, adoption of children by same-race parents is best for the individual child as well as the community, particularly the racial or ethnic community to which they argue the child belongs (Kennedy 2003). The community, they argue, will lose the benefits it may derive from having these transracially adopted children as part of the minority community while the children will not learn to cope with the racism that is inherent in society, that the children will lack self-love, and that the children will be deprived of the wider community's guidance and will not absorb the cultural lessons available in the broader community (Kennedy 2003). Opponents of race matching argue that children need nurturing and capable parents regardless of the race, color, or national origin of either the child or the adoptive parent (Bartholet 1999; Kennedy 2003).

University of Pittsburgh Law Professor David J. Herring has hypothesized, based on research findings in social psychology and behavioral biology, that children placed in racially congruent foster homes may receive more favorable treatment than those placed across racial lines (Herring 2007). By prohibiting the consideration of race, Herring suggested that we may place children at increased risk of maltreatment and poor developmental outcomes. He urged that additional research be done to explore the viability of his hypothesis. While the law generally prohibits consideration of race, color, or national origin in selecting adoptive placements for children in foster care, it addresses the "Indian child" in an entirely different way.

The "Indian Child"

In 1978 Congress passed the Indian Child Welfare Act (ICWA; P.L. 95-608), which is substantive law that governs, among other things, how state courts handle adoption proceedings involving an "Indian child." In this chapter, consistent with the ICWA, *Indian child* refers to a child who is a member of or eligible for membership in an Indian tribe recognized by the government of the United States. In addressing issues regarding the adoption of an Indian child, one must be aware of both issues of race and ethnicity on one hand and sovereignty on the other. That is, federally recognized Indian tribes are sovereign entities with their own laws and legal apparatus. While some commentators have criticized the strength of the evidentiary foundation on which the ICWA was erected (Kennedy 2003), Congress expressed several reasons for adopting the law (25 U.S.C. § 1901). These included the special relationship between the tribes and the federal government, the importance of their children to the continued existence of the tribes, and that "an alarmingly high percentage of Indian families are broken up by the removal, often unwarranted, of their children from them by public and private agencies and that an alarmingly high percentage of such children are placed in non-Indian foster and adoptive homes" (25 U.S.C. § 1901(4)). This displacement of large numbers of Indian children was due, at least in part, to the Indian Adoption Project, which began in the late 1950s and which had as its explicit purpose the placement of Indian children with white adoptive families (Roberts 2002). In adopting the ICWA, Congress sought to protect the interests of not only the child's immediately biological parents but also the interests of the child's tribe.

The ICWA applies only to an "Indian child" as defined in the statute: "an unmarried person who is under age eighteen and is either (a) a member of an Indian tribe or (b) is eligible for membership in an Indian tribe and is the biological child of a member of an Indian tribe" (25 U.S.C. § 1903(4)). Each federally recognized Indian tribe is free to establish its own membership criteria, so it is entirely possible for children to have substantial Native American heritage yet not qualify as an "Indian child" for purposes of the statute. If a child qualifies as an "Indian child," then the statute applies and the child's adoption is governed by the dictates of the federal law even if the case is being heard in a state court. In terms of adoption, unlike the MEPA and IEP which prohibit the consideration of race, the ICWA demands that children be placed in conformity with its provisions, which are unabashedly race conscious. Whenever a qualifying child is to be placed for adoption, the court must place the child pursuant to a statutorily mandated placement criteria, first with a member of the child's extended family, next with members of the child's tribe, and, finally, with other Indian families (25 U.S.C. § 1915[a]).

Because the ICWA seeks to protect tribal interests in their children as well as the interests of the parent, a parent is not free to consummate the direct placement of an "Indian child" under state law for purposes of adoption without taking the steps necessary to protect the tribe's interests (*Mississippi Band of Choctaw Indians v. Holyfield* 1989). In *Mississippi Band of Choctaw Indians v. Holyfield*, the U.S. Supreme Court addressed the separate interests of the tribe when a parent sought to do so. In that case, a woman gave birth to twins born out of wedlock. The mother and father were both members of the Choctaw tribe and were domiciled on the tribe's reservation. When it was time for the mother to deliver the children, she traveled some 200 miles and gave birth off the reservation. She and the father signed consent-to-adoption forms placing the twins with the Holyfields for adoption. Six days after the mother signed the release, the Holyfields petitioned to adopt the children and the court issued a final adoption order 12 days later.

Two months after the final order of adoption was entered, the Choctaw tribe petitioned the court to set aside the orders of adoption asserting that its court had exclusive jurisdiction of the children because they were domiciled on the reservation. The state court denied the tribe's motion for two reasons: 1) the mother traveled away from the reservation and promptly placed the children for adoption; and 2) the children had never resided on the reservation. The tribe appealed the trial court's decision. The Supreme Court of Mississippi affirmed the trial court's decision, holding that the children had been abandoned and that they had never resided on the reservation. The tribe appealed to the U.S. Supreme Court, which reversed that ruling. The Court ruled that the ICWA's jurisdictional provision made clear that the tribal court had exclusive jurisdiction over children who were domiciled on the reservation, that is, that the state court lacked any legal authority over the children. It also ruled that the children were domiciled where the parents were domiciled, on the reservation, despite the fact that the children had never physically been on the reservation. Three years after the children were initially placed with the Holyfields, the Supreme Court vacated the orders of adoption and sent the case back to the tribal court, which it ruled had exclusive jurisdiction over the case. As this case illustrates, although the ICWA applies to relatively few cases, it is crucially important that when it does apply its jurisdictional provisions be carefully considered and followed.

In some circumstances where the Indian child resides off the reservation, the tribe has an absolute right to intervene in the state court proceedings at any point in the case (25 U.S.C. § 1911[c]). In most circumstances where the state court and the tribal court share concurrent jurisdiction over the child, the state court must transfer the case to the tribe's court upon a request by the tribe that it do so (25 U.S.C. § 1911[b]). Even if the state court is required to handle the case, it must do so pursuant to the unique proceedings, higher evidentiary burdens, and the more strenuous demands of the ICWA.

Clinical Issues

As with many of the adoptive families mentioned in this chapter, a major struggle from children's or teens' perspective may come from their need to develop their identity. As with all children and adolescents, the task of developing an identity is one that is challenging, perhaps the most difficult developmental milestone of becoming an adult. When children find themselves looking different from their parents, the pressure that they put on themselves to cope with that difference and the pressure they can receive from the outside world can be quite damaging. Additionally, institutionalized racism in the United States is still a fact of life. For interracial families the bias from schools, day cares, and communities can feel quite hurtful. Forensic evaluators should assess carefully the potential for these types of reactions and the prospective adoptive

parents' capacities to address issues of racial identity when they arise.

As children age into adolescence, it is possible that adopted children may seek to spend more time with communities that reflect their own racial identities. This can be challenging for both the adoptive parent and adopted child, as each part of the family may feel a sense of loss, rejection, and confused sense of reality. The forensic evaluator should consider whether a recommendation for individual and family therapy can assist family members in creating a plan that feels comfortable to all parties and that does not compromise the emerging identity of the adopted child.

Because transracial adoption is a contentious issue, it may impact the objectivity of home studies, evaluations, and recommended services in particular cases. Forensic evaluators should be aware of the parameters of this controversy so that they can assess objectively the quality of information they may receive when asked to evaluate a case in which a child may be adopted by parents of a different race.

Adoption by Gays and Lesbians

As with transracial adoption before the civil rights movement, the adoption of children by gay and lesbian persons and couples was not historically an issue because it was not openly discussed and there were no laws addressing the practice (Wardle 2005a). Lesbians and gay men likely have adopted children for many years by simply failing to disclose their sexual orientation (Mallon 2007). It is unknown how many gay or lesbian individuals or same-sex couples are raising children, although it seems clear that this number is growing, and gay, lesbian, and same-sex headed households are becoming more visible.

Just as the movement for civil rights for African Americans in the 1950s and 1960s included legal challenges to laws prohibiting interracial adoption and marriage (*Compos v. McKeithen* 1972; *In re Gomez* 1967; *Loving v. Virginia* 1967), the gay rights movement, which has its origin in the Stonewall riot of 1969 (D'Emilio 1983), has sought to address the rights of gay, lesbian, bisexual, and transgendered persons to form families by way of marriage and adoption (*Baker v. State* 1999; *Goodridge v. Department of Public Health* 2003; *Lofton v. Secretary of the Department of Children and Family Services* 2004).

Laws Prohibiting Gay and Lesbian Individuals From Adopting

In response to the efforts by gays and lesbians to achieve recognition of their relationships and to establish families, a number of states enacted laws prohibiting members of these sexual minority groups from adopting children. In 1977, Florida enacted a law prohibiting homosexual persons from adopting children (Fla. Stat. § 63.042[3]; *Lofton v. Secretary of the Department of Children and Family Services* 2004). That statute provides that "No person eligible to adopt under this statute may adopt if that person is a homosexual." Although the statute does not contain a definition of "homosexual," Florida courts interpreted the law to apply only to persons who were actively engaged in voluntary homosexual activity (*Lofton v. Secretary of the Department of Children and Family Services*, 2004). A decade later, the New Hampshire legislature was considering a bill that would prohibit gay and lesbian individuals from adopting, becoming foster parents, or operating day care centers. The legislature certified questions regarding the constitutionality of such a bill to the state's supreme court, which held that prohibiting adoption and foster care was permissible and did not offend due process because it was rationally related to the legislature's purpose of providing "appropriate role models for children" (*In re Opinion of the Justices* 1987, p. 1099).[1] While the New Hampshire court ruled that a ban on adoption by gay and lesbian individuals was not unconstitutional, it did so as a hypothetical case rather than in the context of an actual case in controversy. For this reason, the court cautioned "that this opinion makes no attempt to anticipate particular issues that may arise only as the statutory amendments are in fact applied, assuming enactment of the bill" (*In re Opinion of the Justices* 1987, p. 1098).

In *Lofton*, the federal courts were confronted with a challenge to Florida's statutory ban on adoption by ho-

mosexual individuals. Two gay individuals, one gay couple, and one minor brought suit against the State of Florida alleging that its prohibition against homosexual individuals adopting children violated the U.S. Constitution's guarantee of substantive due process and equal protection. The case involved two individuals, each a male nurse and a homosexual, who had acted as foster parents for children for years and who sought to adopt a foster child placed in their care who was available for adoption. Additionally, a gay couple that had been licensed as foster parents filed an application to jointly adopt a child, although none of the children in their care were then currently available for adoption. The care these men provided to the foster children entrusted to their care was by all accounts exceptional. For example, Mr. Lofton, who had considerable experience working with HIV-positive patients, provided care for a child who had tested positive for HIV at birth and was placed in his care immediately. Eighteen months later, the child no longer tested positive for HIV.

Despite the quality of care provided to the children and the years that the children had resided in the foster homes, Florida would not permit these men to adopt because of their homosexuality. The two individual foster parents and the couple filed suit, alleging violations of their right to substantive due process, right to privacy (of their sexual relationships), and equal protection of the laws, and they requested that the statute be declared unconstitutional and that the state be enjoined from enforcing its provisions. The district court dismissed the case for failure to state a claim on which the relief sought could be granted. The plaintiffs appealed, and the United States Circuit Court for the Eleventh Circuit affirmed the district court's decision, holding that the state has an obligation to provide the best possible home for children for whom it is responsible and because there is a rational relationship between the statute's purpose and its bar to homosexuals adopting children. The plaintiffs then sought a review *en banc* and, when that request was denied, appealed to the Supreme Court, which was also denied. Thus, the Florida statute was upheld.

---

[1] The history of this New Hampshire statute provides an interesting example of the fluidity and speed with which the law is changing in regard to adoption by gays, lesbians, and same-sex couples. After the state's supreme court approved the bill, it was enacted into law and gays and lesbians were not permitted to adopt in New Hampshire. Twelve years later, in 1999, the legislature repealed the statute and has now provided gay and lesbian persons the ability to adopt children (N.H. Rev. Stat. Rev. Ann. § 179B:4, 2008; Wardle 2005a, 2005b). Moreover, effective January 1, 2008, New Hampshire recognizes same-sex civil unions (R.S.A. 457-A:1 et seq., 2008). The same-sex parties to a civil union are entitled to all the rights and responsibilities of a heterosexual couple entering marriage, including the right to adopt jointly (R.S.A. 457-A:6).

Law Prohibiting Same-Sex Couples From Adopting

Some states' laws explicitly deny same-sex couples the ability to jointly adopt a child. Mississippi's statutory law, for instance, provides that "[a]doption by couples of the same gender is prohibited" (Miss. Code Ann § 93-17-3(5), 2008). Utah's adoption law establishes a presumption in favor of placing children for adoption only with heterosexual couples. It provides for children to be adopted by persons who are legally married to one another and provides that if the child is in the custody of the state at the time of the adoption proceeding, the authorities "shall place the child with a man and a woman who are married to each other" unless there is no married couple available to adopt the child and adoption by a single person is "in the child's best interests" (Utah Code Ann. § 78-30-1, 2008). As noted above in *Lofton*, Florida's prohibition on adoption by gay or lesbian individuals was upheld against its application to a same-sex couple.

Laws Not Specifically Addressing Sexual Orientation

Most states' laws do not specifically address whether gay or lesbian individuals or same-sex couples may adopt. These states' adoption laws are typically sexual orientation neutral; that is, they are written in a general way that does not explicitly address the sexual orientation of the prospective adoptive parent or parents. Michigan's law is typical of this type of statute and provides that "If a person desires to adopt a child...that person, together with his wife or her husband, if married, shall file a petition with the court" (Mich. Comp. Laws § 710.24, 2008). Since 1990, a number of states' courts have interpreted their sexual orientation–neutral adoption statutes to permit one form or another of adoption by gay or lesbian individuals or by same-sex couples (e.g., *Adoption of B.L.V.B. and E.L.V.B.* 1993; *Adoption of Charles B.* 1990; *Adoption of Tammy* 1993). Meanwhile, courts in other states have declined to read their statutes to permit adoption by either gay or lesbian individuals (e.g., *In re Adoption of T.K.J. and K.A.K.* 1996; *In the Interest of Angel Lace M.* 1994) or same-sex couples (e.g., *In re Adoption of Luke* 2002).

Cases testing the application of sexual orientation neutral adoption laws have most often arisen in the context of second-parent adoption (e.g., *Adoption of B.L.V.B.* 1993; *Adoption of Tammy* 1993). In *Adoption of B.L.V.B. and E.L.V.B.* (1993), the Ver-

mont Supreme Court addressed the question of whether the state's sexual orientation neutral stepparent adoption provision should be applied to a same-sex couple. Under the state's law, a parent was permitted to consent to the adoption of his or her child by a stepparent without the rights of the natural parent having to be terminated. The lesbian couple who were involved in the case had lived together for several years when they decided to begin a family. One of the women became pregnant via artificial insemination by an anonymous donor. Later the couple decided to have a second child, and the same partner became pregnant again using sperm from the same donor. After the birth of the second child, the couple petitioned for the nonbiological mother to adopt the children. A home study by the requisite state agency resulted in a positive recommendation, and an evaluation by a psychologist likewise recommended that the adoption would be in the children's best interests.

Two provisions of the state's adoption law were at issue. The first provided: "A person or husband and wife together, of age and sound mind, may adopt any other person as his or their heir.... A married man or a married woman shall not adopt a person...without the consent of the other spouse. The petition for adoption and the final adoption decree shall be executed by the other spouse as provided in this chapter." The second stated the general rule that when a child is adopted, the child's natural parent no longer has any rights or responsibilities regarding the child. It then made an exception to this rule for adoption by a stepparent: "Notwithstanding the foregoing provisions of this section, when the adoption is made by a spouse of a natural parent, obligations of obedience to, and rights of inheritance by and through the natural parent who has intermarried with the adopting parent shall not be affected" (*Adoption of B.L.V.B and E.L.V.B.* 1993, pp. 1272–1273). Read together, these provisions permitted a natural parent and a stepparent to petition the court for adoption of the child by the stepparent without the rights of the natural parent being extinguished. Although the adoption petitions were uncontested, the trial court denied the petitions because it interpreted the law to require that the parties to a stepparent adoption be married before such a petition could be granted.

On appeal, the Vermont Supreme Court noted that on their face these statutes prohibited only one form of adoption, by one spouse of a married couple. Since the same-sex partners at issue in the case were not married, that provision did not apply. Moreover, the statute provided that "a person" who is unmarried may adopt. Finally, the stepparent adoption provision of the law was adopted in 1947 and it was unlikely that the legislature had contemplated denying same-sex couples the right to avail themselves of stepparent adoption. The court went on to find that while the specific circumstances of the case had not likely been contemplated by the legislature at the time it adopted the statute, its intent was consistent with permitting the same-sex partner of a child's parent to adopt. Finally, because the petitions were uncontested and had been recommended by the state agency, and there was no evidence presented that the adoptions were contrary to the children's best interests, the court approved the adoptions.

Quality of Same-Sex Parenting

As was noted early on in this chapter, the key question in an adoption proceeding is the best interest of the child. In part because of this focus on the best interest of the child in adoption proceedings, and also because of the more general effort to recognize same-sex relations through civil unions and marriage, social science researchers have sought evidence to assess outcomes for children reared by gay or lesbian individuals or by same-sex couples (e.g., Bos et al. 2007; Goldberg 2007; Meezan and Rauch 2005; Stacey and Biblarz 2001). Despite the need for such research, both proponents (Meezan and Rauch 2005) and opponents (Wardle 2005a, 2005b) of gay, lesbian, and same-sex couple parenting have observed that there is insufficient research to speak comprehensively about the impact of gay, lesbian, and same-sex couple parenting on children. Similarly, advocates on both sides of the debate have acknowledged that the research that does exist suffers from various methodological flaws (Meezan and Rauch 2005; Wardle 1997). For instance, Professor Lynn D. Wardle of Brigham Young University Law School, a longstanding opponent of gay, lesbian, and same-sex couple parenting, has stated that the social science research that does exist regarding the impact of these individuals and couples parenting on children is mostly "immature, defective, biased and irrelevant" (Wardle 2005b, p. 515).

Conservative critics of adoption by gays, lesbians, or same-sex couples have argued that the rearing of children by heterosexual married couples is the gold standard, and that children reared by sexual minorities potentially face substantial risks to their well-being (Wardle 1997, 2005a). For these reasons they argue that the burden of proving the fitness of gays, lesbians, and same-sex couples as parents rests with their supporters. Recognizing the limitations of the research,

most researchers have found that although there are differences in various outcomes for children raised by gays, lesbians, and same-sex couples, those differences are not something with which society should be concerned or that concern arises not inherently from those differences but from a normative judgment made about the differences (Bos et al. 2007; Goldberg 2007; Stacey and Biblarz 2001). For instance, Goldberg's (2007) study of 46 adults (36 women and 10 men) who had at least one gay or lesbian parent found that these individuals tended to have less rigid notions about gender and sexuality. On its face there may be nothing concerning about this; however, some would be inclined to be concerned based on a normative judgment that such an outcome is less desirable than the more well-defined understanding of sexuality and gender identity present in adults raised by heterosexual parents.

Indeed, Wardle (2005b) argued that it is precisely the sexual practices of homosexual parents and their partners and their impact, if any, upon the children they are raising that should be the focus of social science research if one is to determine the real impact of gay, lesbian, and same-sex couple adoption on children. He suggested numerous research questions regarding the sexual behavior of gay, lesbian, and same-sex couples that should be addressed before informed policy decisions about permitting them to adopt may be made. While Wardle has focused on the sex lives of prospective homosexual parents, he has not suggested that such research should be conducted regarding heterosexual or single-parent adoptive families. Moreover, Gerald P. Mallon, a professor at the Hunter School of Social Work, an expert in adoption and proponent of adoption by gays, lesbians, and same-sex couples, has observed that "The assessment process for lesbian and gay prospective foster or adoptive parents can become skewed if the assessing worker is either overfocusing on sexuality or totally ignoring it" (Mallon 2007, p. 69). He urged that a prospective adoptive parent's sexual orientation and activities not be ignored and that they not be the primary focus of an adoption assessment. Mallon suggested that sexuality should be considered for every person or couple seeking to adopt, regardless of sexual orientation, but that it not be the focus of the evaluation. He also suggested that the report of an evaluation be written, to the extent possible, just as an evaluation of a heterosexual individual or couple would be written. If a couple is being evaluated, each partner should receive an equal amount of attention within the report, and the evaluation should consider the length of the relationship, its strengths, and its weaknesses (Mallon 2007).

Positions of Major Professional Organizations

Despite the methodological weaknesses in the social science research outlined above, several major professional organizations have taken positions regarding parenting or adoption by gays, lesbians, or same-sex couples based on the existing body of research. First, in November 2002 the American Psychiatric Association's Board of Trustees and Assembly adopted a position statement regarding adoption and coparenting of children by same-sex couples that concludes, "The American Psychiatric Association supports initiatives which allow same-sex couples to adopt and co-parent children and supports all the associated legal rights, benefits, and responsibilities which arise from such initiatives" (American Psychiatric Association 2002).

Next, in 2004 the American Psychological Association's Council of Representatives adopted a policy statement on sexual orientation, parents, and children that concludes, "Overall, results of research suggest that the development, adjustment, and well-being of children with lesbian and gay parents do not differ markedly from that of children with heterosexual parents" (Paige 2005). The American Psychological Association has long held the position that a parent's sexual orientation should not be the primary or main basis on which to make determinations regarding adoption (Conger 1977).

Similarly, the American Academy of Pediatrics (2002) adopted a policy statement in favor of granting adoption rights to gay and lesbian coparents and second parents, which states that "Because these families and children need the permanence and security that are provided by having two fully sanctioned and legally defined parents, the Academy supports the legal adoption of children by coparents or second parents. Denying legal parent status through adoption to coparents or second parents prevents these children from enjoying the psychological and legal security that comes from having two willing, capable, and loving parents."

Clinical Issues

In addition to the basic challenges presented in raising *any* child, the added stressors of not just adoption but adoption into a lesbian or gay household increase the challenges and potential vulnerabilities. When considering the adoption possibilities of a child with a particular gay or lesbian individual or with a same-sex couple, the basic question that underlies all adoption determinations—the best interest of the particular child at issue—should be carefully assessed. As in all other adoption situations, this entails an assessment of the particular child's needs and the capacity and willingness of the prospective adoptive parents to meet those needs.

For children and teens placed into lesbian and gay adoptive households, the pressure faced from peers about the differences of not only their adoptive status but also their status as coming from a lesbian and gay family may be more relevant than some of the other issues mentioned previously. Some children and teens will move through a stage of anger at their adoptive parents for being different from their peers before they are fully accepting of their adopted parents' sexuality. Forensic evaluators should assess the awareness and capacity of gay and lesbian prospective adoptive parents to anticipate these difficulties and to address them in ways that will be supportive of and helpful to the child they wish to adopt.

As described earlier, adoption by gays and lesbians is controversial. This controversy may color the objectivity of professionals working on particular adoption cases. Forensic evaluators who are conducting evaluations of a child and prospective adoptive parents should familiarize themselves with the controversy to discern when homophobia has played a part in home studies and needs assessments.

—Key Points

- All evaluations for the purpose of assessing potential adoptive placements are focused on the best interest of the child.

- No individual or couple has a "right" to adopt a child.

— Forensic evaluators should familiarize themselves with the jurisdiction's criteria for assessing the child's best interest.

— While adoption generally follows a basic process, the specifics of the process will vary from jurisdiction to jurisdiction.

— Forensic evaluators should provide an objective assessment of the needs of the individual child and the capacities of the prospective parents to meet those needs.

— Transcultural adoption poses a number of unique issues for both the child in need of adoption and the prospective adoptive parent. A forensic evaluator conducting an evaluation in a transcultural adoption should become familiar with these issues and assess the needs of the child to be adopted and the abilities of the prospective adoptive parents to meet the child's needs.

— Transracial adoption within the United States is controversial. Forensic evaluators should be aware of the contentiousness of this issue when conducting evaluations as it may influence how issues are presented in reports, home studies, and the like.

— The adoption of American Indian children is governed by the federal Indian Child Welfare Act. Forensic evaluators should be familiar with the rudiments of this statute when evaluating a case in which an Indian child may be adopted.

— A growing number of states permit adoption by single or coupled gays and lesbians. Adoption by individual gay and lesbian persons or by same-sex couples is controversial in some quarters.

— Forensic evaluators should be aware of this controversy and should focus on what is best for an individual child when assessing the ability of a gay or lesbian person or a same-sex couple to meet the child's needs for adoptive parents.

References

Adoption History Project: International Adoptions. Updated July 11, 2007. Available at: http://darkwing.uoregon.edu/~adoption/topics/internationaladoption.htm. Accessed June 20, 2008.

Adoption of BLVB and ELVB, 628 A2d 1271 (Vt 1993)

Adoption of Charles B, 552 NE2d 884 (Ohio 1990)

Adoption of Tammy, 619 NE2d 315 (Mass 1993)

Adoption of Vito, 728 NE2d 292 (Mass 2000)

Ainsworth M, Bowlby J: Child Care and the Growth of Love. London, Penguin Books, 1965

American Academy of Pediatrics: Policy statement: coparent or second-parent adoption by same-sex parents. Pediatrics 109:339–340, 2002

American Psychiatric Association: Position Statement: Adoption and Co-parenting of Children by Same-Sex Couples. November 2002. Available at: www.psych.org/Departments/EDU/Library/APAOfficialDocumentsandRelated/PositionStatements/200214.aspx. Accessed June 24, 2008.

Annotated Laws of Massachusetts GL Ch 210, § 3 (2008)

Arkansas Code Annotated § 9-9-212 (2008)

Baker v State, 744 A2d 864 (Vt 1999)

Bartholet E: Nobody's Children: Abuse and Neglect, Foster Drift, and the Adoption Alternative. Boston, MA, Beacon Press, 1999

Bos HMW, van Balen F, van den Boom DC: Child adjustment in planned lesbian-parent families. Am J Orthopsychiatry 77:38–48, 2007

Bowlby J: Separation: Anxiety and Anger, Attachment and Loss, Vol 2. London, Hogarth Press, 1973

Bush v Dietz, 680 SW2d 704 (Ark 1984)

Compos v McKeithen, 341 F Supp 264 (ED La 1972)

Conger JJ: Proceedings of the American Psychological Association, Incorporated, for the year 1976: minutes of the annual meeting of the Council of Representatives. Am Psychol 32:408–438, 1977

Crea TM, Barth RP, Chintapalli LK: Home study methods for evaluating prospective resource families: history, current challenges, and promising approaches. Child Welfare 86:141–159, 2007

Delgado v Fawcett, 515 P2d 710 (Alaska 1973)

D'Emilio J: A new beginning: The birth of gay liberation, in Sexual Politics, Sexual Communities: The Making of a Homosexual Minority in the United States, 1940–1970. Chicago, University of Chicago Press, 1983, pp 223–239

Drummond v Fulton County Department of Family and Children's Services, 563 F2d 1200 (5th Cir 1977)

Farnsworth v Goebel, 132 NE 414 (Mass 1921)

Festinger T: Adoption disruption: rates, correlates, and service needs, in Child Welfare for the 21st Century: A Handbook of Practices, Policies, and Programs. Edited by Mallon GP, Hess PM. New York, Columbia University Press, 2005, pp 452–468

Florida Statutes § 63.042(3) (2008)

Florida Statutes § 63.192 (2008)

Florida Statutes § 744.304 (2008)

General Court of Massachusetts: Massachusetts Adoption of Children Act, Ch 324, 1851. Updated July 11, 2007. Available at: http://darkwing.uoregon.edu/~adoption/archive/MassACA.htm. Accessed June 16, 2008.

Goldberg AE: (How) does it make a difference? Perspectives of adults with lesbian, gay and bisexual parents. Am J Orthopsychiatry 77:550–562, 2007

Goodridge v Department of Public Health, 798 NE2d 941 (Mass 2003)

Gregory JD, Swisher PN, Wolf SL: Understanding Family Law, 2nd Edition. New York, Matthew Bender, 2001

Groza V, Houlihan L, Wood ZB: Overview of adoption, in Child Welfare for the 21st Century: A Handbook of Practices, Policies, and Programs. Edited by Mallon GP, Hess PM. New York, Columbia University Press, 2005, pp 432–452

Herring DJ: The Multiethnic Placement Act: threat to foster child safety and well-being? Univ Mich J Law Reform 41:89–120, 2007

Hollinger JH: A Guide to the Multiethnic Placement Act of 1994 as Amended by the Interethnic Placement Provisions of 1996. Washington, DC, ABA Center on Children and the Law, 1998

Homes for Black Children (HBC) recruits through courtesy and community connections. Available at: http://library.adoption.com/African-American/Homes-for-Black-Children-Recruits-through-Courtesy-and-Community-Connections/article/6045/1.html. Accessed June 17, 2008.

Illinois Compiled Statutes, Adoption Act of 1960, 750 ILCS 50

Immigration and Nationality Act, 8 USC § 1101 et seq (2008)

Indian Child Welfare Act of 1978, PL 95-608, 25 USC § 1901, et seq

In the Interest of Angel Lace M, 516 NW2d 678 (Wis 1994)

In re Adams, 473 NW2d 712 (Mich Ct App 1991)

In re Adoption of Luke, 640 NW2d 374 (Neb 2002)

In re Adoption of Minor, 228 F2d 446 (DC Cir 1955)

In re Adoptions of TKJ and KAK, 931 P2d 488 (Colo 1996)

In re CDM, 39 P3d 802 (Okla 2001)

In re Gomez, 424 SW2d 656 (Tex Civ App 1967)

In re Melanie S, 712 A2d 1036 (Me 1998)

In re Moorhead, 600 NE2d 778 (Ohio App 1991)

In re Opinion of the Justices, 525 A2d 1095 (NH 1987)

In re Smith Estate, 72 NW2d 287 (Mich Sup Ct 1955)

In the Matter of the Adoption of Moore-Tillay, 135 P3d 387 (Oregon 2006)

Intercountry Adoption Act, PL 106-279, 42 USC § 14901, et seq

Interethnic Adoption Provisions, PL 104-188, 42 USC § 670 et seq

Kansas Statutes Annotated § 59-2112 (2006)

Kansas Statutes Annotated § 59-2136 (2006)

Kennedy R: Interracial Intimacies: Sex, Marriage, Identity, and Adoption. New York, Pantheon Books, 2003

Lindley for Lindley v Sullivan, 889 F2d 124 (7th Cir 1989)

Lofton v Secretary of the Department of Children and Family Services, 358 F3d 804; reh en banc den 377 F3d 1275 (11th Cir 2004); cert den 543 US 1081 (2005)

Loving v Virginia, 388 US 1 (1967)

Mallon GP: Assessing lesbian and gay prospective foster and adoptive families: a focus on the home study process. Child Welfare 86(2):67–86, 2007

McConnell J: Standby guardianship: sharing the legal responsibility for children. Maryland J Contemp Legal Issues 7:249–286, 1995/1996

McRoy R, Mica M, Freundlich M, et al: Making MEPA-IEP work: tools for professionals. Child Welfare 86(2):49–66, 2007

Meezan W, Rauch J: Gay marriage, same-sex parenting, and America's children. The Future of Children 15:97–115, 2005. Available at: http://www.futureofchildren.org/information2827/information_show.htm?doc_id=296792. Accessed June 17, 2008.

Michigan Compiled Laws Annotated § 710.22(g) (2008)

Michigan Compiled Laws Annotated § 14.32 (2008)

Michigan Compiled Laws Annotated § 170.5 (2008)

Michigan Compiled Laws Annotated § 710.21b (2008)

Michigan Compiled Laws Annotated § 710.23a (2008)

Michigan Compiled Laws Annotated § 710.24 (2008)

Miller LC, Chan W, Reece RA, et al: Child abuse fatalities among internationally adopted children. Child Maltreatment 12:378–380, 2007

Minnesota Statutes § 259.24 (2007)

Mississippi Band of Choctaw Indians v Holyfield, 490 US 30 (1989)

Mississippi Code Annotated § 93-17-3(5) (2008)

Multiethnic Placement Act of 1994, PL 103-382, 42 § USC 670 et seq

Navarro M: To adopt, please press hold. New York Times, June 5, 2008

New Hampshire Revised Statutes Revised Annotated § 179B:4 (2008)

New Jersey Statutes Annotated § 3B:12-68 (2008)

Olson E: Families adopting in Vietnam say they are caught in diplomatic jam. New York Times, February 11, 2008

Opinion of Michigan Attorney General, #7160, September 14, 2004. Available at: http://www.ag.state.mi.us/opinion/datafiles/2000s/op10236.htm. Accessed June 20, 2008.

Oregon Rev Stats § 109.305 (2007)

Paige RU: Proceedings of the American Psychological Association, Incorporated, for the legislative year 2004. Minutes of the meeting of the Council of Representatives July 28 and 30, 2004, Honolulu, HI. 2005. Available at: www.apa.org/pi/lgbc/policy/parents.html. Accessed June 17, 2008.

Petition of New England Home for Little Wanderers to Dispense With Consent for Adoption, 328 NE 2d 854 (Mass 1975)

Pew Commission on Children in Foster Care: Fostering the Future: Safety, Permanence and Well-Being for Children in Foster Care, n.d.

Roberts D: Shattered Bonds: The Color of Child Welfare. New York, Basic Civitas Books, 2002

Scott v Family Ministries, 135 Cal Rptr 430 (Cal Ct App 1976)

Seymore ML: International adoption and international comity: when is adoption repugnant? Tex Wesleyan Law Rev 10:381–401, 2004

South Dakota Codified Laws § 25-6-2 (2008)

Stacey J, Biblarz TJ: (How) does the sexual orientation of parents matter? American Sociological Rev 65:159–183, 2001

United Nations: Convention on Protection of Children and Co-operation in Respect of Intercountry Adoptions. The Hague, Hague Conference on Private International Law, 1995

Utah Code Annotated § 78-30-1 (2008)

Vermont Statutes Annotated Title 15A § 1-102 (2008)

Wardle LD: The potential impact of homosexual parenting on children. Univ Ill Law Rev 3:833–920, 1997

Wardle LD: A critical analysis of interstate recognition of lesbigay adoption. Ave Maria Law Rev 3:561–616, 2005a

Wardle LD: The "inner lives" of children in lesbigay adoption: narratives and other concerns. St. Thomas Law Rev 18:511–542, 2005b

Webb v Wiley, 600 P2d 317 (Okla 1979)

PART IV

Child Abuse

Charles L. Scott, M.D.

Chapter 16

Reliability and Suggestibility of Children's Statements

From Science to Practice

Sarah Kulkofsky, Ph.D.
Kamala London, Ph.D.

In spring 1985, a 4-year-old student at the Wee Care Nursery School was having his temperature taken with a rectal thermometer when he commented, "That's what my teacher does to me at nap time at school." The child's comment led to an investigation of Kelly Michaels, a young teacher at the nursery school. All children at the nursery school were repeatedly questioned about potential abuse by their parents (who were informed about sexual abuse suspicions in the school), by investigators, and in individual and group therapy sessions. The children eventually made a number of horrendous and sometimes bizarre allegations, including that they were raped with spoons, knives, and Lego blocks; that Kelly Michaels forced them to lick peanut butter off her naked body; that she forced them to eat feces and drink urine; and that she forced them to play games in the nude. Despite the fact that there was no physical evidence in the case and that Kelly Michaels passed a polygraph test, she was indicted on 299 charges and, after an 11-month trial, was sentenced to 47 years in prison. She served 5 years in prison before her case was overturned on appeal, largely as a result of the unreliability of the children's testimony, which was elicited in a highly suggestive manner.

In the United States, more than 4 million cases of child maltreatment are investigated each year (Pipe et al. 2007). Historically, children rarely provided uncorroborated testimony in legal settings. However, because of society's greater recognition of the prevalence and problems associated with child maltreatment, particularly with child sexual abuse (CSA), several judicial reforms were enacted starting in the 1970s and 1980s that brought more children at younger ages into the courts. It is estimated that more than 100,000 children in the United States testify annually in criminal and civil proceedings (Ceci and Bruck 1993).

As children began flooding the legal system, concerns were raised about their ability to provide complete and accurate accounts about past events. Many of these concerns were raised in response to some high-profile sexual abuse cases, such as those involving Kelly Michaels, as well as similar cases involving Gerald and Cheryl Amirault and the McMartin Preschool. These cases were characterized by bizarre allegations of abuse made by multiple children as well as by aggressive and overzealous interviewing techniques. When many of these cases started to come to light, very little research existed regarding the reliability of children's statements or appropriate interview-

217

ing techniques. In the years since, a vast literature has amassed outlining children's abilities to provide reports of past experiences as well as interviewer behaviors that can compromise the integrity of children's statements.

In this chapter, we provide an overview of the literature on the factors that can affect the accuracy of children's statements. In the first major section, we provide a review of the literature on children's accuracy when reporting past events. In the second major section, we address disclosure patterns among sexually abused children, as beliefs about how and when children disclose abuse often influence interviewers' decisions to pursue more aggressive questioning strategies. Finally, we end the chapter with an overview of recommendations for practitioners.

Children's Accuracy When Reporting Past Events

Memory Development

First and foremost, understanding children's ability to provide complete and accurate reports of past events in forensic contexts requires knowledge of the development of memory about personally experienced events. Research has shown that by around age 2 years, children begin to talk about past events (Nelson and Fivush 2004). At this young age, however, children's reports often require a great deal of adult prompting; their responses to open-ended questions such as "Tell me what happened" tend to include very little detail (Fivush 1993). Because many of the studies of children's personal memory focus on naturally occurring events, accuracy is difficult to assess because the researchers do not know what actually happened. However, maternal reports tend to confirm children's statements (e.g., Fivush et al. 1987), and work involving staged events for which statements can be verified also has shown high rates of accuracy (e.g., Leichtman et al. 2000). As such, young children's spontaneous recall of past events is often characterized as accurate but incomplete.

The conclusion that children's spontaneous reports are largely accurate has led some clinicians to conclude that if a child makes a spontaneous statement, it can be assumed to be true (Ceci et al. 2007a). However, it is certainly not the case that all spontaneous statements are accurate. In particular, if the child is interviewed about confusing events or events that run counter to his or her knowledge, accuracy may be

compromised. This is particularly important because in many forensic contexts, such as CSA, children are indeed asked to report about confusing events.

For example, Ornstein et al. (1998) had children experience a mock medical examination in which some common features (such as listening to the child's heart) were omitted and atypical features (such as wiping the child's belly button with alcohol) were added. When children were interviewed about the event after a 12-week delay, 42% of the 4-year-olds and 74% of the 6-year-olds spontaneously reported that at least one of the missing common features had been a part of the examination. In a similar study, Kulkofsky and colleagues (2008) had preschool-age children engage in a pizza-baking activity that included several unusual elements (e.g., the pizza was cut with chopsticks). When interviewed 1 week later, on average, 24% of the children's free-recall statements were classified as incorrect. Furthermore, it is important to note that these errors were not inconsequential in nature. For example, more than a quarter of all children recalled a nonpresent knife in response to an open-ended question, and many children added further detail and embellishment. To illustrate, one child recalled, "A very sharp knife…it cuts us…I telled Aaron 'Don't use that sharp knife!'"

In actual forensic interviews, the interviewer would not know which statements made by a child were inaccurate. Thus, children may be generally accurate about previously experienced events, but the inclusion of key inaccurate details may lead interviewers down a dangerous road. As we outline in the next section, erroneous beliefs on the part of an interviewer about what might have happened can negatively influence the accuracy of children's statements.

Furthermore, although children are able to report memories of childhood experiences and may report memories from younger ages than adults are able to recall (Fivush and Schwarzmueller 1999), there does appear to be a limit to how early in childhood children can remember. Specifically, children show difficulty remembering events that occurred prior to the onset of language. For example, Peterson and Ridehout (1998) interviewed young children about a visit to an emergency department that occurred when children were between 13 and 34 months old. Only children who were 25 months and older at the time of the injury were able to recall verbally any details of the event at later interviews. In a related study, Simcock and Hayne (2002) exposed 2- to 3-year-old children to a novel event and then tested their memories 6 months and 1 year later. At both the initial exposure and the memory interviews, parents reported children's vocabulary, including words that were pertinent to the novel event. At both time points, no child used words to describe the event that had not been part of the child's vocabulary at the time of the original event. Taken together, these results indicate that later verbal recall of an event is, in part, dependent on children's language ability at the time of encoding.

To summarize, the research on memory development in young children suggests that, in general, young children's spontaneous reports of personally experienced past events are largely accurate but can be quite sparse. However, accuracy is impaired when children are asked to recall confusing or ambiguous events, and their errors are not necessarily limited to inconsequential or peripheral details. In addition, there is a limit to how early in childhood children can remember, and thus, the veracity of memories recalled before the onset of language should be considered suspect.

Suggestibility

Ceci and Bruck (1993) defined *suggestibility* as "the degree to which children's encoding, storage, retrieval, and reporting of events can be influenced by a range of social and psychological factors" (p. 404). This broad definition of suggestibility allows for information that is presented both before and after an event to taint children's recall and further allows for the possibility that children's reports may be inaccurate even without any underlying memory impairment.

Although children's spontaneous reports are generally accurate, reports that emerge as a result of suggestive interviewing techniques tend to be quite error-prone. In the classic sense, suggestive interviewing involves asking leading questions. Studies of actual investigative interviews indicate that interviewers frequently ask children leading questions (Ceci et al. 2007b). Moreover, training programs designed to teach best practices for interviewing young witnesses do not appear to be effective in reducing the number of leading questions interviewers ask (Sternberg et al. 2001b). In general, children are less accurate when answering direct questions compared with open-ended questions (Ornstein et al. 1998; Peterson et al. 1999), and young children are less likely than older children and adults to respond to leading questions with "I don't know" (Hughes and Grieve 1980). Leading questions are particularly problematic because the interviewer presupposes that certain events occurred (e.g., "He took your clothes off, didn't he?"); however, without knowing exactly what happened, which is almost always the case in forensic interviews, an interviewer's leading question may actually be *misleading*.

The suggestiveness of an interview goes beyond simply indexing the number of leading questions. Rather, one must consider how *interviewer bias* plays out in the interview. Interviewer bias characterizes those interviewers who hold a priori beliefs about what has occurred and mold the interview to maximize disclosures that are consistent with those beliefs. As such, interviewer bias has a negative effect on the accuracy of child witnesses' statements. Experimental research has shown that when interviewers are misinformed themselves about what has occurred, children's reports are less accurate and tend to incorporate the misinformation given to interviewers (Goodman et al. 1995; White et al. 1997). Table 16–1 provides categories and examples of suggestive interviewing techniques.

Interviewer bias may be communicated through other suggestive techniques in addition to asking leading questions. These include providing positive reinforcement and negative feedback, using peer or parental pressure, creating a negative or an accusatory emotional tone, inducing stereotypes about the accused, and repeating questions or interviews until the child provides the desired answer. Research indicates that, compared with using a single suggestive technique, combining suggestive techniques tends to result in heightened levels of suggestibility. For example, Garven et al. (1998, 2000) examined how the techniques that were used by investigators in the McMartin Preschool case tainted children's testimony beyond that of misleading questions alone. In one study (Garven et al. 2000), the researchers asked kindergarten children to recall details from when a visitor named Paco came to their classroom. Half of the children were given interviews that included misleading questions about plausible events (e.g., "Did Paco break a toy?") and bizarre events (e.g., "Did Paco take you to a farm in a helicopter?"). In this group, children assented to 13% of the plausible questions and 5% of the fantastic questions. A second group of children were given negative feedback to their "no" responses and positive feedback to their "yes" responses. This latter group falsely assented to the plausible items 35% of the time and the bizarre items 52% of the time. Furthermore, these group differences remained when children were interviewed neutrally 2 weeks later. These data indicate that interviewer bias in earlier interviews can taint children's later reports even if these later interviews are conducted in an unbiased manner.

TABLE 16–1.   Examples of suggestive interviewing techniques

Suggestive technique	Example
Leading questions	Interviewer: He took your clothes off, didn't he?
Repeating questions	Interviewer: Where did he touch you? Child: He didn't. Interviewer: Tell me where he touched you.
Positive reinforcement	Interviewer: Did he touch you on your bottom? Child: Yes Interviewer: That's right. You're doing a really good job.
Negative feedback	Interviewer: Did he kiss you? Child: No Interviewer: You're not doing very well.
Peer or parental pressure	Interviewer: The other kids told me he did these things. I just need you to tell me.
Creating a negative or accusatory emotional tone	Interviewer: These are bad guys. We're going to put these bad guys in jail.
Inviting children to pretend or speculate	Interviewer: What do you think it would have been like? What could have happened?

To illustrate how leading questions may be combined with other techniques (such as question repetition), consider the following interview examples from the Bernard Baran sexual abuse investigation.

Child A

Interviewer: Did you play, did you play a game called "The Touching Game" at ECDC?
Child: No.
...
Interviewer: Yeah. So I was remembering, I know a game that I used to play called "The Touching Game." I wonder if you ever played that at school.
Child: I didn't.
Interviewer: You don't remember that game?
Child: We didn't do it.
Interviewer: You didn't?
Child: No.

Child B

Mom: You can't remember anything he said to you? Did he say, "wake up," or he didn't say anything at all?
Child: No.
Mom: He just went and did what?
Child: Nothing.
Mom: And after he pulled, after he pulled on your pee pee, did he tell you anything then? Did he give you anything?
Child: No.

Mom: No. Did he give you a box of donuts?
Child: What?
Mom: Did he give you a box of donuts?
Child: No.
Mom: No. Did he give you anything or say anything?
Child: He gave us a birthday.

The defendant in this particular case was convicted of eight counts of CSA and was sentenced to three concurrent life terms in prison, based almost exclusively on the testimony of the young children in this case.

Although a combination of highly suggestive techniques is more likely to introduce false memory, such highly suggestive techniques are not necessary to taint children's reports. Children can incorporate misleading information into their accounts even after a single suggestive interview (Ceci et al. 2007b). Furthermore, other milder forms of suggestions have been shown to influence the accuracy of children's reports. For example, in a recent set of studies, Principe et al. (2006, 2008) showed that rumors spread among peers can lead to false reports. Principe and colleagues found that many children not only reported false details as a result of rumor transmission but also maintained that they had actually *seen* the false events themselves.

In most typical suggestibility studies, there are reliable age differences, with younger children being more suggestible than older children and adults (Ceci and Bruck 1993). In fact, age appears to be the single best predictor of suggestibility (Geddie et al. 2000).

However, this is not to say that only young children are suggestible. A great deal of evidence indicates that older children and adults can fall prey to suggestive techniques (Finnilä et al. 2003). Furthermore, in some situations, older children actually may be *more* suggestible than younger children. In particular, in some cases, older children's more advanced cognitive capabilities actually led to increased incorporation of false information (Ceci et al. 2007b; Principe et al. 2008).

One argument that is often made against much of the research on suggestibility is that children are only suggestible about inconsequential, peripheral details of events. However, just as is the case with children's spontaneous errors, the effects of suggestive questioning are not limited to irrelevant and peripheral details of unemotional events. Studies showing the deleterious effects of suggestive techniques have included central details to negative and painful events, such as doctor's office and emergency department visits (Bruck et al. 2000; Burgwyn-Bales et al. 2001) and other forms of bodily touching (Poole and Lindsay 1995; White et al. 1997).

Finally, it is important to note that children's false reports that emerge through suggestive techniques may be indistinguishable from true statements. Both Ceci et al. (1994) and Leichtman and Ceci (1995) had legal and psychological experts watch videotapes of children's true and false reports that emerged as a result of suggestive techniques. In both cases, the professionals were no better than chance at distinguishing true from false memories. Furthermore, Bruck et al. (2002) systematically compared children's true and false narratives and found that false narratives contained more spontaneous details, more temporal markers, more elaborations, and more aggressive details than did true narratives (see also Powell et al. 2003). Even when experts attempt to apply more systematic methods to distinguish true from false reports elicited through suggestive questions, their decisions are not reliable. For instance, criterion-based content analysis has been touted as one way to distinguish true from false reports in forensic contexts (Vrij 2005). In criterion-based content analysis, experts code the witness's statement for the presence of specific contents that are expected to occur more frequently in true reports. Although some limited evidence indicates that criterion-based content analysis can sometimes distinguish truthful statements from intentional lies, it cannot reliably distinguish true statements from false statements that were developed as a result of suggestive questioning techniques (Kulkofsky 2008).

Taken together, the literature shows that children are vulnerable to leading questions and other suggestive techniques, including some very mild forms of suggestion. Although young children appear to be the most suggestible, older children are also susceptible to suggestive techniques. Furthermore, children may be suggestible about central details of events and events that involve pain or bodily touch. Finally, children's reports that emerge through suggestive questioning often appear quite credible.

If suggestive techniques are so dangerous, why do interviewers use them? Several possible reasons for their use exist. First and foremost, children come into contact with an interviewer only if there is some reason to suspect that thy have been abused. This suspicion obviously colors the entire interview and may lead to interviewer bias. Given that young children, in particular, often give very scarce reports, forensic interviewers may be tempted to resort to more suggestive techniques in an attempt to verify their suspicions of abuse. Commonly held beliefs about how children disclose abuse during interviews also may influence an interviewer's decision of how to question them. Some interviewers believe that the use of suggestive techniques is necessary because children may be reticent to disclose sexual abuse and may disclose abuse only in a lengthy process, if at all. Belief in this pattern may lead interviewers to aggressively pursue children who they suspect to be victims of sexual abuse. We now turn to the issue of whether this belief in these disclosure patterns is actually warranted.

Disclosure Patterns Among Sexually Abused Children

Child Sexual Abuse Accommodation Syndrome

In 1983, Summit wrote "The Child Sexual Abuse Accommodation Syndrome," a theoretical view based on his clinical experiences with his adult psychiatric patients. He postulated that children who have experienced intrafamilial sexual abuse may be reluctant to disclose abuse because of motivational reasons such as being ashamed, scared, or embarrassed. As a result, he argued that abused children may delay abuse disclosure, deny abuse when asked, make partial disclosures, and retract abuse disclosures. He later extended the theory to include children who have experienced extrafamilial sexual abuse (Summit 1992). Summit's theory (Summit 1983, 1992) has exerted a tremendous influence on forensic interview practices with children and continues to be taught internationally in many contemporary training seminars for child abuse professionals.

Although Summit (1992) later cautioned practitioners that CSAAS is a clinical opinion, not a scientific or diagnostic instrument, some investigators have latched onto the idea that sexually abused children deny abuse or even that denial is diagnostic of abuse. In many instances of alleged satanic ritualistic abuse cases from the late 1980s, themes emerged whereby the investigators reported refusing to believe children despite their repeated denials of abuse (London et al. 2005). Many clinicians and forensic interviewers continue to interpret abuse denials or inconsistencies in children's statements as consistent with the children passing through the stages postulated by CSAAS.

The tenets postulated by CSAAS have undergone little scientific scrutiny to date. This is perhaps because Summit's theory was seen as consistent with forensic interview practices and general beliefs about abuse disclosure (Summit 1992). However, in several recent publications, London and colleagues (2005, 2007, 2008) reviewed the literature on disclosure patterns among sexually abused children. The goal of these reviews was to examine the contemporary empirical findings regarding the nature and timing of children's sexual abuse disclosures. Two main sources of data exist: 1) adults' retrospective accounts of CSA and whether they disclosed the abuse to anyone and 2) case records from children undergoing contemporaneous forensic evaluation. We briefly review the major findings below.

Research on Secrecy and Delayed Disclosure

Data from the retrospective accounts indicate that many adults reported that they never told anyone during childhood about the CSA they experienced. Even fewer reported that the abuse came to the attention of authorities. Across 13 retrospective abuse disclosure studies reviewed, 21%–87% of the participants reported that they disclosed the sexual abuse during childhood (for studies and citations, see London et al. 2008). Of the 13 studies reviewed, 11 found that between 34% and 54% of their adult sample who experienced CSA reported that they ever told anyone about the abuse during childhood. Fewer studies reported data on adults' retrospective reports of whether the abuse disclosure involved authorities such as police or social workers. Across 7 studies to provide data on disclosure to authorities, 5%–18% of the adults who reportedly experienced CSA indicated that the abuse was brought to the attention of authorities, with 4 of the 7 studies reporting rates from 10% to 13%. Although the retrospective accounts are subject to problems inherent in any retrospective account, London et al. (2008) concluded that extant data support Summit's notion of secrecy among sexually abused children: only about one-third to one-half of children ever tell anyone, and even fewer cases come to the attention of authorities.

Many of the retrospective studies reported very long delays between the abusive episodes and children's disclosures, sometimes of several years. Although data are limited at present, the trend seems to be that some children disclose relatively close in time to the abuse (e.g., within the first 6 months), whereas others wait many years or never tell anyone during childhood (London et al. 2008).

Research on Abuse Denials During Formal Interviews

Although victims may not readily report sexual abuse, this does not mean that they will deny abuse if asked directly about it. Studies of children undergoing assessment for suspected CSA provide the second source of data on disclosure patterns of abused children. These studies generally examined archival records from children who were seen by police, social workers, physicians, or assessment teams. Use of samples undergoing forensic assessment allows an exploration of the extent to which children make denials and recantations during forensic assessment.

Unlike the retrospective studies reviewed earlier, London and colleagues (2005, 2007, 2008) reported a wide range of disclosure rates across 21 different studies to examine abuse disclosure during forensic or medical interviews. Disclosure rates ranged from a low of 23% (Sorensen and Snow 1991) to a high of 96% (Bradley and Wood 1996). Methodological features, particularly sample choices and interview methods, appear to play a primary role in accounting for these discrepant rates. Because of its importance, we focus on this issue.

To calculate true rates of disclosures and denials during forensic interviews, information is needed that accurately classifies children as abused or nonabused regardless of whether they make an allegation during the interview. At the same time, the chosen sample should be representative of all children to come before forensic interviewers. For example, sampling methods that eliminate children from their sample who readily disclose to forensic interviewers would not provide accurate estimates of the overall rates of disclosure. At the same time, because abuse substantiation is often reliant on the child's disclosure, samples that include only highly probable or prosecuted cases may exclude possible true cases in which the child denies abuse during interviews.

London et al. (2005) argued that disclosure rates during forensic interviews vary systematically according to the certainty with which children in the study samples were abused. They divided the literature into four major groupings:

> *Group 1*—cases of dubious validity
> *Group 2*—select subsamples
> *Group 3*—all children to come before forensic interviewers
> *Group 4*—cases that come before forensic interviewers that are rated as founded or highly probable

The lowest disclosure rates came from studies in Group 1, with very dubious or overturned cases and documented poor interview techniques (Gonzalez et al. 1993; Sorensen and Snow 1991). In these studies, the abuse denials may have been true denials rather than evidence of reluctant disclosure. Many of the children from Gonzales et al.'s sample were from the McMartin Preschool case. Children in the Sorensen and Snow (1991) study were from a rash of neighborhood ritualistic satanic abuse cases, most of which either were not prosecuted or were later thrown out of court. Because of the documented highly suggestive techniques used in these studies (Schreiber et al. 2006), we argue that these studies do not provide any information about disclosure patterns among abused children.

The second major group of studies reported disclosure rates among select subsamples of children who come before authorities. These studies provide the second tier of disclosure rates—between 43% and 61% of children disclosed abuse when interviewed (for the study citations, see London et al. 2008). Two types of cases are included in this grouping: 1) children undergoing extended evaluation for nondisclosure with high

suspicion of abuse and 2) children coming to the attention of authorities because of strong evidence of abuse (e.g., videotaped abuse evidence or sexually transmitted disease diagnoses). Although these studies yield important information about abuse disclosure among their specific subsamples, caution is warranted in generalizing the results beyond the context under which these interviews occurred. Rather, the disclosure rates in this second major grouping are representative of the minority of children who do not make disclosures during initial interviews.

In the third major grouping of studies, researchers reported data among all children to come before forensic interviewers regardless of abuse substantiation. In several newly published studies among *all children* with CSA suspicions to come before highly trained forensic interviewers who used a specialized interview protocol, between 71% and 83% made disclosures (Hershkowitz et al. 2005; Pipe et al. 2007). Importantly, in these studies, no efforts were made to weed out cases in which suspicions arose but abuse really did not occur. One important caveat to this finding is that most of these children had made disclosures prior to the interviews, which was the impetus to the investigation. This factor probably contributes to the much higher rates found in these studies.

The final grouping of studies report disclosure rates among highly probable cases that come before investigators. In these studies, efforts were taken by abuse assessment teams to rate the certainty of abuse in light of all the case materials available. The highest rates of disclosure, 85%–96%, were found among these studies reporting disclosure rates among cases classified as highly probable. We argue that these rates provide the best estimate of disclosure rates among general samples of abused children who come before forensic interviewers because some effort must be made to determine which children were abused before evaluating disclosure rates among abused children. Table 16–2 summarizes findings from prospective studies of disclosure.

TABLE 16–2. Summary of prospective studies of disclosure

Methodology	Disclosure rates (%)
Children from dubious satanic ritual abuse or large-scale child care cases	24–58
Select subsamples of children to come to the attention of authorities	43–61
All children to come before highly trained interviewers using the National Institute of Child Health and Human Development interview protocol	71–83
Highly probable cases (based on case materials) to come before investigators	85–96

Research on Recantations During Formal Interviews

Once children have disclosed abuse to authorities, how likely are they to recant their allegations? Like abuse disclosure, recantation rates depend on sampling method and abuse substantiation. Two of highest recantation rates were reported by Gonzales et al. (1993) and Sorensen and Snow (1991). As discussed earlier, because of serious concerns about the forensic interview methods used and uncertainty of abuse substantiation in these cases, we argue that these rates are not representative of cases that come before forensic interviewers who have been trained with contemporary interview protocols. Recantation rates of 5%–9% are reported in general samples of highly probable abuse cases. A higher rate was reported by Malloy et al. (2007), who found that 23% of the children with substantiated CSA cases facing dependency hearings (for removal from the home for reasons stemming from the CSA) recanted their abuse allegations.

Overall, extant data on recantation of CSA disclosures suggest that 1) recantation occurs in a minority of cases and does not typify abuse disclosure patterns, and 2) recantation may be more common in certain groups (e.g., one with pressure or motivation to make recantation, such as having a nonsupportive, nonabusing caregiver). When evaluating the minority of cases in which abuse recantation occurs, like evaluating disclosure evidence, all of the evidence in the case, including potential motivators for recantation, should be considered.

Summary of Research on Child Sexual Abuse Disclosure

Taken together, the research on children's disclosure patterns suggests only limited support for CSAAS—namely, that many children delay reporting or fail to report abuse. However, much less empirical support exists for the idea that children who come before forensic interviewers and are asked directly about sexual abuse are likely to deny or recant abuse. The research thus dispels the notion that children who deny abuse must be bombarded with highly suggestive techniques in order to produce disclosures. Rather, as we outline in the next section, with careful interviewing, children can provide detailed information in response to open-ended prompts. We now turn to specific recommendations for forensic investigators to obtain the most accurate and complete reports from suspected victims of abuse.

Recommendations for Practice

Although our first major section painted a somewhat grim picture of the reliability of children's statements, children certainly can provide accurate information about past events. Specifically, when interviews are neutral in tone and little or no suggestive questions are used, children can provide accurate and useful information about past events, including traumatic events (Fivush 1993; Peterson and Bell 1996). Because of this, best practice guidelines that have been in effect for almost two decades encourage forensic interviewers to rely on open-ended questions as much as possible (American Professional Society on the Abuse of Children 1990; "Memorandum of Good Practice" 1992). However, for a variety of reasons outlined earlier, in real-world contexts, forensic interviewers often fail to follow these guidelines, even when they have undergone extensive training (Sternberg et al. 2001a).

Because of this issue, researchers at the National Institute of Child Health and Human Development (NICHD) developed a structured interview protocol for forensic interviewers (Orbach et al. 2000). The interview protocol is not simply a set of best practices or training guidelines. Rather, it provides a script that guides the interviewer through the various stages of the interview. The protocol begins with a truth–lie discussion to orient children toward truth-telling, then moves to non-abuse-related questions about the children's own life as a means to give children practice talking about the past before asking about the target event, and finally moves through a series of open-ended prompts to obtain information about the alleged abuse. Only if key elements are still missing from the child report after going through the open-ended prompts are more specific questions allowed.

The NICHD interview protocol has been shown to be effective even for young children (Lamb et al. 2003; Sternberg et al. 2001b). For example, in one study comparing protocol interviews with standard interviews (Sternberg et al. 2001b), more information was elicited in response to open-ended prompts in protocol interviews, and 89% of allegations were made in response to these prompts, compared with only 36% in standard interviews. Furthermore, although interviewers in both conditions made suggestive statements, interviewers in the protocol condition made significantly fewer. Thus, use of scripted protocols will likely increase the reliability of children's statements in forensic contexts.

However, it is important to keep in mind that children's reports may reflect other contextual factors outside of the formal investigative interview. As noted earlier, children may be inaccurate even without any suggestive influences, and even mild suggestions in the children's environment, such as rumors spread among classmates, can negatively affect the accuracy of children's statements. Furthermore, children often are interviewed multiple times by concerned parents, teachers, therapists, or social workers prior to their first formal forensic interview. Thus, investigators need to consider the full context of the child's disclosure when making judgments about statement reliability. Forensic practitioners should refrain from the temptation to make claims about specialized knowledge that allows them to determine the reliability of a child's statement.

Forensic practitioners should remain aware that simply because a child has been suspected of being maltreated, this does not mean that the child has necessarily been maltreated or that the suspect is necessarily the perpetrator. In other words, practitioners are advised to keep their own biases in check. This includes the bias to assume that if a child denies that abuse has occurred, then the child must have CSAAS. By remaining as neutral as possible and conducting interviews in a neutral manner, forensic interviewers will be able to get the most reliable statements from young witnesses.

—Key Points

- — Children often are able to provide relatively complete and accurate accounts of past experiences, provided that they are interviewed in a neutral, supportive manner.

- — Simply because a statement is spontaneous does not mean that it is accurate. In particular, when young children are reporting about confusing or unusual events, their accuracy may be impaired.

- — Suggestive interviewing techniques can negatively affect the reliability of children's statements. Furthermore, other suggestive influences outside the interview context can also have negative effects. Importantly, false statements that are induced by suggestive interviewing techniques may appear quite credible.

- — Evidence indicates that children often delay or fail to report abuse, but little empirical support currently exists for the notion posited in CSAAS that denial and recantation typify children's reports. Although denial and recantation may occur in a minority of cases that come before forensic interviewers, the scientific evidence does not support a "syndromelike" disclosure pattern. Thus, aggressive questioning techniques designed to obtain disclosures from children who have denied abuse are unwarranted.

- — Forensic interviewers should follow best practice guidelines by relying on open-ended questioning whenever possible. The NICHD interview may be a useful model for obtaining reliable information from children in the most neutral manner possible. However, investigators need to take into account the full context of disclosure, nondisclosure, and recantation.

References

American Professional Society on the Abuse of Children: Guidelines for Psychosocial Evaluation of Suspected Sexual Abuse in Young Children. Chicago, IL, American Professional Society on the Abuse of Children, 1990

Bradley AR, Wood JM: How do children tell? The disclosure process in child sexual abuse. Child Abuse Negl 20:881–891, 1996

Bruck M, Ceci S, Francoeur E: Children's use of anatomically detailed dolls to report genital touching in a medical examination: developmental and gender comparisons. J Exp Psychol Appl 6:74–83, 2000

Bruck M, Ceci SJ, Hembrooke H: The nature of children's true and false memories. Dev Rev 22:520–554, 2002

Burgwyn-Bales E, Baker-Ward L, Gordon BN, et al: Children's memory for emergency medical treatment after one year: the impact of individual difference variables on recall and suggestibility. Appl Cogn Psychol 15:S25–S48, 2001

Ceci SJ, Bruck M: Suggestibility of the child witness: a historical review and synthesis. Psychol Bull 113:403–439, 1993

Ceci SJ, Loftus EF, Leichtman MD, et al: The possible role of source misattributions in the creation of false beliefs among preschoolers. Int J Clin Exp Hypn 42:304–320, 1994

Ceci SJ, Kulkofsky S, Klemfuss JZ, et al: Unwarranted assumptions about children's testimonial accuracy. Ann Rev Clin Psychol 3:311–328, 2007a

Ceci SJ, Papierno P, Kulkofsky S: Representational constraints on children's suggestibility. Psychol Sci 18:503–509, 2007b

Finnilä K, Mahlberga N, Santtilaa P, et al: Validity of a test of children's suggestibility for predicting responses to two interview situations differing in their degree of suggestiveness. J Exp Child Psychol 85:32–49, 2003

Fivush R: Developmental perspectives on autobiographical recall: child victims and child witnesses, in Understanding and Improving Testimony. Edited by Goodman G, Bottoms B. New York, Guilford, 1993, pp 1–24

Fivush R, Schwarzmueller A: Children remember childhood: implications for childhood amnesia. Appl Cogn Psychol 12:455–473, 1999

Fivush R, Gray JT, Fromhoff FA: Two year olds talk about the past. Cogn Dev 2:393–410, 1987

Garven S, Wood JM, Malpass R, et al: More than suggestion: consequences of the interviewing techniques from the McMartin preschool case. J Appl Psychol 83:347–359, 1998

Garven S, Wood JM, Malpass RS: Allegations of wrongdoing: the effects of reinforcement on children's mundane and fantastic claims. J Appl Psychol 85:38–49, 2000

Geddie L, Fradin S, Beer J: Child characteristics which impact accuracy of recall in preschoolers: is age the best predictor? Child Abuse Negl 24:223–235, 2000

Gonzalez LS, Waterman J, Kelly RJ, et al: Children's patterns of disclosures and recantations of sexual and ritualistic abuse allegations in psychotherapy. Child Abuse Negl 17:281–289, 1993

Goodman GS, Sharma A, Thomas SF, et al: Mother knows best: effects of relationship status and interviewer bias on children's memory. J Exp Child Psychol 60:195–228, 1995

Hershkowitz I, Horowitz D, Lamb ME: Trends of children's disclosure of abuse in Israel: a national study. Child Abuse Negl 29:1203–1214, 2005

Hughes M, Grieve R: On asking children bizarre questions. First Language 1:149–160, 1980

Kulkofsky S: Credible but inaccurate: can criterion-based content analysis (CBCA) distinguish true and false memories? in Child Sexual Abuse: Issues and Challenges. Edited by Smith MJ. New York, Nova Science Publishers, 2008, pp 21–42

Kulkofsky S, Wang Q, Ceci SJ: Do better stories make better memories? Narrative quality and memory accuracy in preschool children. Appl Cogn Psychol 22:21–38, 2008

Lamb ME, Sternberg KJ, Orbach Y, et al: Age differences in young children's responses to open-ended invitations in the course of forensic interviews. J Consult Clin Psychol 71:926–934, 2003

Leichtman MD, Ceci SJ: The effects of stereotypes and suggestions on preschoolers' reports. Dev Psychol 31:568–578, 1995

Leichtman MD, Pillemer DB, Wang Q, et al: When Baby Maisy came to school: mothers' interview styles and children's event memories. Cogn Dev 15:99–114, 2000

London K, Bruck M, Ceci SJ, et al: Disclosure of child sexual abuse: what does the research tell us about the ways that children tell? Psychol Public Policy Law 11:194–226, 2005

London K, Bruck M, Ceci SJ, et al: Disclosure of child sexual abuse: a review of the contemporary literature, in Child Sexual Abuse: Disclosure, Delay, and Denial. Edited by Pipe ME, Orbach Y, Lamb ME, et al. Mahwah, NJ, Lawrence Erlbaum, 2007, pp 11–40

London K, Bruck M, Wright DB, et al: How children report sexual abuse to others: findings and methodological issues. Memory 16:29–47, 2008

Malloy LC, Lyon TD, Quas JA: Filial dependency and recantation of child sexual abuse allegations. J Am Acad Child Adolesc Psychiatry 46:162–170, 2007

Memorandum of Good Practice. London, Her Majesty's Stationery Office, 1992

Nelson K, Fivush R: The emergence of autobiographical memory: a social cultural developmental theory. Psychol Rev 111:486–511, 2004

Orbach Y, Hershkowitz I, Lamb ME, et al: Assessing the value of scripted protocols for forensic interviews of alleged abuse victims. Child Abuse Negl 24:733–752, 2000

Ornstein PA, Merrit KA, Baker-Ward L, et al: Children's knowledge, expectation, and long-term retention. Appl Cogn Psychol 12:387–405, 1998

Peterson C, Bell M: Children's memory for traumatic injury. Child Dev 67:3045–3070, 1996

Peterson C, Rideout R: Memory for medical emergencies experienced by 1- and 2-year olds. Dev Psychol 34:1059–1072, 1998

Peterson C, Dowden C, Tobin J: Interviewing preschoolers: comparisons of yes/no and wh- questions. Law Hum Behav 23:539–555, 1999

Pipe ME, Orbach Y, Lamb ME, et al: Seeking resolution in the disclosure wars: an overview, in Child Sexual Abuse: Disclosure, Delay, and Denial. Edited by Pipe ME, Orbach Y, Lamb ME, et al. Mahwah, NJ, Lawrence Erlbaum, 2007, pp 1–10

Poole DA, Lindsay DS: Interviewing preschoolers: effects of nonsuggestive techniques, parental coaching, and leading questions on reports of non-experienced events. J Exp Child Psychol 60:129–154, 1995

Powell MB, Jones CH, Campbell C: A comparison of preschoolers' recall of experienced versus non-experienced events across multiple interviewers. Appl Cogn Psychol 17:935–952, 2003

Principe GF, Kanaya T, Ceci SJ, et al: Believing is seeing: how rumors can engender false memories in preschoolers. Psychol Sci 17:243–248, 2006

Principe GF, Guiliano S, Root C: Rumor mongering and remembering: how rumors originating in children's inferences can affect memory. J Exp Child Psychol 99:135–155, 2008

Schreiber N, Bellah LD, Martinez Y, et al: Suggestive interviewing in the McMartin Preschool and Kelly Michaels daycare abuse cases: a case study. Social Influence 1:16–47, 2006

Simcock G, Hayne H: Breaking the barrier? Children fail to translate their preverbal memories into language. Psychol Sci 13:225–231, 2002

Sorensen T, Snow B: How children tell: the process of disclosure in child sexual abuse. Child Welfare 70:3–15, 1991

Sternberg KJ, Lamb ME, Davies GM, et al: The memorandum of good practice: theory versus application. Child Abuse Negl 25:669–681, 2001a

Sternberg KJ, Lamb ME, Orbach Y, et al: Use of a structured investigative protocol enhances young children's responses to free-recall prompts in the course of forensic interviews. J Appl Psychol 86:907–1005, 2001b

Summit RC: The Child Sexual Abuse Accommodation syndrome. Child Abuse Negl 7:177–193, 1983

Summit RC: Abuse of the child sexual abuse accommodation syndrome. J Child Sex Abus 1:153–164, 1992

Vrij A: Criteria-based content analysis: a qualitative review of the first 37 studies. Psychol Public Policy Law 11:3–41, 2005

White TL, Leichtman MD, Ceci SJ: The good, the bad, and the ugly: accuracy, inaccuracy, and elaboration in preschoolers' reports about a past event. Appl Cogn Psychol 11:S37–S54, 1997

Chapter 17

Interviewing Children for Suspected Sexual Abuse

Kathleen M. Quinn, M.D.

What Is Child Sexual Abuse?

Child sexual abuse (CSA) describes a wide range of acts. In general, CSA is the use of a child as an object of sexual gratification for an adult or a significantly older minor. The Child Abuse Prevention and Treatment Act (CAPTA) of 1974 articulates the minimum standards for defining physical abuse, neglect, and sexual abuse that states must include in their statutory definitions in order to receive federal funds for programs to identify, treat, and prevent child abuse. CAPTA defines CSA as follows:

> [T]he employment, use, persuasion, inducement, enticement, or coercion of any child to engage in, or assist any other person to engage in, any sexually explicit conduct or simulation of such conduct for the purpose of producing any visual depiction of such conduct;
> [T]he rape, and in case of caretaker or inter-familial relationship, statutory rape, molestation, prostitution, or in other form of sexual exploitation of children, or incest with children.

In CAPTA a child is generally defined as someone who is under age 18 years or who has not reached the age of majority specified by the child protection law of the relevant state, whichever is younger. Each state is responsible to provide its own definition of child maltreatment, including CSA, with civil and criminal proceedings incorporating the CAPTA standards.

All states define children as incompetent to consent to sexual activity with an adult (Myers 1997). However, the age of consent may vary. Although the professional literature describes the unequal power relationship between some peers and the possibility of sexual activity forced by one minor against a younger child, the majority of states do not have child-on-child sexual abuse statutes. States vary on whether they address CSA offenses in existing criminal code sections on rape, incest, and sexual battery or in specific CSA statutes.

CSA is usually defined as contact sexual abuse or noncontact sexual abuse. Contact sexual abuse involves touching of the sexual areas of either the child's body or the perpetrator's body. Noncontact sexual abuse may include exhibitionism, voyeurism, or the child's involvement in the production of pornography. The intent of the act must be demonstrated to be sexual stimulation. Contact with the child's genitals for caretaking purposes (e.g., washing or application of ointments for medicinal purposes) is excluded in the definition of CSA.

Controversy continues in the assessment of whether some acts constitute sexual abuse. For example, when is sexual activity between peers abuse? How old must an adolescent be to consent to intercourse? When are overstimulation and exposure to adult sexual acts abuse? A community standard including the age and intellectual difference between participants, the nature of the relationship (coercive or noncoercive), and relevant legal definitions will aid in defining what is abuse (Finkelhor 1979).

Normative sexual play is usually spontaneous, is mutual, and includes pleasure along with embarrassment. Equally important to recognize is that the majority of juvenile sex offenders commit their first sexual offense before age 15 years. Studies indicate that children victimized by other children exhibit similar levels of emotional distress and behavioral disturbances as juveniles abused by adults (Shaw and Lewis 2000).

Grooming behaviors are often preludes to abuse. Although grooming behavior is not direct evidence of a crime, it may demonstrate an alleged perpetrator's motivation and intent. The goal of grooming is to lower inhibitions of possible victims in order to exploit them sexually. Investigatory interviewing has evolved to include inquiries to victims about what has been given to them (gifts) as well as techniques alleged perpetrators have used to gain children's trust and confidence as evidence consistent with grooming. The Internet gives child molesters anonymity, the ability to create a different persona and lifestyle, and access to multiple possible victims (Brown 2001) and can be a powerful grooming tool.

How Frequently Does Child Sexual Abuse Occur?

In 2006, an estimated 3.6 million children were the subject of a Child Protective Services (CPS) investigation pertaining to allegations of abuse or neglect (U.S. Department of Health and Human Services 2006). CPS agencies assign a finding to each allegation after their investigation. A finding of "substantiated" concludes that the allegation was supported by state law or policy. A finding of "indicated" concludes that the allegation could not be substantiated under state law or policy but that there was reason to suspect maltreatment or risk of maltreatment. "Unsubstantiated" or "unfounded" allegations are simply not proven. Intentionally false allegations are rare (approximately 4%) although likely more common in custody and visitation cases (12%), as found by Trocmé and Bala (2005).

Approximately one-quarter (25.2%) of all maltreatment allegations in 2006 were substantiated or indicated. Of these victims, 8.8% were sexually abused. Children with allegations of sexual abuse were nearly twice as likely to be considered victims as children with allegations of physical abuse. In 26.2% of sexual abuse cases perpetrators were parents, whereas 29.1% were relatives other than parents. These statistics indicate that the most commonly reported type of case of sexual abuse is incest—sexual abuse between family members.

Reports of CSA cases nationwide declined 5% from 2005 to 2006, continuing a decline beginning in the early 1990s. In light of the vast majority of states experiencing significant drops in sexual abuse cases, the decline of more than 50% nationwide of the incidence of CSA appears real. State-by-state data about sexual abuse, physical abuse, and neglect from 1992 to 2006 are available at the website of the Crimes Against Children Research Center (http://www.unh. edu/ccrc). Multiple factors have been cited as possible contributors to the decline of CSA since the early 1990s, including the increased number of child sex offenders incarcerated since the mid-1980s, economic prosperity, increased awareness of the risk of victimization and its impact on parenting practices, and a hypothesized benefit of psychopharmacology with improved functioning and fewer individuals acting out aggressively or sexually (Finkelhor and Jones 2006).

Retrospective surveys also continue to be an important source of data about child maltreatment because many victims do not report their abuse to anyone. Using the Juvenile Victimization Questionnaire with a nationally representative sample of children and youth ($N=2,030$) ages 2–17 years, Finkelhor et al. (2005) reported that during the study year, 1 out of 12 children experienced a sexual victimization. Epidemiological estimates of sexual abuse will continue to be informed by both prospective and retrospective data (Kendall-Tackett and Becker-Blease 2004).

Legal Issues

The basis for state intervention in child maltreatment, including CSA, is based on the legal concept of *parens patriae*, the authority of the state to act as a "parent" to protect the interests of children or other vulnerable populations when their basic needs are not met or when their rights have been violated. Child maltreatment including CSA is subject to state laws (both statutes and case law) as well as to administrative regulation. Definitions of child abuse and neglect are found in three places within each state's statutory code:

1. Mandatory child maltreatment reporting statutes.

2. Criminal statutes that define the forms of child abuse and neglect that are criminally punishable. In most jurisdictions child sexual maltreatment is criminally punishable when one or more of the following statutory crimes have been committed: rape, deviant sexual assault, indecent exposure, child pornography, or computer crimes. Criminal statutes continue to evolve in the face of technology. For example, in Ohio adults sending pornographic material to anyone under 18 can be charged with disseminating material harmful to a juvenile, which is a misdemeanor. Adults seeking sexual acts with minors through telecommunications media can be charged with importuning, which is a felony.

3. Juvenile court jurisdiction statutes define when the court has jurisdiction over a child alleged to have been abused or neglected. The court need not have convicted anyone for perpetrating the act.

Mandatory Child Abuse Reporting Acts

The "discovery" of child abuse, accelerated by the 1962 landmark article "The Battered-Child Syndrome" (Kempe et al. 1962), initially focused on physical abuse. Also in 1962, Congress redefined child welfare services under the Social Security Act as services for "the purpose of…preventing or remedying, or assisting in the solution of problems which may result in the neglect, abuse, exploitation or delinquency of children" (Public Welfare Amendments of 1962, P.L. 87-543). Kempe et al. (1962) specifically wrote of child maltreatment being "inadequately handled by the physician because of hesitation to bring the case to the attention of the proper authorities" (p. 17). Pressure mounted for the need of laws requiring physicians to report suspected abuse. In 1963 the Children's Bureau, the first federal agency devoted to children established in 1912, drafted the first model child abuse reporting statute. In 1963 10 states passed reporting laws. By 1967 all states had passed reporting laws (Myers 2004). Initially most of these laws were limited to mandated reporting by physicians of physical abuse, but laws continued to expand in the late 1960s and early 1970s to cover other professionals as well as other forms of maltreatment, including sexual abuse (Kalichman 1993).

Currently all states, the District of Columbia, the Commonwealth of Puerto Rico, and the U.S. territories have mandatory reporting statutes identifying individuals who are required to report child maltreatment under specific circumstances. Nearly all state statutes enumerate numerous professionals who typically have frequent contact with children as mandated reporters. Mandated reporters have expanded to include commercial film or photograph processors (in 11 states, Guam, and Puerto Rico), substance use counselors (in 13 states), and probation or parole officers (in 15 states). Clergy are now required to report in 26 states. In 18 states and Puerto Rico, any person who suspects child abuse or neglect must report, whereas in the remaining states, territories, and the District of Columbia, reporting by nonmandated individuals is voluntary. The standard for mandatory reporters varies from state to state. The usual wording of the mandate is when the individual acting in his or her official capacity suspects or has reason to suspect a child has been abused or neglected (Child Welfare Information Gateway 2008). The following vignette poses a scenario for the potential reporting of suspected child abuse.

Case Example 1

John, age 10 years, returned from a sleepover at Luke's house tired but excited. He later told his older sister that he and his friend Luke, age 11 years, were "playing doctor." The sister immediately reported this news to their mother, who called the pediatrician who saw John later that day. John was well known to the pediatrician as a small boy with a cognitive deficit who was in special education classes.

Each statute will indicate whether the allegation must be directly from the child or whether it can come from a third party, whether the report can be anonymous, and whether any privileged communication (e.g., attorney–client privilege or clergy–penitent privilege) can create an exception from mandatory reporting. In most statutes a mental health professional or named mandatory reporter can be charged with a violation of criminal law for failure to report known or suspected cases of abuse. Failure to report may also make the professional liable for civil damages in a malpractice case. All state statutes provide the mandated reporter with immunity from suits for negligence or defamation if a suspected case of abuse is reported in good faith. In the wake of concerns about false allegations of CSA, some states have passed statutes making it illegal to knowingly make a false accusation of CSA.

Despite legal protection and possible sanctions, many professionals fail to report suspected abuse. Studies have shown more than 30% of clinicians have suspected abuse in one of their cases but failed to report it (Melton et al. 1995). Mandated reporters must follow the child protection laws in their states to avoid both criminal and civil liability. Professionals encountering cases raising issues concerning abuse should consult with knowledgeable colleagues and/or legal counsel to determine their responsibility for reporting. They may also consult with the legal department of the designated human services agency to determine if a hypothetical set of facts meets criteria for reporting. Mandated reporting of abuse is a well-recognized exception to confidentiality. The Health Insurance Portability and Accountability Act (HIPAA) of 1996 recognizes that there is no right to prevent disclosure of personal health information when the disclosure is required by law and the disclosure complies with and is limited to the requirements of mandated duties such as the reporting of child maltreatment (see 45 CFR § 164.152 [a] [1]).

Case Example 1 Epilogue

When seen in the pediatrician's office, John was embarrassed and answered few questions. His physical exam showed no evidence of genital injury or penetration. Upon reflection, the pediatrician recalled a forensic lecture he had recently attended. He recognized his status as a mandated reporter but was unsure if this incident triggered this duty. He called the local Protective Services and gave a hypothetical example matching these events and inquired if this was a mandatory report. The intake social worker stated that these facts did raise a reasonable suspicion of abuse, and the report was accepted. The physician informed John's mother of his duty and the report.

Relevant Case Law

Three major hearsay exceptions have commonly been used in abuse cases permitting admission of an alleged victim's out-of-court statements: 1) "excited utterances" or *res gestae,* 2) statements made to a physician during diagnosis and treatment, and 3) residual hearsay, an exception permitting such evidence when it can be shown to be reliable. For example, in *White v. Illinois* (1992), the U.S. Supreme Court stated that "[t]here can be no doubt" of the medical diagnosis or treatment exception being firmly noted as an exception to the exclusion of hearsay evidence.

However, in *Crawford v. Washington* (2004), the Supreme Court announced a new rule that "testimonial" statements are no longer admissible in court unless the witness testifies and is available for cross-examination. The Court did not define testimonial, but two relevant questions to determine if a statement is testimonial have been proposed: 1) Was a government agent (e.g., police or investigator) involved in preparing the testimony or taking a formal statement from the witness? and 2) Would an objective person in the witness's position reasonably believe the statement would later be used in court? (Philips 2006).

The scope of the *Crawford* rule continues to be defined. Since *Crawford,* courts have overwhelmingly agreed that medical personnel conducting an exam of an alleged victim related to medical diagnosis and treatment can testify to statements made by the victim. However, sexual assault nurse examiners, sexual assault forensic examiners, or other health care personnel working with a child abuse multidisciplinary team engaged in collecting evidence and statements from alleged victims as part of a law enforcement investigation are likely to be seen as gathering "testimonial" data (see *Medina v. State* 2006) requiring that the alleged victim testify and be cross-examined in a criminal case. Whether or not *Crawford* is operative in abuse/neglect family or juvenile court cases will depend on whether or not the state defines these maltreatment cases as quasi-criminal or civil.

Evolution of case law has indicated that the Sixth Amendment (confrontation clause) does not guarantee a defendant the absolute right to face-to-face confrontation. Two U.S. Supreme Court cases, *Coy v. Iowa* (1988) and *Maryland v. Craig* (1990), have clarified that exceptions to confrontation can be recognized but must be based on adequate demonstration of the necessity of finding that the child witness is physically or psychologically unavailable. Several states have statutes authorizing courts to declare witnesses psychologically unavailable. Clinicians may become involved in assessing a child who is refusing to testify before the defendant. The legal standard of declaring a child unavailable for testimony is high and does not include mere discomfort or reluctance.

Testimony of children via closed-circuit television does not violate the right to confrontation or the *Crawford* rule as the child's testimony actually occurs during the trial but is located outside the courtroom and is electronically transmitted into the proceedings.

Clinical Issues

Validation of Complaint

When faced with a case with an allegation of CSA, the clinician is presented with a number of problems in attempting to assess the complaint. First, few of the cases have any physical corroboration. Even when the offender has confessed to sexual acts, including penetration, the physical exam may be normal (Heger et al. 2002; Kerns and Ritter 1992). Findings that were diagnostic of sexual abuse (genital trauma, sexually transmitted diseases or sperm) were found in only 3%–16% of child victims in a review of 21 studies (Bays and Chadwick 1993). Interpretation of physical findings continues to be defined as evidence-based research is published (Adams 2001). Several reasons exist for the lack of physical findings in sexually abused children, including 1) delay in seeking the medical exam; 2) rapid healing of mucosal tissue; 3) sexual acts, such as fondling, deep kissing, oral sodomy and cunniligus that do not leave physical finds; or 4) elasticity of hymen and anal tissue.

A second problem in the validation of CSA is the issue of false negatives and retractions. The publication of Roland Summit's (1983) paper proposing the "child sexual abuse accommodation syndrome" as an explanation for delayed disclosure, denial of abuse, and recantation of abuse profoundly influenced investigating interview practices. However, the child sexual abuse accommodation syndrome has been critiqued as theoretical rather than data based. London et al. (2008) reanalyzed 13 retrospective studies of adults reporting CSA and confirmed that most adults indicated either delayed disclosure or lack of disclosure in childhood. Their estimate of the composite data of the frequency of childhood disclosure ranged from 31% to 45%, with a low frequency of report (5%–13%) to authorities. Their review of 24 studies of minors reporting CSA found a recantation rate of 4%–27%. The credibility of the recantation must also be considered, including an initial false disclosure, highly suggestive interviewing techniques, and/or emotional reactions to a nonsupportive family or risk of out-of-home placement. Data analyses suggest males and non-Caucasians are more reluctant to disclose abuse. Age was also associated with disclosure rates, with older children more likely to disclose abuse. Lower disclosure rates are found in cases in which the suspected perpetrator is a parent or parent figure (Hershkowitz et al. 2005; Pipe et al. 2007).

Third, in attempting to validate an allegation of sexual abuse, the clinician may be confronted with the problem of interviewing children of special populations who have unique needs. These special populations may include those with sensory losses (e.g., deafness), cognitive disabilities (e.g., retardation), and/or communication challenges (e.g., language disabilities); children whose first language is not English; or preschoolers. These children often require interviewing techniques that the average clinician does not possess.

Case Example 2

A 3-year-old boy alleged his teenage stepbrother had touched his bottom. The child was not yet toilet trained, and the intake social worker taking the complaint found that the stepbrother babysat the 3-year-old and assisted him in the bathroom. The mother, who reported the allegation, stated the 3-year-old had immature language skills. The intake worker on hearing this history decided additional expertise would be required to fully evaluate the allegation.

Fourth, the alleged victim may not appreciate the abusive nature of the alleged events. Approximately 40% of victims of substantiated maltreatment are age 5 years and younger. These children may not appreciate that they are indeed victims of abuse.

Fifth, behavioral problems cited as the bases for sexual abuse allegations may overlap with other sources of a child's problem. Children express distress with a wide range of signs and symptoms. In addition, families with multiple problems may expose the children to multiple stressors. The clinician must be cautious in using behavioral indicators as support for sexual abuse allegations. However, sexual behavior continues to be one of the most valid indicators of sexual abuse in children (Kendall-Tackett et al. 1993).

Finally, the alleged perpetrator is often well known to the child. Younger victims are more likely abused by members of their intimate social network. Although these demographics may lessen eyewitness issues, validation is made more complicated by the child's (and family's) divided loyalties. Sexual abuse by strangers is no more than 10%–30%, as reported in adult retrospective surveys.

All of these factors make investigating an allegation of abuse a complex problem—one that deserves the highest degree of care, objectivity, and up-to-date research to provide the clinical and judicial systems the best set of data.

Case Example 2 Epilogue

The intake worker called the local hospital-affiliated sexual abuse team to discuss how to proceed on the 3-year-old's statements. The two professionals decided that a senior member of the sexual abuse team with experience in early childhood development and special needs children would interview the child while social services personnel watched behind a one-way mirror. The two investigatory interviews were consistent with the 3-year-old describing hygienic touching as opposed to abuse. The family readily acknowledged a need to change the handling of the 3-year-old's toileting. No other overstimulating or inappropriate experiences were detailed during the evaluation.

Evolution of Interviewing Practices

The professional history of CSA has been characterized by its "discovery," its at times overzealous investigation methods, and the subsequent polarization and denial in professionals and the public. Freud discovered the origins of neuroses in the seduction theory and then replaced his recognition of CSA with the Oedipus complex. Kempe (1978) wrote of sexual abuse as "another hidden pediatric problem." In the 1980s a series of highly publicized day care CSA cases, which included allegations of satanic and ritualistic acts, utilized interviewing techniques that appeared to create false reports, causing a backlash against such investigatory methods.

The dangers of the backlash included the complete denial or minimization of the existence of sexual abuse. The backlash against child protection was often enunciated in highly critical, often strident materials describing the child protective system as out of control and on "witch hunts" to find abuse at any cost. The positive aspects of the backlash included increased use of scientifically based investigatory techniques; greater appreciation of the impact of development on both the allegations and adequate investigatory techniques; and increased adherence to basic forensic principles, including objectivity and documentation, in the investigation of CSA.

By the 1990s guidelines for practice were developed by two multidisciplinary organizations, the American Professional Society on the Abuse of Children (1995) and the American Academy of Child and Adolescent Psychiatry (1997). Guidelines were not intended to establish a legal standard or a rigid standard of practice; rather, guidelines endorsed support for flexibility based on professional judgment in individual cases.

Recent trends have focused on the overarching importance of the role of the investigator as well as newer interview techniques to improve objectivity and reliability of investigatory interviews (see Chapter 16, "Reliability and Suggestibility of Children's Statements: From Science to Practice").

Role of the Investigator

Objectivity and impartiality are the key aspects of investigatory interviewing. The interviewer must strive to not ally himself or herself with any particular individual involved in the investigation. Similarly, the investigator must be open, honest, thorough, and unbiased in gathering data and hearing the child's account of his or her experience. Interviewers should utilize the same principle as scientific investigators by ruling in or out alternate hypotheses (Ceci and Bruck 1995) as well as acknowledging the limitations of their data. Kuehlne (1998) proposed a scientist-practitioner model, which utilizes empirically derived data including base rates of behavior for understanding differences between nonsexually abused children, sexually abused children, and children who have not been known to be abused.

The primary role of the forensic investigator is to document the chronology, psychosocial context, and consistency of an allegation. The data gathered should be as uncontaminated as possible for use by the mental health and judicial systems. Contamination occurs when the source of the child's memory of the alleged event becomes distorted or falsified by factors inside or outside the interview. Contamination cannot be eliminated, because memory is reconstructive, not reproductive, but it can be minimized by maintaining objectivity, role definition, and appropriate interview techniques.

Interviewers must be careful to avoid role confusion. The interviewer must remember that he or she is a forensic examiner and not a therapist or child advocate in any particular case. Techniques of investigation must not be mixed with therapy during the assessment of CSA. In some states it is a violation of the mental health professional's code of ethics to do both within one case. There needs to be a sharp demarcation between evaluation and therapy.

A second role confusion often exhibited by interviewers is mixing investigation with inappropriate advocacy. Statements to the referent, such as "I'm sure she'll tell me what happened," demonstrate a lack of independence on the part of the interviewer. Promising to the child that "nothing like this will ever happen again" is an empty promise in that the interviewer has no way of providing total protection to the child once he or she leaves the office. In addition, telling a child after a disclosure that "things will be better now" is likewise a potentially empty promise, because the child who experiences the court proceedings may find that things do not get better for a long time. In fact, things may actually get worse for the child.

A third role confusion to avoid is being the judge or jury. Evaluators should not testify that a child has been sexually abused based on the child's past abuse functioning. However, the investigator can detail what is consistent or not consistent with the allegation.

In summary, clinicians receiving a referral of a case involving an allegation of CSA must define their role for themselves and all participants. In addition, clinicians must clearly understand who has hired them and who will see the data they gather. This is the issue of agency. In forensic evaluations, the evaluator may be hired by a parent or parent's attorney to assess the allegation or may be the agent of an institution (Child Protective Services or the court). The agent initiating the evaluation will see the data, may request a report, or may require testimony. The evaluator of a CSA allegation must provide the data in the form requested and structure the evaluation to provide objective, comprehensive data.

Interviews of Children

Clinicians must bring a developmental perspective to interviewing a child about allegations of abuse. There are well-documented age differences in memory, suggestibility, and reasoning (see Chapter 16, "Reliability and Suggestibility of Children's Statements: From Science to Practice"), as well as sexual knowledge, range of experience, and emotional maturity. The evaluator should plan to screen each child developmentally early in the investigatory interview and tailor the interview to the child's level of functioning as well as interpret responses from a developmental perspective.

Consensus based on research of the past several decades emphasizes that as much information as possible should be obtained using open-ended inquiry rather than focused questions because open-ended questions are more likely than focused questions to elicit accurate information (Dale et al. 1978). Despite this knowledge, even highly trained investigators often pose focused or even leading questions in their forensic interviews (Aldridge and Cameron 1999). Often it is necessary to use focused questions, especially with very young children, to elicit critical information. Such focused questions should be delayed until open-ended inquiries are exhausted. Focused questions (e.g., "Were your clothes on or off?") should be followed up with an open-ended inquiry (e.g., "Tell me everything about how they came off"; Lamb et al. 1998). Other research-

based strategies believed to enhance retrieval include the following (Orbach et al. 2000):

1. Having a relaxed, supportive, distraction-free interview environment
2. Empowering children to appreciate that they are unique sources of information because the interviewer was not present when the alleged acts occurred
3. Clarifying the rules of communication to include the obligation to tell the truth and permission for children to say "I don't know" or "I don't understand" to the interviewer's questions.
4. Having children practice responding to open-ended prompts about neutral events
5. Inquiring about the first or last event or unusual episodes if there appear to have been multiple events

Table 17–1 highlights important interview components to be considered when conducting a child abuse evaluation.

The National Institute of Child Health and Human Development (NICHD) investigatory protocol is a structured interview protocol that incorporates these recommended strategies for forensic interviews. Research by Orbach et al. (2000) indicates that when using the protocol, interviewers elicited more details using open-ended question compared with previous nonprotocol interviews by the same investigators. Although the number of details elicited between protocol and nonprotocol interviews did not differ significantly,

---

TABLE 17–1. Basic interview technique

Create the right environment: quiet, private, supportive

Introduce self and role

Build rapport

Screen for developmental level

Emphasize need to tell truth

Give permission for "I don't know" and "I don't remember" responses

Begin with open-ended inquiry

Discuss neutral events initially

Explore who, what, where, when, how

Follow focused questions with open inquiry

Minimize amount of information suggested in questions

more recent studies (Hershkowitz et al. 2005; Pipe et al. 2007) have shown higher rates of disclosure using the NICHD protocol.

Appellate court decisions such as *Commonwealth of Massachusetts v. Amirault LeFave* (1999) and *State v. Michaels* (1994), analysis of the McMartin Preschool case transcripts (Garven et al. 1998), and the professional literature have described what *not* to do. Techniques to be avoided or minimized include the following:

1. Leading or suggestive questions ("George touched your pee-pee, didn't he?"). These questions introduce information into the interview that has not been volunteered by the child in the same interview or indicate an attempt to direct the response by the interviewer.
2. Repetitive questioning and/or interviewing.
3. Questions promoting pretending, speculation, or use of fantasizing, including the use of puppets ("Let's make believe…").
4. Social influence ("Johnny and Lucy have told us about the 'touch-me game.' Can you tell me about the 'touch-me game'?").
5. Positive and negative reinforcement (e.g., "You are doing such a good job telling me about what Joe did to you").
6. Problematic question formats such as those requiring only a yes or no answer, compound questions, or why questions. A child may endorse a question that is not fully accurate or that may be misunderstood. Children often experience why questions as accusatory and may become defensive about their actions or behaviors.

Table 17–2 summarizes interview techniques to avoid or minimize when interviewing children who may be victims of abuse.

Garven et al. (1998) staged a classroom visit of "Manny Morales" to five different day care centers. One week later, they interviewed half of the children (total $N = 66$) with techniques from the McMartin interviews, including suggestive questions, social influence, and reinforcement, as well as questions promoting pretending and speculation including puppet play. In the group subjected to suggestive questions, 17% made false allegations against the classroom visitor, while 58% of those interviewed with all of the McMartin techniques made false allegations. Garven et al. hypothesized that noncognitive factors such as social influence and reinforcement had a strong immediate impact on the children's statements, whereas techniques inviting fantasy or speculation may have a delayed impact on children's memory.

TABLE 17–2. Interview techniques to avoid or minimize

Leading or suggestive questions

Repetitive questions

Use of pretending or fantasy

Social influence questions

"Yes" or "no" questions

Compound questions

Coercive questions

Parental Interviews

There are a number of psychosocial issues that must be clarified either in the intake interview or during the parental interviews. Especially in cases involving divorce, visitation, or custody, a chronology of escalating allegations should be documented to ascertain if previous attempts by the complainant have not been successful in changing the visitation and custody arrangements. The possible utility of the allegation as perceived by the complainant and child should be assessed, especially as it relates to custody and visitation changes. The complainant's potential for deceptive motives should be addressed, including the possibility of that person's having a major mental illness, which may lead him or her to distort reality. The clinician should also be aware of any person involved in the case who repeatedly sexualizes relationships.

The child's baseline sexual behavior and sexual knowledge as well as the presence of overstimulation should be assessed. A listing of those individuals who come in contact with the child should be made. A good history of the child's symptoms should be made, including the date of initial appearance, any increase or decreases in symptom severity, and the coexistence of other stresses that have occurred. The clinician should also investigate the child's fears or alienation, which might be fueling the allegation.

Efforts to obtain a description of the family's daily living patterns, their traditions concerning privacy and nudity, their approach to sexuality and sex education, and the child's exposure to sexually explicit materials and activities need to be made.

When custody and visitation are at issue in addition to a sexual abuse complaint, the child should be seen for additional appointments to observe the child's interaction with each parent. The clinician performing this set of interviews should be the one doing the custody or visitation assessment. The purpose of this set of interviews is not to further determine the credibility of the allegation but rather to observe the quality of the overall relationship between the child and each parent. These data are often helpful in recommending the nature and frequency of any contact between the child and the alleged perpetrator. Much resistance should be anticipated in attempting to set up such appointments, and on occasion the decision may determine such an appointment is contraindicated due to the child's level of distress and/or resistance.

Use of Anatomical Dolls

Controversy continues over when, or if ever, it is appropriate to use anatomical dolls in the course an investigation of a sexual abuse allegation. Some professionals argue that anatomical dolls may serve as a demonstration aid in which the dolls are used as a prop to show what occurred, as an anatomical model to document the child's vocabulary for body parts, or as an external memory cue (Everson and Boat 1994). Other writers, however, have argued that anatomical dolls are suggestive and may encourage play and/or fantasy (Ceci and Bruck 1995).

Recent research clarifies the impact of anatomical dolls on the investigatory process. Thierry et al. (2005) studied tapes of the interviews of alleged sexual abuse victims ages 3–12 years ($N=178$). The children produced as many details when responding to open-ended questions with or without the dolls. The younger children were more likely to reenact behaviorally rather than verbally, whereas the older children responded with more verbal details. These findings were consistent with the hypothesis that the dolls can have a language-substitution function with younger children. However, enactments tend to be more inaccurate than the verbal responses that accompany doll use (Salmon et al. 1995).

With the dolls, the younger children (3–6 years) were more likely to play suggestively and to contradict details provided without the dolls compared with the older group. Children in both groups produced more fantastic details with dolls than without the dolls. Thierry et al. (2005) concluded, "[I]n sum, the doll asserted details produced by younger children should be interpreted with caution" and "the disadvantages with respect to accuracy or perception of credibility are likely to outweigh benefits when dolls are used as memory-retrieved aids when interviewing older children" (p. 1133).

If anatomical dolls are used, the following procedures can address anticipated concerns regarding the impact of the dolls on the child's allegation (Holmes 2000):

1. In most cases, introduce the dolls after the child has made a verbal disclosure.
2. Instruct the child that the dolls are not toys.
3. Present the doll(s) fully clothed.
4. Determine if the child has the developmental capacity to make a representational shift. Children under approximately 3.5 years may not be capable of using the dolls to represent themselves or others (DeLoache 1995). In presenting two or more dolls, ask the child, "Which doll is the little girl (boy) doll, and which is more like (the already identified alleged perpetrator)?" If the child correctly distinguishes between dolls of different ages/genders, ask, "Which doll is most like you?" prior to asking the child to "show" what happened.
5. Set aside or put doll(s) away (with clothes on) to emphasize their use as investigatory aids and not toys.
6. Never make an assumption about what the child is demonstrating. Ask, "What was happening?"
7. Use professionally produced anatomical dolls that are skin-tone appropriate.

Assessing data from doll interviews should be informed by what is known about children's use of the dolls:

1. Explicit sexual positioning of dolls (e.g., penile penetration of orifices) is uncommon in nonreferred, presumably nonabused children. However, it may occur due to prior sexual exposure or in some demographic groups. Four- and 5-year old boys from lower socioeconomic status (SES) families are somewhat more likely to enact explicit sexual acts with dolls compared with younger children, girls, or children from higher SES families (Boat and Everson 1994). A child's explanation of what he or she is demonstrating may clarify the diagnosis of maltreatment versus overstimulation and overexposure.
2. The mouthing or sucking of a doll's penis is very rare before about age 4 and infrequent after age 4 in nonreferred, presumably nonabused children (Boat and Everson 1994).

3. If a child's positioning of the dolls indicated a detailed knowledge of sexual acts, the probability of sexual abuse or overstimulation is increased.

4. Manual exploration of a doll's genitals, including digital penetration of a doll's vagina or anal opening, is rather common behavior in young, presumably nonabused children (Boat and Everson 1994). Diagnostic concern is raised if such a demonstration is associated with negative emotional expression (fear, anxiety, anger), behavioral regression, obsessive repetition (Terr 1981), or verbal disclosure of maltreatment.

The dolls are not a "test" for abuse. Evaluators who use them should possess training or knowledge and experience to conduct forensic interviews of children suspected of having been sexually abused. The evaluator should know the child's history concerning exposure to, and use of, the dolls. The number of dolls presented depends on their specific use in the interview. A formal interview protocol is not required (American Professional Society on the Abuse of Children 1995). Detailed documentation of the interview process should be preserved.

Documentation

Documentation methods should be complete and detailed. Written notes done at the time of the interview or audiotapes can preserve both the questions and replies. Preservation of a verbatim record of all portions of the interview is preferred to demonstrate the methods of interviewing and the child's behavior and verbal statements. The videotape recording of the interview, if available, offers several advantages, including reduction of the number of interviews, preservation of evidence of abuse, and incentives to use proper interview techniques. A videotape may also encourage confession, and the videotape may be used by experts to review methods of investigation (Myers 1997). Opponents of videotaping have argued that videotaping may

be dissected by the defense to show inconsistencies or incompleteness of children's statements or interviewer error. In general, expert testimony concerning the natural history and developmental issues related to disclosure and the adequacy of an investigation are often sufficient to rehabilitate the evidence.

Credibility

The investigating clinician should document and discuss factors that argue for or against the validity of the allegation. The strongest validation criteria are based on documenting explicit sexual experiences with a progression of sexual acts over time described by the child. The interviewer should look for sexual experiences beyond the child's expected knowledge or experience, a description told from the child's viewpoint and vocabulary, and an emotional response consistent with the nature of the abuse. The assessment of a sexual abuse complaint should also include possible motivations for the issuance of a false sexual abuse complaint by either the child or the adult (Quinn 1988).

The two most common reasons to view an allegation of CSA as not credible are 1) a recantation by the child and 2) the existence of improbable elements in a child's disclosure. Recantations rates are variable, from 4% to 27% (London et al. 2008), and should be assessed for their own credibility. Interest in high-profile cases with bizarre and improbable elements has prompted a small literature on these little-studied aspects of CSA allegations. Everson (1997) wrote that the existence of improbable or fantastic elements in a child's account should not prompt an automatic dismissal of the child's account. He detailed possible sources of the implausible accounts: the event, the assessment process, and influences outside the assessment process. He described 24 specific mechanisms to explain implausible elements in a child's account of abuse. Severe abuse produces more implausible and fantastic allegations (Dalenberg 1996).

—*Key Points*

— Child sexual abuse is commonly perpetrated by individuals well known to the child.

— Reports of child sexual abuse have declined 50% in the past decade.

— Many victims of childhood sexual abuse delay or do not describe their victimization.

— Mental health professionals and many other child-serving professionals are mandated to report reasonable suspicion of child maltreatment, including child sexual abuse.

— Failure to make mandated reports of maltreatment may result in criminal and/or civil sanctions.

— No one behavioral indicator or pattern proves an allegation of sexual abuse.

— Objectivity and impartiality are the key aspects of investigatory interviewing of an allegation of sexual abuse.

— Anatomical dolls are not a "test" for abuse.

References

Adams JA: Evolution of a classification scale: medical evaluation of suspected child sexual abuse. Child Maltreat 6:31–36, 2001

Aldridge J, Cameron S: Interviewing child witnesses: questioning strategies and the effectiveness of training. Appl Dev Sci 3:136–147, 1999

American Academy of Child and Adolescent Psychiatry: Practice parameters for the forensic evaluation of children and adolescents who may have been physically or sexually abused. Am Acad Child Adolesc Psychiatry 36 (10 suppl):37S–56S, 1997

American Professional Society on the Abuse of Children: Guidelines for the Psychosocial Evaluation of Suspected Sexual Abuse in Young Children. Chicago, IL, American Professional Society on the Abuse of Children, 1995

Bays J, Chadwick D: Medical diagnoses of the sexually abused child. Child Abuse Negl 17:91–110, 1993

Boat BW, Everson MD: Exploration of anatomical dolls by nonreferred preschool-aged children: comparisons by age, gender, race, and socioeconomic status. Child Abuse Negl 18:139–153, 1994

Brown D: Developing strategies for collecting and presenting grooming evidence in a high tech world. American Prosecutors Research Institute Update 14(11), 2001

Ceci SJ, Bruck M: Jeopardy in the Courtroom: A Scientific Analysis of Children's Testimony. Washington, DC, American Psychological Association, 1995

Child Abuse Prevention and Treatment Act, Pub Law No 93-247, 1974

Child Welfare Information Gateway: Mandatory Reporters of Child Abuse and Neglect: Summary of State Laws. January 2008. Available at: http://www.childwelfare.gov/systemwide/laws_policies/statutes/manda.cfm. Accessed April 12, 2008.

Commonwealth of Massachusetts v Amirault LeFave, 430 Mass 169, 714, NE 2d, 805 (1999)

Coy v Iowa, 487 US 1012 (1988)

Crawford v Washington, 514 US 36 (2004)

Dale PS, Loftus EF, Rathbun L: The influence of the form of the question in the eye witness testimony of preschool children. J Psycholinguist Res 7:269–277, 1978

Dalenberg CJ: Fantastic elements in child disclosure of abuse. APSAC Advisor 9:1, 5–10, 1996

DeLoache JS: Early understanding and use of symbols: the model. Curr Dir Psychol Sci 4:109–113, 1995

Everson MD: Understanding bizarre, improbable and fantastic elements in children accounts of abuse. Child Maltreat 2:134–149, 1997

Everson MD, Boat BW: Putting the anatomical doll controversy in perspective. Child Abuse Negl 18:113–129, 1994

Finkelhor D: Sexually Victimized Children. New York, Free Press, 1979

Finkelhor D, Jones L: Why have child maltreatment and child victimization declined? J Soc Issues 62:685–716, 2006

Finkelhor D, Ormrod R, Turner H, et al: The victimization of children and youth: a comprehensive, national survey. Child Maltreat 10:5–25, 2005

Garven S, Wood JM, Malpass RS, et al: More than suggestion: the effect of interviewing techniques from the McMartin preschool case. J Appl Psychol 83:347–359, 1998

Health Insurance Portability and Accountability Act, 42 USC 1320d et seq (1996)

Heger A, Tieson L, Velasquez O, et al: Children referred for possible sexual abuse: medical findings in 2,384 children. Child Abuse Negl 26:645–659, 2002

Hershkowitz I, Horowitz D, Lamb ME: Trends in children's disclosure abuse in Israel: a national study. Child Abuse Negl 29:1203–1214, 2005

Holmes LS: Using anatomical dolls in child sexual abuse forensic interviews. American Prosecutors Research Institute Update 13(8), 2000

Kalichman SC: Mandated Reporting of Suspected Child Abuse: Ethics, Law and Policy. Washington, DC, American Psychological Association, 1993

Kempe CH: Sexual abuse, another hidden pediatric problem: the 1977 C. Anderson Aldrich lecture. Pediatrics 62:382–389, 1978

Kempe CH, Silverman F, Steele B, et al: The battered-child syndrome. JAMA 181:17–24, 1962

Kendall-Tackett K, Becker-Blease K: The importance of retrospective findings in child maltreatment research. Child Abuse Negl 28:723–727, 2004

Kendall-Tackett KA, William LM, Finkelhor D: The impact of sexual abuse on children: a review and synthesis of recent empirical studies. Psychol Bull 113:164–180, 1993

Kerns DL, Ritter ML: Medical findings in child sexual abuse cases with perpetrator confessions. Am J Dis Child 146:494, 1992

Kuehnle K: Child sexual abuse evaluations: the scientist-practitioner model. Behav Sci Law 16:5–20, 1998

Lamb ME, Sternberg KJ, Esplin PW: Conducting investigative interviews of alleged sexual abuse victims. Child Abuse Negl 22:813–823, 1998

London K, Bruck M, Wright DB, et al: Review of the contemporary literature on how children report sexual abuse to others: findings methodological issues and implications for forensic interviewers. Memory 16:29–47, 2008

Maryland v Craig, 497 US 836 (1990)

Medina v State, 131 P3d, 15 (2006)

Melton GB, Goodman BS, Kalichman SC, et al: Empirical research on child maltreatment and the law. J Clin Child Psychol 24 (suppl):47–77, 1995

Myers JEB: Evidence in Child Abuse and Neglect, 3rd Edition. New York, Wiley Law, 1997

Myers JEB: A History of Child Protection in America. Philadelphia, PA, Xlibris, 2004

Orbach Y, Hershkowitz I, Lamb ME, et al: Assessing the value of structural protocols for forensic interviewers of alleged child abuse victims. Child Abuse Negl 24:733–752, 2000

Philips A: "I have an 'owie'": health care providers' role after Crawford, Davis and Hammon. American Prosecutor's Research Institute Update 19(4–5), 2006

Pipe ME, Lamb ME, Orbach Y, et al: Factors associated with nondisclosure of suspected abuse during forensic interviews, in Child Sexual Abuse: Disclosure, Delay and Denial. Edited by Ripe ME, Lamb ME, Orbach Y, et al. Mahwah, NJ, Lawrence Erlbaum, 2007, pp 77–96

Public Welfare Amendments, Pub Law 87-543, Sec 528, Statutes at Large 76:172 (1962)

Quinn KM: The credibility of children's allegations of sexual abuse. Behav Sci Law 6:181–199, 1988

Salmon K, Bedrose S, Pipe ME: Providing props to facilitate children's event reports: a comparison of toys and real items. J Exp Child Psychol 60:174–194, 1995

Shaw JA, Lewis JE: Child on child sexual abuse: psychological perspectives. Child Abuse Negl 24:1591–1600, 2000

State v Michaels, 625, A2d, 489 (NJ S Ct App Div 1993), Aff'd, 642, A2d, 1372 (1994)

Summit R: The child sexual abuse accommodation syndrome. Child Abuse Negl 7:177–193, 1983

Terr L: Forbidden games: post-traumatic child's play. J Am Acad Child Adolesc Psychiatry 20:740–759, 1981

Thierry KL, Lamb ME, Orbach Y, et al: Developmental anatomical dolls during interviews with alleged sexual abuse victims. J Consult Clin Psychol 73:1125–1134, 2005

Trocmé N, Bala N: False allegations of abuse and neglect when parents separate. Child Abuse Negl 29:1333–1345, 2005

U.S. Department of Health and Human Services: Statistics and Research: Child Maltreatment. 2006. Available at: http://www.acf.hhs.gov/programs/cb/stats_research/index.htm. Accessed April 12, 2008.

White v Illinois, 502 US 346 (1992)

Chapter 18

Forensic Issues in Munchausen by Proxy

Herbert A. Schreier, M.D.
Catherine C. Ayoub, R.N., Ed.D.
Brenda Bursch, Ph.D.

Case Example

A 7-year-old boy, Ian, is brought in by his mother, Mrs. Ferris, to an emergency room at a major medical center with a history of vomiting and diarrhea of 7 days' duration. He does not appear dehydrated or ill, as would be expected by the reported frequency of episodes and lack of oral intake. Mrs. Ferris reports that her son has a long history of feeding difficulties and school absences because of illnesses and multiple workups at a number of medical centers. He is admitted to the hospital, where his condition deteriorates and he has severe episodes of vomiting. Intravenous fluids are started. On the eighth day, he has an unexplained cardiac arrest; 6 days after that, he has a second arrest. His mother first appears calm and attentive to her son. A nurse overhears her "gleefully" describing the medical events to a friend over a phone close to the nurse's station. Though Mrs. Ferris never leaves the hospital, staff later recalls that she seemed more interested in talking with the nurses and other parents than in engaging with her child.

In the second month of Ian's hospitalization, his gastrostomy drainage bag begins filling up with more fluid than he is being prescribed; at one point it reaches a high of 3,600 mL of fluid when he is supposed to be taking 1,200 mL.

Despite being familiar with Munchausen by proxy (MBP) and the peculiarities of this case, Ian's physician confers with colleagues in two other institutions trying to figure out what might be causing the child's symptoms. One gastroenterologist who had experience with more than 15 cases of MBP suggests yet another procedure requiring surgery. The second colleague suggests the presence of MBP. The pediatric team decides to file a child protection report, and the Department of Social Services removes the child to alternative care. The boy improves immediately after being separated from his mother; he appears to embrace his physical wellness. Although Ian states that he wants to return to his mother when asked directly, he does not ask for her and does not seem sad at being separated from her. The mother mounts a campaign of talking to other parents on the unit, trying to convince them that she was being persecuted by the hospital and physicians, whom she claims blamed her when they could not figure out what was wrong with her son.

Mrs. Ferris was involved actively with the juvenile dependency court and the Department of Social Services for a period of time. After a court hearing regarding her son, she was ordered into therapy with a psychologist affiliated with a university clinic. She admitted to having MBP but, oddly, not to harming her child. Her therapist, an experienced clinician with no working knowledge regarding the treatment of MBP perpetrators, reported that Mrs. Ferris was "improved" after 6 months of therapy. The therapist went on to say that he found her to be engaging and a good conversationalist. Therapy was based on a number of encounters between Mrs. Ferris and her therapist, with little contact with collaterals, especially those working with her son.

The judge, against the wishes of Child Protective Services and the district attorney and without asking for either an outside evaluation or a report from an expert familiar with the disorder, returned Ian to his mother. Ian is now wheelchair bound due to the harm caused him from a cardiac arrest. Medical records indicate that Ian only came to the emergency room on one subsequent occasion, whereby it was found that he had a too-high level of an anticonvulsant in his bloodstream.

Six years later, a genetic counselor was trying to assist with the diagnosis of a 7-month-old infant who weighed 7 pounds, the same as his birth weight (failure to thrive). Multiple procedures, including biopsies, were performed to no avail. The counselor wondered if, because the mother had a history of "pseudo seizures," she could be engaging in illness falsification. The child psychiatrist attending the case conference on this child immediately recognized that this was the half brother of the child he had seen 6 years earlier; he recognized the brother's name, Ian. The mother had remarried and now had two children with a different last name. When the infant was hospitalized and separated from the mother, he gained 2 pounds over the weekend. He continued to do well out of his mother's care.

Mrs. Ferris, as noted, was seen for pseudo seizures while pregnant. Her next child exhibited moderately severe failure to thrive but improved once his mother became pregnant with her third child. The third child, described above, was then nearly starved to death over a 7-month period.

Factitious disorder by proxy, popularly known as Munchausen by proxy (MBP), describes the behavior of a parent or caretaker who repeatedly falsifies symptoms or induces illness in another in order to satisfy a psychological need. First described as a form of child abuse by Roy Meadow (1977), there have been hundreds of reports in the scientific literature (Sheridan 2003) and attention paid to it in the popular media. Case studies and literature reviews indicate that this disorder involves persistent or compulsive harm-causing behavior (Rosenberg 1995; Sheridan 2003). The disorder is overwhelmingly found in women, who often present as dedicated and caring mothers, yet while "imposturing" good parenting, they repeatedly cause harm to their children (Schreier 1992). These women's forethought and efforts to conceal what they are doing reveal that their behavior is conscious and purposeful. Common psychological needs that drive the behavior are the need to be perceived as a devoted parent; the need to be in a close relationship with the individuals in authority, such as medical staff or other health care staff; and/or the need to be the center of attention. Long-term suffering, permanent injury, or death has been documented in over 13% of cases reported in the literature (Ayoub 2006; Sheridan 2003). Among those children who had died due to this form of abuse, 25% of their siblings had also died, with over half of them having had similar and/or suspicious symptoms (Sheridan 2003).

Clinical Issues

Definitions

Guidelines proposed by the American Professional Society on the Abuse of Children (APSAC) address some confusion with the DSM-IV diagnosis of factitious disorder by proxy (American Psychiatric Association 1994) and its text revision (American Psychiatric Association 2000). The APSAC definitional guidelines emphasize that there are two components to consider when evaluating this form of child abuse: 1) victimization of the child and 2) psychopathology of the abuser (Ayoub et al. 2002a). The term *pediatric condition falsification* describes the abusive behavior directed at the child, regardless of motivation or psychopathology of the abuser. Factitious disorder by proxy is the psychiatric diagnosis for the abuser when the motivation to falsify illness is to satisfy personal psychological needs. Pediatric condition falsification due to factitious disorder by proxy constitutes the disorder known as Munchausen by proxy.

Methods of condition falsification include exaggeration, fabrication, simulation, and induction. Exaggeration is embellishment of a legitimate symptom or problem. Fabrication refers to false statements made by the abuser about the child's medical history or symptoms. Simulation can take many forms, including the falsification of records, medical tests, or symptoms. Examples include moving a pH probe during a gastrointestinal evaluation, introducing bacteria into a urine sample, removing a page from a medical record, or inserting one's own blood into a diaper. Induction is directly causing a new problem or aggravating a preexisting problem. Examples include poisoning, suffocation, or manipulation of medications. Evaluations for illness falsification must take into account these four forms of falsification. Any illness can be feigned; any symptom can be falsified; any medical test can be misleading or misinterpreted. Older children are sometimes coached to participate in the deception.

Differential Diagnosis

There are forms of parental psychopathology that are not related to intentional falsification of illness but can be endangering in other ways. It is sometimes difficult to determine the motivation driving abusive parent behavior. Consequently, initial decisions regarding child safety must not depend on parent *intentions* but on parent behaviors, including evidence of victimization/abuse in the child. Excessive parental anxiety may cause parents to have distorted perceptions about the health of a child or danger of a symptom. Their motivation may be to obtain appropriate care for their child, but their distorted perceptions may endanger the child. They may focus on (or avoid) medical care, but they do not repeatedly exaggerate or falsify illness. For example, a parent who has experienced the fear that her baby may not survive may erroneously view the child as more vulnerable than other children and may be more concerned than needed. This is called *vulnerable child syndrome* and can lead to excessive use of health care services and interference with normal development. Parental mood disorders and parental psychotic disorders can also cause distorted perceptions about the health of a child or danger of a symptom. An example is a mother with a circumscribed delusional belief that her son's brain is abnormal and in need of surgical examination. Limited parental cognitive ability or specific unalterable belief systems may interfere with decision making regarding child health and medical needs. Such parents may have good intentions for their children but have difficulty understanding abstract concepts such as a functional gastrointestinal disorder or the importance of evidence-based treatment. Malingering is the psychiatric diagnosis for the abuser when the primary motivation is to obtain external rewards, such as money, shelter, food, drugs, or custody. These motivators are sometimes present as secondary factors in MBP.

Prevalence

Although it is often described as rare, little is known about prevalence of MBP. No epidemiological studies have been conducted in the United States. Extrapolation from a carefully designed study in the United Kingdom (McClure et al. 1996) suggests that at least 130 new cases of falsified acute life-threatening events (e.g., apnea) or nonaccidental poisoning would be expected to occur each year in the United States. Additionally, the literature suggests that as many as 1% of asthma clinic attendees (Godding and Kruth 1991) and 5% of allergy clinic patients (Warner and Hathaway 1984) are victims of falsification. Repeated false allegations of sexual abuse (Schreier 1996), psychiatric presentations (Schreier 1997), and MBP in school settings have also been described (Ayoub et al. 2002b).

Summary of Cases in the Literature

In a review of the literature, Sheridan (2003) found that 76.5% of the MBP perpetrators were birth mothers and 6.7% were fathers. Adoptive and foster parents and other caretakers have also been identified as perpetrators. Almost 30% of the perpetrators appeared to have falsified symptoms in themselves. The perpetrator actively induced symptoms in 57.2% of the cases, and at least half of those who induced symptoms did so while in the hospital. The most common symptom induction methods were suffocation and poisoning with prescribed medications or other agents. Victims averaged 3.25 medical problems (range = 0–19). In her prospective study of 30 legally confirmed MBP families, Ayoub (2006) found that abusing mothers were often very knowledgeable about their children's reported conditions, had a higher-than-expected rate of substance use, and had mixed character disorders. Frequently these mothers reported a childhood trauma such as a serious illness, abuse, serious conflict, separation, or death of a person close to them.

The following are *warning signs related to the illness cited in the literature:* the illness (or test result) does not make medical sense, is oddly difficult to treat, is rare, and/or does not follow a normal illness or recovery trajectory. *Family history warning signs* include the caregiver being involved in or showing great interest in the medical field, and the caregiver or the family having an extensive history of illness. *Behavioral warning signs of a suspected abuser* are also important to note and are outlined in Table 18–1. These behavioral warning signs can be present in nonabusing parents and, therefore, should not be used as the basis for diagnosis. However, as the number of warning signs increases, falsification must be considered in the differential diagnosis.

Medical Record Review

Thorough assessment requires a detailed medical record review and chronological summary (Sanders and Bursch 2002). This is often a time-consuming and tedious task that normally cannot be accomplished during an inpatient admission and that is not reimbursed by billing codes used by clinicians. Nevertheless, an expert should be hired in legal cases to conduct this part of the evaluation before a child is declared safe. Clinicians involved in one aspect of the child's health care and who are not privy to all of the records

TABLE 18–1. Behavioral warning signs suggestive of Munchausen by proxy
Symptoms occur only in the caregiver's presence or after the caregiver has been present.
The caregiver is oddly or excessively attentive to medical issues.
The caregiver's level of alarm differs from that of medical staff (the parent appears less or more worried about child's illness than medical staff).
The caregiver is medically knowledgeable or attempts to appear so.
The caregiver requests unnecessary or dangerous medical procedures.
The caregiver has a pattern of lying.

TABLE 18–2. Inconsistencies suggestive of possible Munchausen by proxy
Reported symptoms do not match objective findings (a caretaker reports severe diarrhea and vomiting for 5 days; however, the child appears well hydrated).
Reported medical history does not match previous medical records (false report of a premature birth or abnormal test result).
A pattern of frequent diagnoses does not match objective findings (a toddler with a diagnosis of severe reflux eats ravenously, with no symptoms, during hospitalizations).
Behavior of a parent does not match expressed distress or reports of symptoms.
Other false or troubling history is provided by a parent.
Medical record names and numbers do not match.

may not have the necessary perspective to make recommendations regarding risk and safety issues.

Medical records requested should include all outpatient appointments, hospitalizations, home visits, emergency response records, and emergency department visits. If there have been unusual illnesses in other family members, suspected abuse in a sibling, or a sibling death, it is useful for the forensic clinician to obtain their records as well. School records can also be helpful.

Diagnoses that are based solely on verbal reports from the suspected parent/caregiver should be identified, and the records should be assessed for warning signs, inconsistencies, exaggerations, signs of simulation, episodes of induction, and other patterns of illness falsification. Chronologically summarizing the medical contacts into a table can reveal patterns of health care utilization, illness and medical treatment trajectories, and behaviors of family members (Sanders and Bursch 2002). If the caregiver is actively inducing illness, the medical record summary can be used to evaluate the logic and likelihood of the medical presentation and to search for signs of induction. If illness falsification is not present, the chronological summary may aid in determining a correct diagnosis. Evaluators should review the summary for the following: 1) recurrent illness that appears unusual, for example, persistent and severe vomiting with no other signs or symptoms of illness; 2) symptom occurrence, for example, symptoms occurring on particular days or during particularly stressful times for the parent, or unexpected similar symptoms in multiple family members; 3) lack of continuity of care, for example, false representation of health care contacts or refusal to release records; and 4) inconsistencies (examples of common inconsisten-

cies to consider are highlighted in Table 18–2). Collateral records and/or interviews with others can be helpful to determine the truth of inconsistencies.

Assessment in the Medical Setting

The complaints and medical history described to the clinician form the cornerstone of medical diagnosis. Diagnoses are often made by the health care provider on the basis of verbal history from the mother alone. If incorrect information is purposely or inadvertently provided, the clinician may understandably misinterpret physical findings, test results, or treatment responses. Slightly abnormal test results or physical findings, considered a normal variation among healthy children, tend to be considered pathological within the context of an illness history. Because it is not common practice to request all past medical records of a patient, some patterns of falsification are missed for extended periods of time. Most clinicians do not regularly suspect that the information presented to them may be false or consider ways in which a symptom may be simulated or induced. As a result, one of the biggest obstacles to the identification of abusive symptom falsification, especially in cases of MBP, is considering it as a possibility.

A multidisciplinary team approach is helpful in developing and conducting a systematic, safe, thorough, and objective assessment without unduly alarming the family or team members. Clinical team composition might include attending physicians and residents, nurses, the hospital child protection team, social workers, psychiatrists/psychologists, the child life team, hospital security, and others interacting with the family. Safety issues to consider for inpatients include location of the child, level of monitoring, and emergency response plans. An objective evaluation requires that the clinician consider how one could simulate or induce a particular symptom and then assess for evidence of such behavior as part of a differential diagnosis. Because it is not the normal process for determining a diagnosis and because it can be highly stressful, it is helpful to discuss the assessment plan with an experienced consultant. Medical claims can be challenged under close supervision, and medications can be systematically removed if it is suspected that they are not needed. If feasible, a systemic medical record review (as described earlier) can be completed. If induction is suspected, lab specimens should be obtained at the time of hospital admission and during increases in symptoms for toxicology. A chain of evidence must be preserved to establish that specimens were not contaminated. This requires protection of the specimen as well as documentation of who handled the specimen at each transition from the point of origin to the person conducting the lab tests, and if relevant, to the time it is presented in court as evidence.

Psychiatric or psychological assessment of a parent alone is rarely useful for identification of illness falsification and typically is not feasible during the hospitalization of the child (since the parent is not the registered patient). There is no consistent psychological profile of someone who has engaged in this behavior, and psychiatric warning signs are not specific to this type of abuse (Parnell 1998). In fact, with a psychiatric interview, a subset of abusers appear "normal." Nevertheless, mental health input from a clinician with experience in the diagnosis of MBP can be helpful in assisting the team in understanding the behaviors of both the parent and the child and in assessing for emotional and behavioral disorders in the child.

Separation

Separation of the child from the suspected abuser is a powerful way to determine if falsification has occurred. However, it is important to note that persistent symptoms do not rule out past falsification. Continued symptoms indicate that some or all of the symptoms are legitimate, that the child has been permanently injured, or that the child is not being sufficiently protected. Older children are sometimes coached to collude. Finally, if medical treatment is altered at the time that separation occurs, it can be impossible to discern the cause for a change in health.

Child Protective Issues

Risk Assessment

MBP abusers engage in falsification compulsively; identification of the behavior is not an effective intervention to prevent it. Additionally, treatment for the abuser is frequently ineffective. McGuire and Feldman (1989) followed six victims of illness falsification and found that all six children were abused during and after the abuser had participated in psychotherapy. Additionally, five of the six children continued to be abused after referral to Child Protective Services. Parents have been known to attempt to abuse their children on supervised visits and during hospitalizations. Serial victimization, including serial suffocation, has been documented (Alexander et al. 1990). One might expect that parents genuinely interested in the health and safety of their child would agree to ongoing monitoring and support. However, in classic and extreme cases, it is most common to see the following behaviors by the abuser when confronted with evidence of illness falsification: entrenched denial; hostility; attempts to remove the child from the medical setting; threats of lawsuits; and a search for individuals, personal and professional, willing to support and strengthen the abuser's position of denial (Kinscherff and Famularo 1991).

Generally, predictors associated with poor outcome among parents seeking reunification after committing any form of child abuse include parental history of severe childhood abuse, persistent denial of abusive behavior, refusal to accept help, severe personality disorder, mental handicap, psychosis, and alcohol/drug abuse (Jones 1987). Severe abuse, including nonaccidental poisoning and illness falsification, is associated with poor prognosis and mortality (Jones 1987).

Among those who have been victims of MBP abuse, predictors associated with poor psychiatric outcome are outlined in Table 18–3.

A prospective study suggests that only the children removed very early in their victimization process and protected from subsequent maternal contact escaped major psychiatric symptoms (Ayoub 2006). Children seem to fare the best psychologically when they are removed from their biological homes at a young age, are placed in permanent safe alternative homes as soon as possible, and have little or no contact with the mother

TABLE 18–3. Predictors of poor psychiatric outcome for Munchausen by proxy victims

Victimization that lasted more than 2 years

Delayed permanent placement

Unsupervised contact with mothers

Contact with mothers who had received insufficient treatment

Contact with fathers who are unable to care for them due to dependency on mothers.

Source. Ayoub 2006.

(or individuals she significantly influenced). The exception to this rule appears to be when abusing mothers fully admit their perpetration early and are sincere and committed in their work to change their behavior. Ayoub (2006) found that such women benefited from an integrative treatment process lasting from 5 to 7 years that included all of the treatment providers for the child and family, Child Protective Services, and a court-designated expert in MBP. Sanders (1996) reported the possibility of success when the parent has admitted the abusive behaviors and demonstrated empathy for the victim.

As mentioned earlier in the chapter, it is not always possible to determine the primary motivation or comorbid psychopathology of an individual engaged in illness falsification. Denial is the typical defense, and perpetrators sometimes appear "normal" to the primary health care provider and inexperienced evaluator. To determine risk, one might compare the child's health status and medical care contacts prior to separation from the suspected abuser with the child's health status and medical care contacts after separation and stabilization/rehabilitation. The larger the discrepancy and the greater the improvement after separation, the greater is the risk for future abuse. This technique is not reliable if there has not been complete separation and stabilization/rehabilitation. Children who have been victims of symptom induction (such as poisoning or suffocation) appear to be at greatest risk for death, but there are iatrogenic deaths as well as significant physical and psychological morbidity due to procedures and treatments provided to children based on exaggeration and fabrication alone. Assessing risk may be challenging when the victim has a legitimate chronic illness that has been manipulated by the parent to create excessive symptoms and/or disability (e.g., an ex-preterm infant may

present with falsified apnea, a medical problem commonly seen in preterm infants).

Placement

Child placement is challenging when it is unclear if family reunification is possible. Successful family reunification can be achieved in a few cases only if the abuser and family members acknowledge the pattern of illness falsification, benefit from effective treatment, and accept and utilize a monitoring and support system. This generally requires a prolonged period of time and necessitates an interim placement plan. In high-risk cases and cases with poor prognostic indicators, a long-term placement plan should be considered. Ensuring the victim's continuing safety requires careful planning by professionals knowledgeable of this condition.

Friends or family members may be caregivers if they genuinely believe the child must be protected from the suspected abuser and if they have the ability to protect the child from the suspected abuser. Caregivers who accept care of the child must also accept responsibility to follow all court orders, which may include the need to prohibit parental access to the child or to closely monitor visits. Caregivers must have a realistic expectation regarding any pressure or hostility they may need to endure in order to abide by the court orders. In her study of mothers who engaged in MBP, Ayoub (2006) found that 55% of fathers acknowledged the allegations of MBP as opposed to only 10% of the mothers. However, a majority of fathers equivocated about the veracity of the abuse allegations for a considerable period of time. Some hesitated to get involved because their wives strongly opposed any increased contact between the fathers and their children. Some fathers (who were able to separate both physically and emotionally from mothers, restructure the family system to acknowledge MBP, and actively work to protect the children) have been able to safely parent following a lengthy intervention period. In Ayoub's study, one-third of the relative placements failed because of extended pressure on family members by the mother and her representatives. In cases of severe abuse that is met with denial by the confirmed abuser and other family members, adoption or placement in foster care without family access to the foster family is warranted.

Treatment of Abuser

A complete treatment team includes child protection professionals, caregivers, physicians, and therapists.

This team must be familiar with the details of the case and have open and regular communication. The suspected abuser should not serve as the primary source of observations and information regarding the medical history and health of the child. Likewise, the suspected abuser should not be present during medical procedures or tests. While increasing levels of involvement may be indicated with successful treatment of the abuser, the goal is to have knowledgeable physicians and other family members always involved in the care of the child. Treating therapists, who are also vulnerable to being misled by someone who has factitious disorder, must demonstrate full knowledge of the condition of MBP and its challenges in therapeutic situations or be willing to accept supervision from a consultant with such experience. The best outcomes have been reported among those parents who fully admit their abusive behavior, engage in meaningful integrated therapy (Ayoub 2006), are committed to changing their behavior, and demonstrate altered behavior and empathy for the victims over time.

Treatment of MBP Victims

Efforts should be made to normalize and optimize the child's functioning as much as possible. Psychotherapy is indicated unless the victim is an infant or preverbal toddler. Victims of illness falsification may deny it; have intense anger at the medical team, abuser, or other collusive family members; have residual sickrole beliefs and behavior; suffer from posttraumatic stress disorder (especially in medical settings), self-esteem problems, or difficulty defining family relationships; and experience immense grief (Ayoub 2006; Bools et al. 1993; Bursch 1999). The psychological impact of MBP victimization appears to be significant and chronic. A longitudinal study by Ayoub (2006) revealed ongoing problems with social interaction, attention, and concentration; oppositional disorders; patterns of reality distortion; poor self-esteem; and attachment difficulties with adults and peers. Although these children can present as socially skilled and superficially well adjusted, they often struggle with basic relationships. Lying is a common finding, as is some sadistic behavior toward other children. Children in stable long-term placements in which they were protected from their mothers and supported in their move toward health have fewer long-term difficulties compared with children who have more exposure to their mothers and less stable placements. Even after an ex-

tended recovery, many children remain trauma reactive and are vulnerable to cyclical anger, depression, and oppositionality. Despite maternal legal rights being restricted or terminated due to MBP, Ayoub (2006) found in her study that the mothers contacted all of their children who had reached adulthood (*n* = 8) on or around their eighteenth birthdays. Despite up to 10 years of no contact, mothers who presented themselves to their children typically expressed that they loved their children and that they were not guilty of the MBP victimization. This demonstrates that professionals who treat these children may need to include a plan for the experience of reconnection and possible continued victimization after legal contact restrictions end when the children become adults.

Legal Issues

Reluctance to Consider the Diagnosis

Although MBP was described over 30 years ago, there is little uniformity in how it is treated in different jurisdictions in the United States and even within a particular jurisdiction in a state. It remains extremely difficult for professionals of all disciplines to consider that someone is capable of this form of abuse, especially if he or she does not appear to be overtly psychiatrically impaired. Furthermore, trials related to suspected MBP cases tend to be very expensive, involving multiple experts. Experts who are knowledgeable about the disorder are difficult to find.

Standards of Proof and Admissibility of Evidence

While dependency cases are often cumbersome and complex, the higher standard of proof (beyond a reasonable doubt) and inclusion of a jury in criminal trials increase the challenge in attempts to criminally prosecute. Ideally these cases belong first and foremost in dependency courts. This is the section of the judiciary that specifically addresses child abuse issues. When allegations of MBP are raised in the context of a divorce or primary custody case in family court, it is much more difficult to obtain a focus on parental fitness, as fitness is often assumed in these proceedings.

MBP in the Courtroom

Judges in criminal proceedings have varied enormously in their decisions on whether to allow testimony that a mother has been diagnosed with factitious disorder by proxy. Jurisdictions often seek to balance relevance against the prejudicial nature that testimony about factitious disorder and MBP may incur. Prior to 1993, the standard for admissibility of expert witness testimony in federal courts originated from the D.C. Circuit Court of Appeals case of *Frye v. United States* (1923). In this case, the court held that expert witness testimony must originate from well-recognized principles that are sufficiently established to have gained general acceptance in the scientific community. This standard is often referred to as the *Frye standard.* The *Frye* standard has also been applied to determine the admissibility of testimony about MBP across a number of states as early as 1981 (*People v. Phillips* 1981). In this 1981 California murder trial, the court admitted evidence related to MBP. Furthermore, the trial court was upheld on appeal when it permitted psychiatric testimony about MBP, despite the fact that the psychiatric witness had not directly evaluated the mother or treated a case of MBP. The trial court allowed the psychiatric expert testimony because it went to the defendant mother's motive in her MBP behavior, which was otherwise beyond common experience or understanding. Parenthetically, *Phillips* upheld the ability of a psychiatrist to diagnose the mother with MBP based on his reading of the literature and the records and without interviewing the mother.

Since 1981, MBP has been treated in a variety of ways by criminal courts, including not being admissible unless the mother raised the issue of her good character. The *Daubert* standard has replaced the *Frye* standard in federal proceedings and is applied in a number of state courts as well. According to the U.S. Supreme Court ruling in *Daubert v. Merrell Dow Pharmaceuticals, Inc.* (1993), the trial judge determines if testimony is relevant and reliable, and this determination is based on many factors in addition to whether or not the basis for the expert's testimony has gained general acceptance in the scientific community. Each state can adopt its own standards, but federal courts are required to follow the *Daubert* standard.

Traditionally, an expert opinion on whether a witness is lying is inadmissible because it exceeds the ability and specialized knowledge of an expert, and juries can decide the veracity of a witness for themselves. However, in *United States v. Shay* (1995), the First Circuit Court reversed a lower court's decision to exclude expert testimony on Munchausen disorder (not by proxy) because lying is characteristic of the condition. As in most cases of MBP that come to trial, there is usually only circumstantial evidence, and the mother's appearance can be persuasive of her innocence despite the weight of numerous abuses, especially those "accomplished" by doctors. The jury should be able to hear that this very picture is not at all uncommon and has been repeatedly documented through confessions. Without this understanding, even the most horrendous reported abuse of a child may lead a jury to doubt the mother's agency when she appears loving and caring (Schreier 2002).

These issues are also important to consider in dependency and family court, where the scientific foundation of MBP has been contested as well. MBP has been upheld as a sound, scientifically based disorder (using the APSAC definitions) in many states, and there is case law backing the validity of the disorder (*Adoption of Keefe* 2000). For example, dependency and family courts have cited MBP alone or as part of a broader pattern of factors to find grounds for state child protection or transfer of custody from one parent to another. Courts are more likely to act where there is direct evidence or very strong circumstantial evidence. However, at least one New York court invoked a statute embodying the doctrine of *res ipsa loquitur* ("the thing speaks for itself") in finding circumstantial evidence of MBP when a child clinically improved upon physical separation from the mother (*In re Jessica Z.* 1987). Despite this particular court's ruling, many courts are averse to considering "profile evidence." As the APSAC guidelines suggest, clinicians and evaluators should be careful not to base their opinions on checklists of maternal characteristics (e.g., being a health care professional) or limited references to simplistic DSM criteria.

Preparation for Court

Once the most difficult problem in MBP—that of suspecting it to begin with—is overcome, the issue of gathering data sufficient to first protect the child and then adjudicate the case poses major (and in some ways unique) issues for medical and legal personnel. These cases most often involve indirect evidence, and the medical and social services people involved as well as the prosecutors must be ready to present a believable *res ipsa loquitur* argument (i.e., given the weight of the evidence, the only possible conclusion is that the mother is causing the symptoms). Peculiar illnesses or unexpected deaths in siblings or others in a mother's care, lack of symptoms in the index child when the mother is absent, and the appearance of symptoms only in the mother's presence require careful documentation. Legal personnel will often be called on to ask the courts for enforced separation from the sickly child, in order to note changes in his or her condition away from the suspected perpetrator, as few mothers will volunteer to this "separation test." The test must be for a sufficient length of time to be valid. All tests must be done with the utmost of care in fairness to the mother and the child. The possibility of false positives, such as food causing a reading in a stool sample that might be mistaken for a laxative, or the child having a rare disease, must be carefully considered.

As professional opinions and hearsay are often admissible evidence in dependency and family courts, these must be gathered with great care, either through direct contact with physicians or hospitals or through a careful review of their records. It is often helpful to speak with clinicians and other caretakers, because MBP mothers frequently misquote what has been told to them. For example, they may utilize a letter written by a doctor that may be somewhat exaggerated by the physician because it was requested to prod a social agency. Furthermore, clinicians may have been misinformed by a false family history given by the mother or may have recorded symptoms in the child that were reported as if they were actually witnessed. Although tedious, a careful review of prior charts can ultimately be the most important aspect in a case.

The U.S. Supreme Court, in a pre-MBP case in 1972, upheld evidence of prior criminal behavior, which is evidence usually excluded from criminal prosecution. The Court said that in "the crime of infanticide...evidence of repeated incidence is especially relevant because it may be the only evidence to prove the crime" (DiMaio and Bernstein 1974, p. 748). The introduction of other incidents of abuse appears to be rarely contested in the cases we have participated in or reviewed.

Covert Video Surveillance

Some institutions use covert videotape to evaluate illness falsification (Hall et al. 2000). Legal concerns include the violation of the Fourth Amendment right to privacy and the related potential for lack of court admissibility. Clinical concerns include safety and financial issues related to who will monitor the video, how it will be monitored (real time, continuously, intermittently, delayed), and how to determine when emergency intervention is indicated. For example, how long does one allow suspected abuse to continue in order to ensure the behavior is correctly interpreted? Is a parent

clearing an airway or inducing emesis? Video surveillance has been found to be effective at identifying episodes of illness induction and has been successfully used in prosecuting a murder in a California case. In one study, covert video surveillance (CVS) was successful in documenting abuse in 33 of 39 cases (Southall et al. 1997). It should be noted that of 41 siblings of these cases, 12 had unexpectedly died, with 11 of the deaths attributed to sudden infant death syndrome (SIDS). After CVS, four parents admitted deliberately suffocating 8 of their children (Southall et al. 1997). It should also be noted that in one series, CVS was useful in making a bona fide medical diagnosis in cases that aroused suspicion of MBP (Hall et al. 2000).

Despite the effectiveness of CVS when induction is present, it is unpredictable how helpful the evidence will be in court. In the United States, CVS in a child's hospital room may be permissible in specific situations, such as for protection of the child, for assistance in diagnoses and treatment, or for the protection of the facility from allegations of negligence. To increase legal protection, some have recommended having a clause in admission consent forms and warning signs posted in the hospital regarding the possibility of covert videotaping, using specific consent forms and/or overt video monitoring, and/or obtaining a warrant prior to covert surveillance. Videotaping without audio may be equally effective and less intrusive. If video surveillance is used, guidelines regarding monitoring and emergency intervention should be developed prior to its initiation. Finally, video surveillance should not be the only technique used to assess for falsification. Behavior captured on videotape is sometimes difficult to interpret. The larger medical context and falsification assessment data can be used to better understand the visual images, decrease the chances of inaccurate conclusions, and may be all that is allowed into evidence in a legal setting. While some hospitals have set up protocols and a committee to monitor investigations when suspected MBP is reported to them, few hospitals have been willing to tackle the thorny issue raised by CVS. In the United States there are no standards for monitoring the videos.

Liability Issues

There are, of course, mandated reporting demands on professionals to protect children, as well as the related possibility of a lawsuit by the nonabusing parent of a child victim against a hospital and staff for not vigorously protecting a child. The danger of false diagnosis has received deserved attention, and the number of such cases may increase. MBP accusations have now appeared in divorce proceedings involving custody. Given the contentious bent of people with this disorder, clinicians have come under fire as well. Physicians have been sued for malpractice for misdiagnosing MBP (both in the positive and in the negative), as well as for violating a mother's constitutionally protected right to have access to her family. In a 1999 federal court case, reporting doctors and an expert hired by the prosecution were sued for violating the mother's civil rights to due process through their court testimony. However, Judge Wexler of the U.S. District Court for the Eastern District of New York stated, "[I]t is without question that these doctors are entitled to absolute witness immunity with respect to their testimony in court regarding Ellen Storck's MBP. That such testimony is alleged to have been without basis and contradictory to acceptable medical practice is irrelevant" (*Storck v. Suffolk County et al.* 1999, p. 22).

Case Example Epilogue

At both the dependency and criminal trials, Mrs. Ferris's husband testified that he believed his wife. There was a community outpouring of support for the family, particularly from their church. The mother's original therapist testified that she did not have MBP and did not harm her children. In the dependency court case, Mrs. Ferris's lawyer argued unsuccessfully for the return of the children to her. At her criminal trial, in which the issue of MBP was permitted to be raised in a hypothetical question as to what might motivate a woman to engage in this kind of abuse, factitious disorder was not accepted as a diagnosis for Mrs. Ferris. She was sentenced to 90 days in a state psychiatric forensic unit for evaluation and then ordered into therapy with a local MBP expert. Mrs. Ferris then became pregnant by another man. The baby was immediately placed into custody pending the outcome of an evaluation of her relationship during visitations over a 6-month period. She will continue to be on probation and see her therapist, who believes that she is making progress.

This case presentation highlights many features of MBP cases: the intense and compulsive nature of the mother's actions, even in the hospital; cognitive slippage in the mother's thinking as she increases the child's fabricated stomach drainage to impossible amount; the likelihood of professionals, such as inexperienced therapists and court personnel, to be fooled by MBP perpetrators; the sometimes supportive role of spouses, despite grave risk to their own children by the stance they take; and the ability of these women to gather community support. Table 18–4 highlights the pitfalls in work related to MBP.

TABLE 18–4. Pitfalls in work related to Munchausen by proxy (MBP)

Failure to suspect/consider MBP and lack of familiarity with the disorder.

Unawareness of the ability of MBP perpetrators to convincingly con professionals

Failure to recognize that this form of abuse can co-occur with true medical problems and that induction is not the only form of dangerous illness falsification

Minimization of parental psychopathology and unwarranted optimism about prognosis

Failure to systematically review all obtainable medical records

Failure to simultaneously consider that the parent may have been accurately or inaccurately suspected of child abuse

Placement of the child with a family member who does not believe the suspected abuser is capable of harming the child and/or who is not capable of protecting the child

Allowing the suspected abuser unsupervised visits or other unsupervised contact (e.g., telephone calls, e-mails)

If the visits are supervised, failure to caution visit supervisors about what to expect and failure to require supervisors to keep careful written observations

Failure to prepare for the possibility of going to court either as witness or defendant

—*Key Points*

— Include illness falsification on the differential diagnosis if the illness (or test result) does not make medical sense, is oddly difficult to treat, is extremely rare, or does not follow a normal illness or recovery trajectory.

— Use a multidisciplinary team to conduct a systematic, safe, thorough, and objective assessment. Ensure there is a team member with knowledge and experience with illness falsification.

— Attempt to obtain and systematically review all past medical records. Sometimes it is helpful to request insurance claims histories to ensure as many records as possible are obtained.

— Initially refrain from altering factors that one would expect might impact symptoms, such as feeding techniques, medications, or diet.

— Closely observe and clearly document observations, including precisely what was observed (e.g., the child vomiting, the emesis on the bed after the mother called the nurse, or the mother's report of emesis that was unwitnessed by the nurse).

— Rely on direct observations and on closely monitored medical tests rather than parent report of symptoms. Consider how one could simulate or induce a symptom and then assess for evidence of such behavior. Systematically challenge medical claims under close supervision. Systematically remove medications if it is suspected that they are not needed. If induction is suspected, lab specimens should be obtained at the time of hospital admission and during increases in symptoms. Consider separation of the child from the suspected abuser.

— When severe abuse is met with denial by the confirmed abuser and other family members, consider placement in foster care without family access to the foster family.

— Adhere to strict guidelines for visitation with parents who have falsified illness.

— Consider the option of termination of parental rights and protection of the child for an extended period of time.

References

Adoption of Keefe, 99-P-1923 (Mass 2000)

Alexander R, Smith W, Stevenson R: Serial Munchausen syndrome by proxy. Pediatrics 86:581–585, 1990

American Psychiatric Association: Diagnostic and Statistical Manual of Mental Disorders, 4th Edition. Washington, DC, American Psychiatric Association, 1994

American Psychiatric Association: Diagnostic and Statistical Manual of Mental Disorders, 4th Edition, Text Revision. Washington, DC, American Psychiatric Association, 2000

Ayoub C: Munchausen by proxy, in Mental Disorders for the New Millennium, Vol 3: Biology and Function. Edited by Plante TG. Westport, CT, Praeger Press, 2006, pp 149–159

Ayoub C, Alexander R, Beck D, et al: Definitional issues in Munchausen by proxy. Child Maltreat 7:105–111, 2002a

Ayoub C, Schreier H, Keller C: Munchausen by proxy: presentation in special education. Child Maltreat 7:149–159, 2002b

Bools C, Neale B, Meadow R: Follow-up of victims of fabricated illness: Munchausen syndrome by proxy. Arch Dis Child 69:625–630, 1993

Bursch B: Presentations, treatment findings, what to do when a new child is born. Paper presented at the annual meeting of the American Academy of Child and Adolescent Psychiatry, Chicago, November 1999

Daubert v Merrell Dow Pharmaceuticals Inc, 509 US 579 (1993)

DiMaio VJM, Bernstein CG: A case of infanticide. J Forensic Sci 19:745–754, 1974

Frye v United States, 293 F 1013 (DC Cir 1923)

Godding V, Kruth M: Compliance with treatment in asthma and Munchausen syndrome by proxy. Arch Dis Child 66:956–960, 1991

Hall DE, Eubanks L, Meyyazhagan S, et al: Evaluation of covert video surveillance in the diagnosis of Munchausen syndrome by proxy: lessons from 41 cases. Pediatrics 105:1305–1312, 2000

In re Jessica Z, 135 Misc 2d 520, 521, 515 NY S2d 370, 371 (Fam Ct 1987)

Jones DPH: The untreatable family. Child Abuse Negl 11:409–420, 1987

Kinscherff R, Famularo R: Extreme Munchausen syndrome by proxy: the case for termination of parental rights. Juvenile Fam Court J 40:41–53, 1991

McClure RJ, Davis PM, Meadow SR, et al: Epidemiology of Munchausen syndrome by proxy, non-accidental poisoning, and non-accidental suffocation. Arch Dis Child 75:57–61, 1996

McGuire TL, Feldman KW: Psychological morbidity of children subjected to Munchausen syndrome by proxy. Pediatrics 83:289–292, 1989

Meadow R: Munchausen syndrome by proxy: the hinterland of child abuse. Lancet 2:343–345, 1977

Parnell TF: The use of psychological evaluation, in Munchausen by Proxy Syndrome: Misunderstood Child Abuse. Edited by Parnell TF, Day DO. Thousand Oaks, CA, Sage, 1998, pp 129–150

People v Phillips, 122 Cal App 3d 69, 86–87, 175 Cal Rptr 703 (Ct App 1981)

Rosenberg D: From lying to homicide: the spectrum of Munchausen by proxy, in Munchausen Syndrome by Proxy: Issues in Diagnosis and Treatment. Edited by Levin AV, Sheridan MS. New York, Lexington Books, 1995, pp 13–37

Sanders MJ: Narrative family therapy with Munchausen by proxy: a successful treatment case. Fam Syst Health 14:315–329, 1996

Sanders MJ, Bursch B: Forensic assessment of illness falsification, Munchausen by proxy, and factitious disorder, NOS. Child Maltreat 7:112–124, 2002

Schreier HA: The perversion of mothering: Munchausen syndrome by proxy. Bull Menninger Clin 56:421–437, 1992

Schreier HA: Repeated false allegations of sexual abuse presenting to sheriffs: when is it Munchausen by proxy? Child Abuse Negl 26:985–991, 1996

Schreier HA: Factitious presentation of psychiatric disorder by proxy. Child Psychol Psychiatry Rev 2:108–114, 1997

Schreier HA: On the importance of motivation in Munchausen by proxy: the case of Kathy Bush. Child Abuse Negl 26:537–549, 2002

Sheridan MS: The deceit continues: an updated literature review of Munchausen syndrome by proxy. Child Abuse Negl 27:431–451, 2003

Southall DP, Plunkett MC, Banks MW, et al: Covert video recording of life-threatening child abuse: lessons for child protection. Pediatrics 100:735–760, 1997

Storck v Suffolk County et al, 97 Civ 2880, 1999

United States v Shay, 57 F3d 126 (1st Cir 1995)

Warner JO, Hathaway MJ: Allergic form of Meadow's syndrome (Munchausen by proxy). Arch Dis Child 59:151–156, 1984

Supplemental Reading

Artingstall K: Tactical Aspects of Munchausen Syndrome by Proxy and Munchausen Syndrome Investigation. Boca Raton, FL, CRC Press, 1998

Firstman R, Talen J: The Death of Innocents: A True Story of Murder, Medicine, and High-Stakes Science. New York, Bantam Books, 1997

Parnell TF, Day DO (eds): Munchausen by Proxy Syndrome: Misunderstood Child Abuse. Thousand Oaks, CA, Sage, 1998

Plum HJ: Legal considerations, in Munchausen Syndrome by Proxy: Issues in Diagnosis and Treatment. Edited by Levin AV, Sheridan MS. New York, Lexington Books, 1995, pp 341–354

Schreier HA, Libow JA: Hurting for Love: Munchausen by Proxy Syndrome. New York, Guilford, 1993

Yorker B: Legal issues in factitious disorder by proxy, in The Spectrum of Factitious Disorders. Edited by Feldman M, Eisendrath S. Washington, DC, American Psychiatric Press, 1996, pp 135–156

Chapter 19

Forensic Issues and the Internet

Charles L. Scott, M.D.
Humberto Temporini, M.D.

The virtual world of the Internet presents a dangerous world in reality. When conducting evaluations of referred youth, forensic evaluators must be familiar with the potential impact of cyberspace on the lives of children and teenagers. Situations in which a detailed understanding of Internet activity may be important for legal purposes range from an assessment of posted online threats to the emotional and legal consequences of various Internet interactions a youth may encounter while online. This chapter addresses four areas to consider when conducting forensic evaluations that involve a youth's Internet activity: 1) taking an Internet use history; 2) the Internet and violence; 3) the Internet and sexual behaviors; and 4) the Internet and suicide.

Taking an Internet Use History

According to the University of California at Los Angeles (UCLA) Center for Communication Policy, 98% of teenagers ages 12–15 years and 97% of teenagers ages 16–18 years describe using the Internet at least once a week (UCLA Internet Report 2004). The predominant Internet activity of teenagers involves e-mailing and instant messaging (Beebe et al. 2004). Youth also communicate with others through text messaging, posting and responding to messages on websites, blogging, playing online games, and participating in social networking websites. Commonly used social networking websites include MySpace, Facebook, Friendster, Bebo, and Xanga, though the popularity of these interactive sites fluctuates with rapidly changing fads and trends. Although each of these social websites has its own unique characteristics, they also have important similarities, including the ability to share pictures and videos, to post messages that can be viewed by others, and to provide member interaction through instant messaging or e-mail services. Fifty-five percent of those online have created profiles on social networking sites, and approximately 80% have included photos of themselves. While most teenagers indicate that they use these sites to stay in contact with people they already know, approximately half also report using social networking sites to make new friends. In addition, nearly 30% of those teens with profiles on social networking sites have friends in their network whom they have never met in person (Lenhart et al. 2007). Table 19–1 includes general screening questions an evaluator should consider when investigating a youth's Internet use.

Evaluators must understand an evolving cyberspace language when examining online conversations. Acronyms serve the function of abbreviating words for rapid communication as well as disguising the actual content from naïve third parties (such as parents). For

TABLE 19–1. Internet use screening questions

What are the various locations where you access the Internet?

Can you access the Internet via a cell phone?

What activities do you engage in while online? (e.g., chatting, instant messaging, blogging, posting messages, etc.)

How much time do you spend each day on the Internet?

Do you belong to an online social networking site?

Do you use the Internet primarily to communicate with known friends?

How often do you communicate with strangers on the Internet?

Do you use the Internet as your primary source of socialization?

Do you participate in online gaming?

Are there any parental controls on your primary source of Internet access?

TABLE 19–2. Emoticon examples	
Anger	>:(
Crying	:,(
Death	8-#
Drunk	:*)
Experiencing a hangover	%-/
Furious	>-<
Got beat up	%+{
Sadness	:-(
Shocked	:-0
Smoking	:-Q~
Tremendously sad	:-C
Wiped out, partied all night	#-)

```
ohionetfin:    ?
spacedude102:   :-C, want 8-#
```

Knowledge of acronyms and emoticons allows the forensic investigator to translate that "spacedude102" was reporting he was drunk and smoking marijuana, had partied all night, and was feeling extremely sad and wanted death (i.e., suicide).

The Internet and Violence

Case Example 1

Joe is a 16-year-old male who was reported to the juvenile authorities because he was identified as the perpetrator on an Internet video that shows him physically assaulting a 14-year-old boy with a bat. An associated message posting reads, "LMAO [Note: laughing my ass off] re this wimp ass!" In addition to a standard violence risk assessment, you are asked to consider Internet issues that may be relevant to your forensic evaluation.

The Internet allows an unknown source to send an unwelcome communication to an unwilling victim with unknown consequences. Precise definitions of online aggressive behaviors have yet to emerge. Terms used to describe these behaviors include online bullying, cyberbullying, Internet harassment, and online harassment. Patchin and Hinduja (2006) defined *online bullying* as "bothering someone online, teasing in a mean way, calling someone hurtful names, intentionally leaving persons out of things, threatening

example, adolescents who wish to hide their Internet sexual communications with an adult stranger from their parent who walks into the room may suddenly type "POS," signaling that there is a "parent over shoulder," followed by the letters "LMIRL" (let's meet in real life), indicating a decision to meet the adult stranger. Likewise, teenagers may decrease their risk of being detected when chatting with a friend about their daily cannabis use by typing "420," the cyberspace code for marijuana. An emoticon is a sequence of keyboard symbols, letters, and numbers used to convey an emotion in a written format. A sample of emoticons that may appear in text is provided in Table 19–2.

Situations in which a forensic evaluator may be asked to interpret cyberspace communications by a child or adolescent include potential threat assessments, evaluation of potential suicidality, or following an unexpected death when a retrospective analysis of the youth's writings is requested to help understand the deceased's state of mind. Consider the following text messaging exchange between two teenagers ("spacedude102" and "ohionetfin") that occurred 1 hour before the 14-year-old boy with the moniker "spacedude102" committed suicide:

```
ohionetfin:    whatup?
spacedude102:   *) and :-Q~ 420
ohionetfin:    :-0
spacedude102:   #-)
```

someone and saying unwanted, sexually related things to someone." Using this definition, these authors found that 29% of an online convenience sample of youth reported being bullied online. When the concept of cyberbullying is expanded to include the "use of the Internet, cell phones, or other technology to send or post text images intended to hurt or embarrass another person," over 40% of youth report being cyberbullied in the past year (Moessner 2007).

Internet bullying appears to increase dramatically after the fifth grade (K. R. Williams and Guerra 2007). Smith et al. (2006) described seven subcategories of cyberbullying: text message bullying, picture/video clip bullying (through mobile phones), phone call bullying via mobile phones, e-mail bullying, chat room bullying, bullying through instant messaging, and bullying via websites. The use of the Internet to post videos of assaults on unsuspecting victims captured by cameras or phones is an emerging and serious concern. This phenomenon, which originated in the United Kingdom in 2005, is known as "happy slapping" and includes videos of serious assaults, some of which have resulted in death (King et al. 2007).

The term *online harassment* as used by Finkelhor et al. (2000) in their telephone surveys of youth Internet users has many similarities to cyberbullying as defined above. These authors define *online harassment* as "threats or other offensive behavior (not sexual solicitation) sent online to the youth or posted online about the youth for others to see" (Filkelhor et al. 2000, p. x). In contrast to the findings of other researchers, Wolak et al. (2006) found that only 9% of a national sample of 1,500 youth ages 10–17 years surveyed described being victims of online harassment. The majority (65%) were harassed in one-on-one exchanges with the harassers, and 35% had been harassed through the posting of messages about the victim that others could see. According to this same survey, nearly 90% of youth harassed were between the ages of 13 and 17 years, the majority of victims were female (58%), and the majority of harassers (55%) were unknown to the victims and outside of the victims' Internet interactions. It is interesting to note that victims of online harassment were also more likely to harass others online (Wolak et al. 2006; Ybarra et al. 2006).

Is the concept of cyberbullying the same as bullying conducted offline such as in a school setting? *School bullying* has been defined as including three components: 1) physically or verbally aggressive acts made with the intent to harm someone, 2) repetition, and 3) a power differential between the perpetrator and his or her target (Smith et al. 2002). Although online communications can certainly include verbal aggression and postings of physically aggressive acts, hands-on physical aggression is precluded (Wolak et al. 2007). Unlike bullying that occurs on school grounds or in person, bullying through the Internet allows the bullies to be physically removed from their victims, thereby freeing them from experiencing any emotional impact of their behavior on the victims (Ybarra and Mitchell 2004). In addition, cyberbullying can occur 24 hours a day, 7 days a week, with no relief for the children even when they are in the safety of their own home, unlike the more traditional offline bullying that occurs in a school environment (Raskauskas and Stoltz 2007).

Cyberstalking involves the use of the Internet or some other type of electronic device (such as a cell phone or global tracking device) to stalk another person (Glancy et al. 2007). Electronic harassment, such as cyberbullying, may qualify as cyberstalking if there is repeated harassment that communicates a threat likely to result in a reasonable person being afraid. Issues specific to cyberstalking are discussed in more detail in Chapter 24, "Juvenile Stalkers."

Forensic evaluators may be requested to evaluate both victims and perpetrators of online harassment or bullying. When interviewing potential victims, the evaluator should be aware that many youth have not told others about their online victimization, and therefore they must be specifically asked about this experience (Smith et al. 2006). Specific questions that should be considered when evaluating possible online victimization include the following:

- Have you told anyone before that you have been harassed online?
- Have you been harassed by people you know, have met online, or both?
- What forms of online harassment have you experienced?
- Have you ever been victimized offline?
- Have you also used the Internet to harass others?

The majority of youth report that they are harassed by people they have met online rather than by people they know in their offline life (Wolak et al. 2007). One-third of youth harassed online describe feeling very or extremely upset by this experience and report at least one symptom of stress (Wolak et al. 2006). Posting of personal pictures or videos has been reported as having the highest negative emotional impact of all types of online bullying (Slonje and Smith 2008).

In situations involving an alleged perpetrator of Internet harassment or bullying, the evaluator must likewise conduct a detailed inquiry of both the person's online and offline behavior. Because youth may be reluctant to fully disclose their activities through self-report, the evaluator should also attempt to obtain collateral records (such as any police reports, victim statements, computer hard-drive printouts, and prior juvenile records) and conduct collateral interviews of individuals who know the youth. Social history is important because perpetrators of aggressive online behaviors are twice as likely to report a history of experiencing sexual abuse, physical abuse, or high parent conflict in the past year (Wells and Mitchell 2008), and in at least one study harassers were more likely to be age 15 years or older (Ybarra and Mitchell 2004). In addition to standard approaches to violence risk assessments, additional questions specific to evaluating an online aggressor are outlined in Table 19–3.

Unfortunately, perpetrators of Internet aggression are not limited to individuals acting alone. In particular, street gangs such as the Crips, Bloods, MS-13, and 18th Street have extended their "gangbanging" street activities to "webbanging" activities, including bragging about their violent exploits, publicly taunting rival gangs, and recruiting other Internet users to join their gang. In a survey of gang members' online habits, 25% of gang members reported that they used the Internet 4 hours per week, and nearly half were able to access the Internet at a local community center. Furthermore, of those gang members who describe themselves as frequent users of the Internet, approximately 75% report that they have developed their own website to demonstrate their respect for their particular gang (King et al. 2007; National Assessment Center 2007).

Case Example 1 Epilogue

During your evaluation of Joe's Internet activity, you learn that he has participated in multiple types of online harassment, including posting videos of other youth being harassed or assaulted, sending threatening text messages, making repeated threatening cell phone calls, bullying others in chat rooms, and sending e-mails with threatened violent acts. He has numerous Internet victims who report that the embarrassing videos and pictures that he has taken of them have caused them significant emotional distress.

A review of Joe's computer hard drive indicates that he frequents gang-related websites and has downloaded information regarding how to make explosive devices. Like many Internet harassers, he has also physically threatened others offline. He has a significant history of physical abuse by his father,

TABLE 19–3. Sample questions for evaluating a perpetrator of Internet aggression

Has the youth used the Internet to harass someone known to him or her?

Has the youth used the Internet to harass someone he or she knows only online?

Has the youth ever made a specific online threat to harm someone?

Has the youth been involved in gang postings on the Internet?

Has the youth ever been threatened or harassed online?

Has the youth ever bullied someone offline?

Has the youth been bullied offline?

and he was sexually abused by a maternal uncle from the ages of 5 through 9. Due to multiple risk factors for both offline and online violence, Joe was recommended for an intense residential treatment facility with severe restriction of his Internet access.

The Internet and Sexual Behaviors

Internet Sexual Perpetrators

The Internet has become a major source of information, entertainment, and social connectivity for teenagers. While parents of teenagers still report a positive view of the Internet (Lenhart et al. 2007), the proportion of parents who describe the Internet as a positive influence in their children's lives has decreased from 67% in 2004 to 59% in 2006. During this same period, the media has reported a high frequency of Internet-initiated sexual crimes against children. In 2004, one of the U.S. television networks aired 1-hour shows that depicted sting operations aimed at arresting adults attempting to meet underage boys and girls for sexual purposes. These programs drew large audiences (Stelter 2007) and contributed to the image of the Internet child molester as someone who uses deceit to lure children into unwanted sexual activities.

Research into these types of crimes indicates that the characteristics of this offender type are far from the projected stereotype (Wolak et al. 2004, 2008). In a study by the National Juvenile Online Victimization (NJOV) study conducted between 2001 and 2002, most of the Internet-initiated sexual crimes involved adult men using the Internet to seduce adolescents into sexual encounters (Wolak et al. 2004). Only 5% of the offenders pretended to be teenagers while communicating with their victims, and 79% of the offenders were open about their sexual motivations, thus refuting the notion of widespread deceit in the commission of these offenses. While some cases of Internet-related crimes involved "hook-ups" (i.e., the rapid progression to a sexual encounter after an online meeting), 64% of offenders communicated online for more than 1 month prior to a face-to-face meeting. Approximately 74% of the relationships progressed to face-to-face sexual encounters, the vast majority of which resulted in illicit sexual activity between the parties. Finally, 73% of the underage victims who met offenders face to face did so more than once, including 20% who actually lived with the offender for some time. Victim characteristics related to Internet sexual crimes are summarized in Table 19–4.

Types of Online Sexual Victimization

Exposure to Pornography

Case Example 2

Harold is a 15-year-old boy who was brought in by his mother after she discovered that he had been using her credit card to pay for access to an X-rated website for approximately 4 months. After the initial shock, Harold's mother found out that her son had also amassed a collection of approximately 50 pornographic clips that were stored in the hard drive of his computer. Harold reluctantly admitted to downloading clips using Bit Torrent, a peer-to-peer file-sharing tool. She contacted the police, who in turn seized his computer for forensic analysis and subsequently indicated that Harold could face criminal charges for using his mother's credit card without permission. Very concerned, Harold's mother made an appointment with a psychiatrist to evaluate any potential behavioral issues that might arise from his sexual behavior on the Internet. As the forensic evaluator, what steps would you take in assessing Harold, and what recommendations would you give his mother?

Research has suggested that involvement with pornography during adolescence might have negative consequences. For example, surveys of students from junior high to college indicate that exposure to sexual media correlates with sexual permissiveness, liberal attitudes toward premarital sex, increased acceptance

TABLE 19–4. Characteristics of victims of Internet sexual crimes

Are ages 13–17 years

Were aware of the age and/or sexual intentions of the offender

Were not typically coerced into sexual activity with force or violence

Often engaged in sexual activities with the offender, including intercourse, more than once

Knew the offender through extensive online communications that frequently resulted in romantic relationships

of aggression against women in both sexual and nonsexual interactions, and the potential development of sexual callousness (Greenfield 2004; Malamuth and Huppin 2005; Ybarra and Mitchell 2005). In addition, teens with high-risk factors for aggressive behavior (such as impulsivity, hostility to women, and promiscuity) appear to have a higher likelihood of sexual aggression in the context of frequent use of pornography (Malamuth et al. 2000).

The number of websites dedicated to pornography is reportedly in the millions. The vast quantity of pornography available online, as well as the ease with which it can be accessed, has been a source of concern for parents, lawmakers, and mental health professionals. This concern appears justified given youth's extensive and skilled Internet use, the fact that exposure to sexually explicit material usually occurs during adolescence, and the normal propensity of adolescents to be curious about sexuality and sexual stimulation (Peter et al. 2006).

The information available regarding teenagers' pattern of exposure to online pornography comes from two studies conducted in the United States and one from the Netherlands. The Youth Internet Safety Survey (YISS) was conducted between fall 1999 and spring 2000 to quantify the Internet experiences of Internet-using teens, ages 10–17 years (Finkelhor et al. 2000). The results of this study indicated that only 15% of regular youth Internet users reported intentional exposure to pornographic material in the year before the survey and that the exposure had occurred both online and offline (e.g., pornographic magazines). The majority of these users were males ages 14 through 17 years, who were more likely to report poor emotional relationships with their caregivers and to engage in delinquent behavior and substance use than their non-pornography-seeking counterparts. An interesting finding of this study was that individuals who reported unintentional exposure to online sexual content were approximately two and a half times as likely to report that they had also sought pornography compared with those who reported no incidental exposure (Ybarra and Mitchell 2005). This suggests that accidental exposure to pornography online may result in purposeful pornography-seeking behavior later on.

The second Youth Internet Safety Survey (YISS-2) was conducted in 2005 (Wolak et al. 2006). With an aim similar to that of its predecessor, this study reported that 42% of teenage Internet users had been exposed to online pornography in the year prior to the survey. Of those exposed, 66% reported only unwanted exposure. The proportion of male teens who had been exposed to pornography, whether wanted or unwanted, increased with age, with approximately two-thirds of those ages 16–17 reporting exposure versus 18% of those ages 10–11. Girls were significantly less likely to seek out pornography or come across pornography accidentally, with only 8% of girls ages 16–17 reporting wanted exposure to pornographic material. Factors that increased the likelihood of unwanted exposure to pornography included 1) using peer-to-peer or file-sharing programs to download images, 2) reporting interpersonal victimization offline, and 3) having symptoms of depression and social withdrawal. Factors that decreased the risk of exposure to pornography included 1) using filtering or blocking Internet software and 2) attending an Internet safety presentation by a law enforcement official.

Teens who had actively sought out pornographic material were nine times more likely to be males in the 13- to 17-year-old age group. They were also more likely to use file-sharing software, to be harassed or solicited online, and to talk online with unknown people about sex. Teens who had been victimized offline, had symptoms of depression, and/or had rule-breaking histories were also more likely to have wanted exposure to online pornographic material.

The third study of teens and exposure to online pornographic material took place in the Netherlands in 2005 (Peter et al. 2006). Unlike the YISS, which conducted telephone interviews with teens and their parents, the Dutch study used an online survey. The results were fairly similar to those from the YISS studies, although the proportion of teens who reported wanted exposure to pornographic material was higher: 71% of males and 41% of females reported seeking out sexually explicit material, whether it was pictures, movies, or erotic contact sites. Factors such as parental control, religiosity, or relationship status did not have an impact on whether teens accessed sexually explicit materials or not. Some personality characteristics, on the other hand, did. Teens who were sensation seeking, those who were dissatisfied with their lives, and those who had elevated sexual interests were significantly more likely to access sexually graphic material online. Finally, teens were also more likely to access pornographic material if they connected to the Internet using a broadband (fast) connection.

Overall, the evidence currently available indicates that teens have frequent exposure to pornography on the Web, that the exposure is both wanted and unwanted, and that some teens are more likely to engage in this type of behavior than others. Although sexual curiosity and exploration is a normal phase of adolescent development, mental health professionals should carefully consider less benign possibilities when evaluating adolescents involved in pornography-seeking behavior. Research has shown that adolescents who demonstrate symptoms of depression, offline victimization, delinquency, and substance use are more likely to seek out online pornography. In addition, because most of the users appear to be male teens ages 13–17 years, the clinically significant consumption of pornography by female teens or much younger children should raise additional concerns regarding the appropriateness of such behavior.

Case Example 2 Epilogue

During the psychiatric examination, Harold disclosed that he had been viewing pornography daily for approximately 2 years. He indicated that he had escalated its use over the 6 months prior to the evaluation. Harold described an overall dissatisfaction with life, talked about feeling awkward because he did not have a girlfriend, and admitted to smoking marijuana occasionally. On further questioning, Harold became tearful and reported that he had been "sad" for approximately 1 year and that his grades had started to decline. A thorough assessment of Harold's risk for self-injurious behavior and a more comprehensive detailed sexual history were recommended in addition to standard treatment approaches for his depression. His parents were instructed to install Internet-filtering software and to carefully monitor his Internet use.

Online Sexual Interactions

Case Example 3

As a busy forensic psychiatrist, you receive a referral to evaluate Stephen, a 15-year-old high school sophomore. Stephen's laptop had crashed, and he took it into a computer repair shop to be fixed. A store employee contacted police after he discovered two movies on Stephen's laptop that depicted graphic sexual behavior between a prepubescent male and an adult. Stephen was subsequently arrested for possession of child pornography. Stephen's parents report that Stephen has been less social for the past 10 months, that he has dropped out of the wrestling team, and that his grades were "not what they used to be." Stephen's attorney requests your opinion on whether there are any mitigating factors to report to the court.

Socialization is an important aspect of children's and adolescents' activity when they are online. It is common for youth to be contacted via instant messaging (IM), messages posted to their social networking site web page, or e-mail by individuals whom they have never met before. While most of these unsolicited contacts are benign, the media consistently reports the dangers that arise from social networking sites (P. Williams 2006) and chat rooms (Hansen 2007), with lurid portrayals of males lurking online and waiting for their next unsuspecting victim. As previously described, online sex offenders typically operate by engaging susceptible adolescents in conversations that begin on the Internet, where sexual topics are brought up. These contacts may progress to telephone calls and eventually culminate in face-to-face meetings. The vast majority of these face-to-face meetings result in nonforcible sexual contact (Wolak et al. 2008).

Not all adolescents, irrespective of whether they reply to an instant message from an unknown individual, are at risk for online sexual victimization. In fact, in a survey of 1,588 teens ranging from age 10 to 15 years conducted in the United States in 2006, only 15% reported being the target of unwanted sexual solicitation (Ybarra and Mitchell 2008). Unwanted sexual solicitation occurs when teens are asked to engage in sexual talk or sexual behavior or to provide sexual information when they do not want to do so, or when the person asking is older than 18 years. These solicitations range from sexually inappropriate questions (e.g., "What is the color of your underwear") to more serious requests to engage in masturbation or to send sexually explicit pictures. A subgroup of solicitations, known as aggressive solicitations, involve individuals who establish or attempt to establish offline contact by asking the teens to meet them in person, calling the teens on the phone, or sending post mail, money, or gifts (Mitchell et al. 2007b).

The rate of "regular" online sexual solicitation in the United States showed a downward trend between 2000 and 2005, in both boys and girls of all age groups. The rate of aggressive solicitations, those that are also potentially more likely to develop into sexual assault cases, has not similarly decreased and continues to involve between 3% and 4% of youth online. Risk factors that increase the likelihood of sexual solicitation are described in Table 19–5 (Mitchell et al. 2007a).

It also appears that a teen's risk for sexual solicitation online partially correlates with his or her willingness to engage in conversations with strangers. In a 2002 U.S. survey, approximately 39% of adolescents interviewed indicated that they had communicated more than once with someone they met online (Wolak et al. 2002). Entertainment, social inclusion, maintaining relationships, meeting new people, and social compensation have been identified as reasons that influence an adolescent's online talk with others. In one survey of 412 adolescents ages 12–18 years recruited from the Dutch school system, teens who talked to strangers online tended to be younger boys and girls (ages 12–14 years) and to have less frequent but intensive chat sessions. They described talking to strangers as a result of needing entertainment, being curious about others, and feeling too inhibited to participate in face-to-face meetings (Peter et al. 2006). The most common venue in which teens interact with strangers is via chat rooms. Not surprisingly, in the NJOV study most of the individuals charged with sexual molestation met their victims in chat rooms. As with IM, chat rooms allow immediate communication between individuals who chose to enter the virtual room. Chat rooms usually have names that tend to illustrate a particular interest of those inside and are known for their graphic sexual content.

TABLE 19–5. Risk factors that increase the likelihood of youth online sexual solicitation

Being of female gender

Using chat rooms

Talking with people met online

Talking about sex with someone met online

Having a history of physical or sexual abuse

Sending personal information about oneself to someone met online using the Internet from a cell phone

Having depressivelike symptoms

Source. Mitchell et al. 2007a.

The risk for online victimization does not appear to increase when teens post information on social networking sites (Mitchell et al. 2008). However, if the information posted includes sexually provocative picture of themselves, an indication of sexual risk-taking behavior, the likelihood of sexual solicitation increases. Furthermore, while many teens have pictures of themselves and their friends posted on social networking sites, a quantitative analysis of publicly viewable adolescent profiles posted to MySpace revealed that only 5.4% of them included pictures that depicted the teens in swimsuits or underwear (Hinduja and Patchin 2008). Teens who show traits of sexual risk-taking behavior, however, may have histories of sexual abuse, which may also put them at higher risk for engaging in sexual activities with adults they meet online.

While the majority of victims of Internet-related sexual contact offenses are female (61%), this number also indicates that a large number of victims are male (Walsh and Wolak 2005). Adolescents who identify as gay or who question or are curious about their sexual orientation appear to be at increased risk of sexual victimization by adults they meet online: the majority of male victims in the NJOV study had met the perpetrators in gay-themed chat rooms. Teens may be reluctant to discuss their sexual orientation with peers or responsible adults because they fear being shunned or made fun of, and they may search the Internet looking for advice, entertainment, or relationships. In doing so, they may fall prey to savvy adult offenders who use a pattern of grooming to increase the comfort level of adolescents.

The offenders are mostly men who are much older than the victim: in 51% of the cases reviewed in the NJOV study, the age difference was at least 21 years. In addition, 30% of defendants held positions that brought them in contact with minors, such as teachers or coaches. While the majority of the victims met the offender in Internet chat rooms, 38% of the cases involved a perpetrator who was known to the victim from the community. In approximately half the cases, the victims appeared to have formed a close bond with or developed a romantic attachment to the perpetrator. More than half the cases involved sexual penetration, 27% involved producing child pornography by taking pictures of the victim, 39% involved showing the victim adult or child pornography, and 34% involved giving the victim drugs or alcohol (Walsh and Wolak 2005).

Case Example 3 Epilogue

During the interview Stephen appears depressed and somewhat anxious about the prospect of incarceration. He describes receiving the movies from someone with the online name "CoachDad19" using an instant message tool that allows peer-to-peer file transfer. When you ask about his Internet activities, Stephen reports that he often enters a chat room called "teen m4m," a gay-oriented room. He tells you that he has several "friends," including CoachDad19, a 29-year-old man who lives in a nearby town and who has been calling and texting him. Stephen appears to have an increased risk for online victimization as he has engaged in several high-risk behaviors, appears to have some preoccupation with his sexual orientation, and has developed an ongoing relationship with an adult who has shared child pornography with him.

The Internet and Suicide

Suicide is the third most common cause of death among adolescents (Bae et al. 2005). Forensic evaluators may be asked to identify risk factors for potentially suicidal youth and for youth who have taken their own life. With the emergence of the Internet as a common source of both information and communication, concerns have arisen that interactions in cyberspace could facilitate a youth's suicidal thoughts or behaviors.

A particularly alarming teen suicide that has been linked to a young teenager's Internet exchanges involves a 13-year-old Missouri girl named Megan Meier. Through her MySpace posting, Megan met a teenage boy named Josh Evans. In reality, "Josh" was a fictional cybercharacter created by one of Megan's female neighbors who knew Megan and who decided to play a hoax on her. Megan became very excited about this online friendship and highly valued her interactions with this new cyberfriend. On October 16, 2006, Megan became suddenly emotionally distressed after logging onto her MySpace page. Later that same evening, Megan's mother discovered her dead daughter hanging from a cloth belt in Megan's bedroom closet. Megan's father subsequently found the final message that Megan had received from Josh that same afternoon, which read, "You're a shitty person, and the world would be a better place without you in it" (Collins 2008).

Although this case involves the impact of a perceived Internet rejection on a vulnerable teenager, there are other potential areas a forensic evaluator should explore when evaluating the potential influence of the Internet on suicidal thoughts or behaviors. First, inquire if the youth has been a victim of online harassment and/or sexual solicitation (as described in the above sections regarding online victimization).

Second, evaluate whether the child or adolescent has visited any website that provides information on how to successfully kill oneself. Numerous websites have been described that address various methods of how to commit suicide (Dobson 1999). Third, ask if the youth has obtained information regarding suicide through chat rooms or other methods of online contact. Fourth, determine whether any suicide pact has been discussed or made by the youth. A phenomenon known as "net suicide" or "cybersuicide" has recently been described wherein individuals who meet on the Internet and are strangers to each other enter into an agreement to commit suicide (Naito 2007). Munro (2001) described the case of two Norwegian teenagers who met online, agreed they would commit suicide through a lethal jump, and eventually enacted their cybersuicide pact.

Fifth, ask if the child or adolescent has learned of any other suicides or been exposed to suicidal statements on the Internet. An individual feeling more suicidal after exposure to someone else's suicidality has been referred to as the "contagion" or "copycat effect." This effect has shown its strongest influence among adolescents (Jobes et al. 1996). Finally, investigate any attempts by the youth to receive treatment for his or her symptoms online or to obtain medications for the purpose of treating depressive symptoms or taking an overdose. Various websites offer quick access to a variety of psychotropic medications with minimal, if any, meaningful mental health screening or monitoring.

—Key Points

In today's rapidly changing cyberspace society, the Internet has an ever-increasing impact on the lives of children and adolescents. In certain types of forensic evaluations, the mental health evaluator should carefully consider investigating a youth's Internet activities as an important potential source of information. The following are key areas to explore:

— Computer hard drives, including visited websites, instant messaging exchanges, and phone text messages

— Exposure to online victimization, with particular focus on victimization through posted videos or embarrassing pictures

— Evidence of Internet harassment and any online gang postings or involvement

— Sexual interactions on the Internet, such as the viewing of pornography, participation in Internet chat rooms with sexual content exchanged, sexual solicitation by others on the Internet, and offline sexual contacts through individuals met online

— Internet information seeking regarding mental health diagnoses and treatment, with a particular focus on a youth's attempts to gain information about methods to commit suicide

References

Bae S, Ye R, Chen S, et al: Risky behaviors and factors associated with suicide attempt in adolescents. Arch Suicide Res 9:193–202, 2005

Beebe TJ, Asche SE, Harrison PA, et al: Heightened vulnerability and increased risk-taking among adolescent chat room users: results from a statewide school survey. J Adolesc Health 35:116–123, 2004

Collins L: Friend game: behind the online hoax that led to a girl's suicide. The New Yorker, January 21, 2008

Dobson R: Internet sites may encourage suicide. BMJ 319:337, 1999

Finkelhor D, Mitchell K, Wolak J: Online Victimization: A Report on the Nation's Young People. Washington, DC, National Center for Missing and Exploited Children, U.S. Department of Justice, 2000

Glancy GD, Newman AW, Potash MN, et al: Cyberstalking, in Stalking: Psychiatric Perspectives and Practical Approaches. Edited by Pinals DA. Oxford, England, Oxford University Press, 2007, pp 212–224

Greenfield PM: Inadvertent exposure to pornography on the Internet: implications of peer-to-peer file-sharing networks for child development and families. J Appl Dev Psychol 25:741–750, 2004

Hansen C: Expensive Home Rich With Potential Predators. July 25, 2007. Available at: www.msnbc.msn.com/id/19961209. Accessed June 10, 2008.

Hinduja S, Patchin JW: Personal information of adolescents on the Internet: a quantitative content analysis of MySpace. J Adolesc 31:125–146, 2008

Jobes DA, Berman AL, O'Carroll PW, et al: The Kurt Cobain suicide crisis: perspectives from research, public health, and the news media. Suicide Life Threat Behav 26:260–269; discussion 269–271, 1996

King JE, Walpole CE, Lamon K: Surf and turf wars online: growing implications of Internet gang violence. J Adolesc Health 41:S66–S68, 2007

Lenhart A, Madden M, Rankin-Macgill A, et al: Pew Internet and American Life Project: Teens and social media: the use of social media gains a greater foothold in teen life as they embrace the conversational nature of interactive online media. December 19, 2007. Available at: http://pewinternet.org/pdfs/PIP_Teens_Social_Media_Final.pdf. Accessed June 10, 2008.

Malamuth NM, Huppin M: Pornography and teenagers: the importance of individual differences. Adolesc Med Clin 16:315–326, 2005

Malamuth NM, Addison T, Koss M: Pornography and sexual aggression: are there reliable effects and can we understand them? Annu Rev Sex Res 11:26–91, 2000

Mitchell KJ, Finkelhor D, Wolak J: Youth Internet users at risk for the most serious online sexual solicitations. Am J Prev Med 32:532–537, 2007a

Mitchell K, Wolak J, Finkelhor D: Trends in reports of sexual solicitations, harassment and unwanted exposure to pornography on the Internet. J Adolesc Health 40:116–126, 2007b

Mitchell KJ, Wolak J, Finkelhor D: Are blogs putting youth at risk for online sexual solicitation or harassment? Child Abuse Negl 32:277–294, 2008

Moessner C: Cyberbullying. Trends Tudes 6:1–4, 2007

Munro R: Want to know how to behead yourself? Just go online. Nurs Times 97:12–13, 2001

Naito A: Internet suicide in Japan: implications for child and adolescent mental health. Clin Child Psychol Psychiatry 12:583–597, 2007

National Assessment Center: Survey of gang members' online habits and participation. Paper presented at the i-SAFE Annual Internet Safety Education Review Meeting, Carlsbad, CA, 2007

Patchin JW, Hinduja S: Bullies move beyond the schoolyard: a preliminary look at cyberbullying. Youth Violence Juvenile Justice 4:148–169, 2006

Peter J, Valkenburg PM, Schouten AP: Characteristics and motives of adolescents talking with strangers on the Internet. Cyberpsychol Behav 9:526–530, 2006

Raskauskas J, Stoltz AD: Involvement in traditional and electronic bullying among adolescents. Dev Psychol 43:564–575, 2007

Slonje R, Smith PK: Cyberbullying: another main type of bullying? Scand J Psychol 49:147–154, 2008

Smith PK, Cowie H, Olafsson RF, et al: Definitions of bullying: a comparison of terms used, and age and gender differences, in a fourteen-country international comparison. Child Dev 73:1119–1133, 2002

Smith PK, Mahdavi J, Carvalho M, et al: An investigation into cyberbullying, its forms, awareness and impact, and the relationship between age and gender in cyberbullying (Research Brief No. RBX03-06). London, Department of Education and Skills, 2006

Stelter B: To catch a predator is falling prey to advertisers' sensibilities. New York Times, August 27, 2007

UCLA Internet Report: The Digital Future Report: Surveying the Digital Future—Year Four, 2004. Available at: http://www.digitalcenter.org/downloads/DigitalFuture-Report-Year4-2004.pdf. Accessed June 10, 2008.

Walsh WA, Wolak J: Nonforcible Internet-related sex crimes with adolescent victims: prosecution issues and outcomes. Child Maltreat 10:260–271, 2005

Wells M, Mitchell KJ: How do high-risk youth use the Internet? Characteristics and implications for prevention. Child Maltreat 13:227–234, 2008

Williams KR, Guerra NG: Prevalence and predictors of Internet bullying. J Adolesc Health 41:S14–S21, 2007

Williams P: MySpace, Facebook attract online predators. February 3, 2006. Available at: www.msnbc.msn.com/id/11165576. Accessed June 10, 2008.

Wolak J, Mitchell KJ, Finkelhor D: Close online relationships in a national sample of adolescents. Adolescence 37:441–455, 2002

Wolak J, Finkelhor D, Mitchell K: Internet-initiated sex crimes against minors: implications for prevention based on findings from a national study. J Adolesc Health 35:424–433, 2004

Wolak J, Mitchell K, Finkelhor D: Online victimization of youth: five years later. Washington, DC, National Center for Missing and Exploited Children, U.S. Department of Justice, 2006

Wolak J, Mitchell KJ, Finkelhor D: Does online harassment constitute bullying? An exploration of online harassment by known peers and online-only contacts. J Adolesc Health 41:S51–S58, 2007

Wolak J, Finkelhor D, Mitchell KJ, et al: Online "predators" and their victims: myths, realities, and implications for prevention and treatment. Am Psychol 63:111–128, 2008

Ybarra ML, Mitchell KJ: Online aggressor/targets, aggressors, and targets: a comparison of associated youth characteristics. J Child Psychol Psychiatry 45:1308–1316, 2004

Ybarra ML, Mitchell KJ: Exposure to Internet pornography among children and adolescents: a national survey. Cyberpsychol Behav 8:473–486, 2005

Ybarra ML, Mitchell KJ: How risky are social networking sites? A comparison of the places online where sexual harassment occurs. Pediatrics 121:350–357, 2008

Ybarra ML, Mitchell K, Wolak J: Risk and impact of Internet harassment: findings from the second Youth Internet Safety Survey. Pediatrics 118:e1–e9, 2006

PART V

Youth Violence

Peter Ash, M.D.

Chapter 20

Taxonomy and Neurobiology of Aggression

R. James R. Blair, Ph.D.
Niranjan S. Karnik, M.D., Ph.D.
Emil F. Coccaro, M.D.
Hans Steiner, M.D.

Aggression, as a psychiatric phenomenon, spans the domains of biology, psychology, and sociology, and one needs knowledge of all of these spheres to plan effective treatment and forensic analysis. Problems with aggression are one of the most common presenting complaints for child mental health professionals and child psychiatrists (Connor et al. 2006; Steiner 1997, 1999; Steiner and Remsing 2007).

Within a developmental psychopathological perspective (Cicchetti and Cohen 2006; Steiner 2004), aggression has a normative developmental role. Along with other emotions of childhood, aggression not only serves as a means to reflect a child's inner emotional state but also is a mechanism through which children learn the limits of the social world and become acculturated to social rules.

When these normative patterns of aggression are exceeded by intensity or when a consistent pattern of aggression emerges, then this may become a focus of clinical attention. It is at this point that possible antisocial patterns may become an area of concern. While almost any childhood psychiatric disorder can present with a pattern of aggression, DSM-IV (American Psychiatric Association 1994) defines several diagnostic categories under the core domain of disruptive behaviors. Excluding attention-deficit/hyperactivity disorder (ADHD) because of its unique set of issues and diagnostic considerations, DSM-IV leaves three diagnoses: oppositional defiant disorder (ODD), conduct disorder (CD), and disruptive behavior disorder not otherwise specified (DBD-NOS).

Although there appears to be a continuity between ODD and CD, the criteria lack a sound basis in the neurobiology of aggression and were developed more from phenomenological and experiential criteria. This chapter reviews the neuroscience of aggression, the implications for taxonomic development, and forensic considerations for the practicing clinician.

Subtypes of Aggression

While multiple nosological divisions of aggression could be made depending on the criteria and characteristics used (Hinshaw and Lee 2003), current research supports at least one key division between a form of aggression that is reactive, affective, defensive, or impulsive (RADI) and another form that is proactive, instrumental, or planned (PIP; Steiner et al. 2003). These two forms correspond to what we term "hot" and "cold" aggression, respectively (Table 20–1).

TABLE 20–1. Associations of emotions and affective states with subtypes of aggression

RADI	PIP
Reactive	Proactive
Affective	Instrumental
Defensive	Planned
Impulsive	Predatory
Stress-responsive	Stress-resistant
Elevated heart rates when acting out	Low resting heart rates
Overt	Covert
Negative emotions (anger, frustration, irritability, fear)	Negative emotions (disgust, contempt)
Unplanned	Positive emotions (interest, pleasure)

Note.   RADI = reactive, affective, defensive, or impulsive aggression; PIP = proactive, instrumental, or planned aggression.

RADI (or "hot") aggression is affectively driven and impulsive. It is often characterized by a rapid response to a perceived threat or slight, and the predominant emotions associated with it are anger and rage, followed by a sense of guilt or remorse. Individuals with this aggressive pattern often describe themselves as unable to contain their anger, and they feel bad afterward and can often reflect, at times of calm, on the fact that their aggression may indeed be maladaptive and problematic.

Conversely, PIP (or "cold") aggression can also be driven by anger, but it is often associated with pleasure or disgust. Individuals with this type of aggressive pattern seem to show little emotionality or response to their acts and will often only exhibit emotions during the act of aggression itself. This form of aggression is much rarer than RADI and is often associated with psychopathy when it exists in a fixed or continuous form of behavior. Individuals often display a calculating nature when it comes to the aggressive acts, and they often see their aggression as adaptive and helpful for their end goals despite consequences that may exist.

The distinction between RADI and PIP aggression has been made by several research groups when examining specific elements of experience (Barratt et al. 1999; Berkowitz 1993; Crick and Dodge 1996; Linnoila et al. 1983). Several teams have also tied these subtypes to specific developmental pathways (Connor 2002; Vitaro et al. 1998), and factor models suggest that although RADI and PIP aggression are strongly correlated, two factors fit the model better than one (Poulin and Boivin 2000).

Research estimates show that the RADI subtype of aggression as measured by components of the Achenbach Youth Self-Report has a prevalence rate of almost 2% in a general high school population, whereas that number rises to over 9% among delinquent youth. Similarly, PIP aggression was found in a little over 1% of a general high school population and 13% among delinquent youth. Finally, the combined condition, in which elements of both RADI and PIP are evident, is present in a little over 1% of high school students and over 48% of delinquent youth (Steiner et al. 2005).

Despite these findings, several critics have challenged the two-factor model (Bushman and Anderson 2001). One group of authors have argued that researchers have confounded two dichotomies of information processing (Norman and Shallice 1986; Shiffrin and Schneider 1977). In automatic processing, responses to stimuli are learned repeatedly and so often that they become routine and therefore automatic. Controlled processing is thought to occur via "executive functions" that select a behavior appropriate to the stimulus. Bushman and Anderson (2001) argued that "hostile" (or what we call RADI) aggression, is unreasoned, whereas "instrumental" (or PIP) aggression is reasoned. They believe that RADI therefore corresponds to automatic processing and PIP to controlled processing and that this dichotomy collapses in most forms of aggression because there are elements of controlled and automatic processing. Although it is possible that investigators have conflated these aggression pathways, it is plausible and likely that despite the automatic-controlled processing dichotomy, RADI and PIP exist as separate aggression pathways that have both automatic and controlled elements. In this way, the subtypes of aggression differentiate through their neural pathways and the relative weighting of automatic and controlled elements through different networks of control that have aggression as a final common pathway. The circuits would be the key point of differentiation, with RADI and PIP as ontological types that lead us to understand these pathways.

Experiences of aggressive subtypes need not be mutually exclusive. We anticipate that while some individuals will have a predominant experience of RADI or PIP aggression, there are also likely to be individuals who present with both subtypes that would be triggered or activated by different social and environmental stimuli or circumstances. Studies among incarcerated juveniles who show a high degree of aggression lend support to the two-factor model and also underscore the presence of individuals who have both phenotypes.

Genetic Studies

Several lines of research, including twin, adoption, and family studies, suggest that there may be genetic influences on aggression. Studies of the related but more narrow phenomenon of CD have found concordance in monozygotic twins to be greater than in dizygotic twins (Raine 1997, 2002). Other studies that have examined biological twins who were adopted later in life found both environmental and genetic factors to be salient (Cadoret et al. 1983; Riggins-Caspers et al. 2003), as has been further explicated in more recent research. Generally, heritability estimates range between 44% and 72% in samples of adults (Rhee and Waldman 2002).

Genetic studies of aggression have generally failed to distinguish aggression based on RADI and PIP subtypes with the exception of work on monoamine oxidase 1 (MAOA). Studies have found MAOA to have a more significant relationship to the RADI form of aggression. Caspi et al. (2002) have shown that a low-activity allele of MAOA requires exposure to social or environmental maltreatment in order to increase the risk of aggression. Recent neuroimaging studies have shown that low-activity MAOA carriers have increased amygdala activity relative to high-activity MAOA carriers when exposed to emotional stimuli (Meyer-Lindenberg et al. 2006). Increased amygdala activity in the face of emotional stimulus is consistent with our emerging model of RADI aggression.

These preliminary lines of evidence suggest that there are genetic factors that contribute to the development of a neurochemical network that when exposed to particular environmental stressors leads to the development and differentiation of PIP and RADI aggressive subtypes. The precise structure of this network is only beginning to become apparent, and much more research from multiple disciplinary perspectives is necessary to understand these complex phenomena.

Reactive Aggression

The roots of RADI aggression lie in the neurophysiology of fear–frustration systems. As an example, we might consider the classic examples of freeze, flight, or fight responses in animal species. When the danger is perceived as being at a distance and at a relatively low level, the animal tends to freeze and attempt to make itself less apparent in the local surroundings. When the danger is more proximate and at a higher level, the animal will attempt to flee the situation. Finally, if escape is impossible and the threat is in the immediate proximity, then reactive aggression emerges and the animal will attempt to fight to save itself (Blanchard et al. 1977).

The neurophysiology of RADI aggression is governed by the basic threat system (Figure 20–1) that begins in the medial amygdala regions, runs downward via the stria terminalis to the medial hypothalamus, and then ends in the dorsal portion of the periaqueductal gray (PAG; Gregg and Siegel 2001; Panksepp 1998). This system has been found to be regulated by areas of the frontal cortex, most especially the orbital, ventrolateral, and medial areas (R. J. Blair 2004).

RADI aggression can be considered as an automatic response of this basic threat circuitry to a threat stimulus. Aggression in this pattern may be normative and an appropriate response to particular situations and stimuli. For example, children who respond to an immediate threat to their life during war or military conflict by harming the person who threatened them or threatened to harm their family might be understood to be responding with adaptive RADI aggression. When such threat responses occur independent of appropriate context or seem disproportionate to the level of threat, then we might consider the RADI aggression to be maladaptive and pathological.

Connor (2002) outlined a set of criteria for delimiting pathological aggression from normative aggression. He argued that maladaptive aggression will be expressed in contexts that are not traditionally seen as sufficiently threatening, that the aggression is disproportionate to the trigger or situation, and that severity and persistence of the aggression are not limited in the ways that they should be.

The transformation of these threat systems from normative to dysregulated can occur in one of two

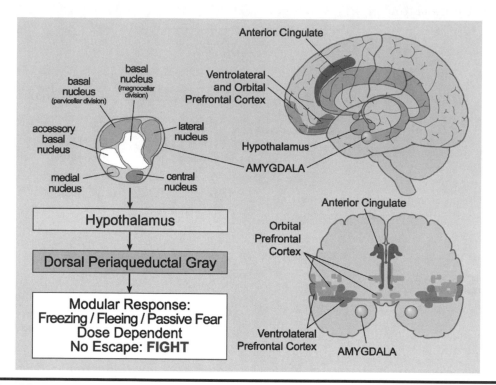

FIGURE 20–1.   Neural systems involved in emotion as well as in reactive, affective, defensive, or impulsive (RADI) and proactive, instrumental, or planned (PIP) aggression.

The response to threat, including reactive aggression, is mediated by a system that runs from medial amygdaloidal areas downward to the medial hypothalamus and from there to the dorsal half of the periaqueductal gray. This system is regulated by the orbital and ventrolateral frontal cortex and anterior cingulate. The amygdala is involved in the formation of stimulus–reinforcement associations (learning whether objects are good or bad). Amygdala dysfunction may be related to an increased risk for instrumental aggression.

ways. First, the system can be overresponsive and reactive to stimuli that should be subthreshold. Second, the regulatory systems that act to keep the threat response from responding inappropriately may not be functioning to reduce the affective response.

Case Example 1

Jack is a 16-year-old male who has a recent history of aggressive patterns in the context of a longer history of academic failure and lack of success. His parents are in the midst of a divorce, and his father has a history of bipolar disorder diagnosed later in life. Jack acts out very aggressively in response to arguments or perceived limit setting and threats by adults in his life. He will often punch holes in walls or direct his aggression toward inanimate objects. His aggression shows a high degree of reactivity and is largely regretted after it has been done. He often finds himself having to fix the damage that he has done, and he displays some degree of guilt about his actions but currently lacks good insight into his actions.

In this case we see a pattern of RADI aggression that is being uncovered by social stressors (the par-

ents' divorce) as well as potential comorbid bipolar disorder, which may be nascent and emergent. Jack has had a number of contacts with local police, who are called when he breaks into one of his aggressive episodes. He is often able to reconstitute himself in the presence of officers and will talk reasonably with them about his actions. His remorse has to this point prevented him from landing in juvenile hall, but he is certainly at risk and would benefit from early intervention or diversion programs with anger management. He is also likely to benefit from a combination of individual therapy, family therapy, and medications to help him reduce his reactivity and teach him some coping strategies.

Basic Threat Response System

The basic threat response system is always active and scanning for threats within one's environment. The degree to which the threat response system is tuned to reach a level of activation to produce RADI aggression is determined by elements of innate biological predispositions and prior environmental experiences. There is some evidence that a biologically overresponsive basic threat system can develop in certain contexts. Studies of depression and anxiety have shown that the amygdala can be primed to overactivity (Drevets 2003; Kagan and Snidman 1999). The overresponsiveness may be partially responsible for the finding that depression and anxiety have a correlation with RADI aggression (Zoccolillo 1992). One of the questions that remains to be fully answered in the neuroimaging research literature is whether biological changes, such as changes in the amygdala, are the result of psychiatric pathology or, conversely, if the psychiatric pathology is a consequence of biological changes. The directionality of these correlations may be highly complex and elements of causation and effect simultaneously.

In concert with these biological predispositions, experiences in the environment can change or modify the basic threat response systems (King 1999) as well as the neurochemical responses to threat (Charney 2003). Such experiences have been shown to make RADI aggression more likely, but we theorize that alternative protective and resiliency experiences can reduce RADI aggression or make it less likely. Environmental experiences can also lead to the creation of associations between physical and sexual abuse and lead to posttraumatic stress disorder (Steiner et al. 1997), thereby also increasing the risk of aggression (Farrington 2000), and more specifically RADI aggression (Steiner 1997).

Elements of the basic threat response system, and more specifically the amygdala, focus attention on environmental threats. Studies have shown that when the threat system is stressed, hypervigilance can emerge in response (King 1999). Along a similar line, children who exhibit RADI aggression tend to show "hostile attribution biases" (Crick and Dodge 1996; Steiner et al. 1997) when they perceive threats in nonaggressive environments. Such systems exist in complex networks with other associative pathways. Thus emotions and experiences such as frustration, which necessarily involve the frontal regions of the brain, likely relate to the basic threat detection circuits and prefrontal regulatory systems. It is interesting that the predominant activating emotions are likely anger or irritability instead of fear when one considers the networks relevant to RADI aggression.

Although our knowledge about the molecular biology of the problems of aggression is far from complete, we include this discussion because of the implications for treatment. Prior environmental threats or innate biological predispositions may exert their influence through neurochemistry and therefore may be amenable to pharmacological intervention (Charney 2003):

- *Norepinephrine.* Norepinephrine has a considerable role in the innervation of the basic threat systems in animals (Pieribone et al. 1994) and humans (Ferry et al. 1999). It is unsurprising that increased noradrenergic activity facilitates aggression in several animal species, including reactive aggression in humans (Coccaro 1996).
- *Arginine vasopressin (AVP).* Animal work suggests that AVP increases the responsiveness of the basic threat systems; it increases anxiety-related behaviors and the neurochemical response to threat (Landgraf et al. 1995). Given this, animal studies suggest a positive relationship between central AVP activity and aggression (Ferris et al. 1997). Work with humans remains in its infancy.
- *Testosterone.* Although androgen receptors are widely distributed in the rat brain, their greatest densities are within the basic threat system: the amygdala, hypothalamus, and PAG (Hamson et al. 2004). Increased testosterone should facilitate reactive aggression, and work with several animal species confirms this suggestion (Book et al. 2001). However, the evidence in humans is not compelling, but the problem here may be methodological. Reactive aggression is a response to environmental threat or frustration and must be provoked; it is not simply spontaneously evoked. Typically, studies using a provocation methodology reported that testosterone administration increased aggression (Pope et al. 2000), whereas studies not using provocation reported that testosterone administration did not increase aggression (O'Connor et al. 2002).

Regulation of the Basic Threat Systems

The current model of the basic threat system implicates the orbital, medial, and ventrolateral frontal cortex regions as being the critical components in the circuitry (R.J. Blair 2004). Neuroimaging studies in adults show that patients presenting with RADI aggression tend to show reduced frontal and temporal cortex functioning (Raine et al. 1998; Volkow et al. 1995). Such findings have not been demonstrated in patients with PIP aggression (Raine et al. 1998) and are consistent with neuropsychology testing of PIP individuals who demonstrate normal performance on tests of frontal lobe functioning. Damage to the basic threat circuits in the relevant frontal lobe regions has been shown to increase the risk of RADI aggression in children (Anderson et al. 1999) and adults (Grafman et al. 1996).

Dysregulation in these systems disrupts processes that are particularly involved in modulating the subcortical systems mediating reactive aggression (R.J. Blair 2004). In particular, they disrupt the alteration of behavior through extinction and response reversal as a function of others' social cues or when reinforcement contingencies have changed (Rolls 2000). Considerable recent neuroimaging work attests to the role of the middle, orbital, and ventrolateral frontal cortex in modifying behavior to social cues and contingency change (e.g., Budhani et al. 2007; Kringelbach and Rolls 2003; O'Doherty et al. 2003; Phelps et al. 2004). Frustration occurs when a behavior is initiated to achieve a reward but the reward does not occur. Frustration has long been linked to the display of reactive aggression (Berkowitz 1993). In short, fear-based or frustration-based reactive aggression will be common in an individual with medial-orbital-ventrolateral frontal cortex dysfunction.

Two psychiatric conditions appear to be related to disruption of these emotion regulatory systems: intermittent explosive disorder or impulsive aggressive disorder (Coccaro 1998) and childhood bipolar disorder (Leibenluft et al. 2003). Patients with these disorders express irritability and are at higher risk for reactive aggression. A third condition is also worth mentioning, although the situation is complex (see J. Blair et al. 2005): ADHD. ADHD has been associated with medial and ventrolateral prefrontal cortex dysfunction (Bush et al. 2005). In line with the regulatory roles of these structures, ADHD is also associated with an increased risk for reactive but not instrumental aggression (Dodge et al. 1997; Kempes et al. 2006).

While the ultimate (environmental/biological predisposition) influences on emotion regulation remain uncertain, it is likely that they will at least partially exert their influence through neurochemistry:

- *Dopamine (DA).*   Dopaminergic influence on reactive aggression is likely to be complex (particularly when the differential impact of various receptor subtypes is considered). There is dopaminergic innervation of the basic threat circuitry (Gregg and Siegel 2001; Panksepp 1998). Consistent with this role, animal studies suggest that increased DA activity facilitates aggressive responding (Coccaro 1996). However, there is also considerable dopaminergic innervation of frontal regulatory systems (Goldman-Rakic et al. 2000). Work with humans has been inconsistent (Coccaro 1996), although dopaminergic blockade does reduce aggression in a

wide variety of psychopathology (Connor 2002; Steiner et al. 2003), probably through innervation of frontal regulatory systems.

- *Serotonin.*   Animal work has shown that serotonin innervates frontal regulatory systems and has a direct inhibitory influence on the PAG (Deakin and Graeff 1991). Consistent with this, considerable animal work and a growing human literature indicate an inverse relationship between serotonergic activity and reactive aggression (Coccaro and Kavoussi 1997; New et al. 2002; Swann 2003). Serotonergic manipulation (fluoxetine treatment) has been shown to have an antiaggressive effect on reactively aggressive individuals (Coccaro and Kavoussi 1997). In line with its role in innervating frontal regulatory systems, serotonergic manipulation (fluoxetine treatment) has been found to increase metabolic activity significantly in the frontal cortex in reactively aggressive individuals (New et al. 2004; see also Connor et al. 2006).

- *Gamma-aminobutyric acid (GABA).*   Although direct stimulation of GABA receptors generally suppresses aggression, considerable animal work has shown that positive allosteric modulators of $GABA_A$ receptors, such as alcohol, benzodiazepines, and many neurosteroids, can all cause increased levels of aggressive behavior (de Almeida et al. 2005; Miczek et al. 2003). Human work also indicates that both alcohol, which is involved in more than half of violent crimes (Pernanen 1991), and benzodiazepines (e.g., Weisman et al. 1998) increase the risk for aggression. These divergent effects seem dose dependent. Although the specific impact of these compounds remains unclear, it is plausible that they disrupt the integrity of the frontal systems involved in the regulation of the basic threat circuitry (see Shah et al. 2004). However, it should be noted that even relatively low dosages of alcohol substantially decrease glucose metabolism in many regions of the human brain in addition to the frontal cortex (Volkow et al. 2006).

RADI aggression has several lines of evidence that are beginning to define its boundaries. It is a form of aggression that likely has a biological and genetic component, but the expression of this phenotype requires particular environmental stimuli that affect the neurochemical pathways related to the experience of aggression and that link key experiential systems to a final common pathway.

Proactive Aggression

There have been suggestions that human PIP aggression might relate to predatory aggression in animals (Gregg and Siegel 2001). However, animal predatory aggression is not displayed toward members of the same species, whereas human PIP aggression almost always is. Moreover, human PIP aggression is goal directed and highly influenced by the individuals' learning history.

Case Example 2

Ben is a 14-year-old male who was recently revealed to have been sexually abusing his adopted 12-year-old sister for the past year. He has a history of a childhood angioma in the right inferior frontal lobe that was successfully resected in infancy. He has not displayed any neurological sequelae of the angioma and has had a normal developmental pattern until his early teens, when he began to exhibit patterns consistent with CD. The violence against his adoptive sister took place whenever the parents left the house for work or short errands, and there were instances when he would stop in response to their early return home. He forced his sister to maintain her silence by use of threats and coercion. He did not exhibit any violence toward other people or other young children in any other context.

Ben was found guilty of sexual violence by a juvenile mental health court, and the opinion of a psychiatrist was requested because of a defense contention that the neurological lesion was the cause of his sexual aggression. The opinion of the psychiatrist was that the lesion was located in an area that was not known to be a part of the aggression circuitry and that the nature of the aggression seemed planned and premeditated in such a way as to be inconsistent with reactive aggression. Given the type of aggression and its highly selective and circumscribed presentation, it seemed highly improbable that the lesion offered any mitigating factor in this case.

We believe that the pathology leading to heightened levels of PIP aggression relates to the decision to utilize antisocial rather than social behaviors to achieve goals. When faced with a goal (e.g., obtain $50), the child has a range of behavioral options (e.g., find a job, mug someone). Choosing between these choices will be a function of, first, availability (e.g., whether a job/potential victim can be found) and, second, action costs (social punishment and the distress of the victims). In short, a child might choose an anti-social behavior because 1) he or she is under social/situational pressure to do so (the antisocial acts are simply the most viable options available), or 2) his or her calculation of the costs related to the actions/empathic responding is deficient.

Parental and peer moral socialization helps the developing child appropriately represent the costs of antisocial behavior. The ease with which a child can be socialized has been positively related to the temperamental variable of fearfulness (Kochanska 1997). The punishment that best achieves moral socialization is the victim's distress; empathy induction, focusing the transgressor's attention on the victim, particularly fosters moral socialization (Eisenberg 2002; Hoffman 1994). Poor empathic responding has been linked to heightened levels of PIP aggression (R.J. Blair 2001).

Given the role of socialization in specifying the costs of antisocial behavior to the developing child, we suspect that dysfunction in either the social processes (which will not be considered here) or the neural systems underlying socialization could lead to an increased risk of instrumental antisocial behavior. We believe psychopathy represents a disorder in which the neural systems underlying socialization are disrupted. As a concept, the modern understanding of psychopathy originates in a monograph by Hervey Cleckley titled *The Mask of Sanity* (1941). Cleckley believed that psychopaths display great charm but lack any ability to have good long-term social relations. He further argued that psychopaths lack any remorse, insight, or affective responses but, interestingly, are not delusional. They are egocentric and have an inability to form meaningful interpersonal relationships.

Psychopathy has behavioral components (e.g., criminal activity and poor behavioral control) but also important affective-interpersonal components (notably a lack of empathy and guilt; Frick et al. 1994; Harpur and Hare 1994). Moreover, while positive parenting techniques are associated with reduced antisocial behavior levels in healthy children, they have a reduced impact on antisocial behavior expressed by children who present with the emotional dysfunction associated with psychopathy (Wootton et al. 1997).

Psychopathy is not currently included in our diagnostic system and is not synonymous with a diagnosis of CD; probably only 10%–25% of those meeting criteria for a CD diagnosis would meet cutoffs for psychopathy (Kosson et al. 2002). While there have been concerns about the extension of this adult-based construct to child and adolescent populations (Edens et al. 2001), these principally concern decisions regarding placements for juveniles on the basis of psychopathy measures. We are sympathetic to these clinical concerns in the absence of a more extensive data set. However, the importance of this construct is its identification of a relatively homogeneous population (at least with respect to causal pathology) that shows a marked propensity for the display of proactive and reactive aggression (Frick et al. 2003). Indeed, the inclusion of the affective and interpersonal deficiencies suggests a pathophysiology that is specific to a subtype of individuals with CD that could refine the DSM criteria.

There appears to be a genetic contribution to the emotional dysfunction seen in psychopathy (Blonigen et al. 2005; Viding et al. 2005), although its impact at the molecular level remains unknown. At the systems level, at least two regions appear to be implicated in psychopathy: the amygdala and the medial orbital/ventrolateral prefrontal cortex.

The amygdala is crucial for moral socialization and empathic responding (R.J. Blair 2003). It allows the formation of stimulus–punishment associations (i.e., learning that an act is bad; Baxter and Murray 2002) and responds to the fear and sadness of others (Adolphs 2002). In short, the integrity of the amygdala is crucial for moral socialization and empathic responding (R.J. Blair 2003). Functional imaging studies in adults with psychopathic traits have found reduced amygdala activation in response to facial expressions (Gordon et al. 2004) and during the performance of emotional memory (Kiehl et al. 2001) and aversive conditioning tasks (Birbaumer et al. 2005). Moreover, considerable neuropsychological work shows that functions reliant on the amygdala's role in stimulus–reinforcement association are dysfunctional in children and adults with psychopathic tendencies (for reviews of this literature, see R.J. Blair 2003, 2006).

The amygdala provides stimulus–reinforcement information to the orbital and middle frontal cortex as expectancy information to guide behavioral choice (R.J. Blair 2006; Schoenbaum and Roesch 2005; Schoenbaum et al. 1999). It has been argued that the interaction between these regions is the basis of an individual's "moral intuitions" (Luo et al. 2006; see also Greene et al. 2004; Moll et al. 2002). Disruption in the interaction of these regions prevents the appropriate guiding of behavioral choice; individuals with psychopathy are less able to use information regarding the costs–benefits of their actions.

As noted above, the ability to change behavior following reinforcement contingency change is extremely important in avoiding frustration and consequent frustration-based reactive aggression (R.J. Blair 2004). Adolescents with psychopathic tendencies show impairment on response reversal paradigms (Budhani and Blair 2005). Response reversal requires the detection of the change in reinforcement schedule as well as the ability to activate the new alternative response. The amygdala and middle frontal cortex/orbitofrontal cortex (see Figure 20–1) appear crucial for detecting the contingency change, whereas the dorsomedial frontal and ventrolateral frontal cortex are important for selecting the new alternative response (Budhani et al. 2007). Behavioral work indicates that the problem children with psychopathic tendencies face is with the detection of the contingency change (Budhani and Blair 2005). Provisional neuroimaging work supports the implication that it is the response of the amygdala and middle frontal cortex/orbitofrontal cortex to punishment information that is particularly anomalous in this patient group. In short, we believe that disruption in the interaction of the amygdala and middle frontal cortex/orbitofrontal cortex is implicated in the increased risk for frustration-based reactive aggression seen in this population.

Forensic Implications

As the neuroscience of aggression evolves and develops, we can expect that there will be implications for the field of child and adolescent forensics. There are several clinical and judicial implications of the current scholarship on aggression and particularly on the emerging taxonomy of these disorder. First, our current nomenclature that is captured in DSM-IV-TR (American Psychiatric Association 2000) and the International Classification of Diseases, 10th Edition (ICD-10; World Health Organization 1992) does not fully consider the neuroscience of aggression in its classification of disruptive behaviors and disorders of aggression. RADI and PIP forms are largely conflated and combined under broader, less differentiated rubrics.

In criminology and jurisprudence, a parallel set of issues emerges wherein offenses are categorized by the nature of the act rather than the type of aggression presented. For example, killing another person in one setting might be a RADI-driven aggressive act that had an impulsive and angry response secondary to a wide range of factors (drugs, psychiatric illness, or self-defense), and in another setting the same act may be driven by PIP aggression that is premeditated and planned by the perpetrator. These two acts share the same result but differ remarkably in their etiology. Courts and prosecutors will consider differences by defining the act as either manslaughter or murder or by considering mitigating circumstances when it comes to sentencing, but the etiology of the aggression does not currently have a clear place in the adult criminal jurisprudence.

While juveniles charged with murder are typically prosecuted in adult criminal court where type of aggression has little to do with adjudications of guilt, for lesser crimes more typically prosecuted in juvenile court, such as aggravated assault or robbery, the nature of the aggression involved is more relevant. Juvenile courts are concerned with rehabilitation and treatment, in addition to punishment, and understanding of a juvenile defendant's violent act is highly relevant to juvenile court interventions.

RADI aggression, due to its nature, relationship to threat response circuits, and generally well-circumscribed pattern, offers some potential for providing a mitigating explanation of the aggression. Knowledge of the potential family, genetic, and environmental stressors in the aggressor's life might help to explain how this individual came to develop a pattern of RADI aggression. Such explanation would not provide a good basis for understanding a single aggressive act, but certainly in individuals with a consistent pattern of this type of aggression, forensic psychiatrists need to keep this consideration in mind because it can be a means to get these individuals into treatment, ideally with a combination of medications and psychotherapy.

In contrast, PIP aggression is far less likely to lead to an emphasis on treatment. The very nature of PIP aggression and its premeditated pattern make it far less defensible. Our present understanding of this form of aggression is very limited, but current treatment options focus on using highly structured settings such as prisons, group homes, and state hospitals as a means of trying to rehabilitate these individuals.

The neuroscience of juvenile aggression is a field that will continue to make contributions to our understanding of psychopathology among children and adolescents. To the extent that we can draw on this knowledge to reconceptualize our taxonomic structures, the greater the potential to create effective and targeted prevention, intervention, and treatment programs. These understandings also have the potential to help us reconsider the social and legal policies that impact these youth.

—Key Points

- — The neuroscience of aggression is a recent development, and the coming years will likely yield more insights and further understandings of relevance to forensic child and adolescent psychiatry and psychology.

- — The neurobiology of aggression can only be understood by also looking at contextual factors. We expect that gene expression–environmental processes will become more important.

- — There seem to be two functional pathways to aggression. One is characterized as reactive, affective, defensive, and impulsive (RADI), and the other is proactive, instrumental, and planned (PIP).

- — Mixed phenotypes with elements of both RADI and PIP aggression are possible.

- — Particular brain regions and neuronal pathways seem to associate with RADI and PIP forms of aggression.

- — Some instances of RADI aggression may provide mitigation for criminal behavior when examined from a forensic perspective.

- — PIP aggression likely requires longer-term treatment in highly structured settings.

References

Adolphs R: Neural systems for recognizing emotion. Curr Opin Neurobiol 12:169–177, 2002

American Psychiatric Association: Diagnostic and Statistical Manual of Mental Disorders, 4th Edition. Washington, DC, American Psychiatric Association, 1994

American Psychiatric Association: Diagnostic and Statistical Manual of Mental Disorders, 4th Edition, Text Revision. Washington, DC, American Psychiatric Association, 2000

Anderson SW, Bechara A, Damasio H, et al: Impairment of social and moral behavior related to early damage in human prefrontal cortex. Nat Neurosci 2:1032–1037, 1999

Barratt ES, Stanford MS, Dowdy L, et al: Impulsive and premeditated aggression: a factor analysis of self-reported acts. Psychiatry Res 86:163–173, 1999

Baxter MG, Murray EA: The amygdala and reward. Nat Rev Neurosci 3:563–573, 2002

Berkowitz L: Aggression: Its Causes, Consequences, and Control: McGraw-Hill Series in Social Psychology. New York, McGraw-Hill, 1993

Birbaumer N, Veit R, Lotze M, et al: Deficient fear conditioning in psychopathy: a functional magnetic resonance imaging study. Arch Gen Psychiatry 62:799–805, 2005

Blair J, Mitchell DR, Blair K: The Psychopath: Emotion and the Brain. Malden, MA, Blackwell, 2005

Blair RJ: Neurocognitive models of aggression, the antisocial personality disorders, and psychopathy. J Neurol Neurosurg Psychiatry 71:727–731, 2001

Blair RJ: Neurobiological basis of psychopathy. Br J Psychiatry 182:5–7, 2003

Blair RJ: The roles of orbital frontal cortex in the modulation of antisocial behavior. Brain Cogn 55:198–208, 2004

Blair RJ: The emergence of psychopathy: implications for the neuropsychological approach to developmental disorders. Cognition 101:414–442, 2006

Blanchard RJ, Blanchard DC, Takahashi T, et al: Attack and defensive behaviour in the albino rat. Anim Behav 25:622–634, 1977

Blonigen DM, Hicks BM, Krueger RF, et al: Psychopathic personality traits: heritability and genetic overlap with internalizing and externalizing psychopathology. Psychol Med 35:637–648, 2005

Book AS, Starzyk KB, Quinsey VL: The relationship between testosterone and aggression: a meta-analysis. Aggress Violent Behav 6:579–599, 2001

Budhani S, Blair RJ: Response reversal and children with psychopathic tendencies: success is a function of salience of contingency change. J Child Psychol Psychiatry 46:972–981, 2005

Budhani S, Marsh AA, Pine DS, et al: Neural correlates of response reversal: considering acquisition. Neuroimage 34:1754–1765, 2007

Bush G, Valera EM, Seidman LJ: Functional neuroimaging of attention-deficit/hyperactivity disorder: a review and suggested future directions. Biol Psychiatry 57:1273–1284, 2005

Bushman BJ, Anderson CA: Is it time to pull the plug on the hostile versus instrumental aggression dichotomy? Psychol Rev 108:273–279, 2001

Cadoret RJ, Cain CA, Crowe RR: Evidence for gene-environment interaction in the development of adolescent antisocial behavior. Behav Genet 13:301–310, 1983

Caspi A, McClay J, Moffitt TE, et al: Role of genotype in the cycle of violence in maltreated children. Science 297:851–854, 2002

Charney DS: Neuroanatomical circuits modulating fear and anxiety behaviors. Acta Psychiatr Scand Suppl (417):38–50, 2003

Cicchetti D, Cohen DJ: Developmental Psychopathology, 2nd Edition. Hoboken, NJ, Wiley, 2006

Cleckley HM: The Mask of Sanity: An Attempt to Reinterpret the So-Called Psychopathic Personality. St. Louis, MO, Mosby, 1941

Coccaro EF: Neurotransmitter correlates of impulsive aggression in humans. Ann NY Acad Sci 794:82–89, 1996

Coccaro EF: Impulsive aggression: a behavior in search of clinical definition. Harv Rev Psychiatry 5:336–339, 1998

Coccaro EF, Kavoussi RJ: Fluoxetine and impulsive aggressive behavior in personality-disordered subjects. Arch Gen Psychiatry 54:1081–1088, 1997

Connor DF: Aggression and Antisocial Behavior in Children and Adolescents: Research and Treatment. New York, Guilford, 2002

Connor DF, Carlson GA, Chang KD, et al: Juvenile maladaptive aggression: a review of prevention, treatment, and service configuration and a proposed research agenda. J Clin Psychiatry 67:808–820, 2006

Crick NR, Dodge KA: Social information-processing mechanisms in reactive and proactive aggression. Child Dev 67:993–1002, 1996

de Almeida RM, Ferrari PF, Parmigiani S, et al: Escalated aggressive behavior: dopamine, serotonin and GABA. Eur J Pharmacol 526:51–64, 2005

Deakin JFW, Graeff FG: 5-HT and mechanisms of defence. J Psychopharmacol 5:305–315, 1991

Dodge KA, Lochman JE, Harnish JD, et al: Reactive and proactive aggression in school children and psychiatrically impaired chronically assaultive youth. J Abnorm Psychol 106:37–51, 1997

Drevets WC: Neuroimaging abnormalities in the amygdala in mood disorders. Ann NY Acad Sci 985:420–444, 2003

Edens JF, Skeem JL, Cruise KR, et al: Assessment of "juvenile psychopathy" and its association with violence: a critical review. Behav Sci Law 19:53–80, 2001

Eisenberg N: Empathy-related emotional responses, altruism, and their socialization, in Visions of Compassion: Western Scientists and Tibetan Buddhists Examine Human Nature. Edited by Davidson RJ, Harrington A. New York, Oxford University Press, 2002, pp 131–164

Farrington DP: Psychosocial predictors of adult antisocial personality and adult convictions. Behav Sci Law 18:605–622, 2000

Ferris CF, Melloni RH Jr, Koppel G, et al: Vasopressin/serotonin interactions in the anterior hypothalamus control aggressive behavior in golden hamsters. J Neurosci 17:4331–4340, 1997

Ferry B, Roozendaal B, McGaugh JL: Involvement of alpha1-adrenoceptors in the basolateral amygdala in modulation of memory storage. Eur J Pharmacol 372:9–16, 1999

Frick PJ, O'Brien BS, Wootton JM, et al: Psychopathy and conduct problems in children. J Abnorm Psychol 103:700–707, 1994

Frick PJ, Cornell AH, Barry CT, et al: Callous-unemotional traits and conduct problems in the prediction of conduct problem severity, aggression, and self-report of delinquency. J Abnorm Child Psychol 31:457–470, 2003

Goldman-Rakic PS, Muly EC III, Williams GV: D(1) receptors in prefrontal cells and circuits. Brain Res Brain Res Rev 31:295–301, 2000

Gordon HL, Baird AA, End A: Functional differences among those high and low on a trait measure of psychopathy. Biol Psychiatry 56:516–521, 2004

Grafman J, Schwab K, Warden D, et al: Frontal lobe injuries, violence, and aggression: a report of the Vietnam Head Injury Study. Neurology 46:1231–1238, 1996

Greene JD, Nystrom LE, Engell AD, et al: The neural bases of cognitive conflict and control in moral judgment. Neuron 44:389–400, 2004

Gregg TR, Siegel A: Brain structures and neurotransmitters regulating aggression in cats: implications for human aggression. Prog Neuropsychopharmacol Biol Psychiatry 25:91–140, 2001

Hamson DK, Jones BA, Watson NV: Distribution of androgen receptor immunoreactivity in the brainstem of male rats. Neuroscience 127:797–803, 2004

Harpur TJ, Hare RD: Assessment of psychopathy as a function of age. J Abnorm Psychol 103:604–609, 1994

Hinshaw SP, Lee SS: Conduct and oppositional defiant disorders, in Child Psychopathology, 2nd Edition. Edited by Mash EJ, Barkley RA. New York, Guilford, 2003, pp 144–198

Hoffman ML: Discipline and internalization. Dev Psychol 30:26–28, 1994

Kagan J, Snidman N: Early childhood predictors of adult anxiety disorders. Biol Psychiatry 46:1536–1541, 1999

Kempes M, Matthys W, Maassen G, et al: A parent questionnaire for distinguishing between reactive and proactive aggression in children. Eur Child Adolesc Psychiatry 15:38–45, 2006

Kiehl KA, Smith AM, Hare RD, et al: Limbic abnormalities in affective processing by criminal psychopaths as revealed by functional magnetic resonance imaging. Biol Psychiatry 50:677–684, 2001

King SM: Escape-related behaviours in an unstable, elevated and exposed environment, II: long-term sensitization after repetitive electrical stimulation of the rodent midbrain defence system. Behav Brain Res 98:127–142, 1999

Kochanska G: Multiple pathways to conscience for children with different temperaments: from toddlerhood to age 5. Dev Psychol 33:228–240, 1997

Kosson DS, Cyterski TD, Steuerwald BL, et al: The reliability and validity of the Psychopathy Checklist: Youth Version (PCL:YV) in nonincarcerated adolescent males. Psychol Assess 14:97–109, 2002

Kringelbach ML, Rolls ET: Neural correlates of rapid reversal learning in a simple model of human social interaction. Neuroimage 20:1371–1383, 2003

Landgraf R, Gerstberger R, Montkowski A, et al: V1 vasopressin receptor antisense oligodeoxynucleotide into septum reduces vasopressin binding, social discrimination abilities, and anxiety-related behavior in rats. J Neurosci 15:4250–4258, 1995

Leibenluft E, Blair RJ, Charney DS, et al: Irritability in pediatric mania and other childhood psychopathology. Ann NY Acad Sci 1008:201–218, 2003

Linnoila M, Virkkunen M, Scheinin M, et al: Low cerebrospinal fluid 5-hydroxyindoleacetic acid concentration differentiates impulsive from nonimpulsive violent behavior. Life Sci 33:2609–2614, 1983

Luo Q, Nakic M, Wheatley T, et al: The neural basis of implicit moral attitude: an IAT study using event-related fMRI. Neuroimage 30:1449–1457, 2006

Meyer-Lindenberg A, Buckholtz JW, Kolachana B, et al: Neural mechanisms of genetic risk for impulsivity and violence in humans. Proc Natl Acad Sci USA 103:6269–6274, 2006

Miczek KA, Fish EW, De Bold JF: Neurosteroids, GABAA receptors, and escalated aggressive behavior. Horm Behav 44:242–257, 2003

Moll J, de Oliveira-Souza R, Bramati IE, et al: Functional networks in emotional moral and nonmoral social judgments. Neuroimage 16:696–703, 2002

New AS, Hazlett EA, Buchsbaum MS, et al: Blunted prefrontal cortical 18fluorodeoxyglucose positron emission tomography response to meta-chlorophenylpiperazine in impulsive aggression. Arch Gen Psychiatry 59:621–629, 2002

New AS, Buchsbaum MS, Hazlett EA, et al: Fluoxetine increases relative metabolic rate in prefrontal cortex in impulsive aggression. Psychopharmacology (Berl) 176:451–458, 2004

Norman D, Shallice T: Attention to action: willed and automatic control of behaviour, in Consciousness and Self-Regulation. Edited by Davidson RJ, Schwartz GE, Shapiro D. New York, Plenum Press, 1986, pp 1–18

O'Connor DB, Archer J, Hair WM, et al: Exogenous testosterone, aggression, and mood in eugonadal and hypogonadal men. Physiol Behav 75:557–566, 2002

O'Doherty J, Critchley H, Deichmann R, et al: Dissociating valence of outcome from behavioral control in human orbital and ventral prefrontal cortices. J Neurosci 23:7931–7939, 2003

Panksepp J: Affective Neuroscience: The Foundations of Human and Animal Emotions: Series in Affective Science. New York, Oxford University Press, 1998

Pernanen K: Alcohol in Human Violence: The Guilford Substance Abuse Series. New York, Guilford, 1991

Phelps EA, Delgado MR, Nearing KI, et al: Extinction learning in humans: role of the amygdala and vmPFC. Neuron 43:897–905, 2004

Pieribone VA, Nicholas AP, Dagerlind A, et al: Distribution of alpha 1 adrenoceptors in rat brain revealed by in situ hybridization experiments utilizing subtype-specific probes. J Neurosci 14:4252–4268, 1994

Pope HG Jr, Kouri EM, Hudson JI: Effects of supraphysiologic doses of testosterone on mood and aggression in normal men: a randomized controlled trial. Arch Gen Psychiatry 57:133–140, 2000

Poulin F, Boivin M: Reactive and proactive aggression: evidence of a two-factor model. Psychol Assess 12:115–122, 2000

Raine A: Biosocial Bases of Violence: NATO ASI Series. Series A, Life Sciences, Vol 292. New York, Plenum, 1997

Raine A: Biosocial studies of antisocial and violent behavior in children and adults: a review. J Abnorm Child Psychol 30:311–326, 2002

Raine A, Meloy JR, Bihrle S, et al: Reduced prefrontal and increased subcortical brain functioning assessed using positron emission tomography in predatory and affective murderers. Behav Sci Law 16:319–332, 1998

Rhee SH, Waldman ID: Genetic and environmental influences on antisocial behavior: a meta-analysis of twin and adoption studies. Psychol Bull 128:490–529, 2002

Riggins-Caspers KM, Cadoret RJ, Knutson JF, et al: Biology-environment interaction and evocative biology-environment correlation: contributions of harsh discipline and parental psychopathology to problem adolescent behaviors. Behav Genet 33:205–220, 2003

Rolls ET: The orbitofrontal cortex and reward. Cereb Cortex 10:284–294, 2000

Schoenbaum G, Roesch M: Orbitofrontal cortex, associative learning, and expectancies. Neuron 47:633–636, 2005

Schoenbaum G, Chiba AA, Gallagher M: Neural encoding in orbitofrontal cortex and basolateral amygdala during olfactory discrimination learning. J Neurosci 19:1876–1884, 1999

Shah AA, Sjovold T, Treit D: Inactivation of the medial prefrontal cortex with the GABA_A receptor agonist muscimol increases open-arm activity in the elevated plus-maze and attenuates shock-probe burying in rats. Brain Res 1028:112–115, 2004

Shiffrin RM, Schneider W: Controlled and automatic human information processing, II: perceptual learning, automatic attending, and a general theory. Psychol Rev 84:127–190, 1977

Steiner H: Practice parameters for the assessment and treatment of children and adolescents with conduct disorder. J Am Acad Child Adolesc Psychiatry 36:122S–139S, 1997

Steiner H: Disruptive behavior disorders, in Comprehensive Textbook of Psychiatry, Vol 2. Edited by Kaplan HI, Sadock BJ. New York, Williams & Wilkins, 1999, pp 2693–2703.

Steiner H: Handbook of Mental Health Interventions in Children and Adolescents: An Integrated Developmental Approach. San Francisco, CA, Jossey-Bass, 2004

Steiner H, Remsing L: Practice parameter for the assessment and treatment of children and adolescents with oppositional defiant disorder. J Am Acad Child Adolesc Psychiatry 46:126–141, 2007

Steiner H, Garcia IG, Matthews Z: Posttraumatic stress disorder in incarcerated juvenile delinquents. J Am Acad Child Adolesc Psychiatry 36:357–365, 1997

Steiner H, Saxena K, Chang K: Psychopharmacologic strategies for the treatment of aggression in juveniles. CNS Spectr 8:298–308, 2003

Steiner H, Saxena K, Medic S, et al: Proactive and reactive aggression and psychopathology in high school students. Paper presented at the annual meeting of the American Psychiatric Association, Atlanta, GA, May 2005

Swann AC: Neuroreceptor mechanisms of aggression and its treatment. J Clin Psychiatry 64 (suppl 4):26–35, 2003

Viding E, Blair RJ, Moffitt TE, et al: Evidence for substantial genetic risk for psychopathy in 7-year-olds. J Child Psychol Psychiatry 46:592–597, 2005

Vitaro F, Gendreau PL, Tremblay RE, et al: Reactive and proactive aggression differentially predict later conduct problems. J Child Psychol Psychiatry 39:377–385, 1998

Volkow ND, Tancredi LR, Grant C, et al: Brain glucose metabolism in violent psychiatric patients: a preliminary study. Psychiatry Res 61:243–253, 1995

Volkow ND, Wang GJ, Franceschi D, et al: Low doses of alcohol substantially decrease glucose metabolism in the human brain. Neuroimage 29:295–301, 2006

Weisman AM, Berman ME, Taylor SP: Effects of clorazepate, diazepam, and oxazepam on a laboratory measurement of aggression in men. Int Clin Psychopharmacol 13:183–188, 1998

Wootton JM, Frick PJ, Shelton KK, et al: Ineffective parenting and childhood conduct problems: the moderating role of callous-unemotional traits. J Consult Clin Psychol 65:301–308, 1997

World Health Organization: International Statistical Classification of Diseases and Related Health Problems, 10th Revision. Geneva, World Health Organization, 1992

Zoccolillo M: Co-occurrence of conduct disorder and its adult outcomes with depressive and anxiety disorders: a review. J Am Acad Child Adolesc Psychiatry 31:547–556, 1992

Chapter 21

Assessing Violence Risk in Youth

Randy Borum, Psy.D., ABPP

Most clinicians who work with children and adolescents can easily remember an instance when they were concerned that a young patient might engage in violent behavior. Nearly all forms of youth violence in the United States increased sharply between the mid-1980s and the mid-1990s. The number of juvenile homicides nearly doubled. The rates of juvenile violence and homicide have since dropped considerably, but there is still cause for concern (Borum 2000; Hoge et al. 2008; U.S. Department of Health and Human Services 2001). Violent and aggressive behavior among children and adolescents is vexing, but it is also quite common.

Mental health professionals are often required or called upon to assess and offer an opinion about a young person's risk for future violence. Sometimes risk assessment is the explicit purpose of the evaluation or clinical encounter, but at other times it is not. Treating clinicians in outpatient and inpatient settings regularly face these issues during treatment or discharge planning. Forensic clinicians are asked specifically for risk assessments, particularly when a young person is charged with criminal or delinquent activity. Increasingly, even professionals who work in or consult with schools are asked to assess a student's propensity for violence.

The clinical and professional challenges of assessing violence risk in youth are substantial but not insurmountable. The fluidity of even normal developmental changes in cognition, affect, and physical status complicates any attempt to forecast a specific behavioral outcome. In essence, it makes a difficult as-

sessment even harder. But with a clear understanding of the task, a foundation of specialized knowledge, and a systematic method or plan for the assessment, clinicians can confidently arrive at a decision that serves both therapeutic and public safety interests. This chapter charts a course with those markers in mind.

Context of Juvenile Violence

It does not surprise most child and adolescent mental health professionals to learn that delinquent—even violent—behavior in adolescence is common and that the teen years are the peak developmental risk period for initiating (first episode) an act of serious violence. The extent of the behavior, however, may be surprising. Most young people are not convicted or even arrested for a violent crime, but official arrest statistics offer an overly narrow view of the problem. If one looks at self-report data, for example, estimates are that about one in four girls and nearly half of all boys in high school report being in a physical fight one or more times in the prior 12 months (Kann et al. 1998; U.S. Department of Health and Human Services 2001). These rates certainly exceed what one might expect from estimates of community-dwelling adults. The good news is that most of this youthful aggression and violence does not continue into adulthood. After age 17 years, violence participation rates drop dramatically, and about 80% of those who are violent during adolescence will stop engaging in violent behavior by age 21 years (Elliott et al. 1983; U.S. Department of Health and Human Services 2001).

Having higher rates of violence, however, is only one of the ways in which violence risk is different in juveniles than in adults. Assessing children and adolescents is somewhat like trying to hit a moving target. Change is constant, and the rate and timing of developmental markers are difficult to predict (Borum 2003; Borum and Verhaagen 2006; Griffin and Torbet 2002; Grisso 1998; McCord et al. 2001; Rosado 2000). Because their identity and personality are nascent, young people's behavioral patterns and styles are generally less consistent than in adults (Grisso 1998). The hormonal vicissitudes of puberty, psychosocial immaturity, and not yet fully developed inhibitory brain structures make behavioral forecasting all the more uncertain (Borum and Grisso 2006; Steinberg and Cauffman 1999).

Understanding Youth Violence

Behavioral scientists still have a lot to learn about violent behavior in children and adolescents, but clinicians certainly can benefit from the current state of the art. In particular, it is useful to understand some basic differences among types of aggression and to separate risk factors based on empirical evidence from those based on erroneous lore.

Types of Aggression

There may be as many different definitions for violence as there are people to define it. The nuances of those differences may not be critically important for clinical risk assessments; however, it is important for the evaluator to have some clear working definition so that he or she knows what *kind* of risk is being assessed. The basic point is simple: there are different types of aggression and different types of risk. One useful distinction for the evaluator is that between reactive and proactive aggression (see Chapter 20, "Taxonomy and Neurobiology of Aggression"). Fundamentally, reactive aggression is characterized as an angry, impulsive, retaliatory response to a real or perceived provocation, whereas proactive aggression is unprovoked, deliberate, and goal directed. While the consequences of either type can be serious, different patterns of thought, mood, and behavior tend to drive and sustain each type.

The main cognitive driver of reactive aggression is a marked and pervasive tendency to perceive that others are acting with hostile intent, even when no such motivation is present. In proactive aggression, the troubling cognitions tend to be rooted in a youth's beliefs that aggression will get the youth what he or she wants and that other strategies will probably not work as well. The youth has come to see aggression as effective and, to some extent, legitimate. Affectively, reactive aggression tends to involve a response of angry arousal that is often uncharacteristic of proactive aggression. Finally, episodes of reactive aggression are behaviorally impulsive ("hot"), whereas proactive events tend to be more deliberate ("cold"). This distinction is not meant to imply that there are only two kinds of aggression or two types of offenders but to illustrate how a more nuanced and functional understanding of violent and aggressive behaviors can facilitate better assessment and treatment.

One reason to understand this distinction is that interventions for reactive and proactive aggression are likely to be quite different. For example, it may not be very effective to prescribe anger management training to reduce violence risk in a youngster with an exclusive pattern of proactive aggression. Likewise, interventions to enhance empathy or diminish antisocial attitudes may meet with less success in an impulsive youngster whose only acts of aggression are angry and reactive.

Risk Factors

Evaluators must understand not only the dynamics of interpersonal violence but also what information to gather, how to gather it, and, ultimately, how to make a professional decision about risk. Knowing what information to gather may seem relatively straightforward, but limitations and biases in human judgment and inaccuracies in clinical lore can complicate the process. For example, some clinicians have been exposed to the idea that there is a "terrible triad" of risk factors—bed wetting, fire setting, and cruelty to animals—that uniquely predicts a particularly heinous pattern of violence such as serial murder. There is not, however, good empirical evidence to support the synergy of this triad. Research, however, has revealed an array of clinical, historical, and social contextual factors that may increase (risk factors) or decrease (protective factors) the likelihood of engaging in violence (Borum and Verhaagen 2006; Cottle et al. 2001; Derzon 2001; Hawkins et al. 1998; Jenson and Howard 1999; Howell 1997; Lipsey and Derzon 1998; Loeber and Stouthamer-Loeber 1998). Table 21–1 shows some of the risk factors that have a consistent base of research support.

It is important to note that this list includes both static factors, which are historical or dispositional and not amenable to change, and dynamic factors, which are potentially changeable or subject to modification. Because static factors often are discretely measurable, they tend to receive the most research attention. And because, by definition, they are stable over time, they also tend to show some of the most robust and consistent empirical links to violence. The dynamic factors, however, may be no less important in understanding and mitigating risk in any given case and are a vital part of any clinical or forensic risk assessment. Clinicians might also be aware that the nature and magnitude of risk factors' links to violence also change somewhat over the course of a young person's development. A prime example is in social influences. For young children, parental factors tend to have stronger predictive power than they do for adolescents, whereas for teens the influence of peers is substantially stronger.

One particular risk factor for youth violence that has received a great deal of attention over the past 15 years is the construct of psychopathy. Psychopathy is an antisocial personality syndrome or orientation characterized by a pervasive lifelong pattern of transgressive behavior, deficient emotional experience, and a callous interpersonal style. Most of the existing research on psychopathy has been conducted with adults. Though the syndrome's etiology is multiply determined and not yet completely understood, it is conventionally believed to be a lifelong disorder. This assumption led some researchers to search for early signs and ways to measure the construct in children and adolescents. What ensued was a fairly productive line of research showing that the behavioral, emotional, and interpersonal traits associated with psychopathy in adults could also be reliably measured in youth. Most of those studies also found that these traits were linked empirically to violent behavior. The debate among clinicians and researchers, however, centers on whether that measurable cluster of psychopathy-related behavioral, emotional, and interpersonal traits can be a reliable and valid marker of psychopathy as a disorder when it is assessed in children and adolescents. There are studies showing that the traits fluctuate through adolescence more than they do in adulthood. The issue has not yet reached a clear, empirically based resolution. The traits of antisocial

TABLE 21–1. Research-based risk factors for youth violence from the U.S. Surgeon General's Report on Youth Violence

Early onset (ages 6–11 years) of general delinquent offenses and substance use (has a large effect in predicting *adolescent* violence)

Weak social ties

Antisocial, delinquent peers

Gang membership

Male gender

Low socioeconomic status/poverty

Antisocial parents

Aggression (for males)

Psychological condition

Hyperactivity

Poor parent–child relations

Harsh, lax, or inconsistent discipline

Abusive or neglectful parents

Problem (antisocial) behavior

Exposure to television violence

Poor attitude toward or poor performance in school

Low IQ

Broken home/separation from parents

Antisocial attitudes and beliefs

Risk taking

Source. The U.S. Surgeon General's Report on Youth Violence (U.S. Department of Health and Human Services 2001).

behavior and low empathy/remorse do appear to be risk factors for violence in youth, but whether psychopathy per se is discernible at such a young age remains to be seen.

Protective Factors

Although there are thousands of studies on risk factors for juvenile violence and at least hundreds on antisocial personality traits in youth, there is remarkably little empirical study of protective factors for violence and antisocial behavior (McCord et al. 2001; U.S. Department of Health and Human Services 2001). A protective factor is not simply the absence of a risk factor (e.g., no history of violence). Rather, it is the positive presence of some person, characteristic, or circumstance that can act to reduce the negative impact of one or more risk factors or otherwise directly buffer risk (Jessor et al. 1995). Howell (1997) identified three classes of protective factors: 1) factors inherent in the individual, 2) factors related to the development of social bonding, and 3) healthy beliefs and clear standards for behavior. The topic of resilience (i.e., having good outcomes despite exposure to bad risk factors) has started to generate some interest among researchers, but too often a youth's potential strengths, supports, and positive attributes are overlooked or undervalued when the issue of violence risk is considered. Studies that have examined the role of protective factors in youth violence risk have found them to have significant predictive value. They certainly deserve clinical attention and due consideration when appraising a young person's potential for violence.

Case Example

Justin was a 17-year-old boy who had been dating Emma for nearly 2 years. She was his "first." As they approached decisions about attending college, however, Emma expressed a desire to "go away to school," while Justin wished for them both to attend a local community college. They argued about the issue for a couple of months before Emma concluded they were "different people" and decided to break up with him. Justin felt "crushed" and emotionally devastated, even contemplating (and threatening) suicide. His parents made an appointment for him to see Dr. Williams for counseling. After a while, Emma began dating another boy. Justin seethed with jealous anger. He would secretly follow them on dates and would then ruminate about her "betrayal." In one of the counseling sessions, Justin told Dr. Williams that he had taken a knife with him when he followed them and would sometimes close his eyes and "imagine what it would be like to kill them both in the act."

Dr. Williams faced a troublesome but not uncommon dilemma, first in deciding whether Justin posed an actual risk of imminent harm, and second, if so, in deciding what to do about it. For many child and adolescent clinicians, this kind of situation evokes memories of the now-famous *Tarasoff* case. While most remember hearing about the case at some point, many are understandably unclear about what—if anything—it means for them.

In the facts leading up to the *Tarasoff* case, a psychologist at a university counseling center was counseling a male student who informed the psychologist of his wish or intent to harm a woman whose name he did not mention but who was ostensibly identifiable as Tatiana Tarasoff. At the time, Ms. Tarasoff was in Brazil. The psychologist and his supervising psychiatrist called the campus police, who questioned the student-client and released him because he seemed rational and reportedly promised them that he would not harm Ms. Tarasoff. When Ms. Tarasoff returned to California 2 months later, however, the student-client killed her.

This case did not "fall through the cracks." The psychologist clearly was concerned about the student-client's potential for violence and took action. The legal question was whether that action was reasonable and sufficient. Although many mental health professionals still associate the *Tarasoff* case with a "duty to warn," the ultimate duty recognized and imposed by the Supreme Court of California (not the U.S. Supreme Court) was actually "a duty to protect" (*Tarasoff II, Tarasoff v. Regents of the University of California* 1976). The essence of the court's ruling was that when a mental health professional determines—or, pursuant to the standards of his or her profession, should determine—that a client presents a serious danger of violence to another, the mental health professional incurs a duty to use reasonable care to protect the victim. The question of what constitutes reasonable care was said to depend on the particular facts of the case. In *Tarasoff*, the Supreme Court of California thought the psychologist did not do enough.

The *Tarasoff* ruling does not apply everywhere. The duty to protect doctrine has been interpreted in a variety of ways in different jurisdictions (Buckner and Firestone 2000). Some states have adopted *Tarasoff*, others have modified the duty (more broadly or more narrowly), and some have rejected completely the notion that a mental health professional should have any duty to protect third parties from harm—foreseeable or not—by a client or patient.

In any event, the *Tarasoff* case was not prompted by an incorrect prediction. Likewise, in the therapy-based encounter with young Justin in the case example, Dr. Williams did not face a "duty to predict." The fundamental preliminary task was to assess the relevant facts to determine whether there was a reasonable basis for clinical concern about Justin's potential for violence. One heuristic device for assessing these facts is represented by the acronym ACTION (Borum and Reddy 2001; see also Borum et al. 1999; Fein and Vossekuil 1998; Fein et al. 1995), which consists of the following elements (Borum and Reddy 2003):

A—attitudes that support or facilitate violence
C—capacity
T—thresholds crossed
I—intent

O—others' reactions

N—noncompliance with risk reduction interventions

Dr. Williams used this framework to gather additional information while maintaining the therapeutic posture of her interaction. Knowing that social psychology research shows that a person's intent to engage in a particular behavior is based, in part, on the nature and strength of attitudes toward that behavior (Ajzen 1985; Jemmott et al. 2001), she asked about whether and how Justin might feel justified in acting violently and if he believed that such action would resolve a particular problem.

Regarding Justin's capacity for violence, Dr. Williams knew that he was cognitively organized and intellectually capable of planning and delivering an attack, and she also heard him describe the knife he had previously taken along while spying on his ex-girlfriend, so she was reasonably sure that he had access to the weapon he had considered using. Dr. Williams also knew that Justin had already crossed certain behavioral thresholds in his consideration of violence. He had acquired and transported a weapon while physically following and mentally rehearsing the act. He had not said that he had a specific plan for when (or even whether) he would attack, but it was clear that his was more than just a transient idea or passing thought.

Dr. Williams sensed a need to better understand whether the attack was something Justin had only thought about and dismissed or whether he intended to act. She wanted to know how committed Justin was in his own mind to taking violent action. She asked Justin what thought he had given to the potential consequences of violence and about what alternative actions or strategies he had considered. Her concern deepened when he said that he didn't care, that he thought he had nothing to lose (since Emma had already rejected him), and that "at the end of it all I might just be dead myself anyway. I might as well be. I feel like it." As Dr. Williams explored the possible influence of others' reactions and responses, she found that some of Justin's friends had been fueling his anger at Emma and "egging him on." Finally, Dr. Williams did not really assess Justin as being noncompliant with risk reduction attempts. They seemed to have a good therapeutic alliance, and Justin kept his appointments and participated willingly, yet she was concerned by his hopelessness and "nothing to lose" mentality. While he was willing to participate in treatment, his demoralization and anger seemed to be clouding his judgment about how things could potentially be better for him in the future.

Dr. Williams judged that she had a reasonable basis for clinical concern about Justin's potential for violence and set to thinking about appropriate options for intervention. Using the ACTION framework helped her calmly and systematically gather the information she needed to make a reasonable professional assessment. It also gave clarity and transparency to the basis for her judgment. She could articulate and document not only that she was concerned but also why, based on a professional assessment, she determined that such concern was warranted. In this circumstance, was the therapist making a categorical "prediction" that the client would be violent? No. Her clinical objective was not to predict per se but rather to assess risk in the current situation.

Dr. Williams's behavior-based approach also helped her to avoid the problem in simply relying on a direct threat as an indicator of risk. It is certainly true that if a young person directly threatens a potential target with violence, the clinician should treat that communication seriously. Threats of violence, however, should not be regarded as a necessary factor for determining risk. Fein and Vossekuil (1998) suggested that, in assessing risk for targeted violence, it is important to distinguish between *making a threat* (i.e., communicating an intent to harm) and *posing a threat* (i.e., engaging in behavior that indicates furthering a plan or building capacity for a violent act, such as discussing attack plans with others or acquiring weapons). Although some people who make threats ultimately pose threats, many do not. Similarly, a client may pose a threat of harm to an identifiable victim, as Justin did, even if he or she has not made a direct threat. Persons judged to pose a threat should provoke the greatest level of concern.

Forensic Risk Assessments

Although risk concerns sometimes emerge in therapy, other times child and adolescent mental health professionals are specifically requested to assess a young person's potential for violence. These assessments also require a thoughtful and systematic approach, although typically the evaluator has more access to collateral information, and the nature of the appraisal and relevant time frame may be broader. The general procedures and professional requirements for conducting a forensic assessment are covered elsewhere in this volume (see Chapter 3, "Introduction to Forensic Evaluations"), but a couple of points specific to assessing risk are worth noting here.

An important first step in any forensic risk assessment is for the evaluator to specify as clearly as possible the purpose of the referral and the nature of the question. If the referral involves relevant legal definitions or thresholds, it is important that the evaluator determine how the referral source interprets those terms and standards. The evaluator should also make clear reference to those definitions in the assessment report. The point here is to establish a good "fit" between the information needed and the assessment provided and also to make any assumptions and legal points of reference as transparent as possible.

The next step is to develop a plan for systematically collecting risk-related information and for making and communicating a decision. Being not just thorough but systematic is essential for success, particularly in forensic risk assessments (Borum and Verhaagen 2006; Hoge 2002; Hoge and Andrews 1996). Unsystematic assessments often result in decisions that are inaccurate, inequitable, and lacking in accountability (Borum 2006; Hoge 2002). This happens, in part, because without proper structure, evaluators tend to rely on factors that do not have a demonstrated relationship to violence recidivism and overlook some of the factors that do (Borum 1996; Borum et al. 1993; Cooper and Werner 1990; Werner et al. 1983, 1989). Wiebush et al. (1995) noted: "Historically, risk assessments and classifications have been informal, highly discretionary procedures carried out by individuals who have varying philosophies and different levels of experience and knowledge, and who use dissimilar criteria in the assessment process" (p. 173).

Risk Assessment Instruments

Within the past decade, several instruments have emerged that help evaluators to structure their assessments and that facilitate more reliable and valid risk judgments. Some of these tools follow a "best practice" trend in applied risk assessment technology by building on the structured professional judgment (SPJ) assessment model (Lewis and Webster 2004). In the SPJ model, an evaluator systematically assesses a set of predetermined risk factors that have demonstrated significant empirical relationships with criterion violence in prior research. Each risk factor is considered and coded for severity, but the ultimate determination of risk level is made on the basis of the examiner's professional judgment, not a particular cutting score derived from summing the items. In this way, the SPJ model increases consistency and draws on the strengths of both the clinical and actuarial approaches

to decision making. The assessment is structured, systematic, empirically based, and yet sensitive to case-specific facts and situational influences. Some studies have found that professional risk judgments made with these tools are more accurate than unstructured clinical judgments, and sometimes even more predictive than the sum of the risk factors themselves (Dempster 1998; Hanson 1998; Kropp et al. 1999; Webster et al. 2002).

Just to be clear, these risk assessment instruments are not conventional psychological tests like the Minnesota Multiphasic Personality Inventory, designed to assess personality or clinical/diagnostic syndromes. Rather, they are guides for structuring the assessment itself. A key advantage of these tools is that they can improve not only assessments but also risk management. Moreover, their use does not require the same degree of clinical or psychometric expertise as do clinical psychological tests. Three of these risk assessment instruments designed specifically for use with children and adolescents are the Structured Assessment of Violence Risk in Youth (SAVRY), the Early Assessment Risk List (EARL), and the Youth Level of Service/Case Management Inventory (YLS/CMI). The SAVRY focuses specifically on violence risk, whereas the EARL (an SPJ instrument) and YLS/CMI focus more generally on delinquency and antisocial behaviors. (See also Chapter 5, "Special Education: Screening Tools, Rating Scales, and Self-Report Instruments," and Chapter 6, "Psychological Testing in Child and Adolescent Forensic Evaluations," in this volume.)

Structured Assessment of Violence Risk in Youth (SAVRY)

The SAVRY (Borum et al. 2005) focuses on violence risk in adolescents. The SAVRY protocol is composed of 24 risk items, divided into three categories (historical, social/contextual, and individual/clinical), and 6 protective items (Table 21–2). The risk items have a three-level coding structure (high, moderate, and low), and the protective items have a two-level structure (present or absent). Specific coding guidelines are provided for each level. The identified risk factors all have been reviewed, analyzed, and well documented in the professional literature. The SAVRY has been translated into Dutch, Swedish, Finnish, German, Spanish, Catalan, and Norwegian. It has been researched and used throughout North America and Europe as well as Singapore. Analyses of the SAVRY's psychometric properties show good to excellent agreement between raters; good concurrent validity with the YLS/CMI (Hoge and Andrews 2002) and the Hare Psychopathy

TABLE 21–2. Items from the Structured Assessment of Violence Risk in Youth (SAVRY)

Historical risk factors

History of violence

History of nonviolent offending

Early initiation of violence

Past supervision/intervention failures

History of self-harm or suicide attempts

Exposure to violence in the home

Childhood history of maltreatment

Parental/caregiver criminality

Early caregiver disruption

Poor school achievement

Social/contextual risk factors

Peer delinquency

Peer rejection

Stress and poor coping

Poor parental management

Lack of personal/social support

Community disorganization

Individual/clinical risk factors

Negative attitudes

Risk taking/impulsivity

Substance use difficulties

Anger management problems

Low empathy/remorse

Attention-deficit/hyperactivity difficulties

Poor compliance

Low interest in/commitment to school

Protective factors

Prosocial involvement

Strong social support

Strong attachment and bonds to prosocial adult

Positive attitude toward intervention and authority

Strong commitment to school

Resilient personality traits

Checklist: Youth Version (Forth et al. 2003); incremental predictive value over both of these other two instruments; and robust, moderate to strong predictive validity for violent offending and general offending (Borum et al., in press).

Early Assessment Risk List for Boys (EARL-20B)

The EARL-20B (Augimeri et al. 2001) is an SPJ tool designed to aid evaluators in making judgments about future violence and antisocial behavior among boys under the age 12 years, particularly those who exhibit behavioral problems and are considered to be at high risk. Each of the 20 risk items is assigned a score of 0, 1, or 2 depending on the certainty and severity of the characteristic's presence in a given case. Items are divided into three categories, including 6 family items (household circumstances, caregiver continuity, supports, stressors, parenting style, and antisocial values and conduct), 12 child items (developmental problems, onset of behavioral difficulties, abuse/neglect/trauma, hyperactivity/impulsivity/attention deficits, likeability, peer socialization, academic performance, neighborhood, authority contact, antisocial attitudes, antisocial behavior, and coping ability), and 2 responsivity items (family responsivity and child responsivity). Preliminary studies show evidence of good interrater reliability and predictive validity (Kogel et al. 2000). A parallel measure—the EARL-21G—exists for assessing risk in young girls. Although the domain names are the same, a few of the risk factors are different from the version for boys. Results of a preliminary unpublished study also show promising psychometric characteristics (Levene et al. 2001).

Youth Level of Service/Case Management Inventory (YLS/CMI)

The YLS/CMI (Hoge and Andrews 2002) is not an SPJ instrument but is a structured quantitative tool for assessing risk, need, and protective factors related to a juvenile's risk for general delinquent reoffending. The instrument is structured as a checklist of 42 items, grouped into eight domains: offense history, family circumstances/parenting, education, peer relations, substance abuse, leisure/recreation, personality/behavior, and attitudes. Items were selected based on their theoretical and empirical support in the literature. Importantly, the YLS/CMI also includes a comprehensive assessment of strengths. Each item is defined and assigned a risk level, but the item coding is somewhat less detailed than with most SPJ instruments. The other significant structural difference between the YLS/CMI and SPJ is that YLS/CMI scores are explicitly linked to decision making. In this way, it operates more like a formal actuarial tool (Grove and Meehl 1996). Scores are tallied and matched to a corresponding percentile ranking based on "norms" from a juvenile sample. The manual suggests that certain score/percentile ranges should correspond to specified levels of relative risk and that those risk levels should guide the nature and intensity of supervision and intervention in the case. Existing research on the YLS/CMI attests to its reliability and validity (Hoge and Andrews 2002; Hoge et al. 1996).

Risk Judgments and Communication

Once the evaluator has collected historical and background information and assessed the relevant risk factors, it is necessary to formulate and communicate a risk judgment. Although having more risk factors generally may increase the likelihood of aggression or violence, there is no "cookbook" approach or generic formula for deciding absolute or relative degrees of risk in all cases. The evaluator must consider and weigh the empirically based historical and dynamic risk factors, the facts of the current situation, and risk indicators that may be specific to the individual case. A systematic consideration of research-based risk and protective factors, however, can help the clinician to anchor a more accurate appraisal of violence risk.

Some clinicians find it useful to use a graphic model or heuristic device as a first step for guiding a judgment of relative risk. Figure 21–1 presents one example of a kind of flowchart (though certainly not an algorithm) with an array of risk factors that might help to guide an appraisal of risk.

In the first step, one determines whether the youth has an "early starter" history of violence and serious antisocial behavior. Early onset of violent offending is one of the strongest markers of likelihood and severity of future violence. Next, the evaluator might consider whether the youth has a co-occurring disruptive behavior disorder (or serious problems related to such a disorder), such as conduct disorder or attention-deficit/hyperactivity disorder, and/or has marked affective deficits resulting in low empathy and impaired capacity for remorse. In the third step, attention is given to whether the youth has engaged in serious violence during adolescence because recency of past violent behavior is associated with risk of future violent behavior.

The next phase of the flowchart is composed of three dynamic risk areas. The first of these considers the presence of delinquent peers/associates, a factor that is particularly robust for teens as opposed to children. The second accounts for the presence of antisocial attitudes, particularly those that would condone or support the use of violence as a legitimate strategy to solve problems or achieve a goal. The third dynamic risk area focuses on the presence of serious problems at home and/or at school.

A second heuristic is drawn from the work of Andrews and Bonta (2003), who have elucidated

> a general personality and social psychology of criminal conduct [i.e., a PCC] that has conceptual, empirical and practical value within and across social arrangements, clinical categories, and various personal and justice contexts....The PCC seeks a rational and empirical understanding of variation in the occurrence of criminal acts and, in particular, a rational empirical understanding of individual differences in criminal activity. (p. 2)

They identified four risk factor domains that have a robust conceptual and empirical relationship to criminal and violent offending: antisocial attitudes, antisocial associates, history of antisocial behavior, and antisocial personality traits. Andrews and Bonta referred to these as the "Big Four." They secondarily recognized the contribution of "problematic conditions in the domains of home, school, work, and leisure" (p. 10). The PCC was developed for criminal conduct more generally and was not designed to apply specifically to juveniles, but the core concepts are quite consistent with the empirical literature on youth violence.

The associated heuristic might be regarded as a theory-based approach that considers the range and severity of clusters of highly robust risk factors. The first step is to determine whether significant problems or risk factors exist in each of the Big Four domains. The next step is to determine their severity and relative importance in the case. As a guideline for gauging risk, if the clinician determines that serious problems exist across all four domains, it may be reasonable to work from the presumption that this indicates a high-risk case. It may not necessarily be one, but this strategy prompts the evaluator to reason carefully and explicitly through the weighty burden of ominous risk factors.

Once the evaluator has reached a decision or derived a clinical opinion about violence risk, there is often a need to communicate that appraisal either to an-

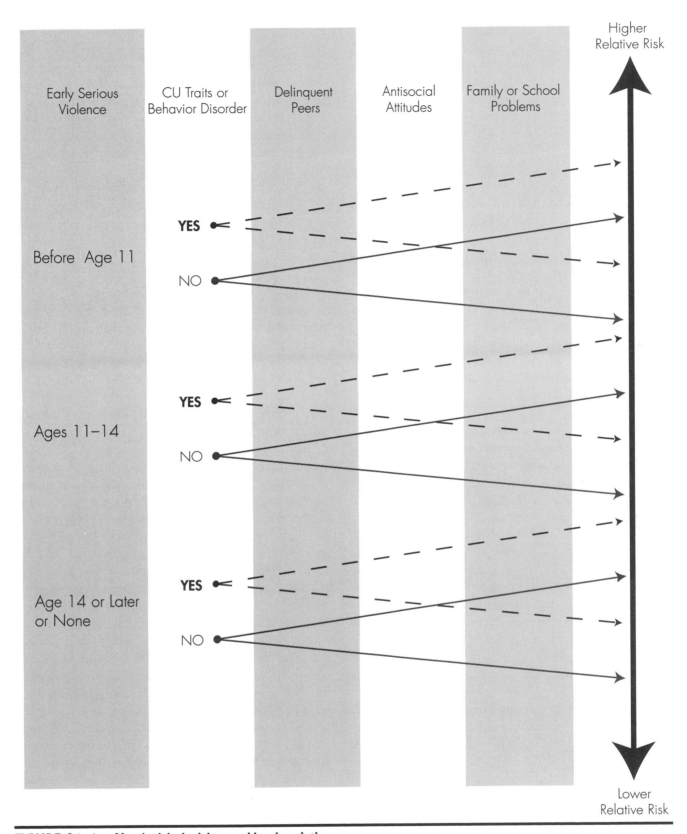

FIGURE 21–1. Youth risk decision-making heuristic.

Note. CU = callous/unemotional.

other clinician or to the legal system in forensic cases. This process is sometimes referred to as *risk communication* (Monahan and Steadman 1996). Heilbrun et al. (2000, p. 138) described risk communication as "the link between risk assessment and decision making about risk." They outlined three common forms of risk communication: descriptive, prediction-oriented, and management-oriented.

With descriptive risk communication, the evaluator identifies and lists the risk factors present in the case but does not go further to draw any inferences about the likelihood of future offending. For example, a descriptive conclusion might say: "Johnny is a 17-year-old male with a history of one prior assault who has no substance abuse problems, shows no major thinking or mood disorders, and demonstrates no significant deficiencies in capacity for empathy."

Prediction-oriented risk communication strategies are commonly used in clinical and forensic practice. These communications do make a direct statement about degree of risk or the likelihood of future violence. The estimates may be framed in either absolute (e.g., 75% likelihood) or relative (moderate risk/likelihood) terms.

Management-oriented risk communication recognizes that risk assessment and management are integrated functions and that the ultimate goal of a risk assessment is to reduce risk and thereby prevent violence (Douglas and Kropp 2002). There is a greater descriptive emphasis not only on the likelihood but also on the nature of that risk and its contingencies. The application of this approach might look something like this: "In my clinical opinion, Johnny's risk of committing an act of violence is dependent on the following factors: (list identified dynamic/situational/ environmental risk factors). In my opinion, Johnny's risk for violence over the next several months may be (slightly/moderately/substantially) reduced by (list interventions that address each risk factor)."

Research has found that clinicians tend to favor the management-oriented form of communication, followed by the descriptive and finally the prediction-oriented approaches. The prediction-oriented style is valued less by clinicians because they question whether the current state of the science can reasonably justify an absolute prediction of future violence. If it does not, then to offer one might be misleading or improper.

It is possible to soften and clarify a relative risk appraisal by anchoring the comparison to a particular reference group or average rate of reoffending, and per-haps even to blend this with risk reduction and management-oriented information. For example, one might say: "In my clinical opinion, relative to other first-time juvenile offenders on community supervision, Johnny is at low/moderate/high risk of committing an act of violence (within the next __ months), and that risk is dependent on the following factors: (list identified dynamic/situational/environmental risk factors). In my opinion, Johnny's risk for violence may be (slightly/moderately/substantially) reduced by (list interventions that address each risk factor)."

Conclusion

Violent and aggressive behaviors are not uncommon among adolescents, and preventing that violence can pose a considerable challenge for clinicians. Mental health professionals are much better equipped to face the question when they have thought through some of the issues in advance and prepared a plan for how to proceed. All adolescents are not alike, however, and neither are all risk assessments. The assessment plan should fit the circumstances and the functional nature of the implicit or explicit risk assessment question. In a routine therapy session, a young person may say something that leads the therapist to believe the client may be thinking of imminently harming someone. There may not be time for making a referral or for gathering collateral information. The clinician will have to think on his or her feet and know how to discern whether there is a reasonable basis for clinical concern about potential violence. In other circumstances, an evaluator may get a referral from the court asking for an appraisal of a person's risk of committing violence in the community within the next 6 weeks while awaiting a hearing. This situation may offer more time, pose a somewhat different functional question, and require a different approach. The state of research and assessment technology for assessing violence risk has advanced considerably since the 1970s. While early studies of violence prediction showed discouraging results, current evidence shows that risk judgments—particularly when structured with evidence-based tools—can be made reliably and with a reasonable level of accuracy. By relying on systematic approaches to assessment, child and adolescent clinicians can help to manage these clinical challenges, perhaps assist legal decision makers, and ultimately help prevent violence and improve outcomes for young people.

—Key Points

— Youth violence in the United States increased sharply between the mid-1980s and the mid-1990s but has dropped considerably since that time.

— After age 17 years, youth violence participation rates drop dramatically, and about 80% of those who are violent during adolescence will stop engaging in violent behavior by age 21 years.

— Reactive aggression is characterized as an angry, impulsive, retaliatory response to a real or perceived provocation, whereas proactive aggression is unprovoked, deliberate, and goal directed.

— In a forensic risk assessment, the evaluator should determine the purpose of the referral and the nature of the question to establish a good "fit" between the information needed and the assessment provided and also to make any assumptions and legal points of reference as transparent as possible.

— Several instruments have emerged that help evaluators to structure their assessments and that facilitate more reliable and valid risk judgments. These include the Structured Assessment of Violence Risk in Youth (SAVRY), the Early Assessment Risk List (EARL), and the Youth Level of Service/Case Management Inventory (YLS/CMI).

— Three common forms of risk communication are descriptive, prediction-oriented, and management-oriented.

References

Andrews DA, Bonta J: The Psychology of Criminal Conduct, 3rd Edition. Cincinnati, OH, Anderson Publishing, 2003

Augimeri L, Webster C, Koegl C, et al: Early Assessment Risk List for Boys: EARL-20B, Version 2. Toronto, ON, Canada, Earlscourt Child and Family Centre, 2001

Ajzen I: From intentions to actions: a theory of planned behavior, in Action Control: From Cognition to Behavior. Edited by Kuhl J, Beckmann J. Heidelberg, Germany, Springer, 1985, pp 11–39

Borum R: Improving the clinical practice of violence risk assessment: technology, guidelines and training. Am Psychol 51:945–956, 1996

Borum R: Assessing violence risk among youth. J Clin Psychol 56:1263–1288, 2000

Borum R: Managing at risk juvenile offenders in the community: putting evidence based principles into practice. J Contemp Crim Just 19:114–137, 2003

Borum R: Assessing risk for violence among juvenile offenders, in The Forensic Assessment of Children and Adolescents: Issues and Applications. Edited by Sparta S,

Koocher G. New York, Oxford University Press, 2006, pp 190–202

Borum R, Grisso T: Forensic assessment from a developmental perspective, in Forensic Psychology: Emerging Topics and Expanding Roles. Edited by Goldstein A. New York, Wiley, 2006, pp 553–570

Borum R, Reddy M: Assessing violence risk in Tarasoff situations: a fact-based model of inquiry. Behav Sciences Law 19:375–385, 2001

Borum R, Verhaagen D: Assessing and Managing Violence Risk in Juveniles. New York, Guilford, 2006

Borum R, Otto R, Golding S: Improving clinical judgment and decision making in forensic evaluation. Journal of Psychiatry and Law 21:35–76, 1993

Borum R, Fein R, Vossekuil B, et al: Threat assessment: defining an approach for evaluating risk of targeted violence. Behav Sciences Law 17:323–337, 1999

Borum R, Bartel P, Forth A: Structured Assessment of Violence Risk in Youth (SAVRY), in Handbook of Mental Health Screening and Assessment in Juvenile Justice. Edited by Grisso T, Vincent G, Seagrave D. New York, Oxford University Press, 2005, pp 311–323

Borum R, Lodewyjks H, Bartel P, et al: Structured Assessment of Violence Risk in Youth (SAVRY), in Handbook of Violence Risk Assessment. Edited by Douglas K, Otto R. New York, Routledge, in press

Buckner F, Firestone M: Where the public peril begins: 25 years after Tarasoff. The Journal of Legal Medicine 21:187–222, 2000

Cooper R, Werner P: Predicting violence in newly admitted inmates: a lens model analysis of staff decision making. Criminal Justice and Behavior 17:431–447, 1990

Cottle C, Lee R, Heilbrun K: The prediction of criminal recidivism in juveniles: a meta-analysis. Criminal Justice and Behavior 28:367–394, 2001

Dempster R: Prediction of sexually violent recidivism: a comparison of risk assessment instruments. Unpublished masters thesis. Burnaby, British Columbia, Simon Fraser University, 1998

Derzon JH: Antisocial behavior and the prediction of violence: a meta-analysis. Psychology in the Schools 38:93–106, 2001

Douglas K, Kropp R: A prevention-based paradigm for violence risk assessment: clinical and research applications. Criminal Justice & Behavior 29:617–658, 2002

Elliott D, Ageton S, Huizinga D, et al: The Prevalence and Incidence of Delinquent Behavior: 1976–1980 (The National Youth Survey Rep No 26). Boulder, CO, Behavioral Research Institute, 1983

Fein R, Vossekuil B: Protective intelligence and threat assessment investigations: a guide for state and local law enforcement officials (NIJ/OJP/DOJ Publ No 170612). Washington, DC, U.S. Department of Justice, 1998

Fein R, Vossekuil B, Holden G: Threat assessment: an approach to prevent targeted violence. National Institute of Justice: Research in Action, July 1995, pp 1–7. Available at: http://www.treas.gov/usss/ntac/ntac_threat.pdf. Accessed June 2009.

Forth AE, Kosson DS, Hare RD: The Hare Psychopathy Checklist: Youth Version manual. Toronto, ON, Canada, Multi-Health Systems, 2003

Griffin P, Torbet P: Desktop guide to good juvenile probation practice. National Center for Juvenile Justice, Pittsburgh, PA [producer]; Washington, DC, Office of Juvenile Justice and Delinquency Prevention, 2002

Grisso T: Forensic Evaluation of Juveniles. Sarasota, FL, Professional Resource Press, 1998

Grove W, Meehl P: Comparative efficiency of informal (subjective, impressionistic) and formal (mechanical, algorithmic) prediction procedures: the clinical-statistical controversy. Psychology, Public Policy and Law 2:293–323, 1996

Hanson RK: What do we know about sex offender risk assessment? Psychology, Public Policy, and Law 4:50–72, 1998

Hawkins J, Herrenkohl T, Farrington D, et al: A review of predictors of youth violence, in Serious and Violent Juvenile Offenders: Risk Factors and Successful Interventions. Edited by Loeber R, Farrington D. Thousand Oaks, CA, Sage, 1998, pp 106–146

Heilbrun K, O'Neill ML, Strohman LK, et al: Expert approaches to communicating violence risk. Law and Human Behavior 24:137–148, 2000

Hoge R: Standardized instruments for assessing risk and need in youthful offenders. Criminal Justice and Behavior 29:380–396, 2002

Hoge R, Andrews D: Assessing the Youthful Offender: Issues and Techniques. New York, Plenum, 1996

Hoge RD, Andrews DA: Youth Level of Service/Case Management Inventory (YLS/CMI): User's Manual. North Tonawanda, NY, Multi-Health Systems, 2002

Hoge R, Andrews D, Leschied A: An investigation of risk and protective factors in a sample of youthful offenders. Journal of Child Psychology & Psychiatry & Allied Disciplines 37:419–424, 1996

Hoge RD, Guerra N, Boxer P (eds): Treating the Juvenile Offender. New York, Guilford, 2008

Howell J: Juvenile Justice and Youth Violence. Thousand Oaks, CA, Sage, 1997

Jemmott JB III, Jemmott LS, Hines PM, et al: Testing the theory of planned behavior as a model of involvement in violence among African American and Latino adolescents. Maternal Child Health J 5:253–263, 2001

Jenson JM, Howard MO: Youth Violence: Current Research and Recent Practice Innovations. Washington, DC, National Association of Social Workers Press, 1999

Jessor R, van den Bos J, Vanderryn J, et al: Protective factors in adolescent problem behavior: moderator effects and developmental change. Developmental Psychology 31:923–933, 1995

Kann L, Kinchen SA, Williams BI, et al: Youth risk behavior surveillance—United States, 1997. MMWR Surveill Summ 47(3):1–89, 1998

Koegl C, Augimeri L, Webster C: Very young offenders: risk factors and outcome. Paper presented at 2000 Biennial Conference of the American Psychology–Law Society, New Orleans, LA, March 2000

Kropp P, Hart S, Webster C, et al: The Spousal Assault Risk Assessment Guide User's Manual. Toronto, ON, Canada, Multi-Health Systems and BC Institute Against Family Violence, 1999

Levene KS, Augimeri LK, Pepler DJ, et al: Early Assessment Risk List for Girls (EARL-21G), Version 1, Consultation Edition. Toronto, ON, Canada, Earlscourt Child and Family Centre, 2001

Lewis A, Webster C: General instruments for risk assessment. Current Opinion in Psychiatry 17:401–405, 2004

Lipsey M, Derzon J: Predictors of violent or serious delinquency in adolescence and early adulthood: a synthesis of longitudinal research, in Serious and Violent Juvenile Offenders: Risk Factors and Successful Interventions. Edited by Loeber R, Farrington D. Thousand Oaks, CA, Sage, 1998, pp 86–105

Loeber R, Stouthamer-Loeber M: Development of juvenile aggression and violence: some common misconceptions and controversies. Am Psychol 53:242–259, 1998

McCord J, Widom CS, Crowell NA (eds): Juvenile Crime, Juvenile Justice. Washington, DC, National Academy Press, 2001

Monahan J, Steadman HJ: Violent storms and violent people: how meteorology can inform risk communication in mental health law. Am Psychol 51:931–938, 1996

Rosado L (ed): Kids Are Different: How Knowledge of Adolescent Development Theory Can Aid Decision-Making in Court. Washington, DC, American Bar Association Juvenile Justice Center, 2000

Steinberg L, Cauffman E: A developmental perspective on serious juvenile crime: When should juveniles be treated as adults? Federal Probation (December):52–57, 1999

Tarasoff v Regents of the University of California, 551 P2d 334, 17 Cal3d 425, Cal Supreme Ct (1976)

U.S. Department of Health and Human Services: Youth Violence: A Report of the Surgeon General. Rockville, MD, U.S. Department of Health and Human Services, Substance Abuse and Mental Health Services Administration, Center for Mental Health Services, National Institutes of Health, National Institute of Mental Health, January 2001. Available at: http://www.surgeon-general.gov/library/youthviolence. Accessed June 2009.

Webster CD, Müller-Isberner R, Fransson G: Violence risk assessment: using structured clinical guides professionally. Int J Forensic Mental Health 1:185–193, 2002

Werner PD, Rose TL, Yesavage JA: Reliability, accuracy, and decision-making strategy in clinical predictions of imminent dangerousness. J Consult Clin Psychol 51:815–825, 1983

Werner PD, Rose TL, Murdach AD, et al: Social workers' decision making about the violent client. Social Work Res Abstracts 25:17–20, 1989

Wiebush RG, Baird C, Krisberg B, et al: Risk assessment and classification for serious, violent, and chronic juvenile offenders, in A Sourcebook: Serious, Violent, and Chronic Juvenile Offenders. Edited by Howell JC, Krisberg BF, Hawkins JD, et al. Thousand Oaks, CA, Sage, 1995, pp 171–212

Chapter 22

Prevention of Youth Violence

Dewey G. Cornell, Ph.D.
Megan Eliot, M.Ed.

Case Example

The conflict between two rival groups of teenage girls escalated dramatically over a period of weeks. Minor incidents, such as a humorous remark that was taken as an insult and joking criticism of unfashionable clothing, were followed by increasingly malicious rumors ("Her boyfriend cheats on her," "Her baby has AIDS") and then threatening remarks ("I'm gonna whip her good"). One night, the girls confronted one another on a downtown street, and harsh words erupted into a brawl that was broken up by the police. One girl was cut with a knife, and her friends vowed revenge.

The conflict expanded when friends of the girls felt compelled to choose sides and the rivals' boyfriends also became involved. The boys introduced guns into the dispute, and a shooting incident at a late-night dance aroused public concern. Nevertheless, police patrols and juvenile court hearings did little to lessen the feud. Many fearful students at the local high school refused to attend school or venture to the local mall, while other students reportedly began carrying weapons in anticipation of the need to defend themselves. Faced with growing tension among students at school and dozens of calls from worried parents, the local school principal observed, "I knew I had a problem, and I knew I needed help."

Violence prevention may seem antithetical to the work of a forensic clinician, who so often deals with an apprehended offender in the aftermath of a violent crime. Nevertheless, knowledge of prevention methods is valuable to forensic practitioners in multiple ca-

pacities. Forensic evaluators are often asked to make recommendations to assist in dispositional or sentencing decisions. Both the defendant and the community benefit when clinicians can make informed recommendations regarding effective interventions. More broadly, forensic practitioners often consult with schools, mental health facilities, juvenile detention centers, and youth services agencies interested in implementing prevention programs for at-risk youth.

Scope of the Problem

Youth violence is a serious problem but one that has declined markedly since its peak years in the early 1990s. Media coverage of sensational cases can generate exaggerated public perceptions of the scope and prevalence of youth violence that must be tempered by careful analysis of more objective evidence (Cornell 2006). Youth under age 18 accounted for about 17% of the violent crime arrests in the United States in 2006, a total of 73,991 arrests that included 956 arrests for murder, 2,519 for forcible rape, 26,092 for robbery, and 44,424 for aggravated assault (Federal Bureau of Investigation 2007). The incidence of violent crime arrests among juveniles has declined 38% since 1993 when there were 119,678 arrests for violent crime, including 3,284 arrests for murder, 5,303 for forcible rape, 43,340 for robbery, and 67,751 for aggravated assault (Federal Bureau of Investigation 1994). The drop in juvenile violence is especially noteworthy because the teenage population increased over this time period. By 2004, the juvenile arrest rate for serious violent crimes was the lowest since 1980 (Snyder 2006).

Less serious forms of youth violence are much more pervasive but harder to measure with precision. According to student self-reports on the Youth Risk Behavior Survey in 2005, approximately 36% of youth in grades 9–12 reported being in a physical fight during the previous 12 months (Dinkes et al. 2007). This included 43% of boys and 28% of girls, with higher rates for students in lower grades. The racial/ethnic breakdown was 33% among white youth, 43% among Black youth, 41% among Hispanic youth, and 22% among Asian youth. Nevertheless, even self-reports show a decline from 42% in 1993 to a low of 33% in 2001.

Youth violence is justifiably recognized as a serious societal concern and public health problem (U.S. Department of Health and Human Services [U.S. DHHS] 2001). Research in the last two decades has brought attention to the value of prevention for youth who are at risk for delinquency and violence (Catalano et al. 2004; Spivak and Prothrow-Stith 2005). Prevention efforts are conceived of as operating at three stages. Primary prevention programs are intended to avoid the initial occurrence of problem behaviors and have universal application to the general population. Secondary prevention efforts are designed to prevent the recurrence of problems that have appeared at an early stage and involve individualized work with youth who are targeted as high risk. Finally, tertiary prevention involves intensive support and intervention with individuals who clearly exhibit problem behavior.

The Surgeon General's 2001 report on youth violence (U.S. DHHS 2001) emphasized the importance of a public health approach to violence prevention that would include greater investment in primary prevention. Primary prevention involves identifying risk and protective factors for violence and then finding strategies to diminish risk and capitalize on protective resources. This approach strives to create a shift in daily behaviors and attitudes: "Central to education and protection is the principle that health promotion is best learned, performed, and maintained when it is ingrained in individuals' and communities' daily routines and perceptions of what constitutes good health practices" (U.S. DHHS 2001, p. 14). Spivak and Prothrow-Stith (2005) contended that effective prevention strategies should be guided by an understanding of the underlying causes of youth violence and directed toward a community-based multidisciplinary approach to intervention.

A good example of primary prevention is the positive youth development approach that emerged in the 1990s (Catalano et al. 2004). Positive youth development programs can take any number of forms but are generally designed to have a broad impact on prosocial and delinquent behavior rather than targeting a single problem such as violence or drug use. They strive to increase resilience and strengthen protective factors, as well as reduce the incidence of negative behaviors. Therefore, these programs have goals such as improving the child's social and behavioral competence, building positive relationships with others, and developing a sense of identity and values. The most effective positive youth development programs offer youth opportunities for prosocial activities and recognition for positive behavior, usually in the context of a structured curriculum or set of activities. They deliver services over an extended period of time, such as a school year. Examples of positive youth development programs (described later in the chapter) are Big Brothers/ Big Sisters (McGill 1997), Life Skills Training (Botvin et al. 2006), and Promoting Alternative Thinking Strategies (PATHS; Domitrovich et al. 2007).

The most significant overarching trend in youth violence prevention is the increasing value placed on evidence-based programs, which have become institutionalized in mental health and educational funding and support practices. For example, in education, the No Child Left Behind Act of 2001 mandates that schools use interventions that have proved effective in improving student outcomes under rigorous experimental conditions. The Safe and Drug-Free Schools Program requires that grant money be awarded to communities that comply with the U.S. Department of Education's (1998) Principles of Effectiveness. These principles include the requirement that schools conduct a needs assessment, choose evidence-based programs with measurable goals to meet identified areas of need, and complete follow-up evaluations of implemented programs. The federal government's Substance Abuse and Mental Health Services Administration developed a compendium of evidence-based practices that can be searched and sorted in the National Registry of Evidence-Based Programs and Practices (http:// www.nrepp.samhsa.gov/). Additional resources on evidence-based programs include the Blueprints for Violence Prevention (http://www.colorado.edu/cspv/blueprints/model/overview.html) and the Collaborative for Academic, Social, and Emotional Learning (http:// www.casel.org). Examples of some well-regarded and widely accepted programs are listed in Table 22–1.

TABLE 22-1. Examples of evidence-based youth violence prevention programs

Barkley Parent Training Program (Antshel and Barkley 2008)
10-step approach for parents of children with severe behavior problems or attention-deficit/hyperactivity disorder
http://www.russellbarkley.org/index.htm

Big Brothers/Big Sisters of America (Tierney et al. 1995)
Nationwide network of mentoring services
http://www.bbbs.org

Boys and Girls Clubs of America (Anderson-Butcher et al. 2003)
4,300 clubs with variety of educational and recreational programs
http://www.bgca.org/

Families and Schools Together (FAST; Keith et al. 2006)
Home- and school-based training for social and academic problems
http://familiesandschools.org/

Incredible Years (Webster-Stratton 2005)
Multifaceted curriculum for parents and teachers to improve child behavior
http://nrepp.samhsa.gov/programfulldetails.asp?PROGRAM_ID=131

Interpersonal Cognitive Problem Solving ("I Can Problem Solve"; Shure 2000)
Program to teach interpersonal problem solving for preschool and middle school students
http://www.colorado.edu/cspv/blueprints/promising/programs/BPP08.html

Multisystemic Therapy (MST) for Juvenile Offenders (Henggeler et al. 2007)
Intensive multimodal home-based therapy to improve family and school functioning
http://www.mstservices.com/

Parent Management Training for Conduct-Disordered Children (Patterson 2005)
Program to help parents modify faulty parenting strategies
http://www.oslc.org

Parenting the Defiant Child (Kazdin 2005)
Comprehensive instruction for parents on defiant child behavior
http://www.alankazdin.com/index.htm

Primary Project (Wohl and Hightower 2001)
Play therapy approach for children with early school adjustment difficulties
http://www.childrensinstitute.net/

Promoting Alternative THinking Strategies (PATHS; Domitrovich et al. 2007)
School-based curriculum to enhance social-emotional development
http://nrepp.samhsa.gov/programfulldetails.asp?PROGRAM_ID=127

Second Step
Classroom-based social skills program for preschool to ninth grade
http://www.cfchildren.org/programs/ssp/overview/

Teaching Students to Be Peacemakers (Johnson and Johnson 1995a)
Program to train students to resolve conflicts and mediate peer disputes
http://www.co-operation.org/index.html

Does Prevention Work?

Effective prevention is difficult to demonstrate. Prevention failures are readily identified when a crime is committed, but successful cases are nonevents, making it difficult for observers to recognize that a prevention effort is working. Only controlled outcome studies, preferably using an experimental design with random group assignment, can offer scientifically convincing evidence of program effects.

Early studies of delinquency prevention and intervention programs found little evidence of success, generating the widely held view that "nothing works" (Elliott 1997). However, more recent reviews of literature refute this pessimistic conclusion. There is now a large body of evidence supporting the effectiveness of many different prevention and intervention approaches (DuBois et al. 2002; Landenberger and Lipsey 2005; Loeber and Farrington 1998; Sherman et al. 1997; Wilson and Lipsey 2007).

Wilson and Lipsey (2007) conducted a meta-analytic study of school-based intervention programs derived from 249 studies concerned with aggressive and disruptive behavior, including fighting, hitting, bullying, and acting out. Overall, well-implemented programs provided a 25%–33% reduction in aggressive and disruptive behavior. DuBois et al. (2002) conducted a meta-analysis of 55 mentoring programs and found a modest effect: the average youth who participated in a mentoring program achieved outcome scores on various measures of adjustment and behavior that surpassed 55% of nonmentored youth.

Interventions are also effective at preventing problems in youth who have already engaged in delinquent or criminal behavior. Landenberger and Lipsey (2005) conducted a meta-analysis of 58 experimental and quasi-experimental studies of cognitive-behavioral therapy (CBT) and found that the odds of recidivism at 12-month follow-up were one and one-half times less likely for offenders who had participated in some form of CBT than for those who had not, amounting to a 25% reduction in repeat offending.

Although meta-analyses show overall positive effects for prevention efforts, it is important to recognize that program success can be quite variable. Carefully supervised programs that adhere to high standards of implementation achieve superior results (Lipsey and Wilson 1998). In the DuBois et al. (2002) meta-analysis of mentoring programs, larger effect sizes ($d = 0.18$ as opposed to $d = 0.06$) were found for programs that monitored implementation. Ongoing training for men-

tors increased effect sizes from $d = 0.11$ to $d = 0.26$. In Landenberger and Lipsey's (2005) analysis of CBT programs, training for treatment providers and monitoring of treatment fidelity were highly correlated with outcomes. Programs that followed best practices reduced recidivism by 50%, which is far superior to the 25% calculated for all programs.

The remainder of this chapter presents a selective overview of empirically validated youth violence prevention strategies. No programs described here are without practical and methodological limitations, and claims of effectiveness must be qualified in many respects. No program is immune to inadequate institutional support, insufficient funding, poorly trained staff, or failure to adhere to program standards.

Effective Prevention Programs

Conflict Resolution

Conflict resolution is the practice of settling disputes by engaging the parties in a problem-solving process in which the disputants collaboratively determine their own solution (Bodine and Crawford 1998). Conflict resolution differs from the more conventional practice of relying on third parties or authorities to arbitrate disputes. In complex cases, mediators may guide the disputants through the negotiation process but refrain from assuming the role of arbitrator or decision maker.

It is clear that conflict resolution is not appropriate in all cases and requires cooperation of both parties; nevertheless, conflict resolution programs can be an effective intervention in schools and other institutions. One potential advantage of conflict resolution is that it results in solutions that are acceptable to both parties so that the conflict is more decisively concluded, thereby reducing the risk of renewed conflict later on. Conflict resolution also teaches the participants skills that they can later utilize to resolve situations in which authorities are not available to intervene.

Peers can learn to adopt the role of mediator. Even primary school students can learn to mediate peer conflicts using structured methods, such as the Teaching Students to Be Peacemakers program (Johnson and Johnson 1995a; Walker 2007). Controlled outcome studies (Johnson and Johnson 1995b) have demonstrated that students can learn conflict resolution skills and apply them to actual conflicts in both school and family settings. Training students as peer mediators has also been found to provide them with skills that they can generalize to home and other settings (Burrell et al. 2006).

Conflict resolution computer games have been developed and are in the initial stages of evaluation. One such program is Students Managing Anger and Resolution Together (SMARTeam; Bosworth et al. 2000), a computer-based multimedia violence prevention intervention designed for sixth through ninth graders. Games, cartoons, and interactive interviews teach conflict resolution skills in three categories: anger management, dispute resolution, and perspective taking.

Social Competence and Problem Solving

Children as young as age 4 can be taught to solve interpersonal problems in an empathic and considerate manner. Social competence generally refers to the ability to get along with others and cope with problems effectively, and so is broader in scope and more foundational in purpose than conflict resolution. There are several well-designed and rigorously evaluated programs that teach social competence (Caplan et al. 1992; Greenberg et al. 1995). One of the best-known programs, Interpersonal Cognitive Problem Solving (ICPS; also known as "I Can Problem Solve"), teaches children to identify problems, recognize the feelings and perspectives of others, consider the consequences of alternative solutions, and then choose the best course of action (Shure 2000). Numerous evaluations, including multiyear follow-up studies, document that training improves children's behavior and generalizes across classroom, home, and peer situations (Shure 2000).

Another well-validated program, the Primary Project (formerly the Primary Mental Health Prevention Project), provides carefully supervised paraprofessional counseling for children with emotional or behavioral problems (Wohl and Hightower 2001). There are specialized components to teach social problem solving, assist children with divorced parents, facilitate peer relationships, and encourage cooperative learning (the Study Buddy program). The Primary Project has a dissemination and training program that has established programs in thousands of schools nationwide (http://www.childrensinstitute.net/programs/primary Project/).

PATHS is a Blueprints for Violence Prevention model program that is also recommended by the Substance Abuse and Mental Health Services Administration (Domitrovich et al. 2007). The PATHS curriculum has been adapted for preschool and elementary school and includes 131 thirty-minute lessons that regular classroom teachers can teach approximately three times a week over the course of the school year. Numerous studies, including randomized, controlled trials, demonstrate an improvement in children's emotional knowledge and social competence and a reduction in aggression and externalizing behavior (Domitrovich et al. 2007). PATHS has been implemented in 38 states and 5 countries; curriculum and parent materials are available in Spanish.

Supervised Recreation

The peak times for juvenile crime occur during the hours immediately after school (Sickmund et al. 1997). The level of juvenile offending at 3 P.M. on school days is more than three times greater than at noon or midnight. These observations alone indicate that many youth are not adequately supervised after school and suggest that after-school basketball is a more promising prevention strategy than midnight basketball (a popular program in some communities).

Several controlled studies have found that well-supervised after-school recreation programs substantially reduce juvenile crime, drug use, and vandalism. A Canadian study of an intensive after-school program (using sports, music, dancing, and scouting) demonstrated a 75% reduction in juvenile arrests, while arrests at a comparison site rose 67% (Jones and Offord 1989). A study of 10 Boys and Girls Clubs by the U.S. Office of Substance Abuse Prevention reported 22% lower levels of drug activity and increased levels of parent involvement (Schinke et al. 1992). A rigorously designed 3-year longitudinal study of 16 Boys and Girls Clubs in eight states also found reductions in alcohol and drug use, particularly in clubs that included active parent involvement (St. Pierre et al. 1997). Anderson-Butcher et al. (2003) compared 150 adolescents who participated in Boys and Girls Clubs with peers in their neighborhood. Although all study information was collected via self-report survey, the researchers found that higher levels of participation were related to lower levels of cigarette use and truancy and increased enjoyment and effort in school. According to the Boys and Girls Clubs of America website, the organization has over 4,000 affiliated clubs serving over 4.8 million children.

Mentoring

Many adolescents today lack parental role models. The proportion of U.S. births by unmarried mothers has grown from just 6% in 1960 to almost 37% in 2005 (Centers for Disease Control and Prevention

2008). Approximately 28% of adolescents in the United States live without one or both parents; among incarcerated juvenile offenders (prior to their arrest), the rate is much higher: 70% for boys and 59% for girls (Cornell et al. 1999). In this context, it is not surprising that mentoring has grown increasingly popular as a means of preventing delinquent behavior. Although parental absence has psychological, social, and economic consequences that cannot be remedied by mentors, most children respond enthusiastically to the prospect of individual attention from a caring adult.

An evaluation of the Big Brothers/Big Sisters of America conducted by Public/Private Ventures (Grossman and Garry 1997; McGill 1997; Tierney et al. 1995) provides support for mentoring. In a controlled experimental study, 959 youth ages 10–16 years from eight cities were randomly assigned a mentor or placed in a wait-list control group. After 18 months, youth who were mentored were 46% less likely than control youth to initiate drug use, 27% less likely to initiate alcohol use, and 32% less likely to hit someone. The study also reported improved relationships with other adults and peers and 52% less truancy.

The results of the Big Brothers/Big Sisters evaluation provide impressive evidence in support of mentoring, but they do not necessarily generalize to the many different sorts of activities and adult–youth relationships currently described as mentoring. The Big Brothers/Big Sisters program has a more structured program than many other mentoring efforts (McGill 1997). Volunteer mentors are screened, trained, and then supervised by case managers. Mentors typically meet with their little sibling an average of 3–4 hours weekly throughout the year. There is no specific set of activities for the mentor pairs; instead, there is an emphasis on befriending the youth and engaging in fun activities that build a positive relationship (McGill 1997).

Mentoring can be challenging work, and as many as half of mentoring efforts may end prematurely because one or both parties decide to discontinue the relationship (Morrow and Styles 1995). A meta-analysis of mentoring programs (DuBois et al. 2002) found that the development of a positive and supportive relationship was the most important factor for improved mentee outcomes. Ongoing training for mentors seemed to be important to the success of the relationship. The study also found that a positive relationship was not dependent on mentors and mentees being from similar racial or ethnic backgrounds. In addition, a positive relationship could be established in an independent mentoring program or one that was part of broader service delivery.

Child and Family Programs

Primary prevention efforts aimed at preschool children can have substantial benefits for families and the quality of a child's social and academic adjustment (Tremblay and Craig 1995; Yoshikawa 1994). The Perry Preschool Program found that children randomly assigned to a preschool and home visit program not only did better in school than control children but had fewer arrests as juveniles and adults (Berrueta-Clement et al. 1984). A strength of the Perry Preschool Program was its emphasis on facilitating parent involvement in children's academic and social development. The RAND report "Investing in Our Children" (Karoly et al. 1998) distinguished between the weak evidence supporting many programs and strong evidence in support of several programs that have verifiable long-term benefits.

For school-age children already exhibiting disruptive or disobedient behavior, secondary prevention in the form of parent education can be highly effective (Hoard and Shephard 2005; Serketich and Dumas 1996). Parent management training for aggressive children improves children's behavior and is a cost-effective means of preventing future crime (McCart et al. 2006). Among the more well-validated approaches to parent education are the following:

- Parent Management Training for Conduct Disordered Children, developed by Patterson (2005) at the University of Oregon Social Learning Center, helps parents recognize discipline strategies that unwittingly promote antisocial behavior and teaches them more effective alternatives.
- Kazdin (2005), at the Yale Child Study Center, also developed a Parent Management Training program that outlines how therapists and parents can work as a team to modify oppositional, aggressive, and antisocial behavior.
- The Barkley Parent Training Program uses an explicit manual to teach a 10-step model to parents of children with severe behavior problems (Antshel and Barkley 2008; Barkley 1997).
- The Incredible Years (Webster-Stratton 2005) is a 24-week program delivered to groups of parents in 2-hour weekly meetings using video vignettes to demonstrate positive parenting techniques.
- Families and Schools Together (FAST) is a comprehensive program that incorporates parent training and home visits along with school-based efforts to improve the social skills and academic performance of elementary school children (Keith et al. 2006; Kratochwill et al. 2004).

For delinquent youth, family therapy can be a useful form of tertiary prevention. Functional Family Therapy (Sexton and Alexander 2002) makes use of cognitive and behavioral methods to improve family relationships and increase reciprocity and cooperation among family members. Outcome studies demonstrated that Functional Family Therapy improved family relationships and reduced recidivism among adolescents referred by juvenile court for offenses such as truancy, theft, and unmanageable behavior (Sexton and Alexander 2002).

Multisystemic Therapy (Henggeler et al. 2007) is one of the most cost-effective and powerful treatments for serious juvenile offenders and their families. In controlled outcome studies, Multisystemic Therapy was superior to standard treatments for chronic juvenile offenders, inner-city at-risk youth, child-abusive families, and other traditionally difficult populations. A hallmark of the multisystemic approach is the therapist's role as a problem solver who works closely with parents to identify and remedy problems in a wide variety of areas, ranging from a child's school attendance to marital discord. Typically, therapists begin treatment by visiting the family several times a week for sessions ranging from 15 to 90 minutes, and later gradually taper contacts over a 4- to 6-month period. Therapists make flexible use of family therapy, parent education, and cognitive-behavioral techniques to improve family relationships, strengthen parental authority and effectiveness, and modify children's behavior.

What Doesn't Work

One of the most common pitfalls in the prevention field is the adoption of unvalidated programs. All too often, programs are selected based on theoretically or philosophically appealing features in the absence of objective evidence of program effectiveness. Once programs are implemented, it becomes increasingly difficult to criticize them or make substantial changes. Objective evaluations of popular programs such as Intensive Supervised Probation (MacKenzie 1997; Petersilia and Turner 1993) and boot camps (Cowles et al. 1995; Cronin and Han 1994; MacKenzie and Souryal 1994) have produced disappointing results that proponents have been unwilling to accept (e.g., see Chapter 27, "Assessment and Treatment of Juvenile Offenders").

D.A.R.E.

No prevention program is more popular, or more controversial, than Drug Abuse Resistance Education

(D.A.R.E.). D.A.R.E. began in 1983 as a collaborative effort between the Los Angeles Police Department and the Los Angeles Unified School District and has been adopted in over 80% of the nation's school districts, as well as 52 foreign countries (U.S. Government Accountability Office 2003). The original core curriculum was designed for uniformed police officers to teach a specific drug prevention curriculum to students in their last (fifth or sixth) grade of elementary school, although there are D.A.R.E. programs for other grade levels that are less widely used.

In 1994, Ringwalt and colleagues released an evaluation of the D.A.R.E. program based on a meta-analysis of eight methodologically rigorous studies involving 9,300 students and 215 schools (Ringwalt et al. 1994). All eight studies assessed students before and after completion of the core D.A.R.E. curriculum and included control groups of students not receiving D.A.R.E. The results indicated that D.A.R.E. was most effective at increasing knowledge about drug use and in improving social skills and that there was a small improvement in attitudes toward police, attitudes about drug use, and self-esteem. Unfortunately, however, the effect size for reported drug and alcohol use was not statistically significant. These results helped generate a storm of criticism and often contentious debate concerning the merits of D.A.R.E. Some researchers and reporters who presented unfavorable findings about D.A.R.E.'s effectiveness were the recipients of harsh criticism and even harassment (Glass 1998; Rosenbaum 1998).

In defense of D.A.R.E., one limitation of most outcomes studies was that they examined drug and alcohol use shortly after completion of D.A.R.E., when students are age 11 or 12 years and the baseline rates of drug use are so low that the effects of D.A.R.E. might not be evident. To overcome this limitation, Rosenbaum and colleagues (Rosenbaum 1998; Rosenbaum and Hanson 1998) reported results of a 6-year longitudinal study of 1,798 students from 36 schools. This methodologically rigorous study used randomized control groups and corrected for many statistical and methodological problems of previous studies. There were expectations that this study would salvage D.A.R.E.'s reputation and demonstrate conclusively that it was effective. Unfortunately, this study again found that D.A.R.E. did not reduce drug use, and in suburban schools, D.A.R.E. was associated with a 3%–5% increase in drug use. A 10-year follow-up study again found D.A.R.E. to be ineffective (Lynam et al. 1999).

To its credit, D.A.R.E. has made changes to its curriculum and focused more efforts on older students who are most likely to use drugs. Twenty-four schools in Minnesota participated in a study of a revised D.A.R.E. program for seventh-grade students conducted by researchers at the University of Minnesota School of Public Health (Komro et al. 2004; Perry et al. 2003). The seventh-grade program included 10 sessions on character and citizenship, as well as specific skills for resisting peer pressure to use drugs and strategies for avoiding potentially violent situations. The Minnesota D.A.R.E. program also investigated an augmentation of the standard curriculum called "D.A.R.E. Plus." The D.A.R.E. Plus component included after-school activities and the creation of neighborhood action teams that planned bullying prevention seminars, community forums, and neighborhood cleanups. Both programs were evaluated in comparison with a control group at baseline and 1-year follow-up through the self-report of 4,976 students.

In 2003, the Minnesota researchers reported that the standard D.A.R.E. curriculum had no effect on seventh graders in reducing tobacco, alcohol, or other drug use (Perry et al. 2003). The D.A.R.E. Plus program did show small, but statistically significant, reductions in tobacco, alcohol, and drug use for boys, but not for girls. The scales showing the reductions were self-report scales that measured "behavior and intentions" combined rather than behavior alone, so it is not certain whether there were reductions in actual drug use or simply attitudes toward drug use.

Efforts have also been made to utilize the resources dedicated to D.A.R.E. more effectively. For example, the Adolescent Substance Abuse Prevention Study (Stephens et al. 2007) developed a new drug education curriculum for seventh and ninth graders that could be delivered by D.A.R.E. officers. A 5-year longitudinal outcome study of this new program (Take Charge of Your Life) is nearing completion.

Despite the substantial evidence against the D.A.R.E. program, it continues to be well received in communities. The Drugs and Organized Crime Awareness Service (2007), a division of the Royal Canadian Mounted Police, conducted a survey of over 5,000 students who had participated in D.A.R.E., as well as their parents, teachers, and principals. Ninety-six percent of parents and school staff believed that D.A.R.E. had a positive impact on students, and 95% of students reported that D.A.R.E. had helped them decide not to use drugs. D.A.R.E. also remains politically popular. In 2008, President Bush continued a presidential tradition by declaring April 10 National D.A.R.E. Day (http://www.dare.org/home/tertiary/default1b34.asp). Presidential recognition of D.A.R.E. would seem to be inconsistent with the U.S. Department of Education's (1998) Principles of Effectiveness that require schools to use programs that are supported by scientific research.

There is evidence for the effectiveness of other drug education programs. Interactive programs that emphasize interpersonal skills to counter peer pressure and use a participatory teaching approach are more effective than programs that rely on moral exhortation, fear arousal, or self-esteem building (Gottfredson 1997; Ringwalt et al. 1994). Life Skills Training (Botvin et al. 2006) is one of the most effective and well-documented drug education programs. Unlike D.A.R.E., Life Skills Training is taught by teachers in the sixth or seventh grade, with 15 sessions in the first year and booster sessions the following 2 years. The program emphasizes self-management and social skills, as well as skills specifically related to dealing with peer pressure to use drugs. Outcomes averaged from a dozen studies indicate that Life Skills Training reduces tobacco, alcohol, and marijuana use 50%–75% and that treatment effects are sustained 6 years later.

Scared Straight

One of the earliest and most influential "scared straight" programs was the Juvenile Awareness Project of New Jersey's Rahway State Prison (Finckenauer 1982). In 1976, Rahway officials began bringing youth into the maximum-security prison to meet with inmates who offered what they called "shock therapy" to frighten and intimidate the youth. The program became a favorite of criminal justice officials and law enforcement officers and was popularized in a widely acclaimed documentary (Finckenauer 1982).

Petrosino et al. (2003) identified nine rigorous studies of the scared straight approach that included a total of 946 youth. In each study, a group of youth was randomly (or alternately) selected to visit a correctional institution or to serve as comparison subjects in a no-treatment control group. Although the young participants, their parents, and their teachers all expressed positive reactions to the program, the program did not reduce subsequent criminal behavior. On the contrary, the researchers concluded that "on average these programs result in an increase in criminality in the experimental group when compared to a no-treatment control. According to these experiments, doing nothing would have been better than exposing juveniles to the program" (Petrosino et al. 2003, p. 5).

Transfer of Juveniles to the Adult Justice System

The juvenile justice system was designed to recognize the developmental needs of juveniles and to make use of rehabilitative alternatives to incarceration in the adult criminal justice system (Scott and Grisso 1997). However, following the increase in juvenile violent crime in the late 1980s and early 1990s, most states modified their laws to facilitate the transfer of juveniles to the adult justice system.

In 2007, the independent nonfederal Task Force on Community Preventive Services conducted a review of published studies on the effectiveness of transferring juveniles to the adult criminal justice system. The review examined specific deterrence, or the reduction in repeat offending rates among individual offenders. Across six studies of specific deterrence, transferred juveniles were 26%–77% more likely to be arrested again compared with nontransferred juveniles. The review also addressed general deterrence, or the reduction of repeat offending in the juvenile population as a whole. Studies of juvenile transfer laws implemented in Idaho, Washington State, and New York demonstrated that the transfer of juveniles was not associated with a reduction in the overall rate of juvenile offending in the general population and, in some cases, was associated with an increase. The task force concluded that aggressive transfer policies were harmful to juveniles and counterproductive as a strategy for deterring subsequent criminal behavior (Task Force on Community Preventive Services 2007).

Case Example Epilogue

The school principal knew that an effective action plan would need to involve multiple levels of intervention. He began by contacting the local social services agency, police department, and juvenile court authorities to develop a coordinated community response, including 1) conflict mediation with the rival groups, 2) individual educational and social services plans to meet the needs of specific group members, 3) a schoolwide violence prevention program, and 4) expanded after-school programs.

To address the individual needs in the immediate problem, a team of professional mediators met with the girls individually and convinced them to attend a day-long mediation session at a neutral secure site. With gentle guidance and minimal direction from the mediators, the girls listened and spoke in turn. For hours the girls aired their grievances, unraveled rumors, and clarified misunderstandings. At an appropriate time, the mediators advised the girls that they could devise their own plan for ending the feud, but the mediators were careful not to take sides or make specific suggestions. It is critical to this form of mediation that solutions are devised by the opposing parties rather than imposed from an outside authority. In this way the girls decided to squash their dispute and settled on terms for reconciliation.

Second, school and community professionals met with individual girls and their parents to devise educational and social services plans. Several of the girls qualified for special education services, whereas others enrolled in vocational or job placement programs. One young woman needed parent support services and child care arrangements for her infant son. Most of the girls received some form of individual and/or family therapy. In several cases, the resolution of juvenile charges was linked to treatment compliance and school attendance.

At the school level, the principal met with a group of student leaders and encouraged their efforts to form an antiviolence organization that initiated a nonviolence campaign in the school. Several hundred students signed a pledge not to engage in fights and to support nonviolent means of resolving conflict. School discipline policies were revised, penalties for fighting were stiffened, and school security was enhanced with the addition of a school resource officer provided by the local police department. The school psychologist established a therapeutic group for at-risk students that emphasized anger control and conflict resolution training.

At the community level, the city council agreed to provide space for a nonprofit organization to establish an after-school recreational program. The program was well staffed and included services to encourage homework completion and school attendance. The previously existing mentoring program was expanded and revamped to emphasize more training and supervision of mentors.

To the surprise and relief of authorities, the girls ended their dispute and engaged in no further acts of aggression or violence toward one another. After 2 years, the agreement was still being honored, and some previous rivals had become friends. Two of the girls obtained a G.E.D., and all of the others graduated with their classmates. The school recorded a marked decline in fights, discipline referrals, and suspensions as a result of their primary, secondary, and tertiary prevention efforts.

Conclusion

Forensic experts consistently deal with a highly skewed sample of the youth offender population—the most serious crimes committed by the most troubled and perplexing youth. They also have little occasion to study successful outcomes, because follow-up information becomes available primarily when a youth is arrested for another crime. Contrary to common perceptions about the chronicity and intractability of juvenile offending, most youth never return to juvenile court after their first referral (Snyder and Sickmund 1995), and many (if not most) aggressive youth desist in their aggressive behavior as they mature (Loeber and Stouthamer-Loeber 1998). Although positive outcomes are commonplace, they are far removed from the experiential knowledge base of the forensic clini-cian, who encounters cases in which prevention efforts have failed. Knowledge of effective, research-validated prevention strategies can deepen the clinician's understanding of violence and broaden his or her expertise as a courtroom advocate and community consultant. Forensic clinicians can play an important role in advancing the field of violence prevention by educating policy makers and practitioners about the availability of a wide array of effective methods of preventing youth violence and by emphasizing the necessity of rigorous program implementation followed by objective evaluation of program outcomes.

—Key Points

— The prevention field has evolved from the view that "nothing works" to the recognition that many programs are effective.

— When implemented properly, evidence-based programs can prevent youth violence and delinquency.

— There is a strong movement to design programs that have an emphasis on positive youth development, as distinguished from a narrow focus on a single problem behavior.

— There are effective programs to teach youth how to resolve conflicts, improve their social competence, and solve problems more effectively.

— Supervised recreation and mentoring programs can reduce youth violence and delinquency.

— Family interventions and parent training can be effective in reducing youth violence and delinquency.

— Some popular, widely used programs, such as scared straight and D.A.R.E., have been found to be ineffective.

References

Anderson-Butcher D, Newsome WS, Ferrari T: Participation in Boys and Girls Clubs and relationships to youth outcomes. Journal of Community Psychology 31:39–55, 2003

Antshel KM, Barkley R: Psychosocial interventions in children with attention deficit hyperactivity disorder. Child Adolesc Psychiatr Clin N Am 17:421–437, 2008

Barkley RA: Defiant Children: A Clinician's Manual for Assessment and Parent Training. New York, Guilford, 1997

Berrueta-Clement JR, Schweinhart L, Barnett W, et al: Changed Lives: The Effects of the Perry Preschool Program. Ypsilanti, MI, High/Scope Press, 1984

Bodine RJ, Crawford DK: The Handbook of Conflict Resolution Education: A Guide to Building Quality Programs in Schools. San Francisco, CA, Jossey-Bass, 1998

Bosworth K, Espelage DL, DuBay T, et al: A preliminary evaluation of a multimedia violence prevention program for early adolescence. Am J Health Behav 24:268–280, 2000

Botvin GJ, Griffin KW, Nichols TD: Preventing youth violence and delinquency through a universal school-based prevention approach. Prevention Science 7:403–408, 2006

Burrell NA, Zirbel C, Allen M: Evaluating peer mediation outcomes in educational settings: a meta-analytic review, in Classroom Communication and Instructional Processes. Edited by Gayle BM. Mahwah, NJ, Lawrence Erlbaum, 2006, pp 113–126

Caplan M, Weissberg RP, Grober JS, et al: Social competence promotion with inner-city and suburban young adolescents: effects on social adjustment and alcohol use. J Consult Clin Psychol 60:56–63, 1992

Catalano RF, Berglund ML, Ryan JAM, et al: Positive youth development in the United States: research findings on evaluations of positive youth development programs. Ann Am Acad Pol Soc Sci 591:98–124, 2004

Centers for Disease Control and Prevention: National Vital Statistics System, U.S. Department of Health and Human Services. 2008. Available at: http://209.217.72.34/VitalStats/TableViewer/tableView.aspx?ReportId=4394. Accessed April 25, 2008.

Cornell DG: School Violence: Fears Versus Facts. Mahwah, NJ, Lawrence Erlbaum, 2006

Cornell DG, Loper AB, Atkinson A, et al: Youth Violence Prevention in Virginia: A Needs Assessment. Richmond, VA, Virginia Department of Health, 1999

Cowles EL, Castellano TC, Gransky LA: "Boot Camp" Drug Treatment and Aftercare Interventions: An Evaluation Review (National Institute of Justice Research Report). Washington, DC, National Institute of Justice, 1995

Cronin R, Han M: Boot Camps for Adult and Juvenile Offenders: Overview and Update. Washington, DC, U.S. Department of Justice, 1994

Dinkes R, Cataldi EF, Lin-Kelly W, et al: Indicators of school crime and safety: 2007 (NCES 2008-021, NCJ 219553). Washington, DC: U.S. Government Printing Office, 2007

Domitrovich CE, Cortes RC, Greenberg MT: Improving young children's social and emotional competence: a randomized trial of the preschool "PATHS" curriculum. J Prim Prev 28:67–91, 2007

Drugs and Organized Crime Awareness Service: National Client Survey, 2007. Available at: http://www.dare.com/home/Resources/documents/RCMP_DARE_Report_FINAL.pdf. Accessed May 12, 2008.

DuBois DL, Halloway BE, Valentine JC: Effectiveness of mentoring programs for youth: a meta-analytic review. Am J Comm Psychol 30:157–197, 2002

Elliott DS (Series ed): Editor's introduction, in Blueprints for Violence Prevention. Boulder, University of Colorado, Institute of Behavioral Science, 1997, pp xi–xxiii

Federal Bureau of Investigation: Crime in the United States 1993. Washington, DC, U.S. Government Printing Office, 1994

Federal Bureau of Investigation: Crime in the United States 2006. Washington, DC, U.S. Department of Justice, 2007

Finckenauer JO: Scared Straight! and the Panacea Phenomenon. Upper Saddle River, NJ, Prentice Hall, 1982

Glass S: Truth and D.A.R.E.: the nation's most prestigious drug prevention program for kids is a failure. Why don't you know this? Rolling Stone, March 5, 1998, pp 42–43

Gottfredson DC: School-based crime prevention, in Preventing Crime: What Works, What Doesn't, What's Promising: A Report to the United States Congress (NCJ 171676). Edited by Sherman LW, Gottfredson D, MacKenzie D, et al. Washington, DC, National Institute of Justice, 1997, pp 125–182

Greenberg MT, Kusche CA, Cook ET, et al: Promoting emotional competence in school-aged children: the effects of the PATHS curriculum. Dev Psychopath 7:117–136, 1995

Grossman JB, Garry EM: Mentoring: a proven delinquency prevention strategy, in Juvenile Justice Bulletin. Washington, DC, U.S. Department of Justice, 1997

Henggeler SW, Sheidow AJ, Lee T: Multisystemic treatment of serious clinical problems in youths and their families, in Handbook of Forensic Mental Health With Victims and Offenders: Assessment, Treatment, and Research. Edited by Springer DW, Roberts AR. New York, Guilford, 2007, pp 315–345

Hoard D, Shephard KN: Parent education as parent-centered prevention: a review of school-related outcomes. School Psychol Q 20:434–454, 2005

Johnson DW, Johnson RT: Teaching Students to Be Peacemakers, 3rd Edition. Edina, MN, Interaction Book, 1995a

Johnson DW, Johnson RT: Teaching Students to Be Peacemakers: results of five years of research. Peace and Conflict: Journal of Peace Psychology 4:417–438, 1995b

Jones MB, Offord DR: Reduction of anti-social behavior in poor children by non-school skill development. J Child Psychol Psychiatry Allied Discipl 30:737–750, 1989

Karoly LA, Greenwood PW, Everingham SS, et al: Investing in Our Children: What We Know and Don't Know About the Costs and Benefits of Early Childhood Interventions. Santa Monica, CA, RAND, 1998

Kazdin AE: Parent Management Training: Treatment for Oppositional, Aggressive, and Antisocial Behavior in Children and Adolescent. New York, Oxford University Press, 2005

Keith W, Moberg DP, McDonald L: FAST and the arms race: the interaction of group aggression and the "Families and Schools Together" program in the aggressive and delinquent behaviors of inner-city elementary school students. J Prim Prevent 27:27–45, 2006

Komro KA, Perry CL, Stigler MH, et al: Violence-related outcomes of the D.A.R.E. Plus project. Health Educ Behav 31:335–354, 2004

Kratochwill TR, McDonald L, Levin JR, et al: Families and schools together: an experimental analysis of parent-mediated multi-family group program for American Indian children. J Sch Psychol 42:359–383, 2004

Landenberger NA, Lipsey MW: The positive effects of cognitive-behavioral programs for offenders: a meta-analysis of factors associated with effective treatment. J Exp Criminol 1:451–476, 2005

Lipsey MW, Wilson DB: Effective intervention for serious juvenile offenders: a synthesis of research, in Serious and Violent Juvenile Offenders: Risk Factors and Successful Interventions. Edited by Loeber R, Farrington DP. Thousand Oaks, CA, Sage, 1998, pp 313–345

Loeber R, Farrington DP (eds): Serious and Violent Juvenile Offenders: Risk Factors and Successful Interventions. Thousand Oaks, CA, Sage, 1998

Loeber R, Stouthamer-Loeber M: Development of juvenile aggression and violence: some common misconceptions and controversies. Am Psychol 53:242–259, 1998

Lynam DR, Milich R, Zimmerman R, et al: Project DARE: no effects at 10-year follow-up. J Consult Clin Psychol 67:590–593, 1999

MacKenzie DL: Criminal justice and crime prevention, in Preventing Crime: What Works, What Doesn't, What's Promising: A Report to the United States Congress. Edited by Sherman LW, Gottfredson D, MacKenzie DL, et al. Washington, DC, National Institute of Justice, 1997

MacKenzie DL, Souryal C: Multisite Evaluation of Shock Incarceration. Washington, DC, National Institute of Justice, 1994

McCart MR, Priester PE, Davies WH, et al: Differential effectiveness of behavioral parent-training and cognitive behavioral therapy for antisocial youth: a meta-analysis. J Abnorm Child Psychol 34:527–543, 2006

McGill D: Big Brothers/Big Sisters of America. Boulder, University of Colorado, Institute of Behavioral Science, 1997

Morrow KV, Styles MB: Building Relationships With Youth in Program Settings: A Study of Big Brothers/Big Sisters. Philadelphia, PA, Public/Private Ventures, 1995

Patterson GR: The next generation of PMTO models. Behav Ther 28:27–33, 2005

Perry CL, Komro KA, Veblen-Mortenson S, et al: A randomized controlled trial of the middle and junior high school D.A.R.E. and D.A.R.E. Plus programs. Arch Pediatr Adolesc Med 157:178–184, 2003

Petersilia J, Turner S: Intensive probation and parole. Crime and Justice 17:281–335, 1993

Petrosino A, Turpin-Petrosino C, Buehler J: Programs for preventing juvenile delinquency: a systematic review of the randomized experimental evidence for Scared Straight and other juvenile awareness programs. Ann Am Acad Pol Soc Sci 589:41–62, 2003

Ringwalt C, Greene J, Ennett S, et al: Past and Future Directions of the DARE Program: An Evaluation Review: Draft Final Report (Award No 91-DD-CX-K053). Washington, DC, National Institute of Justice, 1994

Rosenbaum D: Assessing the effects of school-based drug education: a six-year multi-level analysis of project D.A.R.E. J Res Crime Delinq 35:381–412, 1998

Rosenbaum D, Hanson G: Assessing the effects of school-based drug education: a six-year multi-level analysis of project DARE. Unpublished manuscript. Chicago, University of Illinois, Department of Criminal Justice and Center for Research in Law and Justice, 1998

Schinke SP, Orlandi MA, Cole KC: Boys and Girls Clubs in public housing developments: prevention services for youth at risk. J Comm Psychol 28 (OSAP Special Issue):118–128, 1992

Scott ES, Grisso T: The evolution of adolescence: a developmental perspective on juvenile justice reform. J Crim Law Criminol 88:137–189, 1997

Serketich WJ, Dumas JE: The effectiveness of behavioral parent training to modify antisocial behavior in children: a meta-analysis. Behavior Therapy 27:171–186, 1996

Sexton TL, Alexander JF: Functional family therapy: a mature clinical model for working with at-risk adolescents and their families, in Handbook of Family Therapy: The Science and Practice of Working With Families and Couples. Edited by Sexton TL, Weeks GR, Robbins MS. New York, Brunner-Routledge, 2002, pp 323–348

Sherman LW, Gottfredson D, MacKenzie D, et al: Preventing Crime: What Works, What Doesn't, What's Promising: A Report to the United States Congress. Washington, DC, National Institute of Justice, 1997

Shure MB: Raising a Thinking Preteen: The I Can Problem Solve Program for Eight- to Twelve-Year-Olds. New York, Henry Holt, 2000

Sickmund M, Snyder H, Poe-Yamagata E: Juvenile Offenders and Victims: 1997 Update on Violence. Washington, DC, Office of Juvenile Justice and Delinquency Prevention, August 1997

Snyder HN: Juvenile Arrests 2004. Washington, DC, U.S. Department of Justice, Office of Juvenile Justice and Delinquency Prevention, 2006

Snyder HN, Sickmund M: Juvenile Offenders and Victims: A National Report. Washington, DC, Office of Juvenile Justice and Delinquency Prevention, 1995

Spivak H, Prothrow-Stith D: Murder is no accident: violence prevention through public health and youth development. Appl Dev Sci 9:2–4, 2005

St. Pierre IL, Mark MM, Kaltreider DL, et al: Involving parents of high-risk youth in drug prevention: a three-year longitudinal study in Boys and Girls Clubs. J Early Adolesc 17:21–50, 1997

Stephens RC, Thibodeaux L, Sloboda Z, et al: An empirical study of adolescent student attrition. J Drug Issues 37:475–488, 2007

Task Force on Community Preventive Services: Effects on violence of laws and policies facilitating the transfer of juveniles from the juvenile justice system to the adult justice system: a systematic review. Am J Prev Med 32 (4 suppl):S7–28, 2007

Tierney JP, Grossman JB, Resch NL: Making a Difference: An Impact Study of Big Brothers/Big Sisters. Philadelphia, PA, Public/Private Ventures, 1995

Tremblay, RE, Craig W: Developmental crime prevention, in Building a Safer Society: Strategic Approaches to Crime

Prevention. Edited by Tonry M, Farrington DP. Chicago, University of Chicago Press, 1995, pp 151–236

U.S. Department of Education: Safe and Drug-Free Schools: Principles of Effectiveness Document. June 1, 1998. Available at: http://www.ed.gov/offices/OSDFS/nrg-fin.pdf. Accessed April 30, 2008.

U.S. Department of Health and Human Services: Youth Violence: A Report of the Surgeon General. Rockville, MD, U.S. Department of Health and Human Services, 2001

U.S. Government Accountability Office: Youth Illicit Drug Use Prevention: DARE Long-Term Evaluations and Federal Efforts to Identify Effective Programs (GAO-03-172R). Washington, DC, U.S. General Accounting Office, January 15, 2003. Available at: http://www.gao.gov/htext/d03172r.html. Accessed May 25, 2009.

Walker CE: Teaching students to be peacemakers: implementing a conflict resolution and peer mediation training in a Minneapolis K–6 charter school. Unpublished doctoral dissertation, University of Minnesota. [Dissertation Abstracts International A: Humanities and Social Sciences 68(2-A), 2007]

Webster-Stratton C: The Incredible Years: a training series for the prevention and treatment of conduct problems in young children, in Psychosocial Treatment for Child and Adolescent Disorders: Empirically Based Strategies for Clinical Practice. Edited by Hibbs ED, Jensen PS. Washington, DC, American Psychological Association, 2005, pp 507–555

Wilson SJ, Lipsey MW: School-based interventions for aggressive and disruptive behavior. Am J Prev Med 33:130–143, 2007

Wohl N, Hightower AD: Primary mental health project: a school-based prevention program, in School-Based Play Therapy. Edited by Drewes AA, Carey LJ, Schaefer CE. New York, Wiley, 2001, pp 277–296

Yoshikawa H: Prevention as cumulative protection: effects of early family support and education on chronic delinquency and its risks. Psychol Bull 115:28–54, 1994

Chapter 23

Prevention of School Violence

Dewey G. Cornell, Ph.D.

Sharmila Bandyopadhyay, M.Ed.

Case Example

A ninth-grade student reported to his teacher that he was worried about a classmate named Johnny who had threatened to kill three other students. This student told the teacher that Johnny has been complaining about these students and recounted several incidents in which they teased and mocked Johnny on the bus and in the locker room at school. The teacher questioned Johnny, and he admitted that he had told a group of students that he would like to kill them, but said he wasn't serious. The teacher informed the principal. What should the principal do?

In response to a series of high-profile school shootings in the 1990s, school authorities became highly sensitive to student behaviors that suggested aggressive intentions or potential dangerousness to others. American schools implemented numerous violence prevention programs, enacted stricter disciplinary standards, and developed more extensive security procedures (Cornell 2006; Osher et al. 2004). The widespread enforcement of zero tolerance policies (American Psychological Association 2006) results in thousands of students being suspended or expelled each year because of concerns about the danger they seemingly pose to others. Often these disciplinary actions generate a referral for a risk assessment or an evaluation of treatment needs. In other cases, schools may request assistance in developing or implementing a violence prevention program or in training their staff to identify warning signs or indicators of potential violence in their students. These concerns make it important for forensic clinicians to be knowledgeable about school violence prevention.

Although high-profile school shootings have brought attention to the important issue of school safety, they have also prompted unrealistic fears and beliefs among parents, teachers, and school administrators about the incidence of student-perpetrated homicide (Cornell 2006; Reddy et al. 2001). The perception of school homicides as a frequent and seemingly likely event can skew perceptions of risk. For example, after the 1999 Columbine shooting, a Gallup Poll found that two-thirds of Americans believed that a similar incident could occur in their community (Saad 1999).

On the contrary, the risk of a school homicide is much lower than the public perceives, and the risk of serious violent victimization is much greater outside of schools than in schools. Within a population of nearly 55 million students (ages 5–18 years) in the United States, there were 14 homicides and 3 suicides of school-age youth at school during the 2005–2006 school year (Dinkes et al. 2007). The probability of a student being murdered or committing suicide at school that year was approximately 1 in 3.2 million. Youth are over 50 times more likely to be murdered away from school than at school (Dinkes et al. 2007), yet murders at school make national news and stimulate fears that schools are not safe.

A rough calculation indicates that the risk for individual schools is also low. From the 1992–1993 to 2006–2007 school years, there were approximately 118 schools that experienced a student-perpetrated homicide (one or more fatalities on school grounds) over these 15 years, generating an average of 7.9 school cases per year (cases tallied from National School Safety Center 2008). The number of schools in the United States during this time period averaged about 117,000. Thus the average school can expect a student-perpetrated homicide about once every 14,810 years (117,000 divided by 7.9).

While school shootings have captured the nation's interest, less serious but more pervasive forms of juvenile aggression, such as bullying and fighting, have received comparatively little attention (Cornell 2006). Data compiled by the National Center for Education Statistics (Dinkes et al. 2007) indicate that 78% of public schools reported at least one violent crime at their school during the 2005–2006 school year. In 2005, 8% of high school students reported being threatened or injured with a weapon in the previous 12 months, and 28% of students ages 12–18 years reported being bullied at school in the previous 6 months.

Research findings consistently contradict the common perception that school violence is on the rise. As indicated in Figure 23–1, the annual rate of violent crime victimization in schools declined from 13 incidents per 1,000 students in 1994 to 5 per 1,000 students in 2005 (Dinkes et al. 2007).

The decline in violence at school mirrors an equally dramatic drop in juvenile violent crime, as shown in Figure 23–2. Arrest records from the Federal Bureau of Investigation (FBI) Uniform Crime Reports indicate that, from 1994 to 2006, juvenile arrests for homicide dropped 74% (from 3,710 to 956) and juvenile arrests for aggravated assault dropped 48% (from 85,300 to 44,424), despite an increase in the underlying juvenile population (Federal Bureau of Investigation 1994–2007).

Legal Issues

Forensic clinicians conducting student risk assessments or consulting with schools should be familiar with relevant education law. State and federal laws restrict how schools can share information and influence what kinds of interventions they can take in response to student behavior. Clinicians must be mindful of these parameters in making their recommendations.

Family Educational Rights and Privacy Act

The federal government's Report to the President on Issues Raised by the Virginia Tech Tragedy (Leavitt et al. 2007) revealed a great deal of uncertainty and misunderstanding across the nation regarding the sharing of information about potentially dangerous students. The Family Educational Rights and Privacy Act (FERPA) was originally enacted in 1974 and was amended for the ninth time as part of the USA PATRIOT Act of 2001. FERPA, as well as many state laws and regulations, place restrictions on the sharing of information between schools and on the release of information to others, including mental health and law enforcement agencies. Often educators and mental health profes-

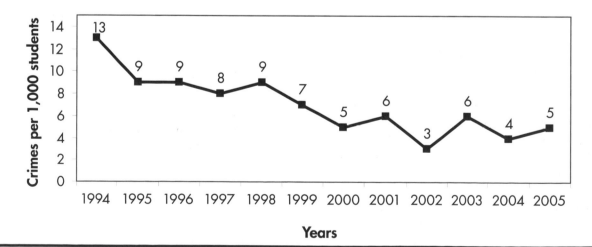

FIGURE 23–1. Annual rate of serious violent crime in U.S. schools.

Source. Data from Indicators of School Crime and Safety 2007.

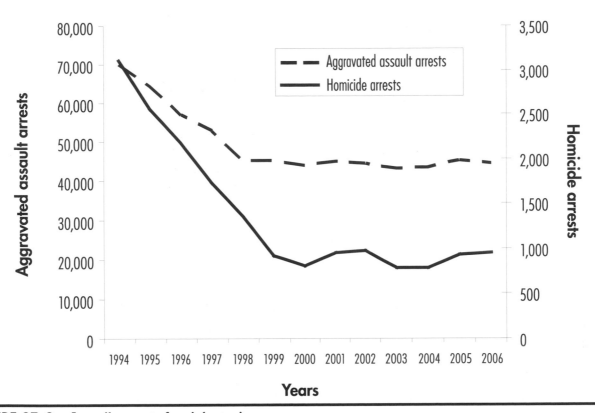

FIGURE 23–2. Juvenile arrests for violent crime.

Aggravated assault arrests *(dashed line)* are graphed on the western axis, ranging from 0 to 80,000. Homicide arrests *(solid line)* are graphed on the eastern axis, ranging from 0 to 3,500.

Source. Arrest statistics obtained from annual Federal Bureau of Investigation Uniform Crime Reports (1994–2007).

sionals alike err on the side of withholding information that might violate legal and professional standards. As a result, high schools typically do not inform postsecondary institutions about the special education status or mental health needs of their entering students. Moreover, concerns identified about these students in the course of their studies might not be shared within organizations, such that teachers, student services personnel, mental health professionals, and law enforcement officers may have their own silos of information that are not integrated and analyzed to gain an overall picture of the students' needs.

Mental health professionals may be more familiar with the restrictions on information sharing under the Health Insurance Portability and Accountability Act (HIPAA) of 1996 and wonder how HIPAA relates to FERPA. Although school nurses, psychologists, and other school personnel provide health care services, according to the HIPAA privacy rule, educational records are largely excluded from HIPAA requirements because they are regulated by FERPA (Dinkes et al. 2007). This exclusion covers information such as health records maintained by the school nurse and diagnostic information on students receiving special education services.

In October 2007, the U.S. Department of Education released a series of documents intended to clarify the limitations of FERPA in situations involving student health or safety (U.S. Department of Education 2007b). Here are some of the main points of clarification that forensic clinicians should keep in mind:

1. FERPA applies only to education records, not to all information about a student that may be known to school authorities. As a result:

   • School personnel can disclose information about a student that is obtained from personal knowledge or observation. For example, a school administrator who has interviewed a student about his or her threatening behavior would not be prohibited under FERPA from sharing that information with a mental health professional who is conducting an assessment.
   • Schools may have "law enforcement units" that maintain investigative reports and other records that are not part of the student's education record. For example, the school resource officer or a school security office can maintain a record of an investigation of a student threat.

2. Disciplinary action taken against a student for conduct that posed a significant risk to the safety or well-being of that student or others can be disclosed to other school staff, including the staff of other schools, who have a legitimate educational interest in the behavior of that student (FERPA 1974). For example, if a student is disciplined for fighting or making threats of violence, the school can share this information with the student's future teachers or school administrators, even if the student moves to a new school.

3. In an emergency, FERPA permits schools to release any information in a student's education records that is necessary to protect health or safety (FERPA 1974). For example, if a student has made a serious threat to injure others, the school might release mental health or disciplinary information that is relevant to intervention or prevention efforts with the student.

4. Staff at postsecondary institutions may be under the impression that they cannot release information to parents because the student is at least 18 years old. However, there are two notable exceptions to this assumption (U.S. Department of Education 2007a):

   • If a student under the age of 21 has violated any law or policy concerning the use or possession of alcohol or a controlled substance, the college or university can contact the student's parents.

   • The U.S. Department of Education has advised that schools may release information to parents without the student's consent if the student is a dependent for tax purposes. This means that if the dean of students or some other college official has concerns about a student's behavior, he or she is not automatically prohibited from consulting with the student's parents and, in the case of undergraduate students, likely is not prohibited. It behooves college and university administrations to determine which students are financially dependent on their parents.

These observations make it clear that FERPA does not impose an impenetrable communication barrier between school officials and those they might wish to contact in seeking assistance to help a troubled student. Mental health clinicians are advised, however, that there may be state laws or school regulations that further complicate the release of information. In the wake of the Virginia Tech shooting, Virginia and other states have initiated legislative actions to review and diminish such restrictions.

Individuals With Disabilities Education Act

The Individuals With Disabilities Education Act (IDEA) of 2004 guarantees all American children with disabilities access to a free appropriate public education (FAPE). This seemingly straightforward guarantee has complex implications for how schools must educate, discipline, and protect students who qualify for special education services. IDEA was reauthorized in 2004 to align with the requirements of the No Child Left Behind Act of 2001 (see also Chapter 5, "Special Education: Screening Tools, Rating Scales, and Self-Report Instruments").

Students who suffer from an emotional disturbance are particularly at risk for discipline violations (Conroy et al. 2002). Students who receive special education services for learning disabilities (LD), as well as children diagnosed with attention deficit/hyperactivity disorder (ADHD) who may receive services under the "other health impaired" classification, also have elevated rates of disciplinary infractions (Skiba et al. 1997; Sprague et al. 2001). A study of the Virginia threat assessment guidelines (Kaplan and Cornell 2005) found that students receiving special education services, particularly those receiving services for emotional disturbance, LD, or ADHD (classified under "other health impairments"), were more likely than other students to come to the attention of school authorities for expressing a violent threat.

When a student has engaged in violent or threatening behavior, school authorities may want to suspend the student or move the student to an alternative setting. However, if the student is receiving special education services, schools must comply with provisions in IDEA that govern changes in the student's placement. In brief, special education services, including educational placement, are guided by the student's Individualized Education Program (sometimes called an Individualized Education Plan, or more commonly, an IEP). An IEP is a legally binding document that represents an agreement between the school and the child's parents designed to meet the child's educational needs (IDEA 2004). Parents are guaranteed the right to participate in the meeting of school personnel who develop the IEP, and if they object to the plan, they can ask for mediation or can file a complaint that leads to a due process hearing. IEPs are subject to review at least once a year but can be reviewed and revised anytime there is concern that the plan is not working or that the child's educational needs have changed.

Violent or threatening behavior is often grounds for reviewing a student's IEP. The IEP might already include specific plans for dealing with disruptive or aggressive behavior, and if the plans do not appear to be working, they must be revised. If the violent or threatening behavior is a new concern, it might be appropriate to develop plans for dealing with it. Such plans can range widely, from options such as the provision of counseling aimed at improving the student's ability to manage anger to specific teacher tactics for reinforcing the student's behavior in the classroom.

A frequent problem arises when school authorities want to suspend a student who is receiving special education services. If the suspension, including previous suspensions, exceeds 10 days, then the suspension may be considered to constitute a change in placement. Ordinarily, a change in placement must be approved at an IEP meeting. When a student has engaged in aggressive or threatening behavior, school authorities may not have time to convene an IEP meeting, or if the meeting takes place, they may find that the parents will not agree to the change in placement. Previously, students had a "stay put" right in many circumstances that permitted parents to insist that their children remain in the current setting until all appeals were exhausted, but the new regulations for IDEA eliminate this provision.

In a clearly dangerous or emergency situation, such as when a student has made a serious threat to kill someone, school authorities are advised to make safety their top priority (Cornell and Sheras 2006). School authorities have at least four options for removing a dangerous student from school:

1. School authorities should attempt to persuade the parents to agree to a voluntary change in placement (such as homebound instruction or transfer to an alternative school). It is always preferable to strive for a cooperative and collaborative relationship with parents and to avoid adversarial situations. Often the most valuable function of a mental health professional is to help school authorities and parents engage in a problem-solving relationship focused on the best interests of the child.
2. If the parents are uncooperative, school authorities can go to a hearing officer and obtain a 45-school-day removal from school for a student who has inflicted serious bodily injury on someone or has engaged in some other behavior involving weapons or illegal drugs (IDEA 2004).
3. If the circumstances do not meet the criteria for a 45-day removal, school authorities might seek a remedy through the courts. If the student has broken the law and poses a risk to the community, the student might be placed in juvenile detention. If the student is on probation for a previous offense, the student's probation officer might have the authority to have the student detained.
4. If the circumstances do not justify the student's detention, school authorities have the final option of seeking a restraining order to keep the student off campus.

It must be emphasized that school authorities should not pursue any of these options unless there is convincing evidence that the student poses a danger to others, which is often the key question in a mental health referral for a risk assessment or threat assessment, discussed below.

Manifestation Determination

When a student with an IEP is suspended for 10 or more days within the same school year, the school is obligated under IDEA to conduct a "manifestation determination." The purpose of this procedure is to determine whether the student's misconduct met either of two conditions. First, was the misconduct caused by, or did it have a direct and substantial relationship to, the child's disability? Second, was the misconduct the direct result of failure to implement the student's IEP? If either of these questions is answered in the affirmative, the school cannot impose a disciplinary suspension on the student for the misconduct. Furthermore, the school must use the IEP process to develop a plan for dealing with the student's misconduct. This may require revision of the IEP or efforts to make sure that the existing IEP is fully implemented.

The criteria for determining whether a student's misconduct was caused by the student's disability or had a direct and substantial relationship to the disability are ambiguous and subject to debate. A relatively clear-cut case might involve a student who acted upon delusional thinking that is produced by a psychotic disorder, but in less obvious cases, there is little guidance. As of 2004, IEP teams are no longer required to consider whether the disability impaired the child's ability to control or understand the impact and consequences of his or her behavior. Furthermore, the burden of proof that a child's misbehavior was a manifestation of his or her disability has been shifted from the school to the parents. Good resources on IDEA include the website for the Families and Advocates Partnership for Education (http://www.fape.org/) and the IDEA Partnership (http://www.ideapartnership.org/).

Gun-Free Schools Act and Zero Tolerance Policies

The Gun-Free Schools Act (GFSA) of 1994 requires any school division receiving funds under the Elementary and Secondary Education Act to expel, for a period of not less than 1 year, any student found to be in possession of a weapon or firearm at school. This act was reauthorized and amended by the No Child Left Behind Act of 2001 to be consistent with IDEA. Although the law permits schools to impose lesser sanctions on a case-by-case basis, often this provision is overlooked or not used. Instead, the federal law instituted a nationwide practice of *zero tolerance*, which is defined as "a philosophy or policy that mandates the application of predetermined consequences, most often severe and punitive in nature, that are intended to be applied regardless of the seriousness of behavior, mitigating circumstances, or situational context" (American Psychological Association Task Force 2006, p. 2).

The term *firearm* for the purpose of GFSA is defined as a weapon or destructive device that can expel a projectile by the action of any explosive, such as a handgun, rifle, and shotgun, as well as any explosive or incendiary device, such as a bomb or rocket. This definition explicitly excludes items such as toy guns, cap guns, BB guns, and pellet guns; nevertheless, many schools expanded zero tolerance to include other weapons, even toy weapons and objects that resembled weapons. The result was the widespread use of excessive punishment for student acts that are not serious, such as bringing a toy gun to school or shooting a paper clip with a rubber band (Cornell 2006; Skiba and Peterson 1999). In one case described in the *Seattle Times* on January 8, 1997, a 10-year-old boy was expelled from elementary school because he brought to school a 1-inch plastic toy pistol that was an accessory to his G.I. Joe action figure. In other cases, students have been suspended or expelled for making drawings, finger-pointing, wearing a T-shirt depicting guns, and playing "cops and robbers" during recess (Rutherford Institute 2003).

The American Bar Association (2001) issued a statement condemning zero tolerance policies in schools. The primary criticism was that this disciplinary model emphasizes punishment over education and encourages school administrators to consider all infractions as deserving of the same consequences without regard to the circumstances or the student's history. In 2006, the American Psychological Association Zero Tolerance Task Force reported a 10-year review of school discipline records to examine the effects of zero tolerance policies. Results indicated that the one-size-fits-all punishment mandated by zero tolerance policies is not effective in creating safer school environments. In contrast, expulsion practices appear to increase misbehavior and lead to higher dropout rates.

School Liability for Student Bullying and Violence

For many years, courts have ruled that schools cannot be held accountable for injury that one student inflicts on another (*Wood v. Strickland* 1975). However, in the case of *Davis v. Monroe County Board of Education* (1999), the U.S. Supreme Court determined that a school board could be found liable for sexual harassment of one student by another under certain conditions. The case involved a fifth-grade girl who was harassed by a classmate who engaged in sexually suggestive actions, including physical contact, on numerous occasions over a period of months. Despite repeated complaints by the victim and other girls in the class, the teacher and principal did not discipline the boy but simply admonished him and allowed the girl to move to another desk. The girl's grades dropped and she became so distressed that she wrote a suicide note, prompting the parents to file suit. The harassment was deemed a violation of Title IX of the Education Amendments of 1972, which prohibits a student from being "excluded from participation in, being denied the benefits of, or being subjected to discrimination under any education program or activity receiving Federal financial assistance" (Title IX, 20 U.S.C. § 1681(a)–1688, 1972). The Supreme Court determined that a school could be liable if 1) school authorities had knowledge of the harassment; 2) they were deliberately indifferent to it; and 3) the harassment was so severe, pervasive, and objectively offensive that it deprived the victim of access to educational opportunities and benefits.

In recent years, courts have applied the reasoning in *Davis v. Monroe* to many other cases involving bullying. For example, in the case of *Scruggs v. Meriden Board of Education* (2005), the U.S. District Court of Connecticut found the school to be negligent and deliberately indifferent in the case of a middle school boy who was repeatedly bullied and who eventually committed suicide. The case of *L.W. v. Toms River Regional School Board of Education* (2005) involved a boy who was repeatedly teased and physically bullied about his perceived sexual orientation from the elementary grades into high school. The court ordered the school to revise its policies, train its staff, and implement a bullying prevention program.

In recent years, bullying has become recognized as a pervasive problem in the United States, in part because a U.S. Secret Service report identified bullying as a significant factor in rampage school shootings (Vossekuil et al. 2002). Since 1999, at least 16 states have enacted laws to address bullying, intimidation, or harassment in school (National Conference of State Legislatures 2008). One problem is that bullying is a broad concept that can be difficult to define or to distinguish from other forms of peer conflict (Cornell and Bandyopadhyay, in press). Bullying can involve physical, verbal, or social acts that are intended to humiliate a weaker person. Conflict between peers of comparable strength or status is not bullying. Teasing and horseplay are not necessarily bullying either, if the actions are good-natured and there is no humiliated victim.

Bullying prevention is a worldwide movement that originated in Norway in 1983 following two highly publicized cases of middle school students who committed suicide in reaction to bullying. The nationwide Norwegian effort to curb bullying led to Olweus's (1993) pioneering work on bullying and the development of the Olweus Bullying Prevention Program, which is widely used across the world and in the United States (Olweus and Limber 1999). The program involves schoolwide, classroom-level, and individual efforts to educate students and staff about bullying, to enforce rules against bullying, and to work with identified victims and aggressors and their parents. Early studies documented large reductions (up to 50%) in student self-reports of bullying and victimization (Olweus Bullying Prevention Program 2003), but independent reviews of other studies have been less positive (Merrell et al. 2008; Smith et al. 2004). Schools should be advised to take concerted action whenever bullying is identified but to keep in mind that there are no easy solutions, because bullying is a persistent, recurring problem (see also Chapter 33, "Clinical and Forensic Aspects of Sexual Harassment in School-Age Children and Adolescents").

Risk Assessment Approaches to School Violence

School authorities often want forensic clinicians to conduct an evaluation of a student who has aroused concern that he or she might be dangerous. Ideally, school authorities would like to receive a report either affirming that a student is dangerous in order to support a decision to remove the student from school or assuring them that the student is not dangerous as a condition for the student's return to school. Such a request may seem reasonable to the school authorities from a defensive, liability perspective, but it does not reflect modern conceptions of risk assessment and threat management. Static predictions of dangerousness, or slightly more elaborate classifications of a student as low, medium, or high risk, are misleadingly simple, unrealistic, and prone to error. A more appropriate approach is to take a risk management approach, as distinguished from a prediction approach, and to offer recommendations aimed to help school authorities manage and reduce the risk of violence (Borum and Verhaagen 2006; Cornell and Williams 2006; Heilbrun 1997).

Static predictions are unrealistic because dangerousness is not a personal trait or fixed characteristic of a student but a variable condition that depends heavily on situational as well as individual factors. A student who is unsupervised and who uses alcohol or other drugs, associates with antisocial peers, and has access to firearms is much more dangerous than the same student in a structured, supervised, supportive setting. A depressed student who is being antagonized by bullies could decide to take violent action despite no history of violent or disobedient behavior even though prior violence is considered the best clinical predictor of future violence. Accordingly, clinicians should qualify their assessments of students based on environmental factors, recognizing that risk fluctuates over time and circumstances. Although this perspective makes prediction seem even more uncertain, it offers prospects for management strategies that can reduce the risk of violence.

Profiling Versus Threat Assessment

At its 1999 conference on school shootings, the FBI's profiling experts concluded that profiling was not a useful approach to identify potential school shooters:

> One response to the pressure for action may be an effort to identify the next shooter by developing a "profile" of the typical school shooter. This may sound like a reasonable preventive measure, but in practice, trying to draw up a catalogue or "checklist" of warning signs to detect a potential shooter can be shortsighted, even dangerous. Such lists, publicized by the media, can end up unfairly labeling many nonviolent

students as potentially dangerous or even lethal. In fact, a great many adolescents who will never commit violent acts will show some of the behaviors or personality traits on the list. (O'Toole 2000, pp. 2–3)

An important finding from the FBI's study of school shootings was that the students almost always communicated their intentions to harm someone before carrying out their shooting. Furthermore, the FBI identified a number of cases in which school shootings were prevented because authorities investigated a student's threatening statement and found that the student posed a serious threat. These observations suggested that schools should focus their efforts on the identification and investigation of student threats as a violence prevention strategy, a process commonly known as threat assessment.

The U.S. Secret Service developed threat assessment as an explicit process of threat investigation and intervention in its efforts to protect government officials, and it recommended that each school adopt a similar procedure using a threat assessment team composed of mental health and law enforcement professionals (Fein et al. 2002; Reddy et al. 2001). Threat assessment differs from profiling because it does not involve the application of a general checklist or set of warning signs to the entire population of students in hope of identifying a dangerous individual; instead, the process focuses on students who identify themselves by making a threatening statement or engaging in threatening behavior that demands attention. However, all threats are not equally serious, and the task of the threat assessment team is to determine whether the student actually poses a threat, that is, has both the intention and the means to carry out the threat. If the threat appears to be genuine, the team moves into a threat management and risk reduction phase. The team undertakes immediate protective action, such as warning potential victims and removing a student from school, and then develops a longer-term plan for resolving the problem or conflict that generated the threat (Cornell and Sheras 2006).

Threat Assessment Guidelines

Researchers and educators at the University of Virginia developed a set of guidelines for school administrators to use in responding to a reported student threat of violence (Cornell and Sheras 2006). The guidelines followed a decision tree that began with an initial assessment of the seriousness of the threat, followed by a determination whether the case could be easily resolved as a transient threat or would require more extensive assessment and protective action as a substantive threat. In the most serious cases, a multidisciplinary team would conduct a comprehensive safety evaluation that would include both a law enforcement investigation and a mental health assessment of the student.

The multidisciplinary team ordinarily consists of a school administrator (principal or assistant principal), one or more mental health professionals (often a school counselor and a school psychologist), and a school resource officer (or another law enforcement representative). Such teams ensure a coordinated and comprehensive approach to student threats that combines educational, law enforcement, and mental health perspectives.

School-based teams are preferable to teams or individuals working outside the school setting for several reasons. School-based teams help ensure a prompt response to a student threat and have a wealth of information about school climate and student interactions that provides a context for understanding a student's threat. School-based teams are in position to gather information from teachers and classmates that is not readily available to professionals working outside the school. Finally, a school-based team is most knowledgeable in developing workable plans for monitoring and supporting a student who returns to school after a threat assessment. Because threat assessment also involves threat management, a school-based team must be prepared to remain in contact with the student over time as intervention and prevention efforts are implemented.

School threat assessment teams can make good use of outside consultants, such as forensic mental health professionals in the community, in complex cases such as those involving severe or unusual psychiatric disorders. Mental health professionals can also provide a more neutral outsider's perspective in highly charged or controversial cases. However, mental health professionals in the community should refrain from accepting full responsibility for conducting a student threat assessment. As noted above, a community-based mental health professional cannot respond as promptly as is needed when there is a question about immediate safety and cannot gather information from school personnel and other students that may be essential to understanding the circumstances of a student's threat. Community-based mental health professionals might need to educate school personnel about the nature of a threat assessment approach and should be wary of accepting responsibility that exceeds what they can reasonably undertake and accomplish.

When mental health professionals are asked to conduct threat assessments for schools, they should clarify the limitations of their role and define their task as one component of a threat assessment. Threat assessment should be conceptualized as an ongoing threat management and violence prevention strategy rather than an absolute determination that a student is or is not dangerous. From this point of view, the mental health evaluation represents one stage in a process rather than an endpoint. The mental health clinician can best advise school authorities and parents about the student's mental health needs and make treatment recommendations. He or she can help school authorities understand why the student made a threat and give them insight into the student's motives and behavior. In many circumstances, the mental health clinician can also make recommendations regarding strategies for resolving the conflict or problem that stimulated the threatening behavior.

A mental health assessment of a student who has made threats of violence will consist largely of extensive interviews with the student and his or her parents. However, the clinician must have access to additional sources of information and will want to consult with school authorities, who should be able to provide additional perspectives on the student's academic performance, peer relations, and prior adjustment, as well as information about the resources and programs available in the school. Sometimes parents object to the disclosure of information from the school or other sources, such as prior therapists or medical records, because of concern that the clinician will be biased by these views. On the contrary, it is essential to have complete information, and clinicians should explain to parents that it is their professional obligation to take an objective approach and resist biasing influences. The clinician must be prepared to refuse to undertake an evaluation with insufficient cooperation by all parties. When the clinician does conduct an evaluation and for any reason is not able to obtain complete information, then it is best to acknowledge these limitations explicitly and to refrain from offering conclusions that cannot reasonably be made without additional information. Any provisional recommendations that are made should be qualified by cautions about the need for additional information.

The Virginia threat assessment guidelines follow a decision tree that consists of seven steps (Cornell and Sheras 2006; Table 23–1). At step 1, a team member (typically the team leader, often a school administra-

tor) investigates a reported threat by interviewing the student who made the threat and any witnesses to the threat. The guidelines manual includes a basic set of interview questions that consider both the actual threat behavior and questions about the meaning and intent of the threat from each observer's perspective.

At step 2, the team leader decides whether the threat is transient or substantive. A threat is considered transient if it is not a serious threat and can be easily resolved. Examples of transient threats are jokes or statements made in anger that are expressions of feeling or figures of speech rather than expressions of a genuine intent to harm someone. Any threat that cannot be clearly identified as transient is treated as a substantive threat.

If a threat is transient, it is resolved at step 3 through a brief counseling process intended to resolve the conflict or clarify the misunderstanding that might have stimulated the threat. The student might be reprimanded and could receive a disciplinary consequence appropriate to the seriousness of the behavior (e.g., creating a disturbance or being disrespectful to others). If this process is deemed successful by the team, the incident is resolved and no further action is needed.

The first three steps are essentially a triage process designed to address simpler cases without an extended process. If a threat cannot be resolved as transient or appears to be substantive, the process becomes more complex. Substantive threats always require protective action to prevent the threat from being carried out. At step 4, the threat is determined to be serious or very serious. A threat to hit, assault, or beat up someone is serious, whereas a threat to kill, rape, use a weapon, or severely injure someone is considered very serious. Serious threats are addressed at step 5, whereas very serious threats are addressed at step 6.

At step 5, serious substantive threats require protective action to prevent violence, including notification of potential victims and other actions to address the conflict or problem that generated the threat. The response to serious threats is completed at this step.

Steps 6 and 7 are reserved for very serious substantive threats. At step 6, the team takes immediate protective action, including contact with law enforcement followed by a comprehensive safety evaluation. The student may be suspended from school pending completion of a safety evaluation. A safety evaluation includes both a law enforcement investigation and a mental health assessment. The mental health assessment follows a standard list of topics and questions described in the manual (Cornell and Sheras 2006) and may incorporate other assessment procedures,

---

TABLE 23–1. Steps in student threat assessment

Step 1—Evaluate the threat.

A team member investigates a reported threat by interviewing the student who made the threat and any witnesses to the threat. The context and meaning of the threat are more important than the literal content of the threat.

Step 2—Decide whether the threat is transient or substantive.

A transient threat is not a serious threat and can be easily resolved, but a substantive threat raises concern of potential injury to others. For transient threats, go to step 3; for substantive threats, skip to step 4.

Step 3—Respond to a transient threat.

Appropriate responses to a transient threat include a reprimand, parental notification, or other actions that reflect the severity and chronicity of the situation. The incident is resolved at this step.

Step 4—If the threat is substantive, decide whether it is serious or very serious.

If a threat is substantive, the team must decide how serious the threat is and take appropriate action to protect potential victims. A threat to hit, assault, or beat up someone is serious, whereas a threat to kill, rape, use a weapon, or severely injure someone is considered very serious. For serious threats, go to step 5; for very serious threats, skip to step 6.

Step 5—Respond to a serious substantive threat.

Serious substantive threats require protective action to prevent violence, including notification of potential victims and other actions to address the conflict or problem that generated the threat. The response to serious threats is completed at this step.

Step 6—Respond to a very serious substantive threat.

Very serious threats require immediate protective action, including contact with law enforcement, followed by a comprehensive safety evaluation. The student is suspended from school pending completion of a safety evaluation, which includes a mental health assessment.

Step 7—Implement a safety plan.

The threat assessment team develops and implements an action plan that is designed both to protect potential victims and to meet the student's educational needs. The plan includes provision for monitoring the student and revising the plan as needed.

Source.   Cornell and Sheras 2006.

---

such as the Structured Assessment of Violence Risk in Youth, or SAVRY (Borum et al. 2006; see Chapter 21, "Assessing Violence Risk in Youth," for a discussion of SAVRY). Community-based mental health professionals are most appropriately engaged at this stage, particularly when there are unresolved questions about a student's mental health and treatment needs.

At step 7, the threat assessment team uses the results of the safety evaluation to develop and implement an action plan that is designed both to protect potential victims and to meet the student's educational needs. The plan includes provision for the team to monitor the student and revise the plan as needed. From this perspective, threat assessment is a process that evolves into threat management and intervention.

The Virginia threat assessment guidelines were field-tested in 35 public schools where school-based teams evaluated 188 student threats over the course of

1 school year (Cornell et al. 2004). The cases involved threats to hit, stab, shoot, or harm someone in some other way. Most of the cases (70%) were resolved as transient threats, such as comments made in jest or in a moment of anger. The remaining 30% were substantive threats that required protective action to prevent the threats from being carried out. In such cases, the threat assessment teams attempted to understand the context and meaning of the threat in order to develop a plan to address the underlying conflict or problem that drove the student to make a threat.

Unlike a zero tolerance policy, under which most students would be expelled for making threats to kill or injure someone, a threat assessment approach gives school authorities flexibility in choosing the disciplinary consequences for students who make threats. Only 3 students were expelled from school, although half of the students (94) received short-term suspensions (typically 1–3 days). Based on follow-up interviews with school principals at the end of the school year, the threats were satisfactorily resolved and the students who made the threats engaged in few subsequent acts of violence. Approximately 17% of the students engaged in some form of aggressive act, such as a fight or assault, during the remainder of the school year, but none of the students carried out their threat of violence against their intended victims. A second evaluation of the Virginia threat assessment guidelines was conducted in Memphis city schools (Strong and Cornell 2008). This evaluation examined 209 cases resolved by threat assessment with no reported cases of threats being carried out and almost all students returning to their school or an alternative school setting.

Case Example Epilogue

Consider how Johnny's case would be handled under zero tolerance, profiling, and threat assessment models. Under a zero tolerance policy, the principal would simply suspend Johnny from school and recommend him for expulsion. With use of a profiling approach, the principal would compare Johnny against a checklist of risk factors or warning signs, and if he appeared to meet the criteria, the principal would consider this student dangerous.

In contrast, a threat assessment team approach would begin with interviews of Johnny and other relevant witnesses. If there was sufficient concern about the nature of Johnny's statements, the school resource officer would inquire about his access to weapons and investigate whether there were any other indications that Johnny was planning to carry out the threat. Johnny also would be referred for a mental health assessment designed to evaluate his mental state and his amenability to working out a more constructive solution to his problems with his peers. If there was no indication that Johnny was planning and preparing to carry out the threat, and it was evident that Johnny was simply frustrated because he was being teased, then the assessment team might develop a plan to address the bullying, set up a counseling relationship for Johnny, and keep the situation under close observation to make sure that the bullying problem was resolved.

Threat assessment should be considered one component of a comprehensive approach toward maintaining a safe school (Osher et al. 2004). Threat assessment identifies students who may be in need of additional services as well as more general problems in the school environment, such as bullying, that merit broader attention. Wilson et al. (2003) reviewed 221 studies of school-based interventions and found that well-implemented demonstration programs are highly effective and can result in 50% reduction in aggressive and disruptive behavior.

More broadly, the foundation for a safe school rests on the maintenance of a caring community in which students feel safe and secure (Catalano et al. 2004). Safety and security derive from two conditions: 1) an orderly, predictable environment where school staff provide consistent, reliable supervision and discipline; and (2) a school climate in which students feel connected to the school and supported by their teachers and other school staff. A balance of structure and support is essential and requires an organized schoolwide approach that is practiced by all school personnel (Sprague et al. 2001; Sugai et al. 2000). The National Registry of Evidence-Based Programs and Practices (http://www.nrepp.samhsa.gov/) is a good resource for effective programs at all grade levels.

—Key Points

— Forensic mental health clinicians should attempt to counter misconceptions about the danger and severity of school violence with base rate evidence that schools are much safer than commonly believed.

— There are many circumstances in which the Family Educational Rights and Privacy Act (FERPA) does not prevent schools from sharing information relevant to student risk of violence.

— Although the Individuals With Disabilities Education Act (IDEA) ensures the rights of students with handicapping conditions, it does not preclude removing a student from school if he or she poses a threat to others.

— Research evidence does not support zero tolerance discipline practices.

— Threat assessment is preferable to profiling as a means of preventing school violence.

— Threat assessment is a multidisciplinary team-based approach to evaluating the seriousness of a threat and then taking appropriate protective action.

— The purpose of a mental health evaluation as part of a threat assessment is prevention rather than prediction of violence, so recommendations should focus on developing a plan to address the problem that generated the threat rather than static classifications of risk.

References

American Bar Association: Zero Tolerance Policy Report. Washington, DC, American Bar Association, Juvenile Justice Committee, 2001

American Psychological Association Task Force: Are Zero Tolerance Policies Effective in the Schools? An Evidentiary Review and Recommendations. Washington, DC, American Psychological Association, 2006

Borum R, Verhaagen D: Assessing and Managing Violence Risk in Juveniles. New York, Guilford, 2006

Borum R, Bartel P, Forth A: Manual for the Structured Assessment of Violence Risk in Youth (SAVRY). Odessa, FL, Psychological Assessment Resources, 2006

Catalano RF, Berglund ML, Ryan JAM, et al: Positive youth development in the United States: research findings on evaluations of positive youth development programs. Ann Acad Pol Soc Sci 591:98–124, 2004

Conroy MA, Katsiyannis A, Clark D, et al: The IDEA disciplinary provisions: national trends and state practices. Behavioral Disorders 27:98–108, 2002

Cornell D: School Violence: Fears Versus Facts. Mahwah, NJ, Lawrence Erlbaum, 2006

Cornell D, Bandyopadhyay S: The assessment of bullying, in The International Handbook of School Bullying. Edited by Jimerson SR, Swearer SM, Espelage DL. Mahwah, NJ, Lawrence Erlbaum (in press)

Cornell D, Sheras P: Guidelines for Responding to Student Threats of Violence. Longmont, CO, Sopris West, 2006

Cornell D, Williams F: Student threat assessment as a strategy to reduce school violence, in The Handbook of School Violence and School Safety: From Research to Practice. Edited by Jimerson SR, Furlong MJ. Mahwah, NJ, Erlbaum, 2006, pp 587–602

Cornell D, Sheras P, Kaplan S, et al: Guidelines for student threat assessment: field-test findings. School Psychology Review 33:527–546, 2004

Davis v Monroe County Board of Education, 526 US 629 (1999)

Dinkes R, Cataldi EF, Lin-Kelly W, et al: Indicators of School Crime and Safety: 2007 (NCES 2008-021, NCJ 219553). Washington, DC, U.S. Government Printing Office, 2007

Family Educational Rights and Privacy Act of 1974, 20 USC § 99.36–1232g, 34 CFR Part 99 et seq (1974)

Federal Bureau of Investigation: Uniform Crime Reports: Crime in the United States. Washington, DC, U.S. Government Printing Office, 1994–2007

Fein R, Vossekuil B, Pollack W, et al: Threat Assessment in Schools: A Guide to Managing Threatening Situations and to Creating Safe School Climates. Washington, DC, U.S. Secret Service and Department of Education, 2002

Gun-Free Schools Act, 20 USC § 8921 et seq (1994)

Health Insurance Portability and Accountability Act, Public Law 104-191, § 45, 110 Stat 1936 (1996)

Heilbrun K: Prediction versus management models relevant to risk assessment: the importance of legal decision-making context. Law Human Behav 21:347–360, 1997

Individuals With Disabilities Education Act, 20 USC § 1414 (2004)

Kaplan S, Cornell D: Threats of violence by students in special education. Behav Dis 31:107–119, 2005

Leavitt MO, Gonzales AR, Spellings M: Report to the President on Issues Raised by the Virginia Tech Tragedy. Washington, DC, U.S. Department of Health and Human Services, Department of Education, and Department of Justice, 2007

LW v Toms River Regional School Board of Education, US Dist WL 3299837 (NJ Sup AD December 7, 2005)

Merrell KW, Isava DM, Gueldner BA, et al: How effective are school bullying intervention programs? a meta-analysis of intervention research. Sch Psychol Q 23:26–42, 2008

National Conference of State Legislatures: School Bullying: Legislation and Laws. 2008. Available at: http://www.ncsl.org/programs/educ/SchBullyingLegislation.htm. Accessed April 30, 2008.

National School Safety Center: School Associated Violent Deaths. Westlake Village, CA, National School Safety Center, 2008. Available at: http://www.schoolsafety.us/pubfiles/savd.pdf. Accessed May 2, 2008.

No Child Left Behind Act, 20 USC § 6301 (2001)

Olweus D: Bullying at School: What We Know and What We Can Do. Cambridge, MA, Blackwell, 1993

Olweus D, Limber S: Blueprints for Violence Prevention: Bullying Prevention Program. Boulder, University of Colorado, Institute of Behavioral Science, 1999

Olweus Bullying Prevention Program: Evidence of Effectiveness: Research Basis for the Olweus Bullying Prevention Program. 2003. Available at: http://www.clemson.edu/olweus/evidence.html. Accessed May 1, 2008.

Osher D, Dwyer K, Jackson S: Safe, Supportive and Successful Schools: Step by Step. Longmont, CO, Sopris West, 2004

O'Toole ME: The School Shooter: A Threat Assessment Perspective. Quantico, VA, Federal Bureau of Investigation, National Center for the Analysis of Violent Crime, 2000

Reddy M, Borum R, Berglund J, et al: Evaluating risk for targeted violence in schools: comparing risk assessment, threat assessment, and other approaches. Psychology in the Schools 38:157–172, 2001

Rutherford Institute: Tracking and Fighting Zero Tolerance. October 27, 2003. Available at: http://www.rutherford.org/articles_db/legal_features.asp?article_id=71. Accessed July 4, 2005.

Saad L: Public Views Littleton Tragedy as Sign of Deeper Problems in Country. April 23, 1999. Available at: http://www.gallup.com/poll/content/login.aspx?ci=3898. Accessed April 2, 2005.

Scruggs v Meriden Board of Education, US Dist WL 2072312 (D Conn August 26, 2005)

Skiba R, Peterson R: The dark side of zero tolerance: can punishment lead to safe schools? Phi Delta Kappan 80:372–376, 381–382, 1999

Skiba RJ, Peterson RL, Williams T: Office referrals and suspension: disciplinary intervention in middle schools. Educ Treat Child 20:295–315, 1997

Smith JD, Schneider BH, Smith PK, et al: The effectiveness of whole-school antibullying programs: a synthesis of evaluation research. School Psychology Review 33:547–560, 2004

Sprague J, Walker H, Golly A, et al: Translating research into effective practice: the effects of a universal staff and student intervention on indicators of discipline and school safety. Educ Treat Child 24:495–511, 2001

Strong K, Cornell D: Student threat assessment in Memphis City Schools: a descriptive report. Behav Disord 34:42–54, 2008

Sugai G, Horner RH, Dunlap G, et al: Applying positive behavior support and functional behavioral assessment in schools. J Pos Behav Intervent 2:131–143, 2000

Title IX, Educational Amendments, 20 USC § 1681(a)–1688 (1972)

U.S. Department of Education: Disclosure of Information From Educational Records to Parents of Postsecondary Students. Washington, DC, U.S. Department of Education, 2007a. Available at: http://www.ed.gov/policy/gen/guid/fpco/hottopics/ht-parents-postsecstudents.html. Accessed April 28, 2008.

U.S. Department of Education: Safe Schools and FERPA: FERPA Guidance on Emergency Management. Washington, DC, U.S. Department of Education, 2007b. Available at: http://www.ed.gov/policy/gen/guid/fpco/ferpa/safeschools/index.html. Accessed April 28, 2008.

Vossekuil B, Fein RA, Reddy M, et al: The Final Report and Findings of the Safe School Initiative: Implications for the Prevention of School Attacks in the United States. Washington, DC, U.S. Secret Service and U.S. Department of Education, 2002

Wilson SJ, Lipsey MW, Derzon JH: The effects of school-based intervention programs on aggressive behavior: a meta-analysis. J Consult Clin Psychol 71:136–149, 2003

Wood v Strickland, 420 US 308 (1975)

Chapter 24

Juvenile Stalkers

Charles L. Scott, M.D.
Peter Ash, M.D.
Todd S. Elwyn, J.D., M.D.

Stalking is a serious problem in the United States. All 50 states, the federal government, and the District of Columbia classify stalking as a crime. Although precise statutory definitions vary, most stalking statutes incorporate the following elements: 1) there is a course of conduct, 2) the conduct is directed at a specific person, and 3) the conduct results in a reasonable person experiencing fear.

Approximately 1 in 12 women and 1 in 45 men will be stalked at some point in their lifetime. Nearly 90% of stalkers are men, and the majority of female and male victims know their stalker. Women are more likely than men (59% vs. 30%) to be stalked by an intimate partner. Although the average duration of stalking is 1.8 years, the duration increases to 2.2 years when the stalking relationship involves an intimate partner. Over 70% of current or former intimate partners verbally threaten their victim with violence, and 81% of women stalked by a current or prior partner are eventually physically assaulted and over 30% will be sexually assaulted (Tjaden and Thoennes 1998).

Little research has been done regarding the prevalence of stalking by juveniles or how commonly youth are the object of stalking. Some stalkinglike behaviors are common in immature courtship behaviors of children and adolescents, but stalking characterized by repeated unwanted intrusion and communications that elicit fear in the target is relatively rare. In recent years, a number of published case reports demonstrate that some children and young adolescents exhibit stalking behavior, and research on college populations indicates that stalking behavior in late adolescence is not uncommon.

Stalking can occur in a variety of circumstances, including attempts to contact the victim directly or indirectly through the phone, mail, faxes, or personal notes left at a particular location. With the advent of electronic communication, stalkers may use the Internet to maintain contact with their victims, either through e-mails or through gathering information about the victim using common search engines (McGrath and Casey 2002). Such behaviors have been referred to as *cyberstalking* and do not require face-to-face contact. Additional technologies that can be used to cyberstalk include text messaging, computer monitoring software (spyware), and even the placement of Global Positioning System (GPS) devices to pinpoint the location of a potential victim (Southworth et al. 2007).

To best address concerns regarding a potential juvenile stalker, the clinician should be familiar with the following areas: stalking definitions and established typologies, childhood developmental origins of stalking behaviors, developmentally normal "following behaviors" of juveniles and young adults, frequency and characteristics of juvenile stalkers, stalkinglike behaviors among juveniles, and recommended approaches to managing juvenile stalking. We address each of these topics in the following sections.

Stalking Definitions and Established Typologies

Clinical definitions of stalking vary, and there is no consensus definition at this time. Mullen et al. (2000, pp. 9–10) described stalking as "those repeated acts, experienced as unpleasantly intrusive, which create apprehension and can be understood by a reasonable fellow citizen...to be grounds for becoming fearful." Westrup (1998, p. 276) proposed using a DSM-type definition in which stalking was defined as "a constellation of behaviors that 1) are directed repeatedly towards a specific individual (the target), 2) are experienced by the target as unwelcome and intrusive, and 3) are reported to trigger fear or concern in the target." These definitions have been described based on work with adult populations.

Numerous typologies have attempted to classify stalking behavior in adult stalkers, though none of these have been specifically studied in children or adolescents. One of the most commonly referenced typologies was developed by Michael Zona, who initially divided adult stalkers into the following three categories (Zona et al. 1993):

1. *Simple obsessional.* These individuals usually have a prior relationship with the victim and are motivated by a desire to enact revenge on a former partner or to force reestablishment of the lost relationship. This group of stalkers poses the greatest risk of harm to their victims.
2. *Love obsessional.* In contrast to the simple obsessional, the vast majority of love-obsessional stalkers have had no prior relationship with their victim. These perpetrators may become focused on their victim after seeing the person in the media or other public forum. They are commonly viewed by others as an obsessed fan. A significant number suffer from a mental disorder such as schizophrenia or bipolar disorder.
3. *Erotomanic.* Stalkers in this category delusionally believe that their love object also loves them. The typical perpetrator is a female who is convinced that an older male, usually of higher status, returns her affection despite the lack of any rational evidence to support this belief.

Mullen et al. (1999) expanded Zona et al.'s typology of stalking to include five categories of stalkers described by their primary motivation, context in which the stalking developed, and functioning of the stalker's behavior. The primary types described include the rejected, the intimacy seekers, the resentful, the predatory, and the incompetent. Characteristics of each stalker category are noted in Table 24–1.

A more recent typology classifies adult stalkers according to their relationship, if any, with the victim and the private versus public figure context of their pursuit. The acronym RECON was selected for this scheme; it is both relationship (RE) and context (CON) based (Mohandie et al. 2006). The four categories of stalkers described by victim selection are labeled intimate, acquaintance, public figure, or private stranger. An outline of this categorization scheme and associated features is shown in Table 24–2. Research examining the applicability of these various adult typologies to juveniles has not yet been systematically conducted, but they can serve as additional frameworks to help the clinician assess children and adolescents.

The stalking behaviors of youth described in reports of juveniles of high school age and younger (Emer 2001; McCann 1998; Snow 1998; Urbach et al. 1992; Vaidya et al. 2005) appear to follow patterns similar to those of adults. Stalkers are typically male, and their targets are typically female. Stalking behaviors included telephone calls, repetitive letter writing, and physical approach. Threats were found in over half of the cases. In the college-age group, intrusive or unwanted pursuit most commonly followed the breakup of a romantic relationship. In a significant minority of cases, however, the victim was a professor or someone other than a romantic partner.

Childhood Developmental Origins of Stalking Behaviors

How does adult or juvenile stalking develop? A number of dynamic theories regarding the development of adult stalkers have been proposed. Although it is likely that many of these factors also play a role in juvenile stalking, no empirical research has been conducted to date that verifies if developmental factors for adult and juvenile stalking are the same. One theory of stalking suggests that it is a variant of intimate violence. Logan (2000) found a high level of association in victims of stalking with prior physical or emotional abuse victimization.

The development of pathological childhood attachments has also been proposed as a possible etiology of

TABLE 24–1. Mullen stalker typology

Type	Characteristics
Rejected	Majority are males who pursue an ex-intimate Goal is reconciliation or revenge Stalker is usually personality disordered rather than psychotic Stalker's advances are frequently persistent and intrusive
Intimacy seekers	Desired attachment is usually romantic but can involve parent, child, or other close relationship Stalker believes target loves him/her and that intimate relationship will ensue Stalker persists in pursuit despite negative responses from victim Stalker may have underlying psychotic disorder
Incompetent	Stalker feels entitled to a relationship with person of his/her interest Stalker is indifferent to target's preferences Stalker lacks insight regarding target's lack of reciprocity Stalker's advances are persistent and inept
Resentful	Target is person who stalker feels has wronged him/her Stalking behaviors are intended to cause fear Stalker gains sense of power and control from stalking Stalker feels his/her actions are justified retribution for a perceived injustice
Predatory	Majority are men who target unsuspecting women Stalking behaviors are preparation for sexual assault Stalker pursues multiple victims over time

Source. Adapted from Mullen et al. 2000.

stalking behavior (Meloy 1992, 1996), and these theories may also be understood in the context of juvenile stalking. First, Bowlby's (1980) theory of childhood attachment centers on the importance to the child of maintaining the affectional bond to the caregiver. As a result, the child demonstrates a range of behaviors in an effort to preserve this bond and keep the attachment figure readily available. Crying, clinging, temper tantrums, and angry demands serve to attract the caregiver's attention, with the desired reunion following. These infantile behaviors have been compared with those behaviors of adult stalkers who attempt to woo their love objects through the use of letters, phone calls, following, and increasingly angry protests.

Another theory posits that deficits in different subphases of Mahler et al.'s (1975) separation-individuation paradigm contribute to adult stalking behavior (Keinlen 1998). For example, Meloy (1996) theorized that disturbances in the differentiation and practicing subphases are important in the development of obsessional following, whereas Dutton and Golant (1995) proposed that deficits in the rapprochement phase play a significant role.

Kienlen et al. (1997) proposed that disturbed childhood relationships with a parent or caregiver can re-

sult in a preoccupied attachment pattern in adulthood. In some individuals, this preoccupied attachment ultimately erupts into stalking behavior. In their study of childhood relationships among individuals who exhibit adult criminal stalking behavior, Kienlen et al. (1997) found that more than 60% of adult stalkers experienced a loss or change in a primary caregiver during their childhood. Among juvenile and adolescent stalkers, these dynamic contributing factors may also play a role.

Developmentally Normal "Following Behaviors" of Juveniles and Young Adults

Many developmentally appropriate behaviors exhibited by children and adolescents superficially resemble adult stalking behavior. For example, both school-age children and adolescents commonly develop crushes on their teachers and write notes or present small gifts to them in an attempt to garner their attention. Youth frequently idolize celebrity figures such as movie or

TABLE 24–2. RECON (RElationship- and CONtext-based) stalking typology

Stalker type	Relationship category	Characteristics	Risk management
Intimate	Previous relationship (marriage, cohabiting, dating/sexual)	Most dangerous group, many with history of violence Threat can quickly escalate Abuse alcohol and stimulants > one-half physically assault victim One-third use or threaten to use weapons >one-third have suicidal ideation or behavior	Intense probation/parole supervision Intervene to decrease risk of domestic violence before and after separation
Acquaintance	Previous relationship (employment related, affiliative/friendship, customer/client)	Pursuit is sporadic but relentless Strong desire to initiate relationship One-third will assault victim or damage property	Careful diagnostic assessment Work with law enforcement and mental health
Public figure	No previous relationship (pursuit of public figure victim)	Greater proportion of female stalkers and male victims Older with less violence history Increased likelihood of psychosis Unlikely to threaten; low violence risk	Professional protection of target Psychiatric treatment Prosecution with forensic hospitalization as option
Private stranger	No previous relationship (pursuit of private figure victim)	Often mentally ill men 12% are suicidal Communicate directly with victim One-third are violent toward persons or property	Psychiatric treatment Aggressive prosecution

Source.   Adapted from Mohandie et al. 2006.

rock stars and make repeated attempts to be closer to them through writing letters or attending concerts.

Children and adolescents also develop intense romantic feelings toward other peers in their environment, often at school. Following the object of their affections around school is common early adolescent courtship behavior. Behaviors such as calling repetitively on the phone, writing multiple notes, waiting in locations where the loved person is likely to come, and following the love object are generally viewed as a normal part of development. Such behavior is rarely experienced as threatening by the target. The following case example illustrates how an adolescent romantic crush can involve elements of intrusive or unwanted attention that may not qualify as actual stalking.

Case Example 1

J.B. is a 12-year-old girl who idealizes her seventh-grade history teacher, Mr. Davis. She begins leaving him "secret love notes" in his desk drawer that she signs from "your biggest admirer." She finds out his cell phone number and often calls after school "just to hear his voice." Mr. Davis notices a particular number is associated with frequent hang-ups and he calls back the number. When J.B. answers the phone, she is mortified that her number has shown up on her teacher's phone as she thought she was able to block her number from showing up.

J.B.'s behavior is characteristic of a teenage girl who develops a romantic "crush" on an older popular male peer or teacher. Although she has repeated behaviors to establish some type of contact with Mr. Davis, when confronted she is extremely embarrassed and vows to stop all attempts to contact her teacher. Mr. Davis experiences annoyance rather than fear. J.B. does not represent a high risk of continued following behavior, although she may need some emotional reassurance to overcome her personal shame.

College dating behavior has received more attention than earlier-age courtship. One study found frequent forms of intrusion reported by over 60% of an undergraduate sample, including making hang-up telephone calls, calling on the telephone and arguing, watching from a distance, and failing to take hints that one is unwelcome (Cupach and Spitzberg 1998). Less common behaviors in this sample included sending offensive pictures, sending excessive e-mails, making threatening communications, breaking into someone's home, tape-recording conversations without permission, and taking photographs without consent. A second study found that 20% of undergraduate students surveyed had been the target of intrusive contact, and 20% of those had feared for their safety as a result (Haugaard and Seri 2003).

In a study of 120 college students who had experienced a dissolution of a romantic relationship and who had not initiated the breakup (i.e., breakup sufferers), 99% indicated that they had engaged in at least one act of an unwanted pursuit behavior toward their prior partner. The most common pursuit behaviors initiated by the breakup sufferers were unwanted phone messages, phone calls, and unwanted in-person conversations. Men and women breakup sufferers did not appear to have significant differences in their pursuit behaviors. However, women appeared more likely to leave unwanted phone messages, whereas men were more likely to seek in-person contact with their ex-partners (Langhinrichsen-Rohling et al. 2000).

Prevalence of Stalking by Youth and Characteristics of Juvenile and Young Adult Stalkers

Actual pathological stalking by youth younger than 18 years does occur but appears to be uncommon. Isolated case reports of child stalkers as young as 9 and 10 years have been published (Brewster 2003; McCann 2000; Snow 1998). A study of restraining orders issued by a Massachusetts family court over a 10-month period indicated that 757 restraining orders were issued to juveniles exhibiting threatening, abusive, or stalking behavior (National Center for Victims of Crime 2008). Although this study did not separate those restraining orders issued for stalking behavior from other threatening behaviors, this report nevertheless suggests that a significant number of adolescents demonstrate stalkinglike behavior (McCann 2001) that may not rise to the level of criminal or delinquent stalking charges.

In the largest sample of juvenile stalkers published to date, McCann (2000) reviewed 13 cases of stalking by children and adolescents that he obtained from his case files, published literature, and media reports. This particular sample had a mean age of 14.1 years, with ages of offenders ranging from 9 to 18 years. McCann described these youth as "obsessional followers" and noted that the majority of perpetrators were male and the majority of the victims were female. In this same sample, nearly half of the victims were adults and the other half were same-age peers. The most common method of stalking noted was physical approach toward the victim. Other forms of stalking included unwanted sexual advances, telephone calls, letter writing, and vandalism.

McCann's (2000) study found that juvenile perpetrators were more likely to stalk casual acquaintances (64%), followed by strangers (21%) and prior intimate partners (14%). He contrasted this perpetrator–victim pattern to that of Meloy's (1998) study of adult stalkers, which found that the majority of adult stalkers' victims were from prior intimate relationships. McCann (2000) theorized that this difference stems from particular developmental issues faced by adolescents. In particular, he proposed that because adolescents are exploring their self-identity and emerging sexual feelings, their obsessive fixations are more commonly directed toward casual acquaintances rather than prior intimate partners (McCann 2001). This theory would appear to apply better to those in early to mid-adolescence than to those in late adolescence.

For example, in a study examining stalking following the breakup of romantic relationships among college students, Roberts (2002) evaluated 305 female undergraduates who had experienced a breakup of a heterosexual relationship. Nearly 35% were classified as stalking victims, 32% suffered some type of harassment, and only 33% reported experiencing no form of harassment. These findings suggest that stalking and/or harassment behaviors by young adult males toward a prior female intimate partner are not uncommon. Characteristics noted in these undergraduate males who stalked former partners are outlined in Table 24–3.

Stalkinglike Behaviors

Other behaviors that may overlap certain characteristics of juvenile stalking include bullying and sexual harassment. In the United States, the percentage of students who report being bullied ranges from 25% (Duncan 1999) to 75% (Hoover et al. 1992). *Bullying*

TABLE 24–3. Characteristics of young adult males who stalk following a breakup

History of substance use

History of violence and criminal involvement

Mental health problems

Difficulties forming relationships

Tendency to react to rejection with inappropriate emotion and jealousy

Suspiciousness of their ex-partner's relationships with others

Source. Adapted from Roberts 2002.

has been defined as occurring when a person is repeatedly exposed to negative actions on the part of one or more other students (Olweus 1993). *Cyberbullying* involves the use of electronic media to extend the in-person bullying behavior to the victim at any time. The issue of cyberbullying is discussed in more detail in Chapter 19, "Forensic Issues and the Internet."

McCann (2001) noted the following similarities between stalking and bullying: 1) more than one incident of threat, harassment, or intimidation is common; 2) the perpetrator threatens or evokes fear in the victim; and 3) the victim is aware that he or she is being threatened. Differences between bullying and stalking noted by McCann include the following: 1) bullying can be perpetrated by a group rather than an individual; 2) the motivation of bullying centers on dominating the victim, whereas stalking indicates a disturbance of attachment; and 3) a bully's attempt to exclude the victim from a peer group is not a common feature of a stalker. Although there are differences between bullying and stalking, a victim of bullying may nonetheless be allowed to pursue civil protection orders and possible criminal charges of stalking against the perpetrator when the bullying behavior meets a state's legal definition for stalking.

In some cases, stalking may be a component of dating violence. Studies report between 20% and 40% of college-age girls have experienced some dating violence (Neufeld et al. 1999; Straus 2004). Although sexual harassment and stalking are not equivalent, certain types of sexual harassment by youth may closely resemble stalking behavior. In their study of 561 students ages 11 to 16 years, Roscoe et al. (1994) noted that 50% of girls and 37% of boys described having experienced some form of sexual harassment. Of this sample, approximately 20% of students received telephone calls, letters, or notes perceived as sexually harassing. Because these types of behaviors have also been described

in child and adolescent obsessional followers, McCann (2001) suggested that a subset of sexual harassers may also meet the definition of stalking. When considering intervention, the evaluating clinician should recognize the presence of sexual harassment because additional school and legal interventions are available to juvenile victims of sexual harassment.

Management of the Juvenile Stalker

Management of a stalking situation involves interventions with both the stalking victim and the alleged stalker. Key aspects of these interventions are outlined below.

Immediate Interventions With the Stalking Victim

In addition to contacting the police, stalking victims should be told to keep any evidence that could be useful for law enforcement and a possible prosecution of the stalking perpetrator. Victims should also be advised to avoid any type of contact with the stalker as continued contact may serve to reinforce the stalker's behavior (Meloy 1997). The National Center for Victims of Crime (2003) recommendations for victims of cyberstalking are outlined in Table 24–4.

Evaluation of the Alleged Juvenile Stalker

There has been little research conducted regarding the psychiatric assessment of juveniles referred for stalking. Evaluation of a potential juvenile stalker utilizes general violence risk assessment approaches, research from adult stalkers, and data published from McCann's (2000) small samples of adolescent obsessional followers. Based on our own clinical and forensic work, we recommend the use of a comprehensive approach when evaluating a juvenile referred for stalking. Important components of the psychiatric assessment are listed in Table 24–5.

The evaluator should take a detailed history from the youth regarding all alleged verbal or written threats. Other sources of information to consider in evaluating juvenile threats include the victim's account, notes, letters, diaries, pictures of graffiti, recorded audio- and/or videotapes, school records, juve-

TABLE 24–4. National Center for Victims of Crime recommendations for juvenile victims of cyberstalking

1. Tell parent or another adult.

2. When perpetrator is known, communicate in writing to the offender that contact is unwanted and should cease. This communication should occur only once.

3. For continued contact, consider filing a complaint with the stalker's service provider as well as your own service provider.

4. Collect and print all contacts from stalker; include headings, date, and time.

5. Develop log of each communication outlining circumstances as to how and when it occurred.

6. Note steps taken to stop harassment.

7. Consider filing a report with local law enforcement and investigate with local prosecutor what charges, if any, can be pursued.

8. Consider changing Internet service provider, and examine possibility of obtaining encryption software or privacy protection programs.

9. Block e-mails from any addresses of stalker.

10. Contact online directory listing such as www.four11.com, www.switchboard.com, and www.whowhere.com to request removal from their directories.

11. Never agree to meet the perpetrator for any purpose.

Source. National Center for Victims of Crime 2003.

nile arrest records, juvenile probation reports, counseling records, computer website visits, and e-mail correspondence. Collateral interviews with the potential victim, the juvenile's parents/caretakers, peers, counselors, and schoolteachers may yield useful information. In examining these data, the evaluator should consider the following:

- Potential target(s) of the threat
- Relationship of the potential target to the juvenile
- Type and nature of the threat
- Situation(s) that have triggered threat
- Escalation of the threat over time
- Attempts to act on the threat
- Previous interventions to manage the threat
- Involvement of others in making the threat
- Any suggested use of weapons
- Attitude by the juvenile when confronted

Because most juveniles reside with their parents or legal guardians, the clinician should ask about parental and guardian attempts to control or manage the juvenile's behavior. Because some adult stalkers ultimately harm those individuals who prevent them from contacting their victim, parents may be at increased risk from juveniles who stalk.

The evaluating clinician needs to determine peer influences on the youth's behavior. Peer relationships are extremely influential in adolescence, and the evaluator must determine whether peers play a role, either directly or indirectly, in the stalking behavior. In particular, the evaluator should ask whether other peers participate with the juvenile in stalking, and if not, whether peers are providing encouragement to the juvenile to continue the stalking behavior. The evaluator may also wish to explore whether the juvenile has been exposed to stalking behaviors and themes through television, books, and movies. Representations of juvenile and adolescent stalking in the media are not uncommon, and although there are no data linking them directly to stalking behavior, an awareness of these portrayals can be important for assessment of stalking risk and effects for stalking victims (Scott et al. 2007).

TABLE 24–5. Evaluation of potential juvenile stalkers

Detailed history of present behavior

Peer influences

Intent of behavior

Environmental access to target

Fit between behavior and applicable legal definition of stalking

History of prior attachments and prior stalking

Presence of psychiatric disorder

Violence risk assessment

Evaluators should consider the youth's emotional, cognitive, and psychological maturity when determining the juvenile's capacity to form the specific intent for stalking outlined in their jurisdiction (McCann 2001). Some antistalking statutes require that the perpetrator intend to cause fear of harm or injury to the victim. Intent is also relevant for treatment considerations. Therefore, the evaluating clinician must address the juvenile's understanding of and beliefs about the purpose of his or her behavior.

Investigation of a potential autism spectrum disorder (ASD) may be particularly relevant in analyzing the intent of an alleged stalking perpetrator. Stokes et al. (2007) compared social and romantic functioning among 25 ASD adolescents and adults (13–36 years) with 38 "typical" adolescents and adults (13–20 years). Their study found that individuals with ASD were more likely to engage in inappropriate courting behaviors; were more likely to focus their attention on celebrities, strangers, colleagues, and ex-partners; and were more likely to pursue their targets longer than control subjects. These authors noted that individuals with ASD did not appear to know how to discriminate between appropriate and inappropriate behaviors or to be discerning in their choice of target. Furthermore, persons with ASD in their study seemed to have difficulty understanding that their pursuit strategies were inappropriate or that their contact was distressing to their target. These findings are specifically relevant when evaluating the intent of a person accused of stalking who may have ASD.

The evaluator should determine whether the behavior triggering the referral is consistent with the legal definition of stalking. Other behaviors sometimes confused with stalking include bullying, sexual harassment, and general threats to harm others, such as bombing or shooting up a school. Although threats may not technically meet the statutory criteria for stalking, a violence risk assessment may nevertheless be warranted.

The evaluator should carefully review any prior history of stalking behavior or obsessional attachments by the juvenile, including behaviors toward other peers, celebrities, or teachers. The clinician should attempt to determine whether the youth's thoughts are consistent with developmentally appropriate fantasies, which often include unrealistic expectations that a teacher, peer, or other person will return one's love. Indications that the behavior is in excess of expected fantasy includes a youth's persistent fixation despite feedback or intervention, a youth's continued attempts to access the victim in violation of agreements not to do

so, and escalating intrusions (such as making threatening communications or repeatedly following).

The evaluating clinician should carefully screen for the presence of any psychiatric disorder, with particular consideration to the possibility of a first episode of a developing psychotic disorder. In addition, the clinician should review the impact of any other mental disorder, cognitive impairment, or behavioral difficulty on the youth's reported stalking.

The evaluator should explore the various environments familiar to the juvenile to determine the proximity risk to the alleged stalking victim. This inquiry may be particularly important for those youth who target other youth. Common locations where juveniles can easily stalk other peers include school, the local neighborhood, parks, malls, clubs, concerts, and sporting events.

The evaluator should conduct a thorough general violence risk assessment of the youth. McCann (2001) noted that many risk factors for future violence by stalkers appear similar to those associated with violence in general. In his sample of child and adolescent obsessional followers, McCann (2000) found that 31% eventually acted violently after having expressed a threat. In general, risk factors for future violence in juveniles include a past history of violence, early onset of offending, chronicity of offending, diversity of law-violating behaviors, access to weapons, involvement with gangs, cognitive impairment, use of alcohol and drugs, presence of a conduct disorder, and disturbed family relationships (Scott 1999). A possible risk factor for future violence in adolescents with erotomania is a youth's fixations on multiple people. For example, Urbach et al. (1992) described an adolescent male with multiple object fixations who ultimately demonstrated at least one act of violence. McCann (2001) proposed that a youth's fragile developing sense of self-identity may increase the likelihood of his or her developing multiple and changeable object fixations. However, the exact relationship, if any, of multiple object fixations to future violence remains unclear.

Studies differentiating physically violent and nonviolent juvenile stalkers are currently nonexistent. However, recent research has been conducted in adult stalkers to identify characteristics of those stalkers who went on to engage in violent acts. In her review of 103 Canadian cases of "simple obsessional" stalking, Morrison (2008) found that physically violent stalkers were more likely to have the following factors:

- Stronger previous emotional attachment to their victim

- Higher fixation/obsession with their victim
- Higher degree of perceived negative affect toward their victim
- Greater likelihood of engaging in verbal threats toward the victim
- History of battering/domestic abuse of the victim

Although this study was evaluating adult simple obsessional stalkers, these findings may assist in evaluating risk factors for potential physical violence in referred youth.

In the wake of the Columbine and Virginia Tech school tragedies, schools have become highly sensitized to threats of potential violence and may suspend youth whom they suspect of being at risk "pending a psychiatric evaluation." These youth may be brought by school personnel or parents to emergency rooms for "clearance" that they are safe to return to school. Adolescents suspected of stalking are sometimes referred for an evaluation in this manner. One critical limitation in an evaluation conducted in an emergency room is that collateral information, especially from peers, is seldom available. Patients may minimize or conceal their behavior and thoughts. The evaluating clinician should therefore be very cautious in making determinations of risk with such limited information.

Finally, the evaluator should consider the possibility that a victim may make a false allegation of having been stalked. Five contexts involving false claims among alleged adult victims are 1) stalkers who claim to be victims, 2) persons who have delusions of being stalked, 3) persons who have been previously stalked and then misperceive benign acts of others as stalking, 4) persons with factitious disorder who allege stalking to achieve the sick role, and 5) malingerers who fabricate claims for external rewards such as money or to avoid criminal prosecution (Mullen et al. 2000).

Interventions With a Juvenile Stalker

The first intervention step involves explicitly informing the alleged stalker that his or her behavior is not welcomed by the target. The establishment of a moratorium of the alleged stalker's stalking activities is important and may provide useful information as to the willingness of the juvenile stalker to accept recommended boundaries (Mullen et al. 2000). Minimizing contact between the alleged stalker and victim may be useful. When the perpetrator attends the same school as the victim, a change in schools may be necessary to

avoid ongoing interactions between both parties and to minimize the risk of persistent danger to the potential victim. Sometimes, this will mean that the victim may need to change schools. Although this may seem like the victim is being punished, in some cases it may be the safest, quickest, and simplest option. When working with school districts to authorize the transfer of a student to another school, families and mental health evaluators should be familiar with the Unsafe School Choice Option (2004), section 9532 of the Elementary and Secondary Education Act (ESEA) of 1965, as amended by the No Child Left Behind Act. This policy requires that each state receiving funds under the ESEA implement a statewide policy requiring that students who attend a persistently dangerous public elementary or secondary school or who become victims of a violent criminal offense be allowed to attend a safe school (Unsafe School Choice Option 2004). Educating school personnel as to the risk of danger to the stalked youth in their school environment may increase the school's willingness to transfer the student to another school environment to maintain compliance with ESEA.

Scott et al. (2007) outlined a variety of school interventions that can help prevent the stalker from reaching the intended victim should the stalker come to the victim's school. First, the security staff at the school can be educated regarding the identity of the alleged stalker, the importance of early identification and apprehension should the stalker enter campus, and the significance of preventing contact between the stalker and victim. Second, the front desk, reception, and administrative staff can be similarly educated and have an emergency action plan in place should the stalker be noted to enter the school. Third, the intended victim's teachers can be made aware of a potential stalking situation involving one of their students and the importance of minimizing contact with the perpetrator. All the above parties should have a photograph of the alleged stalker to assist in immediate identification. Fourth, emergency contact numbers should be readily available to everyone involved.

A juvenile's parents can also impose restrictions to help decrease activity by a child or adolescent who is stalking. Such restrictions can include limitations on telephone and computer use, denial of car privileges, and close monitoring of after-school and weekend activities. In small communities where youth are often involved in the same activities outside of school, cessation of contact can be very difficult. In designing an intervention plan, it is important to consider the likely situations where the stalker can readily find his or her victim. In those circumstances where the victim is not aware of being stalked and the perpetrator communicates a desire to harm the victim, clinicians should try to protect the victim in a manner that comports with the local jurisdiction's laws regarding confidentiality and duties to third parties.

There is no one-size-fits-all approach to juveniles who stalk; stalkers must be evaluated on a case-by-case basis. Treatment of any underlying psychiatric disturbance represents one general principle that should be implemented. Although some youth will have mental illnesses responsive to psychotropic medication, the vast majority of youthful offenders will also require other types of therapy and intervention. Self-management approaches described by Wexler (1991) represent one potential therapy that may be useful with adolescents whose obsessional following begins after a breakup from an intimate relationship (McCann 2001). The self-management approach includes a combination of cognitive-behavioral and psychoanalytic self-psychology techniques. This approach may be effective in those adolescents who react with anger and jealousy after a breakup. McCann (2001) proposed that juveniles who stalk acquaintances or strangers do so in response to their feelings of depression, anxiety, and envy. He recommended therapies designed to increase the youth's social skills and feelings of competence.

Legal Responses to Juvenile Stalkers

Little is known about how often juveniles are arrested or prosecuted for stalking. One study in Hawaii examined the legal records of youth committed to the state's youth correctional facility during a 1-year period. The study found that none of the incarcerated youth were charged with, or had a history of being charged with, harassment by stalking or aggravated harassment by stalking. However, a small percentage of youth (5.5%) had been adjudicated for harassment, which under Hawaii law may include some stalking behaviors such as making repeated communications after being told to stop (Elwyn et al. 2004). Juveniles who have been charged with stalking may be addressed by the juvenile justice system or by adult criminal courts, depending on applicable state laws. In some states, such as Florida, prosecutors have the authority to prosecute as adults adolescents charged with aggravated stalking who are 14 or older at the time of the offense (Fla. Stat. § 985.227 [1] [a], 2004).

Juveniles who have been adjudicated delinquent for stalking in juvenile court face a variety of consequences

depending on their state's statutes. These consequences can range from outpatient monitoring (probation) to a requirement that the juvenile be placed in a secure residential treatment facility. Outpatient supervision can include special curfews, driving restrictions, no victim contact, ongoing counseling, and periodic risk assessments of violence. A juvenile court judge may also place a youth in intensive residential treatment. For example, in Florida, children who are younger than 13 years of age and are adjudicated delinquent on aggravated stalking are eligible for intense residential treatment programs (Fla. Stat. § 985.03, 2004).

Other restrictions may also be placed on the juvenile. In Washington State, any juvenile who has committed a felony while stalking a family or household member may not lawfully possess a firearm (Rev. Code Wash. Ann. § 9.41.040 [2] [a] [i], 2004). In Arkansas, stalking is included among a list of crimes defined as sex offenses (Ark. Code Ann. § 12-12-903, 2004).

When a youth is adjudicated delinquent for a stalking offense, his or her juvenile court records may lose their traditional confidential status. In Minnesota, if a juvenile has been adjudicated delinquent of stalking, the juvenile's probation officer must transmit a copy of the court's disposition order to the superintendent of the juvenile's school district or the chief administrative officer of the juvenile's school (Minn. Stat. § 260B.171, 2004). In Washington State, when a juvenile adjudicated delinquent for stalking is released from a juvenile facility, written notice is sent to law enforcement agencies and schools where the juvenile intends to reside or the last school attended by the juvenile (Rev. Code Wash. Ann. § 13.40.215, 2004). In addition, if the juvenile resides in a residential facility, the statute authorizes notification of any employer that employs the offender while residing at the residential facility. If requested in writing, any witness who testified against the juvenile as well as any person specified in writing by the prosecuting attorney may also receive notice regarding the release of the juvenile.

A charge of stalking against an adult may also affect the confidentiality of that person's juvenile court records. In Minnesota, a mental health professional evaluating an adult convicted of stalking is granted access to that person's juvenile court records if deemed relevant and necessary for the assessment (Minn. Stat. § 609.749, 2004). In Virginia, the probation officer has the authority to include information from available juvenile court records when a person is tried in a circuit court for stalking (Va. Code Ann. § 19.2-299, 2000).

Some states have enacted legislation that permits issuing restraining orders against juvenile stalking offenders. For example, in Colorado, any municipal or district court can issue a temporary or permanent civil restraining order against a juvenile who is 10 years or older to prevent stalking (Col. Rev. Stat. Ann. 13-14-102, 2004). As with interventions targeting adult stalkers, careful consideration must also be given to the possibility that a restraining order may escalate the behavior of some juvenile stalkers. To date, there is no research that examines the efficacy of restraining orders when applied against children or adolescents.

The following case provides an example of juvenile stalking behavior and potential interventions.

Case Example 2

John is a 16-year-old boy who had been involved for 2 years with Lisa, a same-age peer who attends the same school. Lisa told John that she was no longer interested in dating him after John found Lisa "making out" with his best friend behind the bleachers at a school football game. Although Lisa has told John that "it is over," he continues to call her on her cell phone, send e-mails to her Internet account, and attempt to send text messages to her.

When Lisa does not return John's phone calls or e-mail messages, he begins waiting after class to talk to her to convince her that they should "get back together." He tells her that he "forgives her" and emphasizes that "you are the only one for me." Lisa informs John that their breakup is final and tells him to "get over it."

Over the next month John becomes increasingly depressed and has thoughts of committing suicide combined with fantasies of killing Lisa and her new boyfriend. One evening while watching television with her new boyfriend at his house, Lisa looks out the window and sees John sitting outside in his car watching them. When John sees Lisa looking out the window, he drives away while she calls the police. The police pull John over and find a loaded registered .45 revolver in the glove compartment of the car. John denies any intent to harm Lisa and states that he was just driving by to "see if she was home so that he could talk to her."

John's initial behaviors following the breakup with Lisa are not atypical for a teenager who feels emotionally bruised regarding the ending of a relationship. However, John's increasing depression and inability to stop thinking about Lisa indicate that he has become inappropriately preoccupied with his former girlfriend. John develops suicidal and homicidal fantasies, and as a result, his risk of aggression and violence increases substantially. His driving to Lisa's home to watch her and her new boyfriend indicates that he is taking active steps to monitor her new relationship.

Lisa, her new boyfriend, and both families should consider several interventions to minimize any future risk. First, all parents need to be notified regarding the concern about John's behavior to help enact additional recommendations. Second, Lisa and her new boyfriend must cease all contact with John to prevent any encouragement or escalation of behaviors. Third, John should be taken immediately to a mental health professional to evaluate and treat his depression and suicidality. A decision regarding immediate inpatient hospitalization should be considered. Fourth, all firearms and weapons should be removed from John's environment to minimize the risk of impulsive aggression. Fifth, a determination needs to be made about whether to prosecute John, a 16-year-old, for being in possession of a handgun. Sixth, careful consideration should be given for a restraining order against John. The risks and benefits of such an order would need to be reviewed to determine if the implementation of such an order could potentially further increase violence. Considerations might include any history of prior responses to limit setting or prior restraining orders, antisocial tendencies, and relationship with local police or authority who would be delivering the restraining order and monitoring it. Seventh, Lisa's family may wish to consider notifying the local police so that they are aware of the situation should emergency intervention be required. Eighth, the school should consider transferring John to another school to minimize his contact with Lisa and assist in lessening his obsessive attachment. Less desirable, but occasionally indicated, would be to transfer Lisa to another school. Ninth, appropriate school officials, security, and teachers at Lisa's school should be educated about John's behavior toward Lisa and an emergency preparedness plan devised should John come to the school campus in the future.

Summary

Although important research regarding adult stalkers has been conducted in the past 20 years, juvenile stalkers have received little attention. Recent research on child and adolescent obsessional followers represents an important first step in understanding the characteristics of both juvenile perpetrators and the interpersonal context in which stalking occurs. Future research will help guide not only assessments of such youth but also appropriate interventions for them.

—Key Points

— The legal definition of stalking generally involves a course of conduct that is directed at a specific person and results in a reasonable person experiencing fear.

— An increasing number of adult stalking typologies have emerged, though none have been systematically studied in juvenile stalkers.

— Many behaviors of children and adolescents may resemble stalking but can be developmentally appropriate, depending on the circumstances.

— McCann's (2000) study of 13 juvenile stalkers noted that the majority of stalkers were male, the majority of the victims were female, and the most common method of stalking was physical approach toward the victim.

— Bullying and sexual harassment have similar characteristics to stalking behaviors, although they may not meet the legal definition of stalking.

— A detailed psychiatric history is important in evaluating the juvenile stalker, with a particular focus on examining whether or not the youth intended to cause fear in the alleged victim.

— A violence risk assessment is an important component of a juvenile stalker evaluation.

— The evaluator must be familiar with common clinical and legal interventions for managing juvenile stalking behavior.

References

Arkansas Code Annotated § 12-12-903 (2004)

Bowlby J: Attachment and Loss. New York, Basic Books, 1980

Brewster MP: Children and stalking, in Stalking: Psychology, Risk Factors, Interventions, and Law. Edited by Brewster MP. Kingston, NJ, Civic Research Institute, 2003, pp 9.1–9.22

Colorado Rev Statutes Annotated § 13-14-102 (2004)

Cupach WR, Spitzberg BH: Obsessive relational intrusion and stalking, in The Dark Side of Close Relationships. Edited by Cupach WR, Spitzberg BH. Mahwah, NJ, Lawrence Erlbaum, 1998, pp 233–263

Duncan RD: Peer and sibling aggression: an investigation of intra- and extra-familial bullying. J Interpers Violence 14:871–886, 1999

Dutton DG, Golant SK: The Batterer: A Psychological Profile. New York, Basic Books, 1995

Elwyn TS, Wang E, Goebert D, et al: Youth incarcerated in Hawaii for stalking offenses. Poster presented at the annual meeting of the American Academy of Psychiatry and the Law, Scottsdale, AZ, October 2004

Emer DM: Obsessive behavior and relational violence in juvenile populations: stalking case analysis and legal implications, in Stalking Crimes and Victim Protection: Prevention, Intervention, Threat Assessment, and Case Management. Edited by Davis JA. Boca Raton, FL, CRC Press, 2001, pp 33–68

Florida Statutes § 985.03 (2004)

Florida Statutes § 985.227 (1) (a) (2004)

Haugaard JJ, Seri LG: Stalking and other forms of intrusive contact after the dissolution of adolescent dating or romantic relationships. Violence Vict 18:279–297, 2003

Hoover JH, Oliver R, Hazler RJ: Bullying: perceptions of adolescent victims in the Midwestern USA. School Psychol Intl 13:5–16, 1992

Kienlen KK: Developmental and social antecedents of stalking, in The Psychology of Stalking: Clinical and Forensic Perspectives. Edited by Meloy JR. San Diego, CA, Academic Press, 1998, pp 51–67

Kienlen KK, Birmingham DL, Solberg KB, et al: A comparative study of psychotic and nonpsychotic stalking. J Am Acad Psychiatry Law 25:317–334, 1997

Langhinrichsen-Rohling J, Palarea RE, Cohen J, et al: Breaking up is hard to do: unwanted pursuit behaviors following the dissolution of a romantic relationship. Violence Vict 15:73–90, 2000

Logan TK, Leukefeld C, Walker B: Stalking as a variant of intimate violence: implications from a young adult sample. Violence Vict 15:91–111, 2000

Mahler MS, Pine F, Bergman A: The Psychological Birth of the Human Infant: Symbiosis and Individuation. New York, Basic Books, 1975

McCann JT: Subtypes of stalking (obsessional following) in adolescents. J Adolesc 21:667–675, 1998

McCann JT: A descriptive study of child and adolescent obsessional followers. J Forensic Sci 45:195–199, 2000

McCann JT: Stalking in Children and Adolescents: The Primitive Bond. Washington, DC, American Psychological Association, 2001

McGrath MG, Casey E: Forensic psychiatry and the internet: practical perspectives on sexual predators and obsessional harassers in cyberspace. J Am Acad Psychiatry Law 30:81–94, 2002

Meloy JR: Violent Attachments. Northvale, NJ, Jason Aronson, 1992

Meloy JR: Stalking (obsessional following): a review of some preliminary studies. Aggress Violent Behav 1:147–162, 1996

Meloy JR: The clinical risk management of stalking: "someone is watching over me...". Am J Psychother 51:174–184, 1997

Meloy JR (ed): The Psychology of Stalking: Clinical and Forensic Perspectives. San Diego, CA, Academic Press, 1998

Minnesota Statutes § 260B.171 (2004)

Minnesota Statutes § 609.749 (2004)

Mohandie K, Meloy JR, McGowan MG, et al: The RECON typology of stalking: reliability and validity based upon a large sample of North American stalkers. J Forensic Sci 51:147–155, 2006

Morrison KA: Differentiating between physically violent and nonviolent stalkers: an examination of Canadian cases. J Forensic Sci 53:742–751, 2008

Mullen PE, Pathé M, Purcell R: Stalkers and Their Victims. New York, Cambridge University Press, 2000

Mullen PE, Pathé M, Purcell R, et al: Study of stalkers. Am J Psychiatry 156:1244–1249, 1999

National Center for Victims of Crime: Cyberstalking. Washington, DC, National Center for Victims of Crime, 2003. Available at: http://www.ncvc.org/src/Main.aspx?dbName=DocumentViewer&DocumentID=32458. Accessed November 2, 2008.

National Center for Victims of Crime: School Crime: K–12. Washington, DC, National Center for Victims of Crime, 2008. Available at: http://www.ncvc.org/ncvc/main.aspx?dbName=DocumentViewer&DocumentID=32368. Accessed June 2, 2009.

Neufeld J, McNamara JR, Ertl M: Incidence and prevalence of dating partner abuse and its relationship to dating practices. J Interpers Violence 14:125–137, 1999

Olweus D: Bullying at School: What We Know and What We Can Do (Understanding Children's Worlds). Cambridge, MA, Blackwell, 1993

Rev Code Washington Annotated § 9.41.040 (2) (a) (i) (2004)

Rev Code Washington Annotated § 13.40.215 (2004)

Roberts KA: Stalking following the breakup of romantic relationships: characteristics of stalking former partners. J Forensic Sci 47:1070–1077, 2002

Roscoe B, Strouse JS, Goodwin MP: Sexual harassment: early adolescents' self-reports of experiences and acceptance. Adolescence 29:515–523, 1994

Scott CL: Juvenile violence. Psychiatr Clin North Am 22:71–83, 1999

Scott CL, Ash P, Elwyn T: Juvenile aspects of stalking, in Stalking: Psychiatric Perspectives and Practical Approaches. Edited by Pinals D. New York, Academic Press, 2007, pp 195–211

Snow RL: Stopping a Stalker: A Cop's Guide to Making the System Work for You. New York, Plenum Trade, 1998

Southworth C, Finn J, Dawson S, et al: Intimate partner violence, technology, and stalking. Violence Against Women 13:842–856, 2007

Stokes M, Newton N, Kaur A: Stalking, and social and romantic functioning among adolescents and adults with autism spectrum disorder. J Autism Dev Disord 37:1969–1986, 2007

Straus MA: Prevalence of violence against dating partners by male and female university students worldwide. Violence Against Women 10:790–811, 2004

Tjaden P, Thoennes N: Stalking in America: Findings From the National Violence Against Women Survey (NCJ 169592). Washington, DC, U.S. Department of Justice, National Institute of Justice, April 1998

Unsafe School Choice Option: Non-Regulatory Guidance. Washington, DC, U.S. Department of Education, May 2004. Available at: http://www.ed.gov/policy/elsec/guid/unsafeschoolchoice.pdf. Accessed November 2, 2008.

Urbach JR, Khalily C, Mitchell PP: Erotomania in an adolescent: clinical and theoretical considerations. J Adolesc 15:231–240, 1992

Vaidya G, Chalhoub N, Newing J: Stalking in adolescence: a case report. Child Adolesc Mental Health 10:23–25, 2005

Virginia Code Annotated § 19.2-299 (2000)

Westrup D: Applying functional analysis to stalking behavior, in The Psychology of Stalking: Clinical and Forensic Perspectives. Edited by Meloy JR. San Diego, CA, Academic Press, 1998, pp 275–294

Wexler DB: The Adolescent Self: Strategies for Self-Management, Self-Soothing, and Self-Esteem in Adolescents. New York, WW Norton, 1991

Zona MA, Sharma KK, Lane JC: A comparative study of erotomanic and obsessional subjects in a forensic sample. J Foren Sci 38:894–903, 1993

PART VI

Juvenile Offenders

Charles L. Scott, M.D.

Chapter 25

Overview of Juvenile Law

Eraka P.J. Bath, M.D.
Stephen Bates Billick, M.D.

Laws and legal procedures relating to juvenile offenders have a long history, dating back thousands of years. As far back as 4,000 years ago, the Code of Hammurabi referenced runaways and disobedient children. Even 2,000 years ago, Roman civil and church law used the concept of the "age of responsibility" to distinguish between juveniles and adults (Lawrence and Hemmens 2008). Early Jewish and Muslim laws also established parameters in which age and development were factored into assessing culpability and degree of punishment. Under Jewish law, the Talmud set forth conditions under which immaturity was to be considered in imposing punishment. Under Muslim law, standards of leniency were called upon for punishing youthful offenders, and children younger than 17 years were exempt from receiving the death penalty. Under Roman law, children younger than 7 years received immunity from criminal liability because they were thought to be *doli incapax*, incapable of forming criminal intent (Godfrey and Lawrence 2005). Much of English common law was based on these early principles of Roman law, which formed the basis for the U.S. approach to juvenile justice.

As early as the eighteenth century, legal scholars contemplated the distinction between children and adults with regard to assessing a person's criminal culpability. In 1765, William Blackston, an important legal scholar of his time, published many commentaries on how English common law differentiated "infants" and adults who had committed a criminal act. The concept of *malitia supplet aetaem*, or "malice supplies the age," was rooted in the thought that knowing the difference between right and wrong is an age-related phenomenon and an underlying premise of the resulting "infancy defense." According to the infancy defense, children younger than 7 years were classified as "infants" and were determined incapable of committing a crime secondary to being too young to fully understand their actions. These "infants" were assessed as not having the cognitive capacity to form the requisite criminal intent, or *mens rea*, to commit the crime. In contrast, individuals older than 14 years were classified as adults and were determined to be fully capable of knowing right from wrong and therefore did not require a developmental shield against criminal culpability. As a result, those persons older than 14 who were charged with a criminal act were subject to the full authority of the law and punishment, including death, if found guilty of a crime. The gray zones in this schema were the children between ages 7 and 14 years, who were presumed to lack capacity unless proven otherwise by a prosecutor. These children ages 7–14 years could be found guilty only if prosecutors could prove that the child defendants knew and understood the consequences of their acts (Malmquist 2002).

Historical Origins of Juvenile Law in the United States

The emergence of the American juvenile justice system has its roots in the English common law system. Houses of refuge, or reformatories, were one of the first steps in the evolving U.S. approach in the management of juvenile offenders. The *parens patriae* doctrine has its roots in English common law and granted the inherent power and authority of the state to protect persons who are legally unable to act on their own behalf. The state was considered the supreme guardian of all children within its jurisdiction, and state courts possessed the inherent power to intervene to protect the best interests of children when necessary. Functioning under the model of *parens patriae*, the first step to addressing the differences between adults and children was the creation of reformatories, separate housing facilities for wayward youth. The first house of refuge was established in New York in 1825 by the Society for Prevention of Juvenile Delinquency. The primary challenge for the reformatory was to focus on rehabilitation of wayward youth and to help these youthful offenders avoid recidivism through character development, education, and vocational skills (Malmquist 2002). Important historical aspects that differentiated the management of juvenile offenders from that of adults are outlined in Table 25–1 (Platt 1977; Shepherd 1999).

Although the theory of reform school was rooted principally in the beneficence of wanting to help young offenders, in practice, there were occasionally problems within its operations. Lack of regulatory oversight meant that some youth were assaulted, abused, and victimized. Pisciotta (1982) examined the records, annual reports, and daily journals of superintendents of some facilities and found a significant disparity between the theory and practice of juvenile incarceration. He noted that the disciplinary style was more brutal than parental and that the institutional environment of the school had a corrupting influence on the residents. For a variety of reasons, some reformatories were not able to provide the level of parental care, education, or training that had been promised under the *parens patriae* doctrine, and discriminatory treatment against African Americans, Mexican Americans, American Indians, and poor whites remained a problem in the reformatory schools. Additionally, the involuntary institutionalization of youth in these reformatories was met with constitutional challenges

TABLE 25–1.   Early goals of the juvenile justice system

Segregate young offenders from adult criminals

Imprison the young "for their own good" by removing them from adverse home environments

Minimize court proceedings

Provide indeterminate sentences to last until the youth was reformed

Use punishment only if other alternatives prove futile

Help youth avoid idleness through military drills, physical exercise, and supervision

Use a cottage approach within larger institutions in rural areas

Reform youth by focusing on education, preferably vocational and religious

Teach sobriety, thrift, industry, and prudence

Source.   Platt 1977; Shepherd 1999.

based on infringement of habeas corpus rights. *Habeas corpus*, translated from the Latin phrase as "you shall have the body," represents a legal action where one can seek relief from unlawful detention and serves as an important safeguard in protecting personal freedom from arbitrary state action. Because of these many issues, concern around the efficacy, safety, and constitutionality of the reformatories grew. At the same time, the Progressive Era was beginning to establish roots, and a cohort of like-minded individuals were taking up causes such as women's suffrage, child labor laws, mandatory education, and school lunches aimed at enhancing optimal child development in the industrial city (Schlossman 1983).

The Child Saving movement emerged as one group concerned about the welfare of these young individuals. The Child Savers were a group of individuals largely comprising educated and middle-class professionals and philanthropists who were dedicated to improving child welfare. In addition, the increasing frequency of the practice of jury nullification in dealing with child defendants gave more traction to the movement to change the way in which juvenile cases were handled. Jury nullification, the process by which jurors acquit an apparently guilty criminal defendant rather than impose a disproportionately severe sanction, had become more commonplace as society struggled with how to process juvenile offenders (Shepherd 1999). Through the advocacy efforts of the Progressives and evolving standards of understanding child development as it related to punishment and culpability, the first juvenile court was founded in Illinois in 1899. The Illinois Juvenile Court Act of 1899 authorized this groundbreaking juvenile court and gave the court jurisdiction over abused, neglected, delinquent, and dependent children younger than 16 years. The court's charge was to focus on rehabilitation rather than punishment, and accordingly, the act required separation of juveniles from adults, eliminated the detention of children under the age of 12 years in jails, and kept records confidential to minimize stigma later in life. Proceedings were also held in a nonadversarial manner whereby many judges would engage the youth in a parental way. Other states followed suit, with all but two states establishing juvenile courts by 1925 (Billick and Lubit 2003).

The idea of *parens patriae* expanded, with the state assuming the responsibility of acting in a parental role to facilitate the well-being and development of minors in trouble (Billick and Lubit 2003). Dependency and neglect cases came under the jurisdiction of the juvenile court, and the concept of CHINS/PINS (children/persons in need of supervision) evolved. The courts emphasized guidance, protection, and rehabilitation instead of punishment. Because the courts were seen as nonadversarial and proceedings were held in civil court and not criminal court, juveniles were not afforded due process protections. Due process refers to the concept that laws and legal proceedings must be fair and provide procedural safeguards to ensure fairness. The U.S. Constitution guarantees that the government cannot take away a person's basic rights to life, liberty, or property without due process of law through the Fifth and Fourteenth Amendments. Historically, adults in criminal proceedings have invoked the issue of due process to guarantee that legal proceedings were occurring justly. Judges also had broad discretion in how they handled cases, and since the state was thought to be functioning in the best interest of the child, it was felt that judges needed such wide latitude to rehabilitate juveniles. The role of the court went beyond addressing youth with possible criminal behaviors to include a broader variety of misbehaving children and status offenders. Arguments regarding civil liberties, such as habeas corpus rights, were basically moot because if a juvenile was determined to need confinement, such confinement was viewed as rehabilitation rather than punishment. Soon, this lack of uniformity coupled with the lack of due process protections led to increasing concern. In the 1950s, increasing criticism of both excessive leniency and harshness arose (Billick and Lubit 2003; Tanenhaus 2002).

Key Legal Cases

Between 1966 and 1975, five key cases involving the juvenile court were decided by the U.S. Supreme Court. This period of time is often referred to as "the criminalization of juvenile court" because the legal challenges involved issues of constitutionality concerning due process and loss of liberty rights. As a result of these legal challenges, the constitutional protections provided in juvenile courts became increasingly similar to those found in the adult court system. The first U.S. Supreme Court case concerning the juvenile court system was *Kent v. United States* (1966), which centered on due process rights and protections afforded a juvenile being considered for waiver to adult court from the juvenile justice system. Morris Kent was a 16-year-old who was accused of housebreaking, robbery, and rape, and a waiver hearing was scheduled in juvenile court. Although Kent's defense attorney submitted an affidavit from a psychiatrist stating that Kent required psychiatric hospitalization and juvenile court staff and probation noted that Kent's mental status was deteriorating, the judge did not take this information into consideration and ruled that Kent should be transferred to adult court for his trial. Once in adult court, Kent was found guilty and sentenced to 30–90 years in prison.

On appeal, the U.S. Supreme Court ruled that the waiver hearing represented a critical stage of the juvenile court proceedings and required representation by counsel, inspection of all records by defense, and a statement of reason for the court's decision. The Court commented that the lower court judge abused his discretionary power when he made the decision to send Kent to adult court. Furthermore, Kent had been interrogated and sent to detention without a lawyer present and was not informed of his right to remain silent and right to counsel, vital constitutional rights as stipulated by the Fifth and Sixth Amendments, respectively, thereby violating due process. The Court specifically stated, "We do hold that the leaving must hold up to the essentials of due process and fair treatment" (*Kent v. United States* 1966). In a famous quote, the Court majority expressed their concern regarding the inadequate constitutional protections afforded juveniles, noting that juveniles "receive the worst of both worlds, he gets neither the protection accorded adults, nor the solutions, care and regenerative treatment postulated for children" (*Kent v. United States* 1966).

The *Kent* decision marked a shift in society's approach and understanding as to the purpose of juvenile court. There were increasing concerns regarding the validity of the juvenile court's informality and the substantial risk that a singular focus on treatment may leave due process protections by the wayside. Subsequently, the publication of a task force report titled "Juvenile Delinquency and Youth Crime," which arose from President Lyndon Johnson's Commission on Law Enforcement and Administration of Justice, formally questioned many of the fundamental practices of juvenile court that had traditionally weighted the goals of rehabilitation against the constitutional requirements of due process (Woolley and Peters 1968).

In the very next year (1967), the case of Gerald Gault further addressed many of the due process issues raised by *Kent* and the task force report. *In re Gault* (1967) concerned a 15-year-old boy named Gerald Gault who was on probation at the time when he and a friend made a lewd crank call to a female neighbor, asking her if she had "big bombers." Although Gault was picked up and detained by the police, his parents were not notified until the next day. During the court hearing, Gault was not represented by legal counsel, evidence concerning the charge was not presented, and the victim did not appear in court. Gault was adjudicated a delinquent and committed to a juvenile correctional facility for an indeterminate period, even though the maximum sentence for an adult convicted of the same crime would have been 2 months in jail or a $50 fine. His attorney submitted a writ of habeas corpus, and the case was eventually heard by the U.S. Supreme Court. In his opinion, Justice Fortas wrote, "Under our constitution the condition of being a boy does not justify a kangaroo court" (*In re Gault* 1967, p. 387). His comment signaled a new era for juvenile court—an era that was to more closely follow an adult criminal due process model—in sharp contrast with the historic informality of the juvenile court proceedings. Importantly, the *Gault* Court held that under the Fourteenth Amendment, juveniles have a right to receive notice and obtain counsel, to be protected against self-incrimination, and to question witnesses if the hearing could result in commitment to an institution. The important rights granted to juveniles as a result of the *Gault* ruling include:

- Right to receive notice of charges
- Right to obtain legal counsel
- Right to confrontation and cross-examination
- Right to privilege against self-incrimination

Two areas of rights that were not granted to juveniles by the *Gault* Court included the right to a transcript of the proceedings and the right to an appellate review.

In 1970, *In re Winship* established that the standard of proof to find a juvenile delinquent in juvenile court should shift to the highest standard of "beyond a reasonable doubt." Prior to *In re Winship* (1970), the standard of proof in juvenile court was a preponderance of the evidence standard as these courts were considered civil rather than criminal proceedings (Lawrence and Hemmens 2008). *In re Winship* further moved the juvenile court system into the adult criminal sphere by requiring the highest burden of proof for a finding of delinquency, thereby providing yet another means of ensuring due process protections for juveniles.

In *Breed v. Jones* (1975), Gary Jones, age 17 years, was charged with armed robbery and appeared in juvenile court where he was adjudicated delinquent. At the disposition hearing (the sentencing equivalent in adult court), the judge waived Jones to adult court. Jones's attorney filed a writ of habeas corpus arguing that waiver to adult court was a violation of the Fifth Amendment, which prohibits a person from being tried twice for the same crime (i.e., double jeopardy). Jones's attorney challenged that Jones had already been adjudicated in juvenile court and his waiver to an adult court resulted in his effectively being tried a second time in a second court. The U.S. Supreme Court concluded that adjudication in juvenile court is equivalent to the guilt phase of an adult trial and noted that a court waiver must take place before or in place of an adjudication hearing. Chief Burger stated, "We believe it is simply too late in the day to conclude that a juvenile is not put in jeopardy at a proceeding whose object is to determine whether he has committed acts that violate a criminal law and whose potential consequences include both the stigma inherent in such a determination and the deprivation of liberty for many years" (*Breed v. Jones* 1975, p. 421).

More and more, the Court evolved to include provisions that enabled due process protections for juveniles. Although this era of change in juvenile law is often referred to as the criminalization of juvenile justice, there were limitations to the extent to which the U.S. Supreme Court was willing to provide juvenile court with the same procedural safeguards as those of adult court. In the case of *McKeiver v. Pennsylvania* (1971), the U.S. Supreme Court ruled that trial by jury was not required for children and adolescents in juvenile court. The Court contended that allowing jury trials for minors would turn proceedings into an adversarial situation that was contrary to the original mission of the juvenile court system, whose founding principles were rooted in rehabilitation. Additionally, the Court felt that allowing jury trials would further blur the important distinction between juvenile and adult court.

Legal Issues Related to the Investigation and Detention of Juveniles

Constitutional rights of juveniles in school settings have become an important area of debate with the increasing concern about student violence and drug use. In *New Jersey v. T.L.O.* (1985), the U.S. Supreme Court established a "reasonable suspicion" as enough justification to allow a warrantless search of students by school officials. Although the Court found that juveniles were entitled to protection from an unlawful search and seizure (provided by the Fourth Amendment), the standard of reasonable suspicion differs from the higher standard of probable cause required for law enforcement officials when dealing with adults. The Court emphasized that teachers and administrators have a "substantial need" to "maintain order in the schools" and this important function outweighs the requirement for the probable cause determination granted adults (*New Jersey v. T.L.O.* 1985, p. 341).

Legal issues related to the detention of juveniles are multifold, and the specific question around the constitutionality of preventive detention of juveniles was heard in the 1984 U.S. Supreme Court case of *Schall v. Martin*. From the vantage point of juveniles, preventive detention is experienced as a punishment even though legally it is not viewed as such. The U.S. Supreme Court found that pretrial detention was justified for those who might run away and/or commit another offense and held that pretrial detention was a legitimate state objective in protecting juveniles and society from the hazards of pretrial crime (Malmquist 2002). Legal issues related to investigations and confessions of juveniles relate to cognitive capacity and are affected by child development and maturity. This topic is covered thoroughly in Chapter 26, "Juvenile Waiver and State-of-Mind Assessments."

Recent Trends in Juvenile Justice

During the late 1980s and early 1990s, juvenile crime was increasing, and the level of aggression and severity of these crimes intensified. Society began to "get tough on crime," and tolerance for juveniles involved with the law decreased. More and more youthful offenders were being waived to adult court, and the shift was to a more punitive model. There were chants of "adult crime, adult time" and "do the crime, do the time," which seemed to justify treating juveniles who violated the law in a manner similar to adults. Depending on the severity of the crime (e.g., homicide), some states passed legislation that authorized the automatic transfer of a juvenile from juvenile court to adult court. For additional information regarding emerging laws resulting in juveniles being transferred to adult court, see Chapter 26, "Juvenile Waiver and State-of-Mind Assessments."

In addition to the increasing number of juveniles being waived to adult courts, the concept of the constitutionality of executing defendants who committed crimes as juveniles moved to the forefront of public discourse. This particular issue dovetailed with concerns regarding whether individuals under age 18 years had sufficient cognitive maturity to be held as morally blameworthy as an adult who had committed a similar offense. The United States was the only developed country that continued to allow execution of offenders who committed crimes as minors, and it was joined by Somalia as one of the only United Nations members that had not ratified the U.N.'s Convention on the Rights of the Child, which forbade execution or life imprisonment without parole for offenses committed as a minor (Billick and Lubit 2003). The first landmark case to challenge the constitutionality of executing offenders who committed crimes as minors was *Thompson v. Oklahoma* (1988). In *Thompson v. Oklahoma*, the U.S. Supreme Court held that Oklahoma's statute violated the Eighth Amendment against cruel and unusual punishment because it did not specify any specific age limit for the execution of a juvenile. Though it seemed that a trend may have been developing to restrict the use of capital punishment for juvenile offenders, two 1989 U.S. Supreme Court cases, *Stanford v. Kentucky* and *Missouri v. Wilkins*, held that capital punishment of 16-year-olds did not represent cruel and unusual punishment.

From 1973 to 2004, 228 juvenile death sentences were imposed, 22 (14%) resulted in execution, and 134 (86%) were reversed and commuted (Snyder and Sickmund 2006). It was not until 2005 that this issue was revisited by the U.S. Supreme Court in *Roper v. Simmons*. In 1993, the 17-year-old Christopher Simmons concocted a plan to murder Shirley Crook, bringing two younger friends, Charles Benjamin and John Tessmer, into the plot. Simmons had been known to talk about how much he wanted to kill someone before his eighteenth birthday because he was under the false impression he would not face the death penalty because of his age. His plan was to commit burglary and murder by breaking and entering, tying up a victim, and tossing the victim off a bridge. The three met in the middle of the night; however, Tessmer then dropped out of the plot. Simmons and Benjamin broke into Mrs. Crook's home, bound her hands, and covered her eyes. They drove her to a state park and threw her off a bridge while alive. Simmons confessed to the murder, and the jury recommended the death penalty. His attorney challenged the constitutionality of the death penalty, citing many mitigating factors about Simmons's mental state in addition to citing the Eighth Amendment protection against cruel and unusual punishment. His attorney also hoped to gain more traction by referencing the case of *Atkins v. Virginia*, decided in 2002, which overturned the ruling in *Penry v. Lynaugh* (1989) and held that the evolving standards of decency had made the execution of the mentally retarded cruel and unusual punishment and thus unconstitutional.

Roper v. Simmons (2005) was the third and final ruling by the U.S. Supreme Court on the juvenile death penalty. Although the crime committed by Simmons was heinous and cruel, national and international advocacy groups began applying more and more pressure to abolish the death penalty for youth. Amicus briefs poured in from around the world, including some from major medical associations such as the American Psychiatric Association and the American Academy of Child and Adolescent Psychiatry. Some of the arguments presented by scientific groups included evidence from neuroscience findings that suggested that juveniles had diminished capacity regarding their criminal culpability secondary to immaturity of the brain and cognitive development. In a 5–4 ruling, citing the "evolving standards of decency" test, the Court held that it was cruel and unusual punishment to execute a person who was under age 18 years at the time of the murder. The Court referenced the large body of sociological and scientific research that found that juveniles have a lack of both maturity and sense of responsibility compared with adults. Adolescents were noted to be overrepresented statistically in virtually every category of reckless behavior. The Court in *Roper v. Simmons* also noted most states had provisions and laws to prevent those under age 18 years from voting, serving on juries, or marrying without parental consent, largely in recognition of the comparative immaturity and irresponsibility of juveniles. The studies cited also found that juveniles are more vulnerable to negative influences and outside pressures (including peer pressure), have less behavioral control over their own environment, and lack the freedom that adults have in escaping a criminogenic setting.

In support of the "national consensus" position, the Court noted that there was a dramatic decrease in states that applied capital punishment for juvenile offenders. Many states no longer had a juvenile death penalty, and at the time of the decision, only six states had executed prisoners for crimes committed as juveniles since 1989, and only three states had done so in the past 10 years: Oklahoma, Texas, and Virginia. Furthermore, five of the states that allowed the juvenile death penalty at the time of the 1989 case had since abolished it (Lawrence and Hemmens 2008).

Legislative Trends in Juvenile Justice

In addition to the important landmark cases described earlier, several national legislative acts have targeted juvenile reform. In 1968 Congress passed the Juvenile Delinquency Prevention and Control Act (JDPCA), which was designed to encourage states to develop plans and programs that would receive federal funding and would work on a community level to discourage juvenile delinquency. Upon signing the JDPCA of 1968, President Lyndon Johnson remarked that the bill "will rehabilitate life and renew hope" (Woolley and Peters 1968). Goals of this act were multifold and included building new facilities for rehabilitation, funding allocation for novel intervention programs, and providing training and education at both the community and law enforcement levels. The JDPCA was a precursor to the extensive Juvenile Justice and Delinquency Prevention Act (JJDPA) that replaced the JDPCA in 1974 (Roberts 2004). The JJDPA introduced a strong federal presence to the juvenile justice arena by committing resources and establishing a legislative commitment to certain goals and policies. The Office of Juvenile Justice and Delinquency Prevention was created to institutionalize the federal presence in juvenile justice. Additionally, financial resources such as awards and grants were made available to the public and private nonprofit sectors to operationalize JJDPA's goals. The act also established the National Institute for Juvenile Justice and Delinquency Prevention to conduct research, gather and disseminate information to the field, and provide training and technical assistance. Overall, JJDPA's mission was very important because it emphasized federal–state partnerships and prioritized the identification of national goals for the rehabilitation and reform of the juvenile justice system.

Funding was contingent upon states adhering to core principles. For example, states were required to remove youth from "secure detention and correctional facilities" and separate juvenile delinquents from convicted adults. The rationale was that if youthful offenders were sharing time in facilities with hardened adult criminals, the learned behaviors derived from such associations would undermine the amenability to treatment and therefore impede the rehabilitation efforts. Statistics have shown that youthful offenders who have significant contact with adult criminals have higher rates of recidivism and are more likely to have a life of future crime. Table 25–2 outlines core provisions of the JJDPA.

Another important feature of the JJDPA of 1974 was the establishment of governmental entities that provided monitoring, research, and prevention services. These government agencies included the Office of Juvenile Justice and Delinquency Prevention, the Runaway Youth Program, and the National Institute for Juvenile Justice and Delinquency Prevention.

In 1980, President Jimmy Carter signed the Juvenile Justice Amendments of 1980 into law. The successes of the JJDPA of 1974 provided the impetus and rationale for the amendments of 1980 that continued the authorization of both the JJDPA and the Runaway and Homeless Youth Act for 4 years. In his address, President Carter noted,

The Juvenile Justice and Delinquency Prevention Act is particularly important, because it establishes a program to prevent young people from having that first negative experience with the criminal justice system, rather than reacting to incidents after their occurrence. Six years after its enactment, we can take great pride in its accomplishments. It has demonstrated many new alternatives to traditional methods of dealing with children in the juvenile justice system and contributed to substantial progress in providing fair and effective treatment for our young people. (Woolley and Peters 1980)

Subsequent legislation has largely focused on extending the time, resources, and core protections initiated by the JJDPA of 1974. The Juvenile Justice and Delinquency Prevention Act of 2002 reaffirmed the four core protections of the JJDPA of 1974 (American Bar Association 2009): 1) deinstitutionalization of status offenders, 2) separation of juveniles from adults in institutions, 3) removal of juveniles from adult jails and lockups, and 4) reduction of disproportionate minority contact. *Disproportionate minority contact* is defined as the detention of juveniles from minority groups in secure detention facilities in proportions greater than their representation in the general population. If such disproportionate contact is identified, then this disparity should be addressed. The 2002 act

---

TABLE 25–2. Core provisions of the Juvenile Justice and Delinquency Prevention Act of 1974

Deinstitutionalization of status offenders

Status offenders who have not committed a criminal offense will not be held in secure juvenile facilities for extended periods of time or in secure adult facilities for any length of time. These youth should receive community-based services, such as day treatment or residential home treatment, counseling, mentoring, alternative education, and job development support.

Adult jail and lockup removal

Juveniles may not be detained in adult jails and lockups except for limited times before or after a court hearing (6 hours), in rural areas (24 hours plus weekends and holidays), or in unsafe travel conditions. This provision does not apply to children who are tried or convicted in adult criminal court of a felony-level offense. This provision is designed to protect children from psychological abuse, physical assault, and isolation.

"Sight and sound" separation

When children are placed in an adult jail or lockup, as in exceptions listed above, "sight and sound" contact with adults is prohibited. This provision seeks to prevent children from psychological abuse and physical assault. Under "sight and sound," children cannot be housed next to adult cells; share dining halls, recreation areas, or any other common spaces with adults; or be placed in any circumstances that could expose them to threats or abuse from adult offenders.

Disproportionate minority confinement

States are required to assess and address the disproportionate confinement of minority juveniles in all secure facilities. Studies indicate that minority youth receive tougher sentences and are more likely to be incarcerated than nonminority youth for the same offenses. With minority children making up one-third of the youth population but two-thirds of children in confinement, this provision requires states to gather information and assess the reason for disproportionate minority confinement.

Source. Woolley and Peters 1968.

also provided funding to states that were able to develop and implement a strategy for achieving and maintaining compliance with these four core protections as part of the annual Formula Grants State Plan.

The Juvenile Justice and Delinquency Prevention Reauthorization Act (JJDPRA) of 2008, introduced by Senator Patrick Leahy of Vermont, was passed by the Judiciary Committee with broad bipartisan support on July 31, 2008 (Leahy-Spector-Kohl 2009). This bill reauthorized the juvenile delinquency prevention programs of the JJDPA through fiscal year 2013, stating, "With the reauthorization of this important legislation, we recommit to these important goals but also push the law forward in key ways to better serve our communities and our children" (Leahy-Spector-Kohl 2009). The reauthorization bill was conceived with the understanding that psychiatric illnesses are prevalent among youthful offenders and aimed to address this issue as one of its important goals.

Other important updates provided by the JJDPRA to the original bill include the following:

- Rigorous new procedures before a state can detain a status offender, with strict limitations on the time they may be detained
- The encouragement of states to move away from keeping young people in adult jails
- Prioritization and funding of mental health and drug treatment

- Emphasis on effective training of personnel who work with young people in the juvenile justice system
- Creation of incentives for the use and expansion of programs that are evidence based
- Shifting the juvenile justice focus to prevention programs intended to keep children from ever entering the criminal justice system

Conclusion

The future of the juvenile justice system hinges on developing prevention programs, providing mental health and drug treatment, and keeping youth out of adult jails. There is a significant body of research that demonstrates that youth detained in adult correctional facilities have higher rates of suicide and are 34% more likely to commit more crimes upon release. Despite this statistic, between 1990 and 2004, the number of youth in adult jails increased 208%, and every day in the United States an average of 7,500 youth are incarcerated in adult jails (Leahy-Spector-Kohl 2009). The debate over the best way to handle youthful offenders continues, and psychiatrists and other mental health professionals can play a pivotal role in enhancing the dialogue by generating research and providing standardized treatment and assessment guidelines.

—Key Points

— The focus of the juvenile justice system is on rehabilitation and not punishment.

— Differences between the juvenile justice system and the adult criminal justice system developed secondary to an evolution in the understanding of child development and continue to evolve to this day.

— Child development affects the perception of culpability and therefore affects legal consequences and outcomes.

— Significant legislative and congressional acts have resulted in policy changes that provide federal funding for preventing delinquency and improving the juvenile justice system through research, training, regulation, and advocacy.

— The U.S. Supreme Court has been instrumental in providing the legal framework and upholding constitutional provisions for protecting juveniles through several landmark cases.

— Psychiatric illness is endemic in the juvenile justice population, and psychiatric needs remain largely unmet.

References

American Bar Association, Division for Public Education: History of the Juvenile Justice System. 2009. Available at: http://www.abanet.org/publiced/features/DYJpart1.pdf. Accessed January 16, 2009.

Atkins v Virginia, 536 US 304 (2002)

Billick S, Lubit R: Juvenile delinquency, in Principles and Practice of Forensic Psychiatry, 2nd Edition. Edited by Rosner R. New York, Oxford University Press, 2003, pp 389–395

Breed v Jones, 421 US 519 (1975)

Godfrey B, Lawrence P: Crime and Justice 1750–1950. Cullumpton, UK, Willan Publishing, 2005, pp 128–149

In re Gault, 387 US 1 (1967)

In re Winship, 397 US 358 (1970)

Juvenile Justice Delinquency Prevention Reauthorization Act of 2008, § 3155. Available at: http://www.scribd.com/doc/4285876/S-3155-Juvenile-Justice-and-Delinquency-Prevention-Reauthorization-Act-of-2008. Accessed January 16, 2009.

Kent v United States, 383 US 541 (1966)

Lawrence R, Hemmens C: Juvenile Justice. San Diego, CA, Sage, 2008

Leahy-Spector-Kohl Introduce Juvenile Justice Reauthorization Bill (press release, Washington, DC, March 24, 2009). Available at: http://leahy.senate.gov/press/200806/061808b.html. Accessed June 16, 2009.

Malmquist C: Overview of juvenile law, in Principles and Practice of Child and Adolescent Forensic Psychiatry. Edited by Schetky D, Benedek E. Washington, DC, American Psychiatric Publishing, 2002, pp 259–266

McKeiver v Pennsylvania, 403 US 528 (1971)

Missouri v Wilkins, 492 US 361 (1989)

New Jersey v TLO, 469 US 325 (1985)

Penry v Lynaugh, 492 US 302 (1989)

Pisciotta A: Saving the children: the promise and practice of parens patriae, 1838–1898. Crime Delinquency 28:410–425, 1982

Platt AM: The Child Savers: The Invention of Delinquency, 2nd Edition, Enlarged. Chicago, IL, University of Chicago Press, 1977

Roberts A: Juvenile Justice Sourcebook: Past, Present and Future. New York, Oxford University Press, 2004

Roper v Simmons, 543 U.S. 551 (2005)

Schall v Martin 104 S Ct 2403 (1984)

Schlossman S: Juvenile justice: history and philosophy, in Encyclopedia of Crime and Justice, Vol 3. Edited by Kadish S. New York, Free Press, 1983, pp 961–969

Shepherd RE Jr: Juvenile court at 100 years: a look back. Juvenile Justice 6(2):13–21, 1999. Available at: http://www.ncjrs.gov/html/ojjdp/jjjournal1299/2.html. Accessed January 16, 2009.

Snyder HN, Sickmund M: Juvenile Offenders and Victims: 2006 Status Report. Washington, DC, Office of Juvenile Justice and Delinquency Prevention, 2006

Stanford v Kentucky, 402 US 361 (1989)

Tanenhaus DS: The evolution of juvenile courts in the early twentieth century: beyond the myth of immaculate construction, in A Century of Juvenile Justice. Edited by Rosenheim MK, Zimring FE, Tanenhaus DS, et al. Chicago, IL, University of Chicago Press, 2002, pp 42–71

Thompson v Oklahoma, 487 US 815 (1988)

Woolley JT, Peters G: The American Presidency Project (online). Lyndon B. Johnson: Remarks Upon Signing the Juvenile Delinquency and Prevention Control Act of 1968, July 31, 1968. Santa Barbara, CA, University of California (hosted), Gerhard Peters (database). Available at: http://www.presidency.ucsb.edu/ws/?pid=29054. Accessed January 15, 2009.

Woolley JT, Peters G: The American Presidency Project (online). Jimmy Carter: Juvenile Justice Amendments of 1980, Statement on Signing § 2441 Into Law, December 8, 1980. Santa Barbara, CA, University of California (hosted), Gerhard Peters (database). Available at: http://www.presidency.ucsb.edu/ws/?pid=44384. Accessed January 15, 2009.

Chapter 26

Juvenile Waiver and State-of-Mind Assessments

Charles L. Scott, M.D.

Case Example 1

Joe, a 15-year-old boy, is facing a complaint of first-degree murder. At the time of the crime, Joe was smoking PCP (angel dust) and feeling like a "zombie." As Joe walked down the street eating a piece of pizza, he saw a young woman (unknown to him) in a car. He decided to steal the car. When the woman told him, "You don't want this old car," Joe pulled out a handgun and shot her in the face. Joe told the evaluating psychiatrist that the victim deserved to die because she waited too long to hand over her keys.

At age 8, Joe was placed in a foster home after Child Protective Services substantiated charges of severe physical abuse and neglect. At age 9, he was discovered drowning the foster family's cat in the bathtub. He had severe violent outbursts and was aggressive toward foster family members. A pediatrician diagnosed him with attention-deficit/hyperactivity disorder. Joe was prescribed methylphenidate (a stimulant), without benefit. By age 11 years, he was placed in a group home, where he assaulted staff and peers and ran away on two different occasions. Two years later, he was hospitalized on an inpatient psychiatric unit for 4 weeks after he started a fire in the group home. He was diagnosed with conduct disorder and dysthymic disorder. He was prescribed fluoxetine (an antidepressant) and valproic acid (a mood stabilizer sometimes used to treat aggression), with no change in his behavior noted.

Three weeks after being placed in a secure treatment facility, Joe ran away and joined a street gang. He began smoking marijuana and crack cocaine

daily. He sold crack cocaine to make money. At age 14 years he was detained in juvenile hall after he was caught stealing a car. Two weeks later, he escaped while being interviewed by a social worker. He returned to the streets and began using PCP in addition to marijuana and cocaine. Five days after his escape, he shot the victim. Within hours after stealing her car, he was apprehended and taken to juvenile hall. While in juvenile hall detention, he found a mop handle, which he shoved in the mouth of a peer who had teased him.

Case Example 2

Rob is a 17-year-old adolescent boy who has been transferred to adult court after he was arrested and charged with the murder of an off-duty police officer. Rob has no prior history of arrests or any legal involvement in the juvenile or adult legal system. During his elementary through junior high school years, Rob was an aloof child who was socially isolated and had very few friends. However, he maintained excellent grades up until his junior year in high school (age 16) when his grades of A's and B's dropped to all D's.

At age 17, Rob started locking himself in his room, and his parents had difficulty getting him to shower or maintain his basic grooming. They forced him to go to an outpatient psychiatric evaluation, and the psychiatrist was very concerned that Rob was developing some type of psychotic illness, such as schizophrenia. During the evaluation Rob communicated significant paranoia about "being followed" though he provided minimal information when questioned about these beliefs. When asked, Rob said that he did not have thoughts of hurting anyone else or himself. The psychiatrist referred him for consideration of civil commitment, but Rob was determined not to meet involuntary commitment criteria by the mental health team at the receiving hospital.

Three days later, Rob was at a local convenience store to buy "emergency supplies." Witnesses reported that Rob appeared quiet and suddenly "out of nowhere" ran over to a 28-year-old man who had just entered the store and stabbed him repeatedly in the chest and abdomen. The man died on the scene; it was later learned that this man was an off-duty police officer. Witnesses noted that after methodically stabbing the man, Rob then turned around, picked up his shopping basket, and bought two cans of tuna and some Gummy bears. The cashier and other customers called 911, and in 2 minutes the police arrived, saw their slain colleague, and immediately arrested Rob, who was still in the store. The entire episode was captured on a video surveillance camera and was consistent with the witnesses' accounts.

When interviewed in jail 5 days later, Rob barely spoke to the evaluating psychiatrist. He was noted to mumble to himself throughout the interview and made repeated nonsensical statements. Eventually he communicated to the psychiatrist that as soon as he saw the victim, he realized that this person was "a member of a covert secret organization." He reported that he had been hearing a voice for days telling him that a man had been hired to kidnap him, brutally rape him, and then kill him by setting his body on fire in the middle of a highway so that his burned carcass would then be run over by trucks and cars. Rob stated that when the victim walked into the store, he knew that "he was the one." He added that he specifically saw the victim glance at a package of cigarettes, which was the victim's way of communicating to him that he was going to burn his body. Rob said that at that moment he believed the victim was about to "transfix" him. He related that he had to act immediately to prevent his own death. He volunteered, "At that second, it was either me or him." He described how he quickly went over to the man and pulled out a large knife that he had purchased the day before to protect himself from this perceived persecutor. When asked if he thought at the moment he stabbed the man that his actions were against the law, Rob answered, "Of course not. The law allows you to defend yourself. He was about to kill me. I had no time." When asked if he would have not stabbed the man if a uniformed police officer had walked into the store at the very moment he was about to stab his victim, he responded, "Yes. I couldn't take the chance of any delay."

Introduction

In the United States, juvenile crime increased dramatically during the late 1980s and peaked in 1994 (Snyder 2008). The American public was confronted with graphic images in the media of violent young children, many of whom appeared armed and ready to kill. The belief that our juvenile justice system was effective in managing these violent offenders was rapidly vanishing. In its place was a growing get-tough attitude toward juveniles highlighted by the phrase, "If you do the crime, you do the time." Society was fed up. Something had to be done.

In response to this emerging skepticism about the juvenile court's ability to rehabilitate wayward youth, numerous states passed laws with more punitive approaches to address juvenile delinquent behaviors. A common thread running through the fabric of these new statutes was a push to remove the protective veil of juvenile court and expose youth to the consequences of their acts in both the juvenile and adult criminal justice systems. This chapter highlights two important areas that have resulted from the efforts to have juveniles handled more like adults with regard to their illegal actions: 1) the waiver of youth to adult court and 2) an increasing focus on a juvenile's state of mind during the crime and following the juvenile's arrest.

Waiver of Youth to Adult Court

A significant purpose of waiving, or transferring, a juvenile to adult court is the imposition of more serious consequences for the youth's illegal behaviors. The most common mechanism for transferring a juvenile from juvenile (civil) court to adult (criminal) court involves a juvenile court transfer hearing. Here, a juvenile court judge has the discretion to decide whether a youth is waived to adult court on the basis of each case and the information presented (Griffin et al. 1998). Depending on the jurisdiction, a judicial waiver is also referred to as a discretionary waiver, certification, bind-over, transfer, decline, or remand hearing. Although the state prosecutor normally initiates the request for a judicial waiver, a juvenile or his or her parents may request a waiver in several states (Snyder and Sickmund 1995).

In all states, a discretionary waiver requires a hearing in juvenile court at which time information regarding the juvenile is presented to the judge. There are no nationally mandated criteria for judges to consider when deciding whether to transfer a juvenile to criminal court. The majority of states adopt (in various degrees) criteria delineated by the U.S. Supreme Court in the case of *Kent v. United States* (1966), also discussed in Chapter 25, "Overview of Juvenile Law." Morris Kent was a 16-year-old boy charged with several counts of robbery and rape. Despite a motion for a waiver hearing by Kent's attorney, the juvenile judge waived Kent to adult court without a hearing. Kent argued that the waiver was invalid and sought to have the criminal indictment dismissed on the grounds that the judge had not made a full investigation before waiving him to criminal court. The U.S. Supreme Court held that the failure to provide a hearing violated Kent's Fourteenth Amendment right to due process. The Court held that before a juvenile could be sent by a judge to adult court, the juvenile was entitled to a hearing, access by counsel to records involved in the waiver, and a written statement by the judge outlining reasons for the waiver.

In an appendix to its opinion, the Court listed eight "determinative factors" to be used by the judge in deciding whether to judicially waive a youth. These factors are outlined in Table 26–1. Most state statutes on judicial waiver incorporate factors outlined in the table into two broad categories: a juvenile's risk for future dangerousness and a juvenile's amenability to treatment. The forensic evaluator typically addresses each of these arenas as described below.

Assessment of Future Dangerousness

A mental health professional's ability to predict future violent behavior over an extended period of time has realistic limitations. When conducting an assessment regarding a youth's future dangerousness, the clinician outlines past and current risk factors associated with an increased risk of violence. As with adults, one of the most important factors in determining a juvenile's risk for future violence is a past history of violence. The greater the number of incidents, types, and circumstances of a youth's illegal behavior, the higher the risk of future criminal behavior (Robins and Ratcliff 1980; Snyder and Sickmund 1995). Additional information to assess potential dangerousness includes exposure to violence within the family, carrying of weapons, and participation in gangs (Scott 1999).

TABLE 26–1. "Determinative factors" for judicial waiver consideration

1. The seriousness of the offense
2. The violence of the offense
3. Whether the offense was against person or property
4. Whether probable cause existed
5. The desirability of trying the whole case in one court
6. The juvenile's personal circumstances
7. The juvenile's prior criminal record
8. The likelihood of a juvenile's amenability to treatment

Source. *Kent v. United States* (1966).

More detailed information on assessing a youth's risk of future violence is included in Chapter 21, "Assessing Violence Risk in Youth," and Chapter 27, "Assessment and Treatment of Juvenile Offenders."

Assessment of Amenability to Treatment

Most state statutes require an evaluation to determine whether the youth is amenable to treatment or rehabilitation within the juvenile justice system prior to transfer to adult court. State statutes' definitions of amenability are often vague, with little or no specification regarding how much success in which areas is considered sufficient (Barnum 1987). In general, amenability to treatment focuses on the likelihood that treatment interventions will successfully rehabilitate the youth in his or her remaining time under the juvenile court's jurisdiction. Many state statutes instruct the court to consider the likelihood of rehabilitation through resources available in the community. In other jurisdictions, lack of resources is not justification for deciding that the youth is not amenable to treatment (Grisso 1998).

Several steps are important in assessing a youth's amenability to treatment. First, the clinician should determine the presence, if any, of a psychiatric diagnosis. When reviewing previous treatment, the evaluator should carefully examine the accuracy of any previous diagnosis. Second, the clinician should review types and efficacy of provided treatment. Various interventions include pharmacotherapy, individual psychotherapies, cognitive-behavioral therapy, family therapy, group therapy, inpatient hospital milieu therapy, drug and alcohol treatment, residential placement, vocational rehabilitation, special education interventions, treatment for sex offenders, boot camps, work programs, and response to incarceration. When assessing the adequacy of pharmacotherapy, important factors include the appropriateness of the medication as well as duration and adequacy of dosage. Although the clinician may determine that lost treatment opportunities have occurred in the past, the focus for the transfer evaluation remains on the youth's current likelihood of treatment response.

Third, the evaluator should assess the individual's motivation for treatment and past history of treatment compliance. Evidence of previous poor motivation includes frequently missed scheduled appointments, nonadherence with medication, refusal to participate in individual or group therapy, and recurrent running away from court-ordered placement. One potential indicator for current motivation for treatment is the juvenile's willingness to "admit the crime." However, the examiner must consider the possibility that a juvenile's denial regarding his or her alleged offenses may be appropriately self-protective to prevent statements in the transfer evaluation from being used at a later hearing to convict. To help clarify this issue, the evaluator can examine how much the juvenile uses denial in areas unrelated to the specific offense (Barnum 1987).

Finally, conclusions regarding the likelihood that a youth will benefit from treatment must include statements regarding how much time is necessary for the treatment to be effective. For older adolescents, effective treatment may not be possible if only a short period of time remains before the juvenile court's jurisdiction ends (Barnum 1987).

Nonjudicial Transfer Mechanisms

In reaction to public frustration with youth violence, numerous states have enacted laws that remove or minimize the opportunity for a judge to determine whether a juvenile is transferred to adult court. Although the judicial waiver discussed above is the most common transfer mechanism, a larger number of youth are actually transferred from juvenile to adult court through these alternative legal mechanisms (Griffin et al. 1998). Unlike judicial waivers, these mechanisms do not typically allow consideration of each youth's individual circumstances. Two of the most common methods placing a juvenile in adult court without a judicial hearing include the following (Redding 2008):

1. *Mandatory waiver.* In a mandatory waiver, the state statute requires that juveniles of a specified minimum age who commit a particular offense be sent to adult court. For example, the legislature may pass a law that any 15-year-old who commits a homicide is automatically tried in adult court, regardless of the circumstances or his or her past history.
2. *Direct file waiver.* In a direct file waiver, the prosecutor is granted the authority to file the case in juvenile or criminal court. Because outcomes for juveniles charged with the same offense vary based on the prosecutor in their jurisdiction, this approach has been given the nickname "justice by geography."

Juvenile State-of-Mind Assessments

Juvenile state-of-mind assessments involve focused forensic mental health evaluations of a youth to address his or her thoughts and beliefs related to a particular situation or task. The forensic examiner must carefully clarify the specific type of evaluation(s) requested because the investigation process and forensic analysis will vary depending on the questions posed. Common state-of-mind assessments include evaluation of a juvenile's competency to waive Miranda rights, competency to stand trial, criminal responsibility (sanity), diminished capacity, and pleas of guilty but mentally ill (GBMI).

Competency to Waive Miranda Rights

Legal Background

According to the U.S. Supreme Court holding in *Miranda v. Arizona* (1966), suspects must be informed that they have a constitutional right to avoid self-incrimination (Fifth Amendment) and the right to an attorney during questioning (Sixth Amendment). These rights have been extended to youth involved in juvenile court proceedings (*In re Gault* 1967; *Kent v. United States* 1966). In some states, police officers must arrange for the youth to have contact with a parent, guardian, or other "interested adult" when the youth is advised regarding the waiver of his or her Miranda rights during police questioning. When determining if a constitutional right has been waived, the U.S. Supreme Court articulated in *Johnson v. Zerbst* (1938) that any such waiver must be done "voluntarily, knowingly, and intelligently." Many states also require that a juvenile suspect cannot be questioned without the permission of a parent or guardian.

Is the standard for evaluating a waiver of Miranda rights different for juveniles when compared with adults? The U.S. Supreme Court addressed this question in the 1979 case of *Fare v. Michael C.* Michael C. was a 16-year-old implicated in the murder of Robert Yeager during a robbery of the victim's home. Michael had previously been under the jurisdiction of the local juvenile court for several prior offenses and had served a term in a youth corrections camp. After he was brought to the police station, an officer initiated the interview by informing Michael that he was being questioned about a murder and fully advised him of his Miranda rights. Michael asked to see his probation officer. When the police denied this request, Michael stated he would speak to the officer without consulting an attorney. He proceeded to make statements and drew sketches implicating him in the murder.

Upon being charged in juvenile court with the murder, Michael moved to suppress the incriminating statements and sketches on the ground that they had been obtained in violation of *Miranda* in that his request to see his probation officer constituted an invocation of his Fifth Amendment right to remain silent, just as if he had requested the assistance of an attorney. The court denied the motion, holding that the facts showed Michael had waived his right to remain silent, notwithstanding his request to see his probation officer.

The California Supreme Court reversed, holding that Michael's request for his probation officer by itself (per se) invoked his Fifth Amendment rights in the same way the request for an attorney was found in *Miranda* to be, regardless of what the interrogation otherwise might reveal. This holding was based on the court's view that a probation officer occupies a position as a trusted guardian figure in a juvenile's life that would make it normal for the juvenile to turn to the officer when apprehended by the police, and was also based on the state law requirement that the officer represent the juvenile's interests.

The case was eventually appealed to the U.S. Supreme Court to address whether Michael had invoked his Miranda rights when he asked to speak with his probation officer. The U.S. Supreme Court held that

the California Supreme Court erred in finding that Michael's request for his probation officer represented an automatic invocation of his Fifth Amendment rights under *Miranda.* The Court found that Michael had voluntarily and knowingly waived his Fifth Amendment rights and consented to interrogation. The Court further noted that whether the incriminating statements and sketches were admissible on the basis of waiver was a question to be resolved on the "totality of the circumstances" surrounding the interrogation.

The Court reasoned that a probation officer is not in a position to offer the type of legal assistance necessary to protect the Fifth Amendment rights of an accused undergoing custodial interrogation that a lawyer can offer. The fact that a relationship of trust and cooperation might exist between a probation officer and a juvenile does not indicate that the officer is capable of rendering effective legal advice sufficient to protect the juvenile's rights during police interrogation or of providing the other services rendered by a lawyer. Although the Court commented that a juvenile's age could be considered as a factor in evaluating the youth's wavier of Miranda rights, the Court did not find that a higher standard for competency to waive Miranda rights was required for juveniles (*Fare v. Michael C.* 1979).

Forensic Evaluation of a Juvenile's Waiver of Miranda Rights

The forensic evaluator may be requested to determine whether an alleged juvenile offender has the capacity to waive his or her Miranda rights when giving a statement or confession. If a youth is assessed as not having the requisite ability, his or her statements may ultimately be deemed inadmissible. Two key areas for the evaluator to consider in evaluating a juvenile's waiver of Miranda rights include 1) the circumstances under which the youth made the confession and 2) the characteristics of the particular youth's capacity to make a waiver. In examining the conditions of confinement when the youth waived his or her right, the evaluator should review the length of time the youth was detained without the opportunity to communicate with others; the physical conditions of the holding environment; any contact with other persons, particularly adults; access to food, water, and other basic necessities; and any behaviors by officers that may have resulted in fear or created an environment of coercion (Grisso 1998).

The second component of this forensic evaluation requires the evaluator to carefully examine the juvenile's capacity to waive his or her Miranda rights.

Three important areas suggested by Grisso (1998) to review when assessing this capacity include the youth's ability 1) to comprehend the Miranda warning, 2) to grasp the significance of rights in the context of the legal process, and 3) to process information in arriving at a decision about waiver.

Comprehension of the Miranda warning addresses the youth's ability to understand the warning and to appreciate that he or she is not required to answer police questions. To understand the significance of the Miranda warning, the juvenile must recognize not only that he or she has a right to have an attorney present but also that the defense counsel serves as his or her advocate. The ability to process the warning requires some capacity for abstract reasoning as the youth must weigh short-term and long-term consequences of the decision to waive the right to self-incrimination.

Important collateral records in this assessment may include mental health evaluations, interviews with parents, delinquency records, police investigation reports, and audio- and/or videotapes of the youth's questioning and confession. If the evaluator has concerns regarding the youth's cognitive abilities, cognitive measures of intellectual ability and academic records may be indicated. Four standardized assessment tools to evaluate a youth's ability to comprehend and appreciate the Miranda rights have been developed by Dr. Thomas Grisso in collaboration with the National Institute of Mental Health. These tools include Comprehension of Miranda Rights, Comprehension of Miranda Rights–Recognition, Comprehension of Miranda Vocabulary, and Function of Rights in Interrogation.

Competency to Stand Trial

The substantive standard for competency to stand trial (CST) in the United States was established by the U.S. Supreme Court in *Dusky v. United States* (1960). The *Dusky* Court defined the test of competency to stand trial as "whether the accused has sufficient present ability to consult with his lawyer with a reasonable degree of rational understanding and whether he has a rational as well as factual understanding of the proceedings against him." This standard focuses on two primary areas: 1) the individual's cognitive abilities to understand the trial process and 2) the individual's ability to assist his or her attorney in the individual's defense (Voigt et al. 2002).

While a juvenile must be competent to stand trial in adult criminal court, the Supreme Court has never held that a juvenile must be competent to stand trial

in juvenile court. Historically, with an emphasis on the rehabilitation mission of the juvenile court, minors did not need to be competent in most juvenile jurisdictions. However, with the recognition of the increasing punitive nature of juvenile courts, states began requiring competence to stand trial in juvenile court as well, so that now a majority of states require competency for juvenile proceedings (Redding and Frost 2001). States also vary considerably in the test they apply for juveniles. For example, if a minor does not have the requisite *Dusky* capacities solely on the basis of immaturity (consider a normal 8-year-old arrested for shoplifting), some states would disallow a finding of incompetency, some would find the minor incompetent, and some would allow for modified judicial proceedings that took the minor's limitations into account. It is therefore important for the clinician to be clear on the particular test applicable in the relevant jurisdiction.

Although the federal *Dusky* standard does not specifically state that a mental disease or defect is necessary to find trial incompetency, the vast majority of state statutes require some type of mental disorder as the predicate basis for a finding of incompetency to stand trial. The CST examination focuses on the presence of mental health symptoms at the time of the interview. The presence of a mental illness alone, however, does not automatically render a person incompetent to stand trial. The evaluator must illustrate the relationship of the mental illness to specific deficits in the defendant's understanding of the trial process or ability to cooperate with the defendant's attorney in his or her defense. Four functional areas outlined by Grisso (1998) to consider evaluating a youth's trial competency include the following: 1) understanding of charges and potential consequences, 2) understanding of the trial process, 3) capacity to participate with the attorney in a defense, and 4) potential for courtroom participation.

Detailed questioning of the youth's understanding in each of these areas is important in assessing the youth's trial competency. Although there is no one single protocol or test to determine a youth's competency to stand trial, there are numerous CST assessment instruments that have been utilized in the adult population, and these may also be of some assistance when evaluating a juvenile. The instruments include the Georgia Court Competency Test, the Interdisciplinary Fitness Interview, the Computer-Assisted Competency Assessment Tool, the MacArthur Competency Assessment Tool–Criminal Adjudication, and the Competency Assessment for Standing Trial for Defendants With Mental Retardation. McGarry (1973) highlighted

13 areas to review when assessing trial competency in an instrument known as the Competency Assessment Instrument. The original 13 areas of functioning to assess in the legal process—the "McGarry criteria"—are outlined in Table 26–2.

Grisso et al. (1987) recommended that a juvenile's trial competence be questioned if any one of the following conditions is present: 1) age 12 or younger; 2) prior diagnosis/treatment for a mental illness or mental retardation; 3) borderline intellectual functioning or learning disability; and 4) observations that youth has deficits in memory, attention, or interpretation of reality. In a descriptive review of 136 juveniles ages 9–16 years who were referred for evaluation of trial competency in South Carolina, Cowden and McKee (1995) found that 80% of youth ages 9–12 years were incompetent to stand trial, nearly 50% of those ages 13 and 14 years were trial incompetent, and approximately 25% of 15- to 17-year-olds were incompetent to stand trial. Cooper (1997), in another study of juvenile offenders in South Carolina, found that a majority of juvenile offenders of all ages had significant deficits in their competence-related abilities. Juveniles ages 13 years and younger and those with low-average or below-low-average IQ scores were particularly at risk.

How do juveniles differ from adults with regard to understanding the legal process? Particular concerns involve a youth's naïve views that the judge or probation officer will always be able to determine the truth, even without the youth's involvement; a youth's internalized belief system that one must always admit any mistakes or wrongdoing; and a youth's lack of experience with the criminal justice system (Mossman et al. 2007).

Grisso et al. (2003) compared abilities relevant to adjudicative competence among 927 adolescents in juvenile detention facilities and community settings versus such abilities among 466 young adults in jails and in the community. Key findings from this study were as follows:

1. In general, juveniles ages 15 years or younger performed more poorly than adults.
2. When presented with hypothetical decision-making vignettes, adolescents were more likely than young adults to make choices indicative of compliance with authority figures.
3. Younger adolescents were less likely to recognize the long-term inherent risks in the legal process (e.g., answering questions when interrogated by the police, not consulting with an attorney or evaluating the pros and cons of a plea agreement.

TABLE 26–2. Competency Assessment Instrument: McGarry criteria

1. Appraisal of available legal defenses
2. Level of unmanageable behavior
3. Quality of relating to the attorney
4. Planning of legal strategy
5. Appraisal of role of defense counsel, prosecuting attorney, judge, jury, defendant, witness
6. Understanding of court procedure
7. Appreciation of charges
8. Appreciation of range and nature of possible penalties
9. Appraisal of likely outcome
10. Capacity to disclose to attorney available pertinent facts surrounding the offense
11. Capacity to realistically challenge prosecution witnesses
12. Capacity to testify relevantly
13. Self-defeating versus self-serving motivation

Many of the deficits noted above are due to psychosocial immaturity rather than a specific mental disorder. Because lack of social or emotional maturity does not qualify as a mental disease or defect, what happens if a child is not competent to participate in juvenile proceedings or in adult court due to psychosocial immaturity? In other words, how does the court manage those youth whose trial competency deficits are related to their young age alone rather than to any mental health diagnosis? There is no one consistent approach to address this situation. Interventions vary according to jurisdiction, age of the child, and severity of the crime. Potential options include dismissal of the charges, civil commitment for youth who are a danger to self or others, or social service, educational, and treatment interventions if further adjudication is not feasible (Grisso et al. 2003).

Criminal Responsibility and the Insanity Defense

Forensic practitioners may be asked to evaluate a juvenile's mental state at the time of an alleged offense for the purpose of determining the degree, if any, of criminal responsibility. A criminal act is composed of two components: *actus rea* (guilty act) and *mens rea* (guilty mind or criminal intent). Under English common law, a youth's age played a significant role in whether he or she was considered blameworthy for illegal acts. Children younger than age 7 were deemed incapable of forming criminal intent. This defense, also known as the infancy defense, held that these very young children were not criminally responsible because of developmental immaturity. Juveniles between the ages of 7 and 14 were also presumed to be incapable of committing crimes, although the government had the right to rebut this presumption. In contrast, juveniles age 14 years and older were treated as adults with regard to the law of criminal responsibility (Fitch 1989).

With the emergence of juvenile courts in the United States during the late 1880s, the focus on troubled youth was rehabilitation, not punishment. Because the juvenile court movement emphasized treatment interventions necessary to curb delinquent behavior, legal defenses (such as the infancy defense) to negate or lessen criminal intent were rarely necessary and therefore rarely used. However, with the increasing pressures to transfer youth to adult court and hold juveniles criminally culpable, forensic examiners may likely face requests to evaluate whether a juvenile was criminally "insane" at the time of his or her act.

Insanity is a legal, but not psychiatric, term. The insanity evaluation determines whether the juvenile is so mentally disordered that he or she is not blameworthy or criminally responsible for the behavior. In contrast to CST evaluations that focus on a defendant's present mental capacity as related to his or her understanding and participation in the legal process, an insanity evaluation involves a retrospective evaluation of a person's past mental state at the time of the alleged offense.

The most common test of insanity in the United States is known as the *M'Naghten standard*, which was developed in 1843 following the trial of Daniel M'Naghten. M'Naghten was found not guilty by reason of insanity after he attempted to assassinate the prime minister of Britain and instead shot his secretary Edward Drummond. Queen Victoria, angered by the legal outcome in this case, ordered her 15 Law Lords to draft a new standard of criminal responsibility. The new standard recommended by the Law Lords was as follows:

> To establish a defence on the ground of insanity, it must be clearly proved that at the time of the committing of the act, the party accused was labouring under such a defect of reason, from the disease of the mind, as not to know the nature and quality of the act he was doing, or if he did know it, that he did not know he was doing what was wrong. (*M'Naghten's Case* 1843)

This test is often referred to as the right/wrong test or cognitive test because of its emphasis on the defendant's ability to know, understand, or appreciate the nature and quality of his or her criminal behavior or the wrongfulness of his or her actions at the time of the crime.

A second insanity test used in some jurisdictions is known as the *irresistible impulse test*. In essence, this test asks the evaluator to determine if the juvenile's mental disorder rendered the juvenile unable to refrain from the behavior, regardless of whether the juvenile knew the nature and quality of his or her act or could distinguish right from wrong. A major criticism of this test has been the broadness of its scope. In other words, because a defendant did not refrain from a particular criminal behavior, mental health clinicians could use this as evidence that the defendant could not resist his or her impulse, thereby concluding that all criminal behavior not resisted equaled insanity. Despite its current unpopularity as a measure of criminal responsibility, this test survives, in part, as both Virginia and New Mexico combine the irresistible impulse test with the M'Naghten test (Giorgi-Guarnieri et al. 2002).

A third test used in only two jurisdictions in the United States is known as the *Durham rule* or *product test* (*Durham v. United States* 1954). This insanity test derived from a District of Columbia circuit case in which Judge David Bazelon allowed a finding of insanity if the defendant's unlawful act was a "product of a mental disease or defect." As with the irresistible impulse test, the product test expanded those eligible for a finding of insanity and rapidly fell out of favor. It is currently used in only two jurisdictions in the United States, New Hampshire and the Virgin Islands (Giorgi-Guarnieri et al. 2002).

A final test of insanity was developed in 1955 by the American Law Institute when formulating the Model Penal Code. This test states,

> A person is not responsible for criminal conduct if at the time of such conduct as a result of mental disease or defect he lacks substantial capacity either to appreciate the criminality of his conduct or to conform his conduct to the requirements of the law. (American Law Institute Model Penal Code 1985; Giorgi-Guarnieri et al. 2002)

This test involves both a cognitive arm (ability to appreciate the criminality of one's conduct) and a volitional arm (ability to conform one's behavior to the law).

A mental health professional who is requested to conduct an insanity evaluation of a juvenile should consider the following guidelines. First, the evaluator should request that the attorney or court provide the exact language of the insanity statute because there are subtle yet important differences in the wording among the various states. Second, it is important to understand how mental disorders or defects are defined. The exact definitions of mental disease and mental defect are usually found in case law and/or statutes. The examiner should carefully review whether any disorders are prohibited from consideration for the insanity defense. Diagnoses commonly excluded include voluntary intoxication with alcohol or other drugs, personality disorders, and adjustment disorders. Psychotic disorders, such as schizophrenia, schizoaffective disorder, or mood disorders with psychotic features, are the most common diagnoses that qualify for an insanity defense. Although some youth in early adolescence may demonstrate premorbid symptoms of a significant thought disorder, they may not meet formal diagnostic criteria for a DSM-IV-TR (American Psychiatric Association 2000) thought disorder, thereby making it difficult for them to meet the mental disorder requirement of an insanity defense.

Third, the examiner must closely review all of the defendant's statements regarding the alleged crime as well as available police reports and witness statements regarding the offense. Additional collateral records that may be important include prior mental health and medical records, academic records and any educational testing, and detailed social background history from family members and individuals who know the juvenile.

Even if the juvenile meets the jurisdictional criteria for a mental disorder or defect, having a mental disorder does not equate with the legal definition of insanity. Once the evaluator has determined if the juvenile meets the criteria for a qualifying mental disorder or defect, the evaluator must determine the relationship, if any, between the mental illness or defect and the alleged crime. Understanding the motivation behind the juvenile's actions is a critical component of the insanity evaluation. The evaluator should obtain the juvenile's account of the crime in great detail by asking the youth to describe his or her thoughts, feelings, and exact behaviors before, during, and after the alleged crime. It is important that the evaluator consider all rational, rather than psychotic, motives for the criminal offense. For example, if a juvenile commits an armed robbery to obtain money to buy drugs, the fact that the juvenile is depressed will unlikely establish a sufficient relationship between his or her mental state and criminal behavior for purposes of the insanity defense. The final area the examiner must consider is whether the juvenile's mental state at the time of the crime meets the jurisdictional requirements for an insanity defense. As outlined earlier, there are various tests of insanity, and it is feasible that juveniles may qualify for the insanity defense in one state but not in another.

In those jurisdictions that utilize some form of the M'Naghten test, the examiner should carefully review whether the juvenile meets the criteria for each component of this test according to the precise governing language. In some states, the defendants must be so impaired from a mental illness that they are unable to know the nature and quality of their actions or are unable to distinguish right from wrong. In general, an individual would have to be extremely impaired so as to not be aware of or know his or her actions.

The more easily met component of the M'Naghten test involves whether the juvenile was able to know or distinguish right from wrong at the time of the offense. In general, there are two broad categories related to a defendant's knowledge of the "wrongfulness" of his or her behavior: legal wrongfulness and moral wrongfulness. Jurisdictions vary as to whether both types of wrongfulness are allowed for consideration when determining a defendant's sanity.

An assessment of a person's understanding of the legal wrongfulness of his or her actions involves determining if the person understood *at the time of the crime* that what he or she did was against the law. Resnick (2007) provided examples of potential behaviors that may indicate a person understands the wrongfulness of his or her behavior, and these are outlined in Table 26–3.

Some states allow the trier of fact to evaluate if the person's mental disorder resulted in the person being unable to know or understand that his or her actions were morally wrong, even if the person knew that society would legally sanction the actions. Consider the case of D.C., a 17-year-old girl whose schizophrenic illness causes her to believe that she has been chosen by God to rid the world of evil. She also has the delusional belief that the local librarian is selling hundreds of innocent children into a slave trade where they are raped, tortured, and eventually killed. Despite D.C.'s repeated reports to the police, the librarian remains in her job with ready access to children. Even though D.C. has been told by law enforcement to stay away from the librarian, D.C. continues to fear that more children will be murdered if she does not act quickly. She may have some understanding that the police would view her killing of the librarian as unlawful, particularly as she has been told by local law enforcement to have no contact with the librarian. However,

TABLE 26–3. Evidence that may indicate a juvenile's knowledge of legal wrongfulness

A. Efforts to avoid detection

- Wearing gloves during a crime
- Waiting until the cover of darkness
- Taking a victim to an isolated place
- Wearing a mask or disguise
- Concealing a weapon on the way to a crime
- Falsifying documents (passport or gun permit)
- Giving a false name
- Threatening to kill witnesses
- Giving a false alibi

B. Disposing of evidence

- Wiping off fingerprints
- Washing off blood
- Discarding a murder weapon
- Burying a victim secretly
- Destroying incriminating documents

C. Efforts to avoid apprehension

- Fleeing from the scene
- Fleeing from the police
- Lying to the police

Source. Resnick 2007.

due to her psychosis, D.C. may nevertheless delusionally believe that her actions are morally right. When evaluating whether a defendant's mental disorder rendered the defendant unable to know or understand the moral wrongfulness of his or her conduct, the examiner should specifically ask if there was any reason the defendant thought his or her actions were morally justified at the time of the offense.

The insanity standard in some jurisdictions requires an analysis of the individual's ability to refrain from his or her actions or to conform his or her conduct to the requirements of the law. This analysis focuses on how the person's mental disorder or defect affected, if at all, the person's ability or capacity to control his or her behavior. In this context, the forensic examiner is evaluating if the juvenile had the ability to refrain from the behavior and chose not to. For example, evidence that the juvenile had the ability to refrain could include stopping or delaying an illegal be-

havior when a witness is present or when a police car drives by the scene.

Diminished Capacity Evaluations

Unlike the insanity defense that utilizes a specific test to evaluate one's criminal responsibility, a diminished capacity defense examines whether the defendant had the capacity to form the requisite intent for the crime. To illustrate the difference, a 16-year-old boy with schizophrenia believes that his next-door neighbor is about to start World War III with nuclear weapons because his neighbor's car license tag contains the number 3. As a result, this boy decides that he must kill his next-door neighbor in order to save the entire planet. He carefully loads his .357 magnum, waits for his neighbor to return home, calmly walks over to his neighbor's house, rings the doorbell, and shoots the neighbor directly in the heart when the neighbor opens the door.

At trial, this boy may be found legally insane under a M'Naghten insanity test if it is proved that his schizophrenia resulted in his belief that his actions were morally right, thereby rendering him unable to distinguish right from wrong. This same boy, however, may not meet the standard for diminished capacity, *despite* his mental illness, if proved that he purposefully walked over to his neighbor's house with a loaded shotgun with the specific intent to kill the neighbor. Therefore, diminished capacity defenses are focused on the degree, if any, that a person's mental disorder influenced the person's ability to form the specific intent to commit a crime.

Not all degrees of intent are viewed the same in the eyes of the law. Under a diminished capacity defense, the forensic expert evaluates if the defendant had a particular culpable state of mind. To illustrate, consider the case of J.G., a 16-year-old who becomes intoxicated for the first time from alcohol while drinking with his best friend, M.C. After consuming 10 beers, he starts to argue with M.C. over a seemingly trivial matter, and they become involved in a fistfight. J.G. repeatedly punches his friend in the face, causing M.C. to have an unexpected fall that results in a severe head injury and subsequent death. J.G. is charged with first-degree murder, which in his jurisdiction is defined as the deliberate and purposeful taking of another human's life.

Did J.G. have the level of specific intent as defined by that state's penal code to deliberately and purposely cause his friend's death? A successful diminished capacity defense in this case would demonstrate that due to J.G.'s marked intoxication, his level of consciousness was so impaired that he did not have the capacity to form the requisite intent. Even if his defense is successful, however, J.G. could still face charges that involve a lesser degree of intent, such as a charge of involuntary manslaughter.

The doctrine of diminished capacity is considered controversial, and not all states allow mental health testimony in this regard. A state's decision to bar such testimony as the effects of intoxication has been upheld by the U.S. Supreme Court in the 1996 case of *Montana v. Egelhoff*. In this case, James Egelhoff had been camping and partying with friends in the Yaak region of northwestern Montana. During the course of the day he consumed psychedelic mushrooms and a substantial amount of alcohol. Later that evening, Egelhoff was found severely intoxicated in the back seat of a car with two of his friends dead in the front seat, each as a result of a single gunshot wound to the back of the head. He was subsequently charged with two counts of deliberate homicide. At trial, Egelhoff was not allowed to present evidence regarding the impact of his intoxication on his specific intent to kill. After he was found guilty on both counts, he appealed his case to the U.S. Supreme Court, which upheld the trial court's decision to exclude mental health testimony related to the effects of intoxication on Egelhoff's specific intent (*Montana v. Egelhoff* 1996).

Likewise, testimony on the effects of severe mental disorders on *mens rea* may also be limited. In *Clark v. Arizona* (2006), the U.S. Supreme Court was asked to review an Arizona trial court decision that prohibited mental health testimony regarding the impact of a psychotic disorder on a defendant's ability to form the required specific intent to kill. Eric Clark was an undisputed paranoid schizophrenic who was charged with the first-degree murder of a police officer in the line of duty. At trial, Clark was not allowed to present evidence regarding the impact of his psychosis on his alleged intent to kill. On appeal, the U.S. Supreme Court upheld the trial court's decision to prohibit at the guilt phase any mental health testimony regarding Clark's intent to kill the officer (*Clark v. Arizona* 2006).

Guilty but Mentally Ill

Twelve states have enacted statutes that allow a jury to find a defendant guilty but mentally ill (GBMI). Although precise definitions vary, this verdict recognizes those defendants with a severe mental disorder who are found guilty but do not meet a legal test for insanity. Proponents of GBMI statutes assert that such ver-

dicts protect the public from dangerous offenders with mental illness by allowing longer periods of incarceration that might occur if such defendants were found insane. Several concerns have been raised regarding GBMI statutes. These concerns include the potential for jury confusion regarding the difference between sanity and GBMI, as well as the lack of any meaningful difference in mental health treatment provided to those who receive a GBMI verdict and those who do not (Melton et al. 2007).

Case Example Epilogues

Case Example 1

The court-appointed psychiatrist diagnosed Joe with severe conduct disorder, cannabis dependence, cocaine abuse, and PCP abuse. Identified risk factors for future violence included a lengthy past history and range of aggression beginning in early childhood, using and selling drugs, affiliation with street gangs, continued violence in a locked setting, and familiarity with firearms combined with a comfortable willingness to use them. Joe's prognosis for amenability to treatment was considered poor owing to his previous treatment failures and frequent escapes from secure settings. Substance abuse treatment was felt to be unlikely to ameliorate his violent behavior because his violence predated his use of drugs and continued when he was abstinent. After a judicial waiver hearing, Joe was transferred to adult criminal court, where he was found guilty and sentenced to life in prison.

Case Example 2

Rob's defense attorney requested a criminal responsibility evaluation to evaluate if Rob had a mental disorder, whether Rob had the specific intent to kill the man, and whether Rob met the state's definition for insanity. The forensic psychiatrist requested a copy of the statutory definition of insanity, which read, "The accused is not guilty by reason of insanity if at the time of the alleged offense they were suffering from a severe mental disease or defect that rendered them unable to know or understand the nature and quality of their acts or to distinguish right from wrong." Collateral records indicated no use of any type of illegal substance or alcohol, and all serum and urine drug screens were negative for alcohol or drugs. The psychiatrist diagnosed Rob with schizophrenia, paranoid type. The psychiatrist rendered an opinion that Rob did intend to kill the police officer despite his suffering from symptoms of acute schizophrenia. However, the psychiatrist also opined that Rob was legally insane under that jurisdiction's test of insanity. In particular, the psychiatrist testified that although Rob knew the nature and quality of his actions in stabbing the police officer to kill him, Rob delusionally believed that he was acting in self-defense and therefore did not believe his actions were either legally or morally wrong.

—Key Points

With the increasing focus on juveniles who commit criminal acts, a significant need exists for evaluators who are competent to perform focused forensic evaluations. Key points when conducting these evaluations include the following:

— The evaluator must clearly understand the exact type of forensic evaluation requested.

— Waiver evaluations focus on a juvenile's risk for future dangerousness and amenability to treatment within the juvenile justice system.

— Evaluations of competency to stand trial focus on the youth's present ability to assist his or her legal counsel and the youth's understanding of the legal process.

— Criminal responsibility evaluations focus on the youth's past mental state at the time of the alleged offense.

— Regardless of the evaluation type, the evaluator should always consider the developmental issues relevant to the juvenile.

References

American Law Institute Model Penal Code, § 4.01 (1985)

American Psychiatric Association: Diagnostic and Statistical Manual of Mental Disorders, 4th Edition, Text Revision. Washington, DC, American Psychiatric Association, 2000

Barnum R: Child psychiatry and the law: clinical evaluation of juvenile delinquents facing transfer to adult court. J Am Acad Child Adolesc Psychiatry 26:922–925, 1987

Clark v Arizona, 548 US 735 (2006)

Cooper D: Juveniles' understanding of trial-related information: are they competent defendants? Behav Sci Law 15:167–180, 1997

Cowden VL, McKee GR: Competency to stand trial in juvenile delinquency proceedings: cognitive maturity and the attorney-client relationship. U Louisville J Family Law 33:629–690, 1995

Durham v United States, 94 US App DC 228, 214 F2d 862 (1954)

Dusky v United States, 362 US 402 (1960)

Fare v Michael C, 442 US 707 (1979)

Fitch WL: Competency to stand trial and criminal responsibility in the juvenile court, in Juvenile Homicide. Edited by Benedek EP, Cornell DG. Washington, DC, American Psychiatric Press, 1989, pp 145–162

Giorgi-Guarnieri D, Janofsky J, Keram E, et al: AAPL practice guideline for forensic psychiatric evaluation of defendants raising the insanity defense. American Academy of Psychiatry and the Law. J Am Acad Psychiatry Law 30:S3–S40, 2002

Griffin P, Torbet P, Szymanski L: Trying Juveniles as Adults in Criminal Court: An Analysis of State Transfer Provisions. Washington, DC, Office of Juvenile Justice and Delinquency Prevention, 1998

Grisso T: Forensic Evaluation of Juveniles. Sarasota, FL, Professional Resource Press, 1998

Grisso T, Miller M, Sales B: Competency to stand trial in juvenile court. Int J Law Psychiatry 10:1–20, 1987

Grisso T, Steinberg L, Woolard J, et al: Juveniles' competence to stand trial: a comparison of adolescents' and adults' capacities as trial defendants. Law Human Behav 27:333–363, 2003

In re Gault, 387 US 1 (1967)

Johnson v Zerbst, 304 US 458 (1938)

Kent v United States, 383 US 541 (1966)

McGarry AL: Competency to stand trial and mental illness, in Crime and Delinquency Issues, A Monograph Series

(DHEW Publ. No. HSM 73-9105). Rockville, MD, National Institute of Mental Health, 1973

Melton GB, Petrila J, Poythress NG, et al: Mental state at the time of the offense, in Psychological Evaluations for the Courts: A Handbook for Mental Health Professionals and Lawyers, 3rd Edition. New York, Guilford, 2007, pp 201–268

Miranda v Arizona, 384 US 436 (1966)

M'Naghten's Case, 8 Eng Rep 718 (1843)

Montana v Egelhoff, 518 US 37 (1996)

Mossman D, Noffsinger S, Ash P, et al: AAPL practice guideline for the forensic psychiatric evaluation of competence to stand trial. American Academy of Psychiatry and the Law. J Am Acad Psychiatry Law 35:23–72, 2007

Redding RE: Juvenile Transfer Laws: An Effective Deterrent to Delinquency? Washington, DC, Office of Juvenile Justice and Delinquency Prevention, 2008

Redding RE, Frost LE: Adjudicative competence in the modern juvenile court. Virginia J Soc Policy Law 9:353–409, 2001

Resnick PJ: American Academy of Psychiatry and the Law forensic review course syllabus. Paper presented at the annual meeting of the American Academy of Psychiatry and the Law, Miami, FL, October 2007

Robins LN, Ratcliff KS: Childhood conduct disorders and later arrest, in The Social Consequences of Psychiatric Illness. Edited by Robins LN, Clayton PJ, Wing JK. New York, Brunner/Mazel, 1980, pp 248–263

Scott CL: Juvenile violence. Psychiatr Clin North Am 22:71–83, 1999

Snyder H: Juvenile arrests, 2005 (Juvenile Justice Bulletin NCJ 218096). Washington, DC, Office of Juvenile Justice and Delinquency Prevention, 2008

Snyder HN, Sickmund M: Juvenile Offenders and Victims: A National Report. Washington, DC, Office of Juvenile Justice and Delinquency Prevention, 1995

Voigt CJ, Heisel DE, Benedek EP: State-of-mind assessments: competency and criminal responsibility, in Principles and Practice of Child and Adolescent Forensic Psychiatry. Edited by Schetky DH, Benedek EP. Washington, DC, American Psychiatric Publishing, 2002, pp 297–305

Chapter 27

Assessment and Treatment of Juvenile Offenders

Stephen W. Phillippi, Ph.D.
Debra K. DePrato, M.D.

Case Example 1

Shawn, a 10-year-old boy, was referred by his school to the local juvenile court for status offenses. He was alleged to have broken school rules repeatedly over the past 6 months of the current school year by being truant. The last straw came when he threw a small plastic wastepaper basket at a teacher. The school had previously referred him to "in house" after school intervention programs; however, he did not participate actively or regularly. In addition, his mother, a single working parent, had not attended any school parent–teacher meetings. Shawn had a reported history of poor grades and poor impulse control, and he lived in a community that was known to be "drug-ridden." Shawn was adjudicated a status offender and was referred for an assessment. The clinician performed a thorough assessment of Shawn, which included his mother and his biological grandmother with whom the family resided. The examination assessed the youth's and family's functioning, in addition to risk and protective factors. A psychological assessment was requested by the examiner because of concerns about Shawn's academic decline.

Case Example 2

Shauna, a 15-year-old girl, was arrested for assault and battery after engaging in a fight with another juvenile in her neighborhood. She was already on probation for shoplifting and running away from home. Shauna has missed many of her probation-ordered treatment sessions with a local agency. She is brought to her local detention center and enters the juvenile justice system not trusting any of the staff and with a history of not being engaged in any previous treatment services.

The Juvenile Justice System

The U.S. juvenile justice system was founded over a century ago with the first Juvenile Court Act passed in Illinois in 1899 (Sharp and Hancock 1995). This newly emerging system was a bifurcated process whereby juvenile and adult offenders began to be treated differently. The goal was to divert youthful offenders from what was considered the destructive punishments of criminal courts and to encourage rehabilitation based on the individual juvenile's needs (McCord et al. 2001). This marked a move from penal punishment to prevention and treatment. Even a new argot evolved: "taken into custody" replaced "arrest"; "trial" became "hearing"; "conviction" was now "adjudication"; and "sentence" became "disposition." Juvenile "delinquents" were no longer sent to prison; instead they were remanded to reformatories or trade schools.

For the next 50 years, juvenile court judges were allowed to handle cases informally, with great discretion regarding individualized treatment plans (Snyder and

Sickmund 1999). This trend was challenged in the 1950s and 1960s when, due to lack of public support, the juvenile justice system began moving away from a therapeutic approach to embracing more punitive correctional models. A series of U.S. Supreme Court decisions proffered in the 1960s and 1970s "made juvenile proceedings increasingly legalized and adversarial" (Bishop et al. 1996, p. 172). The U.S. Office of Juvenile Justice and Delinquency Prevention (OJJDP) was established in 1974 and emphasized community-based treatment and greater utilization of prevention services. By the 1990s, the boundaries, initially set to separate the juvenile system from the criminal justice system, further eroded as state policies and practices across the nation resulted in more juveniles transferred to adult criminal courts, harsher sanctions, and increased rates of incarceration (Snyder and Sickmund 2006). This environment set the stage for ongoing tension, particularly in relation to the plight of mentally ill children in the juvenile justice system. The U.S. Department of Health and Human Services Center for Mental Health Services presented documentation to Congress that described inadequate mental health care services for juveniles held in secure confinement (Center for Mental Health Services 1995). In efforts to quell concerns, Congress considered several bills and amendments mandating mental health and substance abuse screening and treatment programs for youth in the juvenile justice system. Now, in the beginning of the twenty-first century, efforts are under way to once again reform a system of punishment to one of rehabilitation and treatment (see also Chapter 26, "Juvenile Waiver and State-of-Mind Assessments").

Currently, over 2.3 million youth are arrested each year in the United States (Sickmund 2004). Of these juveniles, 29% are female and 71% are male (Snyder and Sickmund 2006). The youth population being served by the juvenile justice system has risen from U.S. courts handling 1,100 delinquency cases per day in 1960 to 4,500 delinquency cases per day in 2004 (Office of Juvenile Justice and Delinquency Prevention 2007a; Snyder and Sickmund 2006). A 44% increase in the total number of cases handled by juvenile courts was noted between 1985 and 2004, which included a 159% increase in the number of drug offense cases, a 141% increase in public offense cases, and a 120% increase in person offense cases (Office of Juvenile Justice and Delinquency Prevention 2007b).

Of the youth entering the juvenile justice system, at least one in five suffers from some sort of mental health issue (Howell 1998; Mears and Aron 2003; Otto et al. 1992; Schultz and Mitchell-Timmons

1995). Additionally, research suggests that a subpopulation of the juvenile justice system, those youth who are incarcerated in juvenile correctional facilities, have as many as 60% of males and 70% of females identified with a mental health disorder, and 20% suffer from severe mental illness (Mears and Aron 2003; Shufelt and Cocozza 2006; Teplin et al. 2002). About half of all adolescents receiving mental health services also have a co-occurring substance use disorder (Greenbaum et al. 1996). Teplin (2001) suggested that "nationwide, more than 670,000 youth processed in the juvenile justice system each year would meet diagnostic criteria for one or more substance abuse or mental health disorders that require mental health and/or substance abuse treatment" (p. 2). Of concern is that many of these youth appear to be placed in the juvenile justice system in order to access mental health services that are unavailable by traditional means in the community. A number of studies amplify this issue. The National Alliance for the Mentally Ill (2001) found that 36% of families surveyed reported placing their children in the juvenile justice system so they could have access to mental health services unavailable to them in the community. In a study by the U.S. General Accounting Office (2003), parents reported placing more than 12,700 youth in the child welfare or juvenile justice system setting for access to mental health services. Congress also documented this trend when it reported the inappropriate use of detention for youth with mental health needs in 33 states, where youth were reported to have been held in detention with no charges against them; there was reportedly no place else for these youth to go (U.S. House of Representatives 2004). Either way, current data suggest that youth in the juvenile justice system experience significantly higher rates of mental health disorders than youth in the general population, in which approximately 9%–13% of the nation's youth suffer from a diagnosable mental disorder (Friedman et al. 1996; Otto et al. 1992). Table 27–1 illustrates prevalence rates of psychiatric disorders among detained juvenile delinquents.

Juvenile Justice Processing

Zimring (2000) stated that a central objective of the juvenile court is to protect delinquents from the punishments of the adult criminal justice system; thus the juvenile court acts as a diversion from criminal justice. Youth move through this system as both adjudicated and nonadjudicated individuals. *Adjudication*

TABLE 27–1. Prevalence of psychiatric disorders among detained juvenile delinquents

DSM diagnosis	Male, %	Female, %
Any listed disorder	**66.3**	**73.8**
Any except conduct disorder	60.9	70.0
Any affective disorder	**18.7**	**27.6**
Major depressive episode	13.0	21.6
Dysthymia	12.2	15.8
Manic episode	2.2	1.8
Psychotic disorders	**1.0**	**1.0**
Any anxiety disorders	**21.3**	**30.8**
Panic disorder	0.3	1.5
Separation anxiety disorder	12.9	18.6
Overanxious disorder	6.7	12.3
Generalized anxiety disorder	7.1	7.3
Obsessive-compulsive disorder	8.3	10.6
Attention-deficit/hyperactivity disorder	**16.6**	**21.4**
Any disruptive behavior disorder	**41.4**	**45.6**
Oppositional defiant disorder	14.5	17.5
Conduct disorder	37.8	40.6
Any substance use disorder	**50.7**	**46.8**
Alcohol use disorder	25.9	26.5
Marijuana use disorder	44.8	40.5
Other substance use disorder	2.4	6.9
Alcohol and other drug use disorder	20.7	20.9

Source. Adapted from Teplin et al. 2002.

is defined as the court process that determines (judicial determination) if a juvenile committed the act for which he or she is charged, and adjudicated indicates that the court concluded the juvenile committed the delinquency or status offense charged in the petition (Stahl et al. 2005).

In the U.S. juvenile justice system, a child can commit two categories of offenses: delinquency offenses and status offenses. *Delinquency offenses* mean that a child has been found guilty of at least one crime that, if committed by an adult, could be punishable by law (e.g., theft, rape). *Status offenses* are acts that would not be crimes if committed by adults; truancy, ungovernability, and running away are considered status of-

fenses. In the case of *In re Gault* (1967), the Court ruled that delinquent offenders were to be afforded the same due process rights as an adult charged with a crime with the exception of jury trial. Prior to *Gault*, all offenders (status and delinquent) were treated equally and were offered no legal protections. The Juvenile Justice and Delinquency Prevention Act of 1974 provided status offenders with protection from the harshest form of punishments: incarceration in juvenile correctional facilities. To continue receiving federal funding, states could no longer lock up status offenders in training facilities. Response to the new restrictions resulted in rapid growth of community-based treatment programs and the child mental health movement.

Once a youth is charged as a delinquent, he or she may enter a diversion program, be adjudicated and receive probation, or be sent to a secure training school or a juvenile rehabilitation and correctional facility. Stahl et al. (2005) noted that of the youth who represent the delinquency and status offense cases handled each year by juvenile courts in the United States in 2002, over one-third of the cases involved property crime (e.g., burglary, larceny-theft, arson, vandalism, trespassing, possession of stolen property), followed by approximately one-fourth that involved public order offenses (e.g., obstruction of justice, disorderly conduct, weapons offenses, liquor law violations). Other smaller delinquency cases for courts handling juvenile matters in 2002 included simple assault (16.7%), drug law violations (12.0%), and violent crimes (4.7%), which included murder, forcible rape, robbery, and aggravated assault (Stahl et al. 2005).

Trends in arrest patterns suggest that as of 2003 there is an increase in the proportion of female youth entering the juvenile justice system for law violations, which is attributed to substantial increases in arrests for aggravated and simple assaults by females (Snyder and Sickmund 2006). Arrest trends also show that violent crime arrest rates as well as overall arrest rates have decreased since 1980 for all youth between the ages of 10 and 17 years with the exception of assault and drug abuse arrests, which have seen a steady increase. The trends in arrests and court handling have also demonstrated an increase in the formal handling of delinquency cases. In 1985 juvenile courts formally processed 45% of delinquency cases, and by 2002 formal processing had increased by 13% (to 58%). Of those formally processed in 2002, nearly 7 in 10 youth were adjudicated. The increases in petitioning for formal court process and subsequent adjudication of delinquency cases from 1985 to 2002 were observed for both male and female youth as well as for all races and ages of youth. Of those adjudicated delinquent in 2002, just under two-thirds were ordered to probation, and just under one-fourth were ordered to an out-of-home residential placement. This indicates that there was a doubling in the number of delinquency cases receiving probation between 1985 and 2002 and a 44% increase in adjudicated youth being sentenced to an out-of-home residential placement (Snyder and Sickmund 2006). How these cases are handled is critical as some researchers suggest that by grouping deviant youth together, unforeseen negative side effects may occur (Arnold and Hughes 1999). Social learning theory (i.e., Albert Bandura's research, wherein he showed that children learn through observation [Bandura 1986]) indicates that training schools tend to train additional deviance rather than prosocial behaviors.

Causes and Correlates of Juvenile Offending and Reoffending

In much of the emerging literature, juvenile offending and reoffending have been attributed to a series of events common to delinquents with specific typologies, multiple pathways, and different developmental sequences leading to different outcomes (Huizinga et al. 1991). Siegel (2004) explained that developmental pathways are either based on latent trait theories, which describe delinquent behavior as controlled by traits present at birth or soon after that remain stable and unchanging throughout the lifetime, or based on a life course view, which describes delinquent behavior as a dynamic process influenced by individual characteristics as well as social experiences. Research that examines the individual and psychosocial factors associated with initiation of delinquent offending and subsequent reoffending is supported by two theoretical frameworks. The public health risk and protective factor model offers a structure for the analysis of risk and protective factors associated with both delinquency prevention and the likelihood of youth engaging in delinquent behavior. The developmental theory model provides a structure for examining the progression of delinquent behavior, including reoffending. These two theoretical approaches relate to facets of both delinquency prevention and delinquency intervention, which are keys to observing and understanding participants in the juvenile justice system and predicting possible outcomes.

Public Health Risk and Protective Factor Model

As is the case in public health and specifically its epidemiology components, there are specific factors that influence the incidence, development, and control of problems in populations. In youth, the etiology of delinquent behavior is affected by psychosocial risk and protective factors that either increase or shield the risk of further development. Psychosocial risk factors include individual factors of the youth (e.g., personality, physiology) or those associated with their social environment, such as family, peer group, school, and community (Hawkins et al. 1992). Psychosocial risk factors have a cumulative negative effect such that as the number of risk factors increases, so does the probability that the youth will engage in delinquent behavior (Kazdin et al. 1997). Opposing influences called protective factors reduce the likelihood of problem behaviors either directly or by mediating the effects of exposure to risk factors (Arthur et al. 2002; Fraser 1997; Rutter 1987; Werner and Smith 1992).

The public health risk and protective factor model provides a predictive description of populations at risk in addition to recommendations as to where to interrupt the progression of the problem. In juvenile justice research, psychosocial risk factors predictive of adolescent problem behaviors are noted as promising targets for preventive intervention and understanding juvenile delinquency (Arthur et al. 2002; Hawkins et al. 1992, 1995; Mrazek and Haggerty 1994; Shader 2003). The evidence suggests that promoting protective factors while decreasing delinquency risk factors is effective for preventing and intervening in juvenile delinquent behavior (Hawkins and Catalano 1992).

Developmental Theory Model

The developmental theory model examines the onset of delinquency against a continuum of behaviors and categorizes those behaviors into three pathways leading to delinquency: authority conflict pathway, covert pathway, and overt pathway. The authority conflict pathway is described as having the earliest onset, with stubborn behavior being observed before age 12 and progressing to specific acts of defiance and disobedience. By early to middle adolescence, an avoidance of authority is observed, as are behaviors such as truancy and running away; the youth may then continue into one or both of the other pathways. The covert pathway is described as having its onset at 15 years or younger, with behaviors that are classified as minor and covert (e.g., shoplifting, lying) progressing to more moderately delinquent acts such as stealing and fraud. The covert pathway culminates in late adolescence with serious delinquency such as auto theft, robbery, and burglary. The overt pathway starts with minor aggression (e.g., bullying) and moves to fighting, including physical assaults and gang-related fighting. The overt pathway culminates in violence by late adolescence, including such acts as battery and even rape and murder (Thornberry et al. 2004).

These trajectories to delinquency offer two main courses from which to chart the development of delinquency. The two trajectories have unique causal explanations and are primarily predicted by age at onset and specific conduct problems. Life-course persistent offenders are predicted by DSM-IV-TR (American Psychiatric Association 2000) conduct disorder, childhood-onset type, with associated behaviors such as minor aggression, lying, hurting animals, and biting and hitting by age 4 years; peer rejection; lower cognitive abilities and slower language development; and neurological problems, such as attention deficit or hyperactivity. Adolescent-limited offenders represent the majority of offenders and are observed to stop offending by age 18 years. This trajectory is predicted by DSM-IV-TR conduct disorder, adolescent type, with associated behaviors such as serious aggression, stealing, running away, truancy, and breaking and entering (Moffitt 1993).

The developmental pathways models have been most consistently observed and reported for male youth. Female offenders have varied more and have not yet been described in such orderly progressions (Moffitt 1993). These pathways also need to be taken into consideration with the other delinquency psychosocial risk factors such as poor parenting practices and family violence, both of which also seem to accelerate overall risk for delinquency (Loeber et al. 2003).

Risk and Protective Factors

In youth, the etiology of delinquent behavior is affected by *risk factors*, which are defined in the literature as the characteristics, variables, or hazards that, if present for a given individual, make it more likely that the individual, rather than someone selected at random from the general population, will develop a disorder or problem (Arthur et al. 2002; Hawkins et al. 1992; Mrazek and Haggerty 1994; Rutter and Garmezy 1983). Risk factors exist in multiple psychosocial domains, including individual, family, school, peer, and community

(Hawkins 1995; Hawkins et al. 1992; Howell 1995). The presence of a risk factor predicts an increased probability of offending, and the likelihood of offending and reoffending is compounded with the presence of multiple risk factors that have a cumulative negative effect (Kazdin et al. 1997). The more risk factors attributed to a youth, the greater the probability of his or her engaging in delinquent behavior. Table 27–2 outlines risk factors associated with delinquent behavior.

Protective factors are defined as those factors that reduce the likelihood of a problem behavior directly or indirectly by mediating the effect of exposure to risk factors. These include intelligence, prosocial peers/activities, and family bonding. To adequately address treatment and intervention needs as part of the evaluation of a juvenile offender, the evaluating clinician needs to review all delinquency risk and protective factors to intervene in risk factors while promoting protective factors in a strength-based approach.

Risk Factors

Individual Factors

Individual risk factors for delinquent behaviors include rebelliousness, attitudes favorable toward problem behavior, early onset of problem behavior, and constitutional factors (Hawkins 1995). In reviews of the literature, this translates to a number of specific factors that have been associated with the development of juvenile delinquency. These individual factors include age, gender, impulsivity, aggressiveness, and substance use (Howell 1995; National Research Council and Institute of Medicine 2001). According to Howell (1995), rebellious behaviors are observed in youth who feel disconnected with society and do not want to be bound by its rules. These youth do not view success for themselves as being responsible within societal norms or rules, and they are observed as acting in an opposite posture. Youth who display attitudes favorable toward problem behavior tend to participate in those behaviors, including delinquent acts.

Age. Early age at onset of particular behaviors is commonly associated as a risk factor in the development of delinquency. Studies of official records of criminal activity by age reveal rates of offending beginning to rise in preadolescence and later falling in late adolescence and young adulthood (Farrington 1991). In a review of three of the major longitudinal studies on the impact of age on delinquency, Thornberry and Krohn (2003) and Thornberry et al. (2004) summarized the findings from the Denver Youth Study, Pitts-

TABLE 27–2. Risk factors associated with delinquent behavior

Individual

Low intelligence; cognitive, learning, and language problems

Poor impulse control

Unwillingness to take responsibility for behavior

Admiration for antisocial behavior

Perception of others as hostile

Early onset of delinquency

Job involving working more than 20 hours per week

Poor social skills

Family

Poverty

Low education levels

Conflict and hostility at home

Ineffective parental discipline and monitoring

Physical/sexual abuse

Familial substance abuse and psychiatric problems

Parental criminal history

Lack of warmth and affection between parents and child

Peer

Association with delinquent youth (for older youth/adolescents)

Peer rejection (for younger children)

Association with youth who use drugs or alcohol

Gang membership

School

Poor achievement/grades

Falling behind same-age peers

Sense of isolation or prejudice from peers

Poor attendance

Community

Availability of drugs and weapons

Poor support network

Isolation from neighbors

Living in "dangerous" neighborhoods

Frequent family moves

burgh Youth Study, and Rochester Youth Development Study. These studies involve a cumulative sample of over 4,000 youth and examine how long disruptive behaviors had been apparent in males who were eventually referred to the juvenile court for a delinquent offense. Findings from all three studies suggest that moderately serious problem behavior was evident by age 9.5 years and serious delinquent behaviors by age 12 years, while the average age of first contact with the juvenile court was 14.5 years (Thornberry et al. 2004).

Gender. Gender is shown in the literature to be associated with specific risk for the development of delinquent behaviors. Males have consistently been shown to commit a higher proportion of juvenile crime. In 2003, just under three-fourths (71%) of the juveniles arrested were male and a little under one-third (29%) were female (Snyder and Sickmund 2006). Most studies reflect the characteristics of the male offender, including both the public health risk and protective factor model and developmental theory model described earlier. These male-oriented studies are drastically different compared with recent research about the female offender.

Female youth populations, unlike their male counterparts, are usually in detention earlier for much less significant offenses. Most girls arrive in the juvenile justice system through paths marked by sexual and physical abuse, mental illness, substance abuse, family disconnection, and educational problems (Acoca 1999). The highest percentage (36%) of girls in custody in Acoca's (1999) research were probation violators whose first offense was running away, truancy, curfew violation, or some other status offense. According to Acoca, a typical pattern of progression into the juvenile justice system for female youth was a minor delinquency or status offense committed by the youth; the female youth being placed on probation; and any subsequent offense, even another status offense, leading to a violation of a valid court order, which then became the vector for greater involvement in the juvenile justice system. Acoca's study reveals that even the more serious female offenders' crimes most often fell into the assault category. However, the assault most often came from nonserious, mutually combative situations with parents. Common threads in the research on female youthful offenders are abuse, drug use, status offense, probation violation, single-parent homes, pregnant or with child, sexually transmitted disease, and chronic health problems (Acoca 1999; Acoca and Dedel 1998; Belknap et al. 1997; Chesney-Lind and Pasko 2004).

Impulsivity. Hawkins et al. (1998) reviewed several studies and reported "a positive relationship between hyperactivity, concentration or attention problems, impulsivity and risk taking and later violent behavior" (p. 113). McCabe et al. (2002) studied the association of diagnosable levels of attention deficit and hyperactivity per DSM-IV criteria for attention-deficit/hyperactivity disorder (ADHD) in a sample of adjudicated youth. Using a diagnostic self-report tool (i.e., the Voice DISC-IV), McCabe et al. (2002) reported that 15% of males and 21% of females in their sample recorded responses consistent with diagnostic criteria of ADHD.

Aggression. Of all the individual factors that are linked to delinquency, Tremblay and LeMarquand (2001) noted in their review of the literature that aggression was the best social predictor of delinquent behavior before age 13 years. Thornberry et al. (2004) reported that in both the Denver and Pittsburgh longitudinal youth studies, the majority of youth (85% males and 77% females in Denver and 88% of the males in Pittsburgh) were involved in some form of physical aggression before age 13 years, indicating that aggression in childhood is quite common. In closer examination of the level of aggression that is highly associated with juvenile offending, 47% of the males and 28% of the females in the Denver study and 14% of the males in the Pittsburgh study reported levels of assaults that resulted in serious injuries to the victim. *Serious injury* was defined as cuts, bleeding wounds, or injuries requiring medical treatment.

Aggression toward people, animals, and property accounts for 9 of the 15 diagnostic criteria for conduct disorder (American Psychiatric Association 2000). In both McCabe et al.'s (2002) and Garland et al.'s (2001) studies, conduct disorder was found in sizable portions of the adjudicated juvenile justice samples. McCabe et al. (2002) reported that 33% of the males and 38% of the females in their sample were assessed as meeting the criteria for conduct disorder on self-report. Similarly, Garland et al. (2001) found that 30% of the sample met criteria for conduct disorder in a self-report assessment.

Substance abuse. Research shows that young people who initiate drug use before the age of 15 have twice the risk of developing drug problems as those who wait until after age 19 years (Robins and Przybeck 1985). Robins and Przybeck also found that onset of drug use prior to age 15 years was positively correlated with self-reports of stealing, vandalism, truancy, and arrest. Similarly, McCabe et al. (2002) determined that substance use disorders were found in large percentages of the ad-judicated juvenile justice sample. McCabe et al. (2002) reported that 37% of the males and 28% of the females were assessed as meeting the criteria for substance use disorder on self-report. The minimum threshold for a substance use disorder in this study was defined by DSM-IV-TR diagnostic criteria for substance abuse, which require "a maladaptive pattern of substance use leading to clinically significant impairment or distress, as manifested by one (or more) of the following, occurring within a 12-month period: 1) recurrent substance use resulting in failure to fulfill major role obligations at work, school, or home; 2) recurrent substance use in situations in which it is physically hazardous; 3) recurrent substance-related legal problems; and 4) continued substance use despite having persistent or recurrent social or interpersonal problems caused or exacerbated by the effects of the substance" (American Psychiatric Association 2000, p. 199). Among youth who progress to the next step in the continuum of juvenile justice detention, half of detainees have been shown to have a substance use disorder (Teplin et al. 2002). The prevalence rate of substance use disorders in every segment of the juvenile justice system argues the need for every youth entering the system to be screened for substance use, abuse, or dependence.

Family Factors

Steinberg (1987) examined three family structures, specifically, youth living with both natural parents, with their mother alone, and with one natural parent and a stepparent. Steinberg concluded that youth living in either of the latter family structures were more vulnerable to delinquent activities than those of two-parent households. According to Steinberg (1987), children living with both biological parents were less susceptible to pressure from their friends to engage in deviant behavior than youth in other family structures.

Johnson (1989) also examined family structure in relation to delinquency by looking at general patterns and gender differences and adding a measure of the quality of the parent–child relationship. Family structure was defined by five categories classified by the combination of parents residing in the home of the youth: biological father/biological mother, biological father/stepmother, biological father only, biological mother/stepfather, and biological mother only. These five categories were measured in association with self-reported delinquency. The study also surveyed the youth with regard to the quality of the parent–child relationship. Johnson (1989) found that home type was moderately related to self-reported official trouble (i.e., number of school suspensions, nontraffic police apprehensions, and juvenile court appearances the youth reported having experienced) with both male and female youth. Males from families with mothers and stepfathers were described as having a significantly higher number of self-reported illegal acts than males from other home structures. Both male and female youth from intact families reported a lower amount of illegal behavior; however, for males, and exceedingly so for females, the family structures without a father were associated with higher rates of self-reported illegal behavior. Self-report of the quality of the family relationship showed no significant differences for either gender or any of the five family structure types (Johnson 1989).

Family characteristics such as family management problems, larger family size, and family conflict have been described as being associated with risk of delinquency (Derzon and Lipsey 2000; Hawkins 1995; Phillippi 2007; Wasserman and Seracini 2001). Family management problems include lack of supervision, lack of clear standards or expectations, and severe inconsistent punishment, which have all been associated with delinquency (Farrington 1991; Kandel and Andrews 1987; Patterson and Dishion 1985; Peterson et al. 1994; Thornberry 1994). In a study of male youth, McCord (1979) found that the strongest predictors of a future violent offense conviction up to age 45 years were poor parental supervision, parental conflict, and parental aggression. Additionally, some research has shown that youth from families with four or more children have an increased rate of offending (Wasserman and Seracini 2001; West and Farrington 1973).

School Factors

Children with low academic performance, low commitment to school, and low educational aspirations are at higher risk for delinquency (Herrenkohl et al. 2001). (Note: Children in the juvenile justice system have higher prevalence rates of learning disabilities.) School experience has been associated with a higher risk for delinquency when youth display persistent aggressive antisocial behaviors at an early age in the classroom, when youth experience early onset of academic failure, and when youth have a low commitment to receiving an education (Hawkins 1995). Aggressive behaviors in combination with social withdrawal or hyperactivity in kindergarten, first grade, and second grade have been associated with a high risk of future delinquency (Loeber et al. 2003; Snyder 2001). Youth experiencing frequent relocations or even normal transitions between schools (e.g., middle school to high school) can be at higher risk for delinquent behaviors (Gottfredson 1998; Hawkins 1995).

In a longitudinal study of youth development and behavior, Herrenkohl et al. (2001) followed a sample of fifth-grade children from Seattle public schools. The sample was almost evenly split between male and female participants and was racially diverse. Of the participants, 52% reported being involved in the free school lunch program, indicating low socioeconomic status, and 42% of participants reported living with a single parent. Information gathered from the youth at age 10 years and then analyzed in relation to predictors of violence and delinquency at age 14 years revealed that teacher-rated hyperactivity, low attention, and antisocial behavior, as well as low family income, among others, had strong persistent effects on later violence. School predictors (e.g., low academic performance, hyperactivity, low attention, and antisocial behavior) and peer predictors (e.g., involvement with antisocial peers) of violence were consistently the strongest mediators of the earlier risk factors with the later measures of violence at age 14 years.

Peer Group Factors

Youth who have friends who engage in delinquent behaviors are much more likely to succumb to social pressures and commit delinquent acts themselves (Barnes and Welte 1986; Cairns et al. 1988; Elliott et al. 1989; Farrington 1991; Hawkins 1995). This is one of the most consistent predictors identified in the research. Studies have found a consistent relationship between involvement in a delinquent peer group and delinquent behavior (Lipsey and Derzon 1998; McCord et al. 2001; Steinberg 1987). According to McCord et al. (2001), adolescent antisocial behavior was associated with peers demonstrating delinquent behavior, peer approval of delinquent behavior, allegiance to such peers, peer pressure toward deviance, and time spent with such peers. Furthermore, Steinberg (1987) found that the relationship between the influences of peers on delinquent behavior is magnified when youth have lower rates of interaction with their parents.

In a study of peers and delinquent behavior, Haynie and Osgood (2005) examined survey respondents participating in the National Longitudinal Study of Adolescent Health, which is a nationally representative sample of adolescents in grades 7 through 12. Unlike earlier studies that relied on self-report information regarding peers, this study introduced independent assessment by constructing network-based measures of peer relationships. The study found that adolescent youth engage in higher rates of delinquency when they have delinquent peers or if their time spent with peers socializing is mostly unstructured (Haynie and Osgood 2005). These outcomes reinforce the position that peer influence is one of the most consistent predictors that research has identified. Even when young people come from well-managed families and do not have other risk factors, just spending time with friends who engage in problem behaviors greatly increases the risk of that problem developing (see also Chapter 20, "Taxonomy and Neurobiology of Aggression," and Chapter 21, "Assessing Violence Risk in Youth").

Protective Factors

The more risk factors a youth is exposed to, the higher the risk of delinquency. It is therefore not surprising that one of the key protective factors is the ability to reduce the number of risk factors to which a youth is exposed. As discussed earlier, protective factors reduce the likelihood of a problem behavior directly or indirectly by mediating the effect of exposure to risk factors (Fraser 1997; Rutter 1987; Werner and Smith 1992). Specific factors shown in studies to shield youth from the effects of being exposed to risk factors include social bonding/attachment, clear standards for behavior, and innate individual factors (Hawkins 1995). The effects of risk exposure appear to decrease when youth make prosocial bonds with adults, including family members or someone outside the family like a coach or teacher. Youth also appear protected by participating in environments (e.g., schools, families) that have clear standards and expectations communicated and reinforced for prosocial behavior. Elliott (1994) reported that later violence may actually be curbed by youth spending time with peers who disapprove of delinquent behavior. Lastly, there are individual factors that are innate or inherent to some youth that seem to have a protective factor for limiting their risk of delinquency. These include being intelligent, being female, and having a resilient temperament (Hawkins 1995).

In summary, the literature shows a number of psychosocial risk factors associated with offending as well as causes and correlates related to reoffending. Risk for developing delinquent behaviors exists in multiple domains, including individual, family, school, and peer associations. Individual characteristics such as early age at onset of aggression, male gender, substance abuse, and impulsivity are cumulative factors placing youth at increased risk of offending and reoffending. Family factors associated with the parent configurations defined by divorce and single parenting, high conflict in the home, larger family size, and lower family income are also characteristics placing youth at increased risk of juvenile offending. Failure in school and association with peers who are delinquent have compounding effects that increase risk of offending, according to the literature. The higher the prevalence of any of these risk factors, the greater the risk for juvenile delinquent behavior. Any combination of these factors may also be causally linked to the maintenance and development of further delinquency. Studies show that early age at onset, drug use, school problems, and mental health problems are among the strongest predictors of persistent delinquent behaviors. Furthermore, the influence of risk and protective factors changes at different developmental levels. Peer influence to a preschool youngster is much less important than it is to an adolescent, and parental influence is less important for an adolescent than it is for a preschooler. Therefore, diagnosticians need to carefully assess what risk and protective factors are more salient given a child's developmental stage. It is also critical to note that any combination of risk factors only increases the risk of delinquency and does not provide an absolute prediction that the youth will offend. What the identification of risk factors does best is provide the targets for prevention and intervention services.

Screening and Assessment of Youth in the Juvenile Justice System

A thorough and accurate assessment of a juvenile offender is key to adequately address the treatment needs of the child and his or her family. The evaluator's assessment must target the risk and protective factors for both the youth and his or her environment and identify those factors in which a treatment intervention is possible and realistic. Knowledge of the literature in this area is essential, as is an understanding of which treatments work with this population and which do not.

The results of the clinician's evaluation and treatment recommendations have serious implications for the child's life. An adequate evaluation will direct treatment to reduce risk factors while enhancing protective factors, thus minimizing the possibility of the youth's further involvement in delinquent activities. Inadequate evaluation and treatment will have little impact on the juvenile's situation and often lead to treatment failure, resulting in serious legal consequences for the youth, such as incarceration. These evaluations take the form of screening and/or assessments, which should be differentiated by the clinician.

Screening instruments are used to identify youth at initial points of contact with the juvenile justice system who may require immediate attention for a safety issue (e.g., suicidal thoughts/behaviors) or who may need more in-depth assessment. Screening is a means of sifting through the often large number of youth contacting the system to initially and tentatively identify a subset who may have mental health problems (e.g., anxiety, depression), behavior problems (e.g., suicide, aggression), or problems in functional areas (e.g., school, peer, family) and then to more fully assess those at risk (Vincent et al. 2007). According to Grisso (2005), "[T]he objective is similar to triage in medical settings, where incoming patients are initially classified indicating their level of urgency. Like triage, screening is useful in systems that have limited resources and therefore cannot respond comprehensively or immediately to every individual's particular needs" (p. 13). It is important to note that screening instruments have a short shelf life and are not designed to provide a clinically valid diagnosis, the etiology of behavioral or mental health problems, or enough information for long-range treatment or rehabilitation planning (Vincent et al. 2007). What the screening results can afford is a current portrayal of acute symptoms and potential problem areas that can then be further assessed. Table 27–3 lists screening tools commonly used in juvenile justice settings.

TABLE 27–3.   Screening tools used in juvenile justice settings

Tool	General use
Substance Abuse Subtle Screening Instrument (SASSI)	Unidimensional screen for substance abuse
Trauma Symptom Checklist for Children (TSCC)	Unidimensional screen for trauma
Suicide Ideation Scale (SIS)	Unidimensional screen for suicidal ideation
Massachusetts Youth Screening Instrument–2 (MAYSI-2)	Multidimensional screen for symptoms of mental and emotional disturbance and potential crisis areas
Global Appraisal of Individual Needs–Short Screener (GAIN-SS)	Multidimensional behavioral health screening tool
Problem Oriented Screening Instrument for Teenagers (POSIT)	Problem/needs-oriented self-report that identifies psychosocial functioning in 10 areas
Child and Adolescent Functional Assessment Scale (CAFAS)	Problem/needs-oriented behavioral rating scale that assesses impairment in functioning across different settings and indicates whether functioning is affected by problems that may require specialized interventions
Child and Adolescent Needs and Strengths–Juvenile Justice (CANS-JJ)	Problem/needs descriptive tool that identifies needs or strengths in a variety of areas to guide service delivery for children and adolescents with mental, emotional, and behavioral health needs and juvenile justice involvement
Diagnostic Interview Schedule for Children (DISC)—Present State Voice Version	Multidimensional scale for an accurate and efficient assessment of child and adolescent mental health problems
Practical Adolescent Dual Diagnosis Interview (PADDI)	Comprehensive diagnostic interview to help identify both DSM-IV substance abuse/dependence diagnoses and the most prevalent mental health disorders
Global Appraisal of Individual Needs–Quick (GAIN-Q)	Instrument used to assess various life problems in adolescents to provide background information on factors that may be related to the behavioral health problems, assess the severity and prevalence of the problems, and question an individual's desire for help

Source.   Adapted from Vincent et al. 2007.

In contrast to screening, "the purpose of assessment is to gather a more comprehensive and individualized profile of a youth" (Vincent et al. 2007, p. 275). Most often, the typical assessment of a juvenile delinquent occurs following adjudication and before sentencing or at the time of detention or incarceration. The judge, attorneys, and/or probation and parole officers often desire an assessment to aid in the disposition of the case and to address specific treatment recommendations. The questions often asked by referral sources include how to best protect the community from the child, the child's risk of rearrest, identification of a mental disorder(s), types of treatment recommended and their availability, and the least restrictive environment necessary. To answer these questions, clinicians must approach the evaluation with a broad ecological perspective, including a thorough investigation of the juvenile's behavior in the home, school, workplace, and neighborhood (Melton et al. 1997). The evaluation should address the child's functioning in the environment in which he or she lives, as well as the primary caretaker's ability to effectively parent across a variety of settings, including home and school. By assessing the child within the system in which he or she lives, evaluators can correctly identify areas for needed intervention and the strengths of the child and family that will prompt success of treatment. Guidelines for assessment of juvenile offenders are presented in Table 27–4.

Juvenile Justice Intervention Models

Identification of factors that contribute to chronic delinquency and factors that protect from delinquency, if incorporated into treatment models, may produce programs with improved outcomes for delinquent youth. Youth can be involved in these programs at different points in the court process: preadjudication in diversion programs, while on probation and living in the community, when placed out of the home in a more restrictive environment, and following incarceration if on parole or in an aftercare program. In fact, the juvenile justice system has moved from the conclusion in the latter part of the twentieth century that nothing works with juvenile offenders to being able to repeatedly and visibly demonstrate positive outcomes for youth (Elliott 2007). A growing body of evidence synthesized in a number of meta-analyses of juvenile programs shows that the average juvenile justice program

---

TABLE 27–4. Assessment guidelines

1. Understand the legal question at hand and any relevant statutes.

2. Understand confidentiality rules that apply to the particular assessment, and relate information to youth and guardian.

3. Review the legal records, such as previous charges and current charge, victim's statements, police report of the current charge, and records from detention center such as behavioral reports/screening information.

4. Obtain and review all pertinent records, including medical, mental health, psychiatric, and school records of the child, and if indicated, those of the primary guardian(s).

5. The clinical interview of the child must specifically include the functioning of the child in the family, the functioning of the child within all domains of his or her environment, a thorough mental status examination assessing all cognitive domains, suicidality, premorbid functioning prior to the act, past legal history, acute or chronic stresses in the child's life, a weapons and violence history, substance use, sexual or physical abuse, medical problems, and prosocial skills.

6. The clinical interview must include the primary caretakers of the child, specifically addressing their style of parenting, evidence of mental disorder or substance abuse disorder that interferes with parenting, ability to interact successfully with the child's environment (such as school and peer group), the family's support system, and the strengths of the family system.

7. Collateral interviews should be conducted with individuals familiar with the child, such as a current treatment provider, teacher, probation officer, and detention staff.

8. Psychological assessment may be indicated for specific academic or diagnostic purposes.

9. A thorough opinion should be rendered that includes the child's and family's functioning, risk and protective factors, and DSM diagnoses if present (inclusive of the symptomatology).

10. Specific and realistic treatment recommendations should be made that address the needs of the youth and family in order to reduce risk factors, build on the youth's and family's strengths, and treat medical or psychiatric issues.

reduces recidivism (Lipsey 1992, 1995, 1999; Lipsey and Wilson 1997). In one meta-analysis, Lipsey (1999) studied evaluations of programs serving noninstitutionalized juvenile offenders and found that, on average, the best programs reduced recidivism by about 40%. The best types of interventions for reducing recidivism with noninstitutionalized youth were identified as individualized interpersonal skills training, behavioral programs, and interventions that involved multiple services (Lipsey 1999). Research has also found that community-based treatment programs are generally more effective than incarceration or residential placement in reducing recidivism, even for serious and violent offenders (Lipsey et al. 2001). Figure 27–1 shows results of a meta-analysis conducted by the Washington State Institute for Public Policy of recidivism in various youth and juvenile offender programs.

The juvenile court models discussed in the following sections are intended to focus on types of youthful offenders, including first-time offenders, status offenders, or youth with specialized needs such as mental health and substance abuse issues. They are legal models by which interventions are delivered. Key to the success of these programs and specialty courts are the types of screening, assessment, and treatment provided so that the youth's and family's needs are accurately identified and appropriate treatment is rendered.

Diversion Programs

Informal processing, also called diversion, refers to the practice of diverting youth from the juvenile justice system (i.e., preadjudicatory) and shifting the responsibility of handling them either to social control institutions such as family or schools or to community-based services (Mulvey et al. 1992). The focus of such efforts is to minimize the number of juveniles who proceed further into the juvenile justice system once they have first entered it. Diversion of juvenile offenders from the juvenile justice system evolved in the 1970s, based on the belief that penetration into the juvenile justice system is more harmful than beneficial, the two main reasons being that involvement in the juvenile justice system gives the child a delinquent self-image and that it stigmatizes the child in the opinion of others (such as teachers, parents, and officers) (Lundman 1993). Diversion programs defer the child's adjudication so that the child's charge will be dropped if he or she successfully completes the intervention program or treatment.

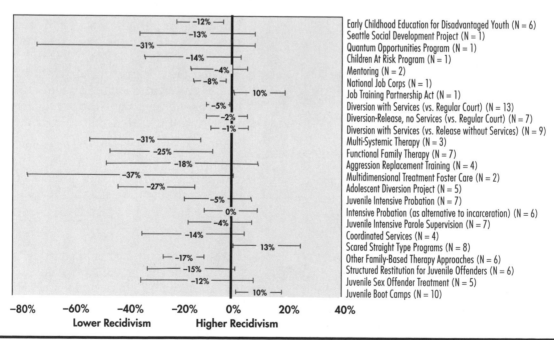

FIGURE 27–1. Estimated effect on criminal recidivism of different types of programs for youth and juvenile offenders.

Note. N = number of studies in program summary. The number in each bar is the effect size of the program, which approximates a percentage change in recidivism rates. The length of each bar is the 95% confidence interval.

Source. Meta-analysis conducted by the Washington State Institute for Public Policy. Reprinted from Barnoski B: Washington State's Experience With Research-Based Juvenile Justice Programs. Paper presented at the Models for Change in Juvenile Justice: Evidence-Based Practice Summit, Baton Rouge, LA, April 2007. Used with permission.

Attributed largely to the heightened awareness of large numbers of youth with mental illness in the juvenile justice system, there has been a resurgence in interest in diversion programs (Skowyra and Powell 2006). Evaluations of these programs yield varied results; however, the potential benefits of diversion remain compelling. These benefits include reducing recidivism, providing more effective and appropriate treatment, decreasing detention center overcrowding, promoting the development of community-based services, increasing the safety of detained youth, facilitating improved working relationships among juvenile justice system–serving groups, expediting court processing and access to services, and promoting family participation in treatment (Arredondo et al. 2001; Cocozza and Skowyra 2000).

Research reviewing a number of major diversion programs reveals several points. Many diversion programs include greater numbers of referrals of juveniles for lesser charges, thereby "net widening," or adding children to the juvenile justice system who would not otherwise be included. In a number of studies supported by OJJDP, four jurisdictions participated in experimentally designed diversion projects in which offenders would have otherwise penetrated further into the system due to their current delinquent charge. Types of treatment involved individual and family therapy, as well as educational, employment, and recreational interventions. Three groups were compared: those released without services, those given diversion services, and those with further involvement in the juvenile justice system. Rearrest rates of the three control groups, 6 and 12 months posttreatment, showed no significant differences. Another study, the Adolescent Diversion Project, revealed that community-based diversion interventions produced lower delinquency rates than did return-to-court intake (i.e., those children who did not receive services but were remanded to court). Taken together, "diversion of juveniles accused of status and property crimes is at least as effective as further penetration into the justice system" (Lundman 2001, p. 302). In other reviews of diversion versus formal adjudication, Smith and Paternoster (1990) found that youth recommended for formal juvenile court processing were significantly more delinquent during a 1-year follow-up period. Additionally, Snyder (1988) found that the rate of re-referral to juvenile court increases with the number of prior juvenile court contacts a youth has, arguing the need for diversion options where appropriate to public safety.

Specialty Courts

In recent years, juvenile justice reform efforts have led to the creation of a number of specialty courts to improve or target the efforts of traditional juvenile courts, which tend to have heavy caseloads and judges who are forced to contend with a broad scope of juvenile issues. These specialty courts include juvenile drug courts, mental health courts, and truancy courts. Many of these courts are so new that evaluations have only begun to yield results, but most argue that the results are promising and include lower recidivism and greater cost-effectiveness. In general, these courts move from the former system of courts judging guilt or innocence and assigning youth to a probation officer to a system in which judges are more involved in working out solutions and following the progress and challenges faced by youth via frequent court sessions (Gest 2007). The motivation for these courts includes concerns about lengthy delays in processing juvenile court cases, the lack of individualized and appropriate treatment, the lack of appropriate sanctioning, and the lack of sustained and consistent monitoring of youth while they are under court supervision (Mears and Aron 2003).

Juvenile Drug Court

A targeted form of diversion for juvenile offenders is the juvenile drug court. Patterned on the adult drug court model first established in 1989, drug courts have led the field of specialty courts. Juvenile drug courts are diversionary for the first-time juvenile offenders charged with a drug-related offense. The primary focus of juvenile drug courts is to expedite youth entering drug treatment and monitor their progress closely (Gest 2007). A drug court team consists of a judge, prosecutor, defense lawyer, treatment personnel, and case management and/or probation staff. As leader of the team, judges are actively involved in the drug court and play a role in coordinating services and drug tests, as well as coaxing young drug abusers to change their behaviors through a system of sanctions and incentives. Participants proceed through phases (detoxification, counseling, educational/vocational assessment and training, and graduation) typically over a period of close to 1 year.

One outcome of drug courts and the frequent court appearances that are required is an increased failure-to-appear rate. Defendants are supervised more closely; thus, their violations are noticed more frequently than when they are on a standard probation. A treatment approach based on a treatment model with relapse expected is extremely important so that the program does not become overly punitive, resulting in higher rates of incarceration. However, all considered, drug courts continue to be seen as a viable alternative to traditional juvenile proceedings. Evidence regarding the effectiveness of drug courts remains largely anecdotal, but studies suggest lower recidivism and drug use by the court's participants as well as an overall cost savings compared with youth not receiving drug court interventions (Butts and Roman 2004).

Mental Health Court

Juvenile mental health courts offer a more responsive process for many youth who meet DSM-IV-TR criteria for a diagnosed mental disorder or developmental disability in an attempt to improve the experience of mentally ill youth in the juvenile justice system and curtail the excessive rates of incarceration. To enter juvenile mental health court, youth undergo initial screening for a variety of mental disabilities upon arrival in detention while awaiting trial. These mental disabilities include serious mental illness such as a primary diagnosis or comorbid condition, including major depression, bipolar disorder, schizophrenia, severe anxiety disorders, or severe ADHD, and developmental disabilities, such as pervasive developmental disorder, mental retardation, autism, and severe head injury. The mental illness must also be identified as having contributed to the youth's delinquent behavior and involvement with the juvenile justice system (Arredondo et al. 2001). All of this is taken into consideration by a multidisciplinary team made up of the district attorney, public defender (or defense counsel), probation staff, school officials, and mental health professionals who must accept the case for mental health court and will also work with the youth and family to develop an individualized treatment plan.

The goal of the mental health courts is to keep youth in their homes, schools, and communities while they are provided comprehensive mental health services during probation, closely monitored by the courts every 30 to 90 days. Program participants are asked to engage in psychological treatment, comply with prescribed medication, and present a general willingness to participate in the process with a positive attitude (Arredondo et al. 2001). Internal program evaluations have suggested lower recidivism rates with participating youth; however, no formal external evaluations have been done on mental health courts to date. Critics of the court suggest these proceedings remove valuable resources from community services that could prevent these youth from ever contacting the juvenile justice system in the first place and that

the concept of the mental health court itself stigmatizes the participants. This latter concept is also fueled by mounting efforts to release the names and records of juvenile delinquents. Some also argue that youth must be adjudicated to receive assessment and treatment because of a lack of community resources.

Truancy Court

Like substance abuse and mental health issues, truancy dockets are a large part of most juvenile court proceedings. Truancy courts seek to bring schools, social workers, mental health treatment agencies, and families to a central place to problem-solve the many issues that contribute to truant behavior. Truancy courts operate out of a system of sanctions and incentives administered by a judge who rewards juveniles for success in overcoming difficulties. Participants waive going through traditional trial processes and volunteer to participate in weekly court monitoring of academic performance, attendance, and behavior. There is limited evidence as to the effectiveness of truancy courts overall; however, early investigations have shown a large proportion of participants increase their school attendance as well as improve their grades. The success has been attributed to the quick response of the court as issues with truancy arise (Gest 2007). Follow-up in traditional juvenile court might take several months as truants are ordered to return for review, whereas in truancy courts the follow-up is often within 2 weeks or less.

Correctional- and Institutional-Based Programs

About 62% of adjudicated juvenile delinquents are given probation, and 23% are placed outside the home (Stahl et al. 2005). Correctional-based programs can be effective in reducing recidivism as long as specific principles are followed throughout incarceration (Andrews et al. 1990; Lipton and Pearson 1996). However, it should be noted that the outcomes are generally poor compared with community-based programs with similar youth. In general, OJJDP found that effective treatment programs share the following principles:

- Target specific characteristics and problems of offenders that can be changed in treatment and that are predictive of future criminality.
- Implement known treatment methods for participating offenders, and use proven therapeutic techniques with educated, experienced staff.

- Allow adequate duration of program time for desired outcome.
- Offer the most intensive programming for offenders with the highest risk of recidivism.
- Utilize individualized cognitive and behavioral treatment methods that maximize positive reinforcement for prosocial behavior.

Foster and Group Homes

Group home treatment of status and delinquent offenders dates back to the early 1900s in Chicago and New York. The programs caught on nationally in the 1960s and 1970s (Piper and Warner 1980; Weber 1981). Group homes typically house from 4 to 12 adolescents. Children generally reside in a family-type setting with houseparents (foster families, trained individuals or couples, counselors, or caseworkers). Residents are usually enrolled in community public schools, may earn the privilege of regular visits with their families on weekends, may hold part-time jobs, and may even enjoy some independent personal time (Krueger and Hansen 1987). Children may benefit from individual and/or family therapy, as well as from behavior management plans (e.g., token economy systems). Group homes are typically cost-effective and provide an alternative to incarceration (Haghighi and Lopez 1993). Specialized services and schools within an institution are not necessary because community resources are available. In general, the effectiveness of foster or group homes varies greatly, as do the models of service delivery; however, models such as multidimensional therapeutic foster care have shown consistent evidence of success (more information is available in Figure 27–1).

Aftercare and Reintegrative Confinement

Effectively transitioning juvenile offenders from incarceration back into the community is critical, especially as numbers of incarcerated juveniles increase and institutions become overcrowded and expensive. In addition, long-term incarceration of juvenile offenders has not been shown to result in reduction of juvenile arrests after release. According to Altschuler et al. (1999), reintegrative confinement emphasizes 1) preparing confined offenders for reentry into the specific communities to which they will return, 2) making the needed arrangements and linkages with agencies and individuals in the offenders' community in direct relation to known risk and protective factors,

and 3) ensuring the delivery of required services and supervision after discharge.

Three OJJDP-funded integrative release/aftercare programs had different results; however, commonalities and recommendations for reform were noted by OJJDP:

1. Aftercare programs must be community based and on a continuum to parallel programs within the correctional institution (i.e., the institution must design services to prepare youth to reintegrate into their communities, with aftercare to follow).
2. Aftercare programs must be sufficiently funded to provide adequate numbers of well-trained, well-supervised staff who can respond to issues of family, education, drug abuse, and employment upon the juvenile's return to the community.
3. Formal assessment must occur to identify high-risk juvenile offenders who require this level of intensive services and supervision.
4. Reduced caseload sizes, greater contact by staff, and clear planning for positive long-term impact are necessary, as is a graduated response regarding sanctions (so that the process is not overly punitive while providing greater supervision).

Juvenile Justice Treatment Models

All treatment for juvenile offenders is not equal, and some are even harmful. It is the obligation of each clinician to be sure he or she is recommending treatment that will address the problems presented by the child and family and also to not recommend treatment that will increase the risk of reoffending. To that end, current science offers clinicians much guidance.

Different types of treatment are offered as part of court-related programs for delinquent and status-offending youth. Treatment prognosis of behavior-disordered and antisocial youth was long considered poor, yet current treatment models have shown successful outcomes. Reviews of delinquency literature of the 1970s gave no indication that treatment worked (Henggeler 1989). Previous forms of treatment focused on a small part of the delinquent youth's behavior; treatment was office based, was often inaccessible, and disregarded environmental factors leading to out-of-home placements (Henggeler 1994). System design and agency interaction often led to fragmented services with lack of coordination of care. For mild forms of antisocial behavior and substance abuse, Kazdin (1995) noted promising treatment with behavioral parent training, cognitive-behavioral therapy, and functional family therapy. Structured skill-oriented treatments described by Lipsey (1992) revealed improvement in delinquents in general. Most individual treatment has not been shown to prevent or improve juvenile delinquency in real-world settings (Lundman 2001) and was not designed for antisocial youth. Family preservation alone has shown no long-term improvement in outcomes for children compared with traditional office-based services. Up to 50% of youth who are hospitalized are admitted for behavioral disorders, even though no studies show that hospitalization is more beneficial than long-term community-based treatments, and youth with antisocial and family pathology show the least benefit (Henggeler 1994).

Teplin et al.'s (2002) study revealed the large percentages of juvenile offenders with psychiatric disorders, which occur at higher rates than in the general population, with female offenders having higher rates of mental disorders than male offenders (see Table 27–1). Disorders that have the highest prevalence rates across studies are depression, posttraumatic stress disorder (PTSD), anxiety, and substance abuse. Many of these disorders are found as co-occurring conditions, which is a critical consideration for both assessment and treatment. In addition, if the youth is housed in a juvenile justice facility, the risk of suicide is three times greater than in the general population (Gallagher and Dorbrin 2006). Therefore it is important to perform a thorough psychiatric evaluation on admission. Appropriate medication management is an important component of treatment and should be an adjunct to interventions that address the overall risk and protective factors of the youth and family. Medications should include those that are indicated for the treatment of the psychiatric disorder diagnosed. Care should be taken in prescribing a medication with addictive properties or medications with high "street" value. Aggressive treatment of ADHD should be considered, because ADHD is highly correlated with the later onset of conduct disorder (Foley et al. 1996) and effective treatment of ADHD may prevent the onset of conduct disorder.

Evidence-Based Practice

Recidivism is an outcome measure frequently used in the juvenile justice system with the limitation that rearrests and new adjudications reflect only those offenses that are brought to the attention of the system (Snyder and Sickmund 2006). The appropriateness of using recidivism as a sole criterion for defining a successful outcome has been questioned in light of empirically tested interventions that target psychosocial factors other than rearrest. The juvenile justice system now has programs with scientific evidence that they reduce out-of-home placements, future delinquency, violence, drug use, and other problem behaviors while often improving family functioning and school performance. This growing number of programs, commonly known as *evidence-based practices*, have program evaluations that use strong research designs, offer evidence of significant deterrent effects, demonstrate sustained effects, and are shown to be cost-effective in multiple site replications.

For example, multisystemic therapy is an evidence-based program delivered in the homes of youth displaying delinquent behaviors that has been shown to be effective with serious, antisocial, substance-abusing, and sex-offending youth without incarceration or hospitalization by demonstrating improvement in the psychosocial functioning of the youth and their families (Borduin et al. 1995; Henggeler 1992; Henggeler et al. 1993). Similarly, functional family therapy is a cognitive-behavioral prevention and intervention program for high-risk youth and their families and has been shown to be effective in reducing not only recidivism but also the cost of treating youth and their families compared with traditional services and other interventions such as incarceration or hospitalization (Alexander et al. 2000; Aos et al. 1998). From an overall rehabilitation perspective, functional family therapy has been shown to be effective in addressing delinquency risk factors such as poor parenting skills, poor relationships with school and community, and low social support and supervision while increasing motivation to change, family communication, positive parenting skills, and compliance with maintaining and generalizing behavioral change (Sexton and Alexander 2000).

The Blueprints for Violence Prevention program at the University of Colorado has led an initiative to review the majority of studies available on programs targeting youth violence and drug abuse. To date, they have reviewed more than 1,200 studies and found most programs have no credible evaluation showing they reduce violence, drug use, and/or delinquency, and a few actually appear to be harmful. However, approximately 30–35 programs have promising outcomes and/or strong empirical support of their effectiveness (Thornberry and Mihalic 2008). A list of the top 11 programs currently supported by extensive evaluations is offered in Table 27–5. According to

Thornberry and Mihalic (2008), the following are commonalities among effective treatment programs:

- They have a sound theoretical rationale with a strong targeting of known risk factors.
- They are intense and clinical.
- They are multimodal and multicontextual.
- They develop social competency and/or have skills development strategies.
- They use cognitive-behavioral delivery techniques.
- They are outside institutional settings.
- They have a capacity for delivery with fidelity.

Furthermore, most successful programs have treatment manuals, structured staff training, written training curricula, methods for monitoring implementation of and fidelity to the treatment process, service delivery documentation procedures, routine structured supervision, outcome monitoring, and quality improvement procedures.

Although these programs are being implemented with great success throughout the United States, many smaller practices and individual providers cannot implement an evidence-based program in its entirety. In those situations, research still offers clear evidence of clinical practices that are effective in working with delinquent youth. Those approaches include motivational interviewing/motivational engagement, cognitive-behavioral treatment, and a systems/ecological approach. For example, substance-abusing youth are now being treated with a combination of these three approaches more successfully than those treated with traditional addictions models (e.g., Alcoholics Anonymous, Narcotics Anonymous, Twelve Steps). In addition, research-based treatments indicated for psychiatric disorders should be utilized because youth in the juvenile justice system have been found to have illnesses such as depression, bipolar disorder, anxiety disorder, and trauma-related disorders, and a small percentage have psychotic disorders.

Motivational Interviewing/ Motivational Engagement

Motivational interviewing emerged from the work of William Miller as a more effective treatment approach to working with highly resistant clients. A central premise of the approach is that most people who drop out of treatment never actually engaged in the treatment in the first place because they never considered the treatment central to achieving their goals. The model emphasizes the consideration of the natural stages in which change occurs while enhancing and supporting individual motivation to consider, attempt, and maintain change. It is a goal-directed model that identifies the youth's ambivalence toward change and then moves toward resolving that ambivalence to promote change.

According to Feldstein and Ginsburg (2006), several studies have shown preliminary data to support motivational interviewing as an effective approach with adolescents in juvenile justice settings. They explained that the success of the model is due to its fit with the adolescent stage of development. Adolescents are largely driven by their individual needs, developing identities, desire for independence, and a competing set of demands for their attention, and motivational interviewing meshes well with these drives as a model that is supportive, flexible, and brief and that promotes autonomy.

Cognitive-Behavioral Treatment

Psychology teaches us that if we can understand behavior, we can predict it, and that if we can predict behavior, we can also change it. There are three possible targets to change behavior: thoughts, feelings, and behaviors. Finding out what drives any of these is the focus of cognitive-behavioral treatment, a model that considers cognitive distortions, triggers/antecedents to behavior, outcomes, and consequences all as critical points of intervention. Interventions typically come in the form of challenging thinking patterns, teaching skills, and establishing a system of reinforcement for desired behavior. Success in intervening and changing one targeted behavior is then generalized to assist in targeting other problems and issues.

To target behavior, the youth and clinician identify and agree to address one or two behaviors that put the youth most at risk. These risk behaviors may result in delinquent offenses or education, occupational, family, and health problems and place the youth at further risk for continued involvement in the criminal justice system. These behaviors become the focus of behavior analysis, skill building, and reinforcement.

Once behaviors are identified and targeted, the next step in cognitive-behavioral intervention is functional analysis of the behavior, which allows the youth and the clinician to carefully scrutinize the behavior in the context in which it occurs. The goal is to determine the function of the behavior, in other words, what drives the behavior. There are a number of cues or antecedents to behavior, and treatment begins with determining the youth's ability to develop new ways of responding to the cues.

This thorough understanding of what drives behavior leads to treatment that takes the form of skill

TABLE 27–5. Blueprints for Violence Prevention model evidence-based programs

Program	Description
Functional Family Therapy (FFT)	Targets youth ages 11–18 years at risk for and/or manifesting delinquency violence, substance use, oppositional defiant disorder, or conduct disorder and their families. Focuses on family relations and communication; builds on strengths as motivation for change. Is flexibly delivered to clients in home, clinic, school, juvenile court, or other community settings.
Multisystemic Therapy (MST)	Targets chronic, violent, and substance-abusing delinquents ages 12–18 years at high risk for out-of-home placement. Focuses on the entire ecology of the youth, including family, school, peer, and community relations. Strives for behavior change in the youth's natural environment, using the strengths of each system (e.g., family, peers, school, neighborhood) to facilitate change.
Multidimensional Therapeutic Foster Care (MTFC)	Targets juveniles ages 12–17 years with histories of chronic and severe delinquent behavior and/or severe mental health problems at risk of incarceration or psychiatric hospitalization who need residential placement. Recruits and supports host families with program goal to return youth to permanency placement (e.g., biological family). Emphasizes behavior management methods with the youth in a structured, therapeutic living environment while also working with the parents during weekly group meetings.
Nurse–Family Partnership (NFP)	Targets first-time-pregnant low-income women. Provides trained nurse home visitors who partner with clients to provide support, counseling, and education from prenatal care through infancy. Is designed to improve prenatal health and the outcomes of pregnancy, infant/toddler care, children's health and development, and the woman's own personal development.
Midwestern Prevention Project (MPP)	Targets 6th- and 7th-grade students. Is initiated in the school setting but reaches out to families and communities. Is described as a comprehensive, multifaceted community-based program to prevent adolescent drug abuse at a time of early adolescence, a critical period for gateway drug use (i.e., alcohol, cigarettes, and marijuana).
The Incredible Years	Targets children ages 2–10 years at risk for and/or presenting with conduct problems. Focuses on parent, teacher, and child training to promote children's emotional and social competence and to prevent, reduce, and treat behavior and emotional problems in young children.
Olweus Bullying Prevention Program (BPP)	Targets 4th- through 7th-grade students. Utilizes trained school staff, and focuses on reduction of victim and bullying problems in school settings.
Life Skills Training	Targets middle/junior high school students (grades 6 and 7). Is implemented over the course of 3 years in school classrooms by schoolteachers and focuses on drug prevention. Includes general self-management skills, social skills, and information and skills specifically related to drug use.
Big Brothers Big Sisters (BBBS)	Targets youth ages 6–18 years from single-parent homes. Focuses on mentoring delivered by volunteers who interact regularly with youth in a one-to-one relationship.
Promoting Alternative Thinking Strategies (PATHS)	Targets children in grades K–5 (regular education and special needs students). Is delivered by educators and counselors in the classroom setting, and focuses on developing social and emotional competence in addition to reducing aggression and behavior problems while simultaneously enhancing the educational process in the classroom. Also includes information and activities for use with parents.

TABLE 27–5. Blueprints for Violence Prevention model evidence-based programs *(continued)*

Program	Description
Project Towards No Drug Abuse (Project TND)	Targets high school youth ages 14–19 years attending traditional or alternative school environments. Focuses on reducing cigarette smoking, alcohol use, drug use, and victimization through motivation, skill development, and decision-making material.

Note. Evidence-based practices are those that have been tested using rigorous research designs, that have demonstrated consistent positive effects in favor of the experimental treatment, and for which there is a high level of standardization (a manual or standardized training materials are available).

development, practice, reinforcement, and generalization. Skill acquisition is a primary method of intervention in cognitive-behavioral treatment, as skills are solutions to problems the youth is encountering. Once skills are taught, cue exposure is essential in affording the youth an opportunity to practice what was learned and to live within the context of his or her environment. Cue exposure will happen naturally or can be intentionally created through well-planned therapeutic situations (e.g., role-plays) in which youth are exposed to stimuli that have elicited problem responses or unskillful behavior in the past.

There are a number of manualized cognitive-behavioral treatment packages to assist clinicians in teaching specific skill sets. This type of treatment has been shown to be effective in treating not only behavior disorders common with juvenile delinquents but also depression, substance abuse, and anxiety disorders.

Systems/Ecological Treatment

Juvenile offenders, like all of us, do not operate in isolation. Juvenile offenders are affected both positively and negatively by their ecology or world around them. These ecological systems can also be key to effectively intervening in the life of troubled youth and typically include family, school, peers, and others. Helping youth to see how their behavior (both desirable and undesirable) fits within the context of the environment is critical. Intervention then takes the form of assisting youth in reshaping their environment to better fit with more prosocial goals and helping their environment support them. In other words, treatment takes place in the youth's ecology (i.e., home, school, and neighborhood). Youth are taught to cope with family and environment problems. Parents and teachers are taught skills to address the current and future problems of the youthful offender.

Interventions with the youth may include increasing prosocial activities with mainstream peer groups while decreasing involvement with antisocial youth, addressing issues of academic performance, and increasing social skills. For the parents, untreated mental illness, substance abuse, lack of knowledge, and lack of social supports are typical targets of treatment. In either case, the goal is for the youth and family to learn successful skills to negotiate the environment in which they live. Clinicians are challenged to collaborate effectively with agencies, schools, courts, probation staff, social services, and others necessary for the youth and family to succeed.

Family Therapy (A Form of Systems/Ecological Treatment)

A literature review by Chamberlain and Rosicky (1995) looked at the various forms of family therapy and their outcomes for treatment. In general, the results of their study reviewed three major categories: 1) social learning family therapy (SLFT), designed to alter dysfunctional patterns of parent–child interactions by building personal skills; 2) structural family therapy (SFT), designed to alter family systems related to poor organization, cohesion, and structure; and 3) multitarget ecological treatment (MET), designed for multistressed families, combining approaches of SLFT and SFT. Compared with individual treatment, SLFT showed long-term improvement up to 1 year after treatment (Bank et al. 1991). In a comparison of parent groups, adolescent groups, and combined parent and adolescent groups, SLFT parent groups showed significantly improved family functioning 1 year after treatment. SFT, when combined with therapeutic foster care versus residential care, showed significantly decreased rates of later hospitalization and incarceration and was more cost-effective. MET is usefully implemented via therapeutic foster care and family preservation approaches, is less costly than other out-of-home placement or hospitalization, and shows improved treatment outcomes. Poor response to family therapy in general was related to three factors:

1. *Attrition.* Families who dropped out tended to be in lower socioeconomic classes, had mothers who were depressed, were agency referred, and had more severe conduct problems in the identified child.
2. *Family areas and lack of social support.* The probability of poor treatment outcome increases as socioeconomic class gets lower and social isolation increases. Stress can be alleviated somewhat by social support, thereby enhancing effectiveness of treatment.
3. *Child variables.* In general, family therapy is more effective for younger children and for teenagers with conduct problems.

In summary, family therapy is a useful mode of treatment. Earlier intervention, service delivery in the community, and agency coordination may further improve family therapy outcomes. Family therapy is generally shown to be beneficial for the following reasons:

1. It targets self-sustaining changes in the family environment.
2. It has shown effectiveness in treating adolescent drug abuse, conduct problems, adolescent associations with antisocial/delinquent peers, and impaired family functioning.
3. It emphasizes family and interpersonal relationships, which appeals to a number of cultural groups in the United States.
4. It is a flexible approach that can be adapted to a broad range of settings such as mental health clinics, treatment programs, and residential treatment.

Group Therapy

There is evidence that grouping delinquent and antisocial youth together for group treatment purposes may produce a negative effect (Arnold and Hughes 1999). The literature shows little evidence of long-term improvement in youth after treatment in groups (Beelmann et al. 1994). As described in the risk and protective factors associated with delinquency, there is a strong association between delinquent youth and their peer groups, which includes evidence that first-time offenders often become worse when grouped with other children with more serious behavior problems. Arnold and Hughes (1999) noted that "homogenous

group treatment of delinquent or at-risk youth opens up the possibility for reinforcement of deviant values, affiliation with peers who model antisocial behavior and values, increased opportunities for criminal activity, [and] stronger identification with a delinquent subculture" (p. 110). Group therapy is often offered in correctional settings; however, better outcomes were noted when family therapy was utilized. More research studying the positive and negative outcomes must be performed in this area.

Although groups may not be the preferred method of treatment, there are some promising group models with specific juvenile justice populations, particularly to treat specific psychiatric conditions. For example, Seeking Safety is a promising manualized treatment model that can be offered in either individual or group settings. Developed by Lisa Najavits under support from the National Institute on Drug Abuse, this treatment is described as a present-focused therapy to address co-occurring trauma/PTSD and substance abuse disorders. Similarly, the Cannabis Youth Treatment Series developed through the support of the Substance Abuse and Mental Health Services Administration combines motivational engagement, cognitive-behavioral treatment, and family therapy approaches to substance abuse treatment that have been shown to be effectively delivered via group methods.

Issues for Consideration

Inadequate Assessment

Evaluators must perform a thorough assessment to best plan intervention and treatment for a juvenile offender. Knowledge of the literature regarding risk and protective factors is essential so that assessment of these factors is included as part of the evaluation of the child and family. Psychiatric disorders, especially those commonly found in juvenile offenders, should be considered, including substance abuse. Collateral information beyond that provided by the child and guardian is necessary to assess the child's and family's functioning within their environment and to assess credibility. Psychological testing should be rendered if clinically indicated. After gathering and assimilating all the data, the evaluating clinician can render a complete diagnostic opinion and make a treatment/intervention plan targeting the child's and family's needs and promoting the child's and family's strengths.

Court Programs Offered as Treatment

Juvenile justice models are not actually treatment but rather are court-related models that attempt to keep children out of the formal court process or attempt to address specific needs of juvenile offenders. Treatment offered within these programs, such as diversion and specialty courts, can range from no treatment to multiple therapeutic interventions to practices that have been shown to have negative effects on youth outcomes. Many types of treatment are offered by institutions, such as medication management, group therapy, family therapy, and individual therapy. The evaluator must be knowledgeable about the treatment of juvenile offenders and which treatment programs are efficacious for the individual offender and his or her family. The evaluator must be able to recommend a treatment plan that is both realistic and useful and that indicates risk level, as courts wish to know which youth can be safely treated within the community. Many children are involved in treatments that have little chance of decreasing recidivism. Unfortunately, these children are seen as treatment failures when they relapse into delinquent behavior, mental illness, or substance abuse, resulting in more punitive sanctions. Frequently, in diversion and aftercare programs, increased supervision and lack of appropriate treatment set the stage for more frequent sanctions.

Case Example Epilogues

Case Example 1

The examiner learned from interviews and record reviews that Shawn had no problems prior to this academic year but was always a marginal student. His parents had recently divorced because of physical abuse that both Shawn and his mother had suffered at the hands of Shawn's father. The family had moved into Shawn's grandmother's home. Shawn was at a new school with no real friends, was isolated, and had become aggressive both at home and at school. Unfortunately, Shawn could have been referred to a status offender diversion program that addressed first-time status offenders prior to adjudication. This would have been appropriate since Shawn was low risk and had previous good functioning. By adjudicating him a status offender, Shawn was now under the supervision of the court. Shawn's mother was struggling to keep two jobs to make ends meet since the divorce, hence her inability to get to the daytime school appointments. Psychological testing of Shawn revealed symptoms of PTSD and a mild

learning disability. Shawn was enrolled in treatment for PTSD, and his family was offered functional family therapy. He was placed in the appropriate programs in school for his learning disability. Shortly after the assessment but prior to the start of treatment, Shawn was once again truant, and the court was considering whether to revoke Shawn's probation due to noncompliance with his "orders."

Case Example 2

Shauna, the 15-year-old mentioned previously who was arrested for assault and battery after engaging in a fight with another juvenile in her neighborhood, was brought to her local detention center not trusting any of the staff and with a history of not being engaged in any previous treatment services. She reports to the assessment staff at the detention center that she doesn't need any help and just wants to get out of detention.

Motivational engagement. Staff response: "So your primary goal sounds like you want to get out of detention. That sounds like a great goal. What kind of ideas do you have to do that?" Shauna responds, "I just need to get the judge off my case." Staff: "That sounds like a good starting point. I've seen a lot of people just like yourself who have worked with us and been able to go to their judge with reasons to get out of here. On a scale of 1 to 10, how bad do you want the judge off your case?" Shauna says, "8." Staff: "That's pretty high. It sounds like you really want the judge off your case, so tell me what kind of things the judge might be on your case about."

Shauna develops some trust with the staff as she feels they have heard her goals and are willing to work with her to achieve them. She then offers more information to the assessment staff that includes a history of substance abuse, family conflict, association with delinquent peers, and a history of assaults, including the assault that resulted in her current arrest and detention.

Behavioral targeting. Behaviors that should be targeted for intervention include assault, which is an immediate issue due to safety and the possibility of further charges if unaddressed (including the possibility of assaulting others in detention). Additionally, Shauna's substance abuse, her association with delinquent peers, and family conflict all constitute critical risk factors for continued delinquent behavior.

Shauna is impulsive and expresses gang values. Prior to her arrest, she spent a great deal of time unsupervised and "hanging out" with delinquent peers and smoking marijuana. Shauna takes pride in her friendships and felt committed to her peers and took aggressive measures to ensure her credibility in her neighborhood. Figure 27–2 outlines how a functional analysis of Shauna's most recent assault can assist the clinician in better understanding her aggression.

Shauna completes her assessment over the course of a few sessions, which includes motivational

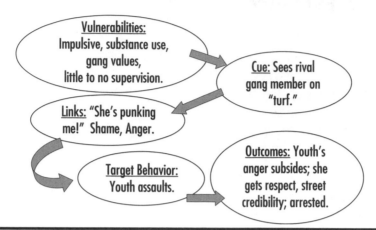

FIGURE 27–2.   Functional behavioral analysis of Shauna's most recent assault.
Vulnerabilities: Impulsivity, substance abuse, gang mentality, lack of parental supervision.
Cues: Shauna sees a rival gang member on her "turf."
Links (cognitive distortions or dysregulated emotions):
  Cognitive distortion: "I must retaliate. She is challenging me."
  Emotions: Anger, shame, fear, anxiety.
  Cognitive distortion: "If I beat her up, she'll leave me alone, she'll know to respect me, and my peers will respect me. No
    one disrespects me."
Problem behavior: Youth assaults the other youth.
Outcomes: Youth's anger subsides; she gets respect, she gets street credibility, and she gets arrested.

engagement techniques to help her identify her goals as well as the pros and cons of continuing her current behaviors. She is considering changes to some limited extent and is at least willing to enter treatment services while in detention. Shauna's treatment includes cognitive-behavioral treatment focused on challenging some of her thinking patterns as well as developing skills to manage and respond to her environment differently. When discharged from detention, she enters a multisystemic treatment program that includes intensive work with both her and her family to work through supervision, substance abuse, and peer association issues. Over the course of the next 6 months, Shauna relapses on marijuana a few times and skips school twice, but she and her family continue to be engaged by her treatment team, and the judge affords some leniency, noting her progress, since these are less serious offenses than originally charged. Shauna completes probation after a year without having to be placed outside her home or school.

Action Guidelines

Understand the Legal Context of the Evaluation

The mental health professional should understand the context in which he or she is to perform the evaluation.

Is it prior to adjudication as part of a diversion program, so that the juvenile must waive confidentiality and agree to treatment in order to participate? Is it following adjudication of a charge, and the court has ordered the evaluation for dispositional recommendations? Is it after the youth is incarcerated and an aftercare plan is being formulated for his or her reintegration into the community as a high-risk offender? The context of the evaluation is extremely important so that the professional can competently provide the recommendations most suited for the individual child's and family's needs, with the goal of decreased recidivism.

Perform a Thorough Assessment and Recommend Appropriate Interventions

A thorough assessment, which evaluates the child and family in the context of the environment in which they live, is necessary. For the child to be successful, he or she will need to be able to negotiate within his or her community. Primary caretakers must be able to function effectively in their parental role. The evaluator must assess for risk and protective factors and recommend interventions that will decrease risk of recidivism while addressing needs of the youth and family.

Use and Promote Evidence-Based Treatment Practices

Treatment outcomes of juvenile offenders range from positive outcomes to no change to increased recidivism rates. Mental health providers need to understand, utilize, and promote those treatment programs for juvenile offenders that actually improve the children's and families' functioning and decrease recidivism rates. Referral sources should inquire as to research-based and evidence-based approaches, as well as outcome data for treatment programs. Juvenile justice systems are moving toward greater accountability. Treatment providers are being required to collect youth outcome data to monitor the effectiveness of their treatment. This information will ultimately improve the quality of care rendered to juvenile offenders by increasing the knowledge base of what actually works, in what context, the cost-effectiveness of the model, and how best to replicate efficacious treatment.

Promote Agency and System Collaboration

For ultimate treatment success, service organizations working with juvenile offenders must effectively communicate, collaborate, and plan both at a local level and at a state level. These include agencies such as the court system, probation, treatment providers, district attorneys, juvenile defenders, corrections, social services, mental health, developmental disabilities, substance abuse, and the school system. Service agencies often have inadequate lines of communication and frequently fight over "who this child belongs to," leaving services fragmented and difficult for the youth and family to either access or negotiate. Youth frequently receive multiple "assessments," but no treatment follows. Oftentimes youth are adjudicated to access services that are not available otherwise in the community. For these reasons many youth penetrate deeper into the juvenile justice system than necessary. Deep-end services should be reserved for those youth who are a risk to public safety, and other mechanisms should be developed for screening and referral of youth to appropriate services within their community. To serve the community best while saving resources, agencies must work more closely in developing a continuum of care, addressing the needs of youth who are at risk of juvenile justice involvement and those who are already involved. This would include data-driven decision making in looking at the needs of youth and families, analyzing treatment allocation, and addressing gaps in the continuum with effective services.

—Key Points

Delinquency Risk

— Developmental models describe delinquent behavior emerging from trajectories defined by traits present at birth and remaining stable throughout the lifetime or a dynamic life course of events influenced by individual characteristics as well as social experiences.

— Public health models describe delinquent behavior as being influenced by established risk and protective factors affecting individual youth. Known individual, family, school, peer, and community factors either increase or decrease the likelihood of a youth becoming delinquent. Many of these are dynamic and changeable factors that should be the focus of effective intervention.

Screening and Assessment

— Valid screening instruments are available to flag issues needing immediate attention by clinicians and to highlight areas in need of further in-depth assessment.

— An in-depth assessment is achieved by clinicians approaching the evaluation with a broad ecological perspective, including a thorough investigation of the juvenile's behavior in the home, school, workplace, and neighborhood, to accurately describe the child's level of functioning in the environment in which he or she lives.

Intervention and Treatment

— Effective intervention programs in the juvenile justice system are often described as incorporating treatments that directly address the established risk and protective factors for delinquency. These treatments most often consist of child and family motivation and engagement practices, cognitive-behavioral treatments, skill development strategies, and social-ecological or systemic approaches (e.g., family, school, peers).

— There are a growing number of evidence-based practices for juvenile justice that, when implemented with fidelity, have been shown to reduce youth out-of-home placement, future delinquency, violence, drug use, and other problem behaviors while often improving family functioning and school performance.

— There is a growing body of literature describing approaches that have limited effect and, in some cases, are even harmful. In general, institutionalization, group therapy modalities, treatments that fail to incorporate the child's social ecology, boot camps, and "scared straight" style interventions have poor outcomes for juvenile offenders.

References

Acoca L: Investing in girls: a 21st century strategy. Juvenile Justice 6(1): 3–13, 1999

Acoca L, Dedel K: No Place to Hide: Understanding and Meeting the Needs of Girls in the California Juvenile Justice System. San Francisco, CA, National Council on Crime and Delinquency, 1998

Alexander JF, Pugh C, Parsons BV, et al: Functional family therapy, in Blueprints for Violence Prevention, 2nd Edition. Edited by Elliott DC. Boulder, CO, Center for the Study and Prevention of Violence, Institute of Behavioral Science, University of Colorado, 2000

Altschuler DM, Armstrong TL, MacKenzie DL: Reintegration, supervised release, and intensive aftercare (Juvenile Justice Bulletin No NCJ 175715). Washington, DC, U.S. Department of Justice, Office of Juvenile Justice and Delinquency Prevention, 1999

American Psychiatric Association: Diagnostic and Statistical Manual of Mental Disorders, 4th Edition, Text Revision. Washington, DC, American Psychiatric Association, 2000

Andrews DA, Zinger I, Hoge RD, et al: Does correctional treatment work? a clinically relevant and psychologically informed meta-analysis. Criminology 28:369–404, 1990

Aos S, Barnoski R, Lieb R: Watching the bottom line: cost-effective interventions for reducing crime in Washington. Unpublished report, Olympia, WA, Washington State Institute for Public Policy, 1998

Arnold ME, Hughes JN: First do no harm: adverse effects of grouping deviant youth for skills training. J School Psychol 37:99–115, 1999

Arredondo D, Kumli K, Soto L, et al: Juvenile mental health court: rationale and protocols. Juven Fam Court J 52:1–19, 2001

Arthur MW, Hawkins JD, Pollard J, et al: Measuring risk and protective factors for substance use, delinquency, and other adolescent problem behaviors: the Communities That Care Youth Survey. Evaluation Rev 26:575–601, 2002

Bandura A: Social Foundations of Thought and Action. Englewood Cliffs, NJ, Prentice-Hall, 1986

Bank L, Marlowe JH, Reid JB, et al: A comparative evaluation of parent-training interventions for chronic delinquents. J Abnorm Child Psychol 19:15–33, 1991

Barnes GM, Welte JW: Patterns and predictors of alcohol use among 7–12th grade students in New York state. J Studies Alcohol 47:53–62, 1986

Barnoski B: Washington State's experience with research-based juvenile justice programs. Paper presented at the Models for Change in Juvenile Justice: Evidence-Based Practice Summit, Baton Rouge, LA, April 2007

Beelmann A, Pfingsten U, Losel F: Effects of training social competence in children: a meta-analysis of recent evaluation studies. J Clin Child Psychol 23:260–271, 1994

Belknap J, Holsinger K, Dunn M: Understanding incarcerated girls: the result of a focus group study. Prison J 77:381–404, 1997

Bishop DM, Frazier CE, Lanza-Kaduce L, et al: The transfer of juveniles to criminal court: does it make a difference? Crime Delinquency 42:171–191, 1996

Borduin CM, Cone LT, Mann BJ, et al: Multisystemic treatment of serious juvenile offenders: long-term prevention of criminality and violence. J Consult Clin Psychol 63:569–578, 1995

Butts JA, Roman J (eds): Juvenile Drug Courts and Teen Substance Abuse. Washington, DC, Urban Institute Press, 2004

Cairns RB, Cairns BD, Neckerman HJ, et al: Social networks and aggressive behavior: peer support or peer rejection? Develop Psychol 24:815–823, 1988

Center for Mental Health Services: Double Jeopardy: Persons With Mental Illness in the Criminal Justice System. Rockville, MD, U.S. Department of Health and Human Services, 1995

Chamberlain P, Rosicky JG: The effectiveness of family therapy in the treatment of adolescents with conduct disorder and delinquency. J Marital Fam Therapy 21:441–459, 1995

Chesney-Lind M, Pasko L: The Female Offender: Girls, Women, and Crime, 2nd Edition. Thousand Oaks, CA, Sage, 2004

Cocozza J, Skowyra K: Youth with mental health disorders: issues and emerging responses. Office Juven Justice Delinquency Prevent J 7:3–13, 2000

Derzon JH, Lipsey MW: The correspondence of family features with problem, aggressive, criminal and violent behavior. Unpublished manuscript, Nashville, TN, Vanderbilt University, Institute for Public Policy Studies, 2000

Elliott DS: Serious violent offenders: onset, developmental course, and termination. Criminology 32:1–21, 1994

Elliott DS: Evidence-based programs and practices: what are they and why are they important. Paper presented at the Models for Change in Juvenile Justice: Evidence-Based Practice Summit, Baton Rouge, LA, April 2007

Elliott DS, Huizinga D, Menard S: Multiple Problem Youth: Delinquency, Substance Use and Mental Health Problems. New York, Springer-Verlag, 1989

Farrington DP: Childhood aggression and adult violence, in The Development and Treatment of Childhood Aggression. Edited by Pepler D, Rubin KH. Hillsdale, NJ, Lawrence Erlbaum, 1991, pp 5–29

Feldstein SW, Ginsburg JI: Motivational interviewing with dually diagnosed adolescents in juvenile justice settings. Brief Treat Crisis Interv 6:218–233, 2006

Fraser MW (ed): Risk and Resilience in Childhood: An Ecological Perspective. Washington, DC, NASW Press, 1997

Friedman R, Katz-Leavy J, Manderscheid R, et al: Prevalence of Serious Emotional Disturbances in Children and Adolescents. Washington, DC, U.S. Department of Health and Human Services, Substance Abuse and Mental Health Services Administration, Center for Mental Health Services, 1996

Foley HA, Carlton CO, Howell RJ: The relationship of attention deficit hyperactivity disorder and conduct disorder to juvenile delinquency: legal implications. Bull Am Acad Psychiatry Law 24:333–345, 1996

Gallagher CA, Dorbrin A: Deaths in juvenile justice residential facilities. J Adolesc Health 38:662–668, 2006

Garland AF, Hough RL, McCabe KM, et al: Prevalence of psychiatric disorders in youths across five sectors of care. J Am Acad Child Adolesc Psychiatry 40:409–418, 2001

Gest T: As specialty courts spread, the jury stays out. Youth Today, January 2007

Gottfredson GD: Issues in Adolescent Drug Use. Baltimore, MD, Johns Hopkins University, Center for Research on Elementary and Middle Schools, 1998

Greenbaum P, Foster-Johnson L, Petrila A: Co-occurring addictive and mental disorders among adolescents: prevalence research and future directions. Am J Orthopsychiatry 66:52–60, 1996

Grisso T: Why we need mental health screening and assessment in juvenile justice programs, in Mental Health Screening and Assessment in Juvenile Justice. Edited by Grisso T, Vincent G, Seagrave D. New York, Guilford, 2005, pp 3–21

Haghighi B, Lopez A: Success/failure of group home treatment programs for juveniles. Fed Probation 57(3):53–58, 1993

Hawkins JD: Controlling crime before it happens: risk-focused prevention. Nat Inst Justice J 3:10–17, 1995

Hawkins JD, Catalano RF: Communities That Care. San Francisco, CA, Jossey-Bass, 1992

Hawkins JD, Catalano RF, Miller JY: Risk and protective factors for alcohol and other drug problems in adolescence and early adulthood: implications for substance abuse prevention. Psychol Bull 112:64–105, 1992

Hawkins JD, Arthur MW, Catalano RF: Preventing substance abuse, in Crime and Justice, Vol 19: Building a Safer Society: Strategic Approaches to Crime Prevention. Edited by Tonry M, Farrington D. Chicago, IL, University of Chicago Press, 1995, pp 343–427

Hawkins JD, Laub JH, Lauritsen JL: Race, ethnicity, and serious juvenile offending, in Serious and Violent Juvenile Offenders: Risk Factors and Successful Interventions. Edited by Loeber R, Farrington DP. Thousand Oaks, CA, Sage, 1998, pp 30–46

Haynie DL, Osgood DW: Reconsidering peers and delinquency: how do peers matter? Social Forces 84:1109–1130, 2005

Henggeler SW: Delinquency in Adolescence. Newbury Park, CA, Sage, 1989

Henggeler SW: Delinquency, in Comprehensive Adolescent Health Care. Edited by Friedman SB, Fisher M, Schonberg SK. St. Louis, MO, Quality Medical Publishing, 1992

Henggeler SW: A consensus: conclusion of the APA Task Force Report on innovative models of mental health services for children, adolescents, and their families. J Clin Child Psychol 23 (suppl):3–6, 1994

Henggeler SW, Melton GB, Smith LA, et al: Family preservation using multisystemic treatment: long-term follow-up to a clinical trial with serious juvenile offenders. J Child Fam Studies 2:283–293, 1993

Herrenkohl TL, Hawkins JD, Chung I, et al: School and community risk factors and interventions, in Child Delinquents: Development, Intervention, and Service Needs. Edited by Loeber R, Farrington DP. Thousand Oaks, CA, Sage, 2001, pp 211–246

Howell JC: Social development strategy, in Guide for Implementing the Comprehensive Strategy for Serious, Violent, and Chronic Juvenile Offenders. Washington, DC, U.S. Department of Justice, Office of Justice Programs, Office of Juvenile Justice and Delinquency Prevention, 1995, pp 23–24

Howell JC (ed): Guide for Implementing the Comprehensive Strategy for Serious, Violent, and Chronic Juvenile Offenders, 2nd Edition. Washington, DC, U.S. Department of Justice, Office of Justice Programs, Office of Juvenile Justice and Delinquency Prevention, 1998

Huizinga D, Esbensen FA, Weiher AW: Are there multiple paths to delinquency. J Crim Law Criminology 82:83–118, 1991

In re Gault, 387 US 1 (1967)

Johnson RE: Family structure and delinquency: general patterns and gender differences. Criminology 24:65–84, 1989

Kandel DB, Andrews K: Processes of adolescent socialization by parents and peers. Int J Addictions 22:319–342, 1987

Kazdin AE: Conduct Disorders in Childhood and Adolescence, 2nd Edition. Thousand Oaks, CA, Sage, 1995

Kazdin AE, Kraemer HC, Kessler RC, et al: Contributions of risk factor research to developmental psychopathology. Clin Psychol Rev 17:375–406, 1997

Krueger R, Hansen JC: Self-concept changes during youth home placement of adolescents. Adolescence 22:385–392, 1987

Lipsey MW: Juvenile delinquency treatment: a meta-analytic inquiry into the variability of effects, in Meta-Analysis for Explanation. Edited by Cook TD, Cooper H, Cordray DC, et al. New York, Russell Sage Foundation, 1992, pp 83–126

Lipsey MW: What do we learn from 400 research studies on the effectiveness of treatment with juvenile delinquents? in What Works: Reducing Offending—Guidelines for Research and Practice. Edited by McGuire J. New York, Wiley, 1995, pp 63–78

Lipsey MW: Can intervention rehabilitate serious delinquents? Ann Am Acad Pol Soc Sci 564:142–166, 1999

Lipsey MW, Derzon JH: Predictors of violent or serious delinquency in adolescence and early adulthood: a synthesis of longitudinal research, in Serious and Violent Juvenile Offenders: Risk Factors and Successful Interventions. Edited by Loeber R, Farrington DP. Thousand Oaks, CA, Sage, 1998, pp 86–105

Lipsey MW, Wilson DB: Effective intervention for serious juvenile offenders: a synthesis of research, in Serious and Violent Juvenile Offenders: Risk Factors and Successful Interventions. Edited by Loeber R, Farrington DP. Thousand Oaks, CA, Sage, 1997, pp 313–345

Lipsey M, Chapman G, Landenberger N: Cognitive-behavioral programs for offenders. Ann Am Acad Pol Soc Sci 578:144–157, 2001

Lipton D, Pearson FS: The CDATE Project: reviewing research on the effectiveness of treatment programs for adult and juvenile offenders. Paper presented at the annual meeting of the American Society of Criminology, Chicago, November 1996

Loeber R, Farrington DP, Petechuk D: Child Delinquency: Early Intervention and Prevention (Child Delinquency Bulletin Series). Washington, DC, U.S. Department of Justice, Office of Juvenile Justice and Delinquency Prevention, 2003

Lundman RJ: Prevention and Control of Juvenile Delinquency, 3rd Edition. New York, Oxford University Press, 2001

McCabe KM, Lansing AE, Garland A, et al: Gender differences in psychopathology, functional impairment, and familial risk factors among adjudicated delinquents. J Am Acad Child Adolesc Psychiatry 41:860–867, 2002

McCord J: Some child-rearing antecedents of criminal behavior in adult men. J Pers Soc Psychol 37:1477–1486, 1979

McCord J, Widom CS, Crowell NA (eds): Juvenile Crime, Juvenile Justice—Panel on Juvenile Crime: Prevention, Treatment, and Control. Washington, DC, National Academy Press, 2001

Mears DP, Aron LY: Addressing the Needs of Youth With Disabilities in the Juvenile Justice System: The Current State of Knowledge. Washington, DC, Urban Institute, 2003

Melton GB, Petrila J, Poythress NG, et al: Psychological Evaluations for the Courts: A Handbook for Mental Health Professionals and Lawyers, 2nd Edition. New York, Guilford, 1997

Moffitt T: Adolescent-limited and life-course-persistent antisocial behavior: a developmental taxonomy. Psychol Rev 100:674–701, 1993

Mrazek PJ, Haggerty RJ (eds): Reducing Risks for Mental Disorders: Frontiers for Preventative Intervention Research. Washington, DC, National Academy Press, 1994

Mulvey EP, Arthur MW, Reppucci ND: The prevention and treatment of juvenile delinquency: a review of the research. Juvenile Delinquency 13:133–167, 1992

National Alliance for the Mentally Ill: Families on the Brink: The Impact of Ignoring Children With Serious Mental Illness. Arlington, VA, National Alliance for the Mentally Ill, 2001

National Research Council and Institute of Medicine: Juvenile Crime, Juvenile Justice—Panel on Juvenile Crime: Prevention Treatment, and Control. Washington, DC, National Academy Press, 2001

Office of Juvenile Justice and Delinquency Prevention: Statistical Briefing Book, Delinquency cases disposed. Washington, DC, U.S. Department of Justice, 2007a. Available at: http://ojjdp.ncjrs.gov/ojstatbb/court/qa06204.asp?qaDate=2004. Accessed March 19, 2007.

Office of Juvenile Justice and Delinquency Prevention: Statistical Briefing Book, Delinquency cases by offense. Washington, DC, U.S. Department of Justice, 2007b. Available at: http://ojjdp.ncjrs.gov/ojstatbb/court/qa06205.asp?qaDate=2004. Accessed March 19, 2007.

Otto R, Greenstein J, Johnson M, et al: Prevalence of mental disorders among youth in the juvenile justice system, in Responding to the Mental Health Needs of Youth in the Juvenile Justice System. Edited by Cocozza J. Seattle, WA, National Coalition for the Mentally Ill in the Criminal Justice System, 1992, pp 7–48

Patterson GR, Dishion TJ: Contributions of families and peers to delinquency. Criminology 23:63–77, 1985

Peterson PL, Hawkins JD, Abbott RD, et al: Disentangling the effects of parental drinking, family management, and parental alcohol norms on current drinking by black and white adolescents. J Res Adolesc 4:203–227, 1994

Phillippi S: Analysis of the association between socio-demographic variables, juvenile offending, and formal vs. informal juvenile justice system handling in a non-urban sample. Unpublished doctoral dissertation, Louisiana State University, Baton Rouge, 2007

Piper E, Warner JR: Group homes for problem youth: retrospect and prospects. Child Youth Serv 3(3/4): 1–12, 1980

Robins LN, Przybeck TR: Age of onset of drug use as a factor in drug and other disorders. NIDA Research Monograph Series 56:178–192, 1985

Rutter M: Temperament, personality and personality disorder. Br J Psychiatry 150:443–458, 1987

Rutter M, Garmezy N: Stress, Coping, and Development in Children. New York, McGraw-Hill, 1983

Schultz C, Mitchell-Timmons J: Prevalence of Mental Disorder in a Juvenile Justice Population. Cleveland, OH, Case Western Reserve University School of Medicine, Department of Psychiatry, 1995

Sexton TL, Alexander JF: Functional family therapy (Juvenile Justice Bulletin). Washington, DC, U.S. Department of Justice, Office of Juvenile Justice and Delinquency Prevention, 2000

Shader M: Risk Factors for Delinquency: An Overview. Washington, DC, U.S. Department of Justice, Office of Juvenile Justice and Delinquency Prevention, 2003

Sharp PM, Hancock BW (eds): Juvenile Delinquency: Historical, Theoretical, and Societal Reactions to Youth. Englewood Cliffs, NJ, Prentice Hall, 1995

Shufelt JS, Cocozza JC: Youth With Mental Health Disorders in the Juvenile Justice System: Results From a Multi-State, Multi-System Prevalence Study. Delmar, NY, National Center for Mental Health and Juvenile Justice, 2006

Sickmund M: Juveniles in Corrections: Juvenile Offenders and Victims National Report Series. Washington, DC, U.S. Department of Justice, Office of Justice Programs, Office of Juvenile Justice and Delinquency Prevention, 2004

Siegel L: Criminology: Theories, Patterns, and Typologies. Belmont, CA, Wadsworth/Thomson Learning, 2004

Skowyra K, Powell SD: Juvenile Diversion: Programs for Justice-Involved Youth With Mental Health Disorders (Research and Program Brief). Delmar, NY, National Center for Mental Health and Juvenile Justice, 2006

Smith D, Paternoster R: Formal processing and future delinquency: deviance amplification as selection artifact. Law Soc Rev 24:1109–1131, 1990

Snyder H: Court Careers of Juvenile Offenders. Washington, DC, U.S. Department of Justice, Office of Justice Programs, Office of Juvenile Justice and Delinquency Prevention, 1988

Snyder HN: Epidemiology of official offending, in Child Delinquents: Development, Intervention, and Service Needs. Edited by Loeber R, Farrington DP. Thousand Oaks, CA, Sage, 2001, pp 25–46

Snyder H, Sickmund M: Juvenile Offenders and Victims: 1999 National Report. Washington, DC, U.S. Department of Justice, Office of Justice Programs, Office of Juvenile Justice and Delinquency Prevention, 1999

Snyder H, Sickmund M: Juvenile Offenders and Victims: 2006 National Report. Washington, DC, U.S. Department of Justice, Office of Justice Programs, Office of Juvenile Justice and Delinquency Prevention, 2006

Stahl A, Puzzanchera C, Sladky A, et al: Juvenile Court Statistics 2001–2002. Pittsburgh, PA, National Center for Juvenile Justice, 2005

Steinberg L: Single parents, stepparents, and the susceptibility of adolescents to antisocial peer pressure. Child Develop 58:269–275, 1987

Teplin LA: Assessing Alcohol, Drug, and Mental Disorders in Juvenile Detainees. Washington, DC, U.S. Department of Justice, Office of Justice Programs, Office of Juvenile Justice and Delinquency Prevention, 2001

Teplin LA, Abram K, McClelland G, et al: Psychiatric disorders in youth in juvenile detention. Arch Gen Psychiatry 59:1133–1143, 2002

Thornberry TP: Violent Families and Youth Violence, Fact Sheet #21. Washington, DC, U.S. Department of Justice, Office of Juvenile Justice and Delinquency Prevention, 1994

Thornberry TP, Krohn MD: Taking Stock of Delinquency: An Overview of Findings From Contemporary Longitudinal Studies. New York, Kluwer/Plenum, 2003

Thornberry TP, Mihalic S: Blueprints for Violence Prevention: Identifying effective prevention programs. Paper presented at the meeting of Models for Change in Juvenile Justice, Alexandria, LA, February 2008

Thornberry TP, Huizinga D, Loeber R: The causes and correlates studies: findings and policy implications. Juvenile Justice 9:3–16, 2004

Tremblay RE, LeMarquand D: Individual risk and protective factors, in Child Delinquents: Development, Intervention, and Service Needs. Edited by Loeber R, Farrington DP. Thousand Oaks, CA, Sage, 2001, pp 137–164

U.S. General Accounting Office: Child welfare and juvenile justice: Federal agencies could play a stronger role in helping states reduce the number of children placed solely to obtain mental health services (Publ No GAO-03-397). Washington, DC, U.S. General Accounting Office, 2003

U.S. House of Representatives: Incarceration of Youth Who Are Waiting for Community Mental Health Services in the United States. Washington, DC, Committee on Government Reform, 2004

Vincent GM, Grisso T, Terry A: Mental health screening and assessment in juvenile justice, in The Mental Health Needs of Young Offenders: Forging Paths Toward Reintegration and Rehabilitation. Edited by Kessler CL, Kraus LJ. Cambridge, MA, Cambridge University Press, 2007, pp 270–287

Wasserman GA, Seracini AG: Family risk factors and interventions, in Child Delinquents: Development, Intervention, and Service Needs. Edited by Loeber R, Farrington DP. Thousand Oaks, CA, Sage, 2001, pp 165–189

Weber RJ: Group Homes in the 1980s. Washington, DC, National Center for the Assessment of Alternatives to Juvenile Justice Processing, National Institute of Justice, 1981

Werner E, Smith R: Overcoming the Odds: High-Risk Children From Birth to Adulthood. Ithaca, NY, Cornell University Press, 1992

West DJ, Farrington DP: Who Becomes Delinquent? London, Heinemann, 1973

Zimring F: The common thread: diversion in juvenile justice. California Law Rev 88:2477–2495, 2000

Chapter 28

Sexually Aggressive Youth

Jon A. Shaw, M.D.
Diana K. Antia, M.D.

Case Example 1

George, a 14-year-old boy, was brought in for treatment after anally sodomizing two younger boys and tying one up with ropes and sticking a knife to his throat. He showed little remorse, regret, or victim empathy. He had a history of sexually victimizing other boys. In his therapy he would reveal and openly acknowledge "violent sexual fantasies." He described how he "seeks out" little boys, wishes to "trap them," and wants "to have control over them." He spoke of the pleasure he derived from having the "power to make anybody I want do anything I want." He enjoyed his victims being "scared, shaking, and cooperative." He coerced them by threatening to cut off their penises or shoot them in the head.

George had a history of aggressive and impulsive behavior and had been called a bully. He reportedly "sexualized" everybody. He grabbed the breasts of his 60-year-old grandmother, and there was a history of sexually touching younger children. When asked about his feelings while sexually molesting children, he responded, "My mother did this to me, and I decided I will do it to them." He reported that in his family, "We would have sex together." He claimed that since he was about age 5, "We would have sex with each other, Mom, Dad, sister, and me." There was a long history of physical abuse, neglect, and abandonment. His mother was sent to jail for sexually molesting his sister. He was ordered into foster care when he was age 7, "based on abandonment and a history of being exposed to deviant sexual behavior." His school and academic record was characterized by behavior problems and poor academic performance in spite of good intelligence.

George recalls how from age 4 to age 7 his mother would come home drunk and make him sleep with her, forcing him down upon her, coercing him to have oral sex with her, and laying on top of him, trying to get him to stick his penis into her. He described these experiences without affect, minimizing their importance. He spoke of "enjoying the scary moment." It was only with continuing therapy that he began to talk about feeling trapped, his repugnance to her drunken breath, her threats to deprive him of food, her slapping him, and her vague threats to castrate him. His mother had a history of being sexually abused by her own father. George stated that he had a "big problem...if I don't get help, I will be doing these things to kids the same way that they did to me, get arrested...maybe the electric chair."

Case Example 2

Tony, a 12-year-old boy, was referred to treatment after being apprehended for sexual assault. He presented with a history of breaking and entering 10 times during the previous year. Although it was initially thought that this was for the purpose of stealing, it became apparent that it was motivated by a wish to molest women as they slept. Tony would peep through the windows, spying on a woman until she went to sleep. He would then sneak into her room and proceed to uncover her and begin to sexually touch her. He had been caught four times for this behavior and had been placed in juvenile detention each time for short periods, with no change in his criminal behavior. He reported that since the age of 11, he felt a compulsion to observe women, ages 20–

30 years, through windows as they were undressing or taking a shower. As this compulsion became stronger, it became associated with the wish to break into the house to sexually touch the women. He had the fantasy that the women would wake up and want to have sex with him. He did not understand the nature of this compulsion and was initially vague when talking about his sexual activities. Tony reported that in kindergarten he was instructed by his teacher to sit under her desk and stroke her legs repetitively, and he recalled moments of sexual arousal and excitement.

On admission to the residential treatment center, Tony was found to be very depressed and suicidal, with symptoms of insomnia, psychomotor retardation, appetite disturbance, and self-recrimination.

Case Example 3

Jorge, a 13-year-old boy, was brought into treatment after repetitively sexually abusing his 7-year-old sister by forcing her to fellate him and vaginally penetrating her. He showed little remorse or regret. Despite her protestations and crying, he would persist in his behavior. His family minimized the behavior, noting that he was just being a boy. In the course of therapy, he described his masturbatory fantasy, which graphically illustrated how one's own sexual victimization gets played over and over again in sexual offending behavior.

He reported the fantasy as follows: "I walk into a small room; there is a girl, 10 to 11 years of age. She is sitting and writing at a desk. I look around to see if there is anybody around. I look twice. I scream at her to stand up. She looks scared and helpless. She is terrified. I tear off her dress. I begin to fondle her. She fights back. I overpower her. I feel strong. I force her to suck my penis. I stick my penis in her vagina. I interrupt the fantasy. I try to intervene. Suddenly the image turns into my father. I remember my father coming into my room. It is a small room. He begins to fondle me, touching my penis. I remember he tore off my clothes and made me suck his penis, and he stuck his penis into my anus. I felt powerless and afraid. I don't like to feel powerless. It's when I feel powerless that I begin to imagine raping a girl. When I tear off her dress, I feel in control." He describes being powerless as meaning that "I can't control other people." Further discussion led to his remembering the sexual excitation, the erection he felt when his father abused him. He had two feelings. He felt scared, helpless, and terrified, but he also had the feeling of sexual excitement. He didn't understand why he was sexually aroused. He felt guilty about the sexual excitement.

Introduction

Youth younger than age 20 years account for approximately 50% of all incidents of sexual aggression in the United States (Lowenstein 2006). Studies of juvenile sex offenders indicate that the majority commit their first sexual offense before age 15 and not infrequently before age 12. There is increasing awareness that children under age 12 may be sexually aggressive toward other children.

Adolescent male sex offenders often have a history of nonsexual antisocial behaviors (Fago 2003). Whereas adolescents (ages 15–18 years) make up only 6% of the population of the United States, they commit 25% of the index crimes, such as arson, homicide, manslaughter, robbery, aggravated assault, and burglary (Siegel and Senna 1988). In 1999, for instance, there were 104,000 arrests of persons under age 18 for robbery, forcible rape, aggravated assault, or homicide (Snyder 2000). The highest risk for the initiation of serious violent behavior occurs between ages 15 and 16 years (Elliott 1994b). In Elliott's (1994a, 1994b) longitudinal study of a national probability sample of 1,725 youth (ages 11–17 years), he found that the prevalence of serious violent offenses, such as rape, that involved a resulting injury or use of a weapon peaked at age 17 years for males and at ages 15 and 16 years for females. It is generally estimated that 20% of all rapes and 30%–50% of all child molestations are perpetrated by male adolescents (Disher et al. 1982).

Sexually aggressive acts perpetrated by youth have become increasingly common. Forcible rapes by juveniles have increased by 20% (Megan's Law 1996; Office of Juvenile Justice and Delinquency Prevention 1995). Ageton (1983) concluded from a probability sample of male adolescents ages 13–19 years that the rate of sexual assault per 100,000 adolescent males ranged from 5% to 16%. A survey of high school students revealed that 20% of the students had been involved in forcing sex on another person and that 60% of the boys found it acceptable in one or more situations for a boy to force sex on a girl (Davis et al. 1993). In their national survey of 1,600 sexually abusive youth, Ryan et al. (1996) reported that the youth came from all racial, economic, ethnic, and religious backgrounds and generally mirrored the population. The youth ranged in age from 5 to 21 years, with a modal age of 14 years, and were predominantly male. Whereas the majority of juvenile sex offenders are adolescents, there is increasing concern about sexually aggressive and exploitative behaviors in prepubescent and latency-age children (Araji 1997; Gil and Johnson 1993).

Various terms are frequently used in reference to sexual behaviors, and definitions of these common terms are highlighted in Table 28–1.

Psychiatric Legal Issues

Waiver

Society is increasingly demanding that juveniles be held more accountable for their criminal acts. Several states have passed legislation redefining the spectrum of crimes and the minimum age at which juveniles may be referred to the adult court. In some states there are no age restrictions for trying a juvenile in the adult court if the crime is perceived as particularly violent or heinous. Although sexual crimes vary in severity and offenders vary as to amenability to treatment, there is a readiness in some jurisdictions to waive all juvenile sex offenders to the adult court. Waiver of juveniles into the adult court system leads to penalties reserved for adult criminals, may lead to incarceration with adults, decreases the probability of appropriate treatment, and lessens the probability of parole (see Chapter 26, "Juvenile Waiver and State-of-Mind Assessments").

Competence

With the increasing readiness to waive juveniles to the adult court, there are increasing concerns regarding competency of juveniles to stand trial in the adult court system (Grisso 2005). A person's cognitive,

TABLE 28–1. Definitions

Sexually abusive behavior[a]	Sexual behavior that occurs without consent, without equality, or as a result of coercion
Sexual offense[a]	Sexually violating/exploiting behavior that breaches societal norms and moral codes, resulting in physical or psychological harm; violation of federal, state, or municipal law, statute, or ordinance
Rape[a]	To seize or take by force for sexual gratification
Sodomy[a]	An act of anal intercourse (may include oral penetration as well)
Sexual harassment[b]	Unwelcome sexual attention that may consist of sexual overtures, requests, advances, and verbal or physical conduct of a sexual nature
Sex offender[a]	Individual who has committed an act of sexual aggression breaching societal norms and moral codes; violating federal, state, or municipal law, statute, or ordinance
Paraphilia[c]	Recurrent, intense sexually arousing fantasies, sexual urges, or behaviors generally involving 1) nonhuman objects, 2) the suffering or humiliation of oneself or one's partner, or 3) children or other nonconsenting persons that occur over at least a 6-month period
Pedophilia[c]	Sexual activities focused on a prepubescent child generally younger than 13 years of age
Sexually reactive child[d]	Child who displays sexually inappropriate behavior as a result of sexual abuse or exposure to explicit sexual stimuli
Equality[a]	Two participants operating with same level of power in a relationship, with neither being controlled or coerced by the other
Coercion[a]	Exploitation of authority through use of bribes, threats of force, or intimidation to gain cooperation or compliance

[a]National Task Force on Juvenile Sex Offending 1993.
[b]Equal Employment Opportunity Commission 1980.
[c]American Psychiatric Association 1994: In order for a youth to be diagnosed as a pedophile, he must be 16 years or older and at least 5 years older than the child.
[d]Gil and Johnson 1993; Yates 1982.

moral, and personality development is still in the process of evolving during the juvenile years. The trend toward trying juveniles in adult courts raises a number of questions. Among them are questions regarding juveniles' capacity to understand the legal case against them, their ability to meaningfully consult with their attorney, and their judgment in making responsible decisions regarding their defense. This is particularly relevant with juvenile sex offenders, who often have comorbid learning and academic-related problems as well as intellectual deficits (see Chapter 26, "Juvenile Waiver and State-of-Mind Assessments").

Record Confidentiality

The clinical records of juveniles referred for clinical assessment of alleged sexual crimes and those in treatment may be made public. The clinician should explain his or her role to the juvenile and the juvenile's family and the limits of confidentiality prior to the clinical interview and before administering assessment instruments. Clinicians who do not inform their clients of the risk of disclosure may themselves be vulnerable to civil suit. Paradoxically, whereas disclosure may enhance the possibility of being judged amenable to treatment, it may increase the severity of legal consequences if further information is uncovered regarding the nature and severity of the sexually aggressive acts. It is generally advisable to conduct the clinical assessment following adjudication with the intent of determining amenability to treatment, required level of care, and estimated risk of recidivism. Table 28–2 summarizes community notification and registration requirements that may apply to juveniles who meet their jurisdictional designation as a sex offender.

There have been recent concerns that current legislation has been counterproductive in that public labeling and shaming of juvenile sex offenders makes it difficult to reintegrate them into the community, isolating them and throwing them together with other sex offenders in the few locations possible (Appelbaum 2008).

Assessment of Recidivism Risk

Clinicians are being asked with increasing frequency by the courts to determine the risk of further sexual offenses. A specific instrument that has been utilized to assess the level of dangerousness is the Juvenile Sex Offender Assessment Protocol II (J-SOAP-II). The J-SOAP-II is a 23-item checklist designed for either adjudicated or nonadjudicated male sex offenders ages 12–18 years to determine the risk of sexual reoffending behavior. The instrument addresses such behaviors as sexual drive, sexual preoccupation, impulsivity, antisocial behavior, and measures of treatability and community adjustment (Prentky and Righthand 2003). Decisions about the risk of reoffending, however, should not be based exclusively on this instrument alone but should be part of a comprehensive clinical evaluation. The decision remains a clinical judgment (Lowenstein 2006).

Clinical Issues

Profile of Sexually Aggressive Youth

Juvenile sex offenders are a heterogeneous population. The overwhelming majority are male. They are represented in every socioeconomic class and every racial, ethnic, religious, and cultural group. Juvenile sex offenders differ from adult sex offenders in that they often have more severe and pervasive adverse developmental and family experiences (Veneziano and Veneziano 2002).

Psychosocial and clinical features frequently found in the history of juvenile sex aggressors include the following:

- Impaired social and interpersonal skills
- Prior delinquent behavior
- Impulsivity
- Academic difficulties
- Family instability
- Family violence
- Abuse and neglect
- Psychopathology

There are essentially four kinds of sex offenders: 1) the offender with a true paraphilia and a well-established deviant sexual arousal pattern; 2) the antisocial youth whose sexual offending behavior is but one facet of his opportunistic exploitation of others; 3) the juvenile compromised by a psychiatric or neurobiological disorder such that he is unable to regulate and modulate his impulses; and, 4) the youth whose impaired social and interpersonal skills result in his turning to younger children for sexual gratification, which is unavailable from his peer groups. Most juvenile sex offenders combine various features of each.

TABLE 28–2.   Community notification and registration requirements

Violent Crime Control and Law Enforcement Act of 1994	The law mandates that states establish registries for individuals convicted of sexual crimes.
Megan's Law (1996)	The 1996 amendment to the law requires state and law enforcement agencies to release relevant information regarding dangerous sexual offenders in order to protect the community.
PROTECT Act of 2003	This directive was enacted mandating all states to place sexual offender information on a public website[a] available to the community.
Adam Walsh Child Protection and Safety Act of 2006	The act expanded the crimes covered by the registries, making failure to register a federal crime; lowered the age requirements for registering sex offenders to 14 years and older; and mandated that states report to a national database by 2009 (Appelbaum 2008).

[a]Dru Sjodin National Sex Offender Public Website, U.S. Department of Justice (http://www.nsopw.gov/Core/Conditions.aspx).

Spectrum of Sexual Offenses

Sexual offending behavior ranges from sexual behavior without physical contact (e.g., obscene phone calls, exhibitionism, voyeurism, lewd photographs) to varying degrees of child molestation involving direct sexual contact (e.g., frottage, fondling, digital penetration, fellatio, sodomy, and various other sexually aggressive acts). There is a considerable range of diversity and severity of sexual offending behavior that in some instances may be related to social and emotional immaturity, curiosity, and experimentation. In other instances, the sexually aggressive acts are but one facet of a pattern of aggressive and violent acts against others or a manifestation of severe emotional, behavioral, and developmental psychopathology.

The most common sexual crimes are those associated with indecent liberties or sexual touching. A national survey of sexually aggressive youth, ages 5–21 years, from a diversity of outpatient and residential programs found that 68% of the sexual offenses involved penetration and/or oral–genital behavior: vaginal or anal penetration without oral–genital contact, 35%; oral–genital contact, 15%; and penetration and oral–genital contact, 18% (Ryan et al. 1996). The typical juvenile sex offender younger than 18 years has committed eight to nine sexual offenses with six to eight victims.

Victim Profile

The victims of juvenile sex offenders are younger children. Ninety percent of sexual abuse victims are between the ages of 3 and 16 years. The majority of the victims are younger than age 9, and approximately 25% to 40% are younger than age 6. Most victims of male sex offenders are females. Adolescent sex offenders commit most of the sexual assaults against boys. Boys, when victimized, tend to be younger than their female counterparts.

Role of Coercion

It is generally recognized that even though juveniles usually employ coercion in the process of committing sexual offenses, they are less likely to harm their victims when compared with adult sex offenders (Fehrenbach et al. 1986; Knight and Prentky 1993; Ryan et al. 1996). The coercion is usually expressed as bribery, intimidation, threats of harm or violent injury, physical force, and, rarely, the use of a weapon. Most victims report higher levels of coercion and force than are self-reported by offenders. Fehrenbach and colleagues (1986) found that 22% of the offenders continued their sexually aggressive acts even when the victims expressed "hurt or fear."

The Role of Sexual Victimization

Reports of sexual victimization in the history of adolescent sex offenders vary from 19% to 82% (Becker et al. 1986; Dhawan and Marshall 1996; Fehrenbach et al. 1986; Longo 1982; Kahn and Chambers 1991; Ryan et al. 1996; Shaw et al. 1993; Zgourides et al. 1994). Boys and girls exposed to sexual abuse and deviant sexual experiences are at risk for early erotization and precocious sexualization. They may experience their first sexual arousal during the victimization. Sexually abused boys are more likely to be sexually aroused at the time of sexual victimization and to subsequently exhibit more sexual behaviors as compared with sexually abused girls (Friedrich 1995; McClellan et al. 1997).

The victims of sexual abuse may internalize the aggressive and erotic facets of the sexual experiences into preferred pathways of sexual gratification through a process of social learning, imitation, modeling, and identificatory pathways. Boys who have been sexually abused often demonstrate higher rates of aggression, impulsivity, sexual preoccupations, and sexually inappropriate behaviors. They tend to have an earlier onset of sexual offending behavior, to have more victims, and to manifest greater psychopathology and interpersonal problems. The younger the child when he commits his first sexual offense, the more likely that the child has been sexually victimized. The factors related to the sexual abuse experience thought to increase the risk for inappropriate sexual behaviors are sexual arousal at the time of the sexual abuse, uncertainty and confusion about sexual identity, compensatory hypermasculinity, and a readiness to reenact the sexually victimizing experience (Friedrich 1995; Watkins and Bentovim 1992).

As important as sexual victimization is in the history of juvenile sexual abusers, it is not exculpatory. Most victims of sexual abuse do not grow up to be abusers. As a form of child maltreatment, it is only one of a number of critical factors that may contribute to the risk of becoming sexually abusive (Prentky et al. 1997). Nevertheless, it is essential to understand the role of sexual victimization in the patterning of sexual offending behavior and as a critical factor in the planning of therapeutic interventions.

Psychopathology

Sexually aggressive behavior is associated with a matrix of behavioral, emotional, and developmental problems. Juvenile sex offenders manifest a range of psychopathological and personality disturbances. Comparisons of juvenile sex offenders with delinquent juveniles whose violence is nonsexual and those who are nonviolent have generally found few significant differences between the groups. Compared with non–sexually abusive delinquents and conduct-disordered youth, sexually aggressive youth are twice as likely to have been sexually abused and to perform less well on academic achievement tests (Lewis et al. 1979; Shaw et al. 1993). Psychiatric comorbidity has been found in approximately 60%–90% of adolescent sexual abusers. The most prevalent comorbid psychiatric disorders are conduct disorder, 45%–80%; mood disorders, 35%–50%;

anxiety disorders, 30%–50%; substance abuse, 20%–30%; and attention-deficit/hyperactivity disorder (ADHD), 10%–20% (Becker et al. 1986, 1991; Kavoussi et al. 1988; Shaw 1999; Shaw et al. 1993). The younger the child when he first committed his sexual offense, the higher the number of coexisting psychiatric diagnoses (Shaw et al. 1996).

Juvenile sex offenders often manifest severe personality traits that include narcissistic, borderline, conduct-disordered, and antisocial behaviors. The younger the age at onset of sexual offending behavior and the younger the adolescent was at the time of his own sexual victimization, the more likely the adolescent is to exhibit personality trait disturbances. The high prevalence of narcissistic and borderline psychopathology among sex offenders is consistent with histories of severe emotional, physical, and sexual abuse. Sexual offending behavior is strongly linked to core antisocial psychopathology with severe character disturbances (Ageton 1983; Hastings et al. 1997; Lewis et al. 1979; Shaw et al. 1993).

Delinquency

Sexual offending behavior is often one facet of a long and sometimes multifaceted history of delinquent behavior. The great majority of sexually aggressive youth have a history of prior nonsexual delinquent behavior ranging from cruelty to animals, vandalism, and theft to aggravated assault. Twenty-five percent of sexually aggressive youth have committed three or more nonsexual criminal offenses. Rape is often the final step in an escalating sequence of violent criminal activity. It is evident that there is a subset of sexually aggressive offenders characterized by core antisocial features in which the sexual aggression is only one facet of a lifestyle in which the individual opportunistically exploits others for personal gain.

Family and Social Environments

Most juvenile sex offenders live at home when committing their sexual offenses. The family environment is frequently characterized by family conflict, poor family cohesion, family instability, family dysfunction, exposure to violence, harsh and inconsistent parenting, and physical and sexual maltreatment. Juvenile sex offenders usually manifest impaired social and interpersonal skills. Two-thirds have been described as socially isolated, one-third do not have any friends, and approximately one-half are reported to be loners. There is some evidence that juvenile sex offenders unable to relate to their own peer group may turn to younger children for the gratifications denied to them by their own peer group (Awad and Saunders 1989; Schoor et al. 1966).

School and Academic Problems

Juvenile sex offenders usually present with a history of academic and school-based behavior problems such as learning problems, learning disabilities, and truancy. Awad and Saunders (1989) evaluated 29 adolescent sex offenders and found that 83% had serious learning problems and 65% had repeated a grade. Adolescent sex offenders generally perform less well on tests of academic skills and are below grade level in such tasks as reading and arithmetic. Not infrequently, there are learning deficiencies and vulnerabilities associated with neurobiological and cognitive impairments that have often compromised the juvenile's capacity to do well in school and to assimilate and integrate complex social information.

The Female Juvenile Sex Aggressor

There have been few studies of female sexual aggression. Anderson (1996) surveyed young college women and found that 29% had engaged in sexual coercion (verbal pressure, lying, threatening to end a relationship), 21% had committed sexual abuse (sex with a minor 5 or more years younger), and 43% reported initiating sexual contact by using sexually aggressive strategies. Female adolescent sex offenders are generally thought to have engaged in less antisocial behaviors and to have experienced more severe and pervasive child maltreatment experiences (Lowenstein 2006; Mathews et al. 1997). Vandiver and Teske (2006) noted that female adolescent sex offenders were younger at the time of arrest and were more likely to choose female and male victims proportionately, whereas male adolescent sex offenders were more likely to choose females as victims. Female juvenile aggressors were more likely than a matched group of male juvenile sex offenders to have been sexually abused at a young age (50%–95%) and to have had multiple abusers, and they were three times more likely to have been sexually abused by a female (Mathews et al. 1997). Studies of female juvenile sexual aggressors indicate they are most likely to commit their sexual offenses while babysitting.

The Developmentally Disabled Juvenile Sexual Aggressor

There is some suggestion that developmental disabilities are overrepresented in juvenile sex offenders. The prevalence of sexual offending behavior is at least as common, if not more common, in the developmentally disabled population. Low verbal IQ has been correlated with sexually inappropriate behavior (McCurry et al. 1998). Fago (2003) evaluated 72 sexually aggressive youth (ages 6–17 years) and found that 59 (82%) of the subjects had evidence of ADHD or other neurodevelopmental deficits and that these findings were more frequent the younger the child was. The clinical characteristics, spectrum of sexual offenses, and victim profiles of developmentally disabled sex offenders are not demonstratively different from those of non–developmentally disabled sex offenders. It has been suggested, however, that sex offenders with learning disorders may be more opportunistic and less gender specific in their choice of victims (Fyson et al. 2003).

Clinical Assessment

The American Academy of Child and Adolescent Psychiatry has published "Practice Parameters for the Assessment and Treatment of Children and Adolescents Who Are Sexually Abusive of Others" (Shaw et al. 1999). These guidelines describe how clinical assessment should be conducted.

Review of Records

Important sources of information include medical and psychological reports, police and offense reports, victim statements, Protective Services reports, and probation reports. The collateral information should be obtained before the individual interview; otherwise, the clinician is left relatively unprepared to deal with the offender's normal proclivity to minimize and deny.

Clinical Interview

The cornerstone of assessment and evaluation of the sexual abuser is an extensive and comprehensive individual clinical interview. The following sections explore major issues to be addressed in the clinical interview.

Minimization and Denial

The clinician should assess the sex offenders' capacity for cooperation, honesty, and forthrightness, and their acceptance of responsibility for their sexual offense as well as sense of remorse and regret. It is known that half of all juvenile sex offenders will deny the sexual offending behavior at the time of referral and that this denial is usually supported by the offender's family. Only one in five will accept full responsibility for the sexual offense. Most sexually aggressive youth exhibit little empathy or remorse, and one-third will blame the victims, stating that the victims consented to the sexual activity despite all evidence to the contrary.

Nature of the Sexually Aggressive Behavior

It is often a difficult task to explicate and uncover the details of the sexually abusive behavior. Because specific laws have been transgressed, the offender is often less than forthcoming. Issues of shame, guilt, and fear of punishment impede disclosure. Most offenders are not motivated to disclose the circumstances of their sexually aggressive behavior until they are confronted or fear the consequences if they do not talk.

The clinician attempts to answer a number of questions regarding the sexually aggressive episode:

- Was the sexually aggressive act planned or impulsive?
- What was the relationship with the victim, the age difference between perpetrator and victim, and the precipitating factors that led to the sexually aggressive behavior?
- What was there about the victim that attracted the perpetrator?
- What was the nature of the sexually aggressive offense(s), the frequency and duration of the sexually aggressive behavior, and the characteristics of the coercive behavior?
- How did the sex offender attempt to avoid detection?
- What was the juvenile offender's understanding of the effects of his sexual behavior on the victim, the consequences of his behavior, and his insight into the wrongfulness of his sexual behavior?

Sexual History

The interviewing clinician should assess the juvenile's sexual knowledge and education, sexual development, and sexual experiences. The clinician will need to explore the history of sexually aggressive behaviors; the pattern and spectrum of previously committed sexually aggressive acts; the victim profile; the internal and external triggers that preceded the sexually aggressive behavior; the role of aggression and sadism in the sexual offense; the need to dominate, control, and humiliate the victim; the erotization of the aggression; the history of sexual victimization, physical abuse, and emotional neglect; the history of exposure to inappropriate and sexually explicit behavior; and the history of prior nonsexual delinquent behavior.

Developmental and Psychosocial History

Other areas of the assessment process are those associated with a comprehensive developmental and psychosocial history of the juvenile sex offender: family history of psychiatric disorder, nature of the pregnancy, prenatal history, developmental milestones, family relationships, early identifying models, capacity for relationships, school experiences, social skills, substance abuse, and prior medical and psychiatric history. The family assessment provides an opportunity to understand the early developmental and environmental context within which the juvenile sexual abuser developed.

Legal History

Is there a history of arrests, convictions, incarcerations, use of weapons, or cruelty to animals?

Medical and Psychiatric History

It is important to obtain a comprehensive medical and psychiatric history, with specific attention to sexually transmitted diseases, HIV infection, psychopathology, and psychiatric comorbidity.

School and Academic History

A specific area of concern is the evaluation of intellectual capacities and academic performance. Information is obtained from the school and from formal psychoeducational and psychological assessments.

Mental Status Examination

A comprehensive mental status examination is carried out to assess the presence of psychopathology, personality disturbances, organicity, and substance abuse and to acquire an understanding of adaptive, coping, and defensive strategies. Suicidal thoughts and risk should be specifically assessed. Apprehension by judicial authority and the associated shame of exposure, embarrassment, stigmatization, fear of punishment, and incarceration are risk factors for suicidal behavior (see Chapter 3, "Introduction to Forensic Evaluations").

Psychological Testing

There are no specific empirical measures or psychometric tests that can identify, diagnose, or classify sexual abusers. Psychological tests are used adjunctively as part of an overall comprehensive evaluation to understand the personality, motivations, ego strengths, intelligence, defense and coping strategies, psychopathology, sexual knowledge, and sexual behaviors of the offender. Neuropsychological testing and psychoeducational assessment may be required when the clinician suspects neurologically based deficits and/or learning disabilities. Measures of learning are an essential part of the assessment procedure. When indicated, family assessment measures may be administered to more fully unravel family dynamics and family process. (See also Chapter 5, "Special Education: Screening Tools, Rating Scales, and Self-Report Instruments," and Chapter 6, "Psychological Testing in Child and Adolescent Forensic Evaluations," in this volume.)

Phallometric Assessment

Phallometric assessment of sexual arousal in response to depictions of children is usually reserved for the most severe and recidivist sexual aggressors. This procedure has generally been used with caution with minors because of the lack of empirical studies, problems of obtaining informed consent, and a reluctance to expose children and adolescents to further sexual stimulation through the portrayal of deviant sexual activities. Caution should be employed in the use of phallometric measures, as there are maturational and developmental factors that may affect the patterns of sexual arousal and erectile measures (Kaemingk et al. 1995).

Use of Visual Reaction Time Assessment Tools

Visual reaction time involves the amount of time a person looks at a particular stimulus and has been proposed as an alternate evaluation tool to assess the sexual interest of male adolescent child molesters (Abel et al. 2004). In theory, persons who are responding honestly generally look longer at those sexual stimuli in which they are most interested. One specific measure of visual reaction time to assess sex offenders is the Abel Assessment for Sexual Interest (AASI). The AASI measures the visual reaction time of an offender to 22 categories of inappropriate sexual stimuli and subjective ratings of sexual interest. In a study of 1,704 adolescent males undergoing evaluation or treatment for paraphilias using the AASI, Abel et al. (2004) found that the amount of time male adolescent child molesters viewed slides of children was significantly longer than that for nonmolesters and was correlated with the number of victims and the frequency of molestation. This instrument may assist the evaluator in providing an objective, nonintrusive measure of male juveniles' sexual interest, in addition to the clinical evaluation.

Evaluation of Dangerousness

An essential element in treatment planning is evaluating the severity of the sexual offending behavior and the risk of recurrence of sexual offending behavior. Because the majority of juvenile sex offenders have a prior history of nonsexual delinquent acts, the clinician is concerned about recidivism not only for the sexual offenses but also for nonsexual delinquent acts. There is evidence that the recidivism rate is higher for nonsexual delinquent acts than it is for the sexual offenses. Considerations in evaluating the risk of further sexual offenses include the frequency and diversity of the sexual offenses; severity of the aggressive and/or sadistic behavior; premeditation or impulsivity of the sexual offending behavior; psychopathology; neurological impairment; prior antisocial or violent behavior; motivation for treatment; intelligence and psychological mindedness; capacity for empathy; and family, community, and social support systems.

Treatment

The average untreated adolescent sex offender will commit over 380 sex crimes in his lifetime (Barbaree et al. 1993). Because most juvenile sex offenders grow up to be adult sex offenders, it is imperative to develop prevention and intervention programs to forestall the course of the sex offending behavior. The first task is to protect the community (Shaw et al. 1999). There is evidence that a significant percentage of adolescent sex offenders respond to a multidisciplinary and multimodality intervention ranging from outpatient to sustained residential placements (Becker and Hunter

1997; Dwyer 1997). Borduin (1999) suggested some efficacy for multisystemic therapy for young sex offenders. The recidivism rate for sexual offenses for treated adolescent sex offenders is estimated to vary from 5% to 15% (Shaw et al. 1999; Veneziano and Veneziano 2002).

Initial intervention is characterized by confronting the sex offender's denial and minimization, assisting with values clarification, correcting cognitive distortions, and elucidating the internal and external cues that precede the sexual offending behavior. Treatment interventions include psychoeducational modules that focus on increasing empathy, problem-solving skills, anger management, sex education, and dating and social skills training; decreasing deviant sexual arousal; and resolving traumatic consequences associated with the sex offender's own history of victimization (Shaw et al. 1999; Veneziano and Veneziano 2002).

Group therapy is the preferred intervention for sex offenders. Peer-related group therapy mobilizes peer pressure as a powerful agent of change and facilitates relatedness, development of interpersonal and social skills, and capacity to work together with others. Most important, group therapy is the venue through which psychoeducational, behavioral, and relapse prevention modules are implemented. Psychoeducational modules provide information and instruction regarding victim empathy, anger management, sex education, anxiety management techniques, and social skills. Relapse prevention techniques stress the importance of understanding the cognitive distortions, antecedents, and contextual factors that trigger the sexually aggressive fantasies and behavior (Shaw et al. 1999; Veneziano and Veneziano 2002).

Psychopharmacological interventions generally target the psychiatric comorbidities that coexist with sexual offending behavior and are guided by the same principles that relate to the treatment of emotional and behavioral problems in other adolescents. Selective serotonin reuptake inhibitors (SSRIs) have been used to mitigate obsessive-compulsive sexual ruminations and for their derivative effects on decreasing sexual urges, fantasies, and behaviors (Kafka and Prentky 1992). Because of the apparent relationship between testosterone and sexually aggressive behaviors, antiandrogens or androgen-depleting drugs (cyproterone acetate, medroxyprogesterone acetate, and luteinizing hormone–releasing agonists) have been used with adult sex offenders to mitigate sexual arousal, sexual fantasies, and sexual predatory behavior (Bradford and Pawlak 1993; Prentky et al. 1997). These drugs carry a considerable risk of side effects including gynecomas-

tia, weight gain, hypertension, cardiovascular disease, gall bladder stones, depression, fatigue, and sleep disturbances (Katz 1999). The use of antiandrogen and hormonal medications for juvenile sex offenders is not recommended before the adolescent has completed puberty (Katz 1999) as there is a lack of evidence to justify their use except in rare instances (Sajith et al. 2008). The lower limit for the use of these medications is usually considered to be about 17 years, and their use is considered only for severe sexual offending behaviors in which there is a high risk of reoffending or for those offenders who have been unresponsive to other treatment interventions or who represent sex offenders with severe developmental disabilities (Katz 1999).

Case Example Epilogues

Case Example 1

George remained generally unresponsive to treatment within a residential setting for adolescent sex offenders and was subsequently transferred to another residential program for continuing therapy.

Case Example 2

Tony responded well to a therapeutic residential program for adolescent sex offenders. He subsequently attended a public school during the daytime and was slowly integrated back into the home environment, where he made a good adjustment with continuing outpatient supportive therapy.

Case Example 3

Jorge was able, with some insight, to develop some empathy not only for his own victimization but also for his sexual victims, and he subsequently showed a good response and was reintegrated back into his family.

Pitfalls

Lack of Information

The readiness of the sex offender to minimize and deny his sexually aggressive behavior, the frequency and severity of his sexually aggressive acts, and his reluctance to discuss his inner sexual life, sexual fantasies, and deviant sexual arousal patterns and motivations may lead to only a superficial knowledge base on which to consolidate clinical judgment and recommendations.

Clinical Assessment Focused Exclusively on the Sexually Aggressive Acts

The proclivity to focus only on the sexually aggressive acts may preclude a careful assessment of the comorbid psychiatric, neurological, and psychological conditions that may have contributed significantly to the sex offender's behavior.

Countertransference

The readiness to experience a spectrum of feelings, ranging from forgiveness and expiation (associated with unrealistic fantasies of rescue) to horror and disgust, may compromise an intellectually honest and comprehensive evaluation regarding the offender's amenability to treatment.

—Key Points

— Sexually abusive behavior is any sexual behavior "which occurs without consent, without equality, or as a result of coercion" (National Task Force on Juvenile Sex Offending 1993).

— A sex offender is an individual who has "breach[ed] societal norms and moral codes [and] violated federal, state, municipal law, statute, and ordinance" (National Task Force on Juvenile Sex Offending 1993).

— Youth younger than 20 years of age account for approximately 50% of all incidents of sexual aggression in the United States.

— The majority of juvenile sex offenders commit their first sexual offense before age 15 and not infrequently before age 12.

— A history of sexual victimization is not uncommon among juvenile sex offenders, and reports vary from 20% to 80% depending on the population studied.

— Juvenile sex offenders present with a spectrum of emotional, behavioral, and developmental problems.

— Juvenile sex offending behavior is often one facet of a history of delinquent behavior.

— Female sex offenders make up approximately 10%–20% of juvenile sex offenders.

— The family of the juvenile sex offender is frequently characterized by conflict, divorce, instability, inconsistent parenting, domestic violence, and child maltreatment.

— Group therapy, with a focus on peer pressure as a powerful agent of change, is the preferred intervention for sex offenders. Psychoeducational, cognitive-behavioral, and relapse prevention strategies are also used.

— Juvenile sex offenders generally respond well to treatment with a surprisingly low rate of recidivism.

References

Abel GG, Jordan A, Rouleau J, et al: Use of visual reaction time to assess male adolescents who molest children. Sex Abuse 16:255–265, 2004

Adam Walsh Child Protection and Safety Act, Public Law 109-248 (1996)

Ageton SS: Sexual Assault Among Adolescents. Lexington, MA, Lexington Books, 1983

American Psychiatric Association: Diagnostic and Statistical Manual of Mental Disorders, 4th Edition. Washington, DC, American Psychiatric Association, 1994

Anderson PB: Correlates of college women's self-reports of heterosexual aggression. Sex Abuse 8:121–133, 1996

Appelbaum PS: Sex offenders in the community: are current approaches counterproductive? Psychiatr Serv 59:352–354, 2008

Araji SK: Sexually Aggressive Children. Thousand Oaks, CA, Sage, 1997

Awad GA, Saunders EB: Adolescent child molester's clinical observations. Child Psychiatry Hum Dev 19:195–206, 1989

Barbaree H, Hudson S, Seto M: Sexual assault in society: the role of the juvenile offender, in The Juvenile Sex Offender, 2nd Edition. Edited by Barbaree H, Marshall W, Hudson S. New York, Guilford, 1993, pp 10–11

Becker JV, Hunter JA: Understanding and treating child and adolescent sexual offenders, in Advances in Clinical Child Psychology. Edited by Ollendick TH, Prinz RJ. New York, Plenum, 1997, pp 177–197

Becker JV, Cunningham-Rathner J, Kaplan MS: Adolescent sex offenders. J Interpers Violence 1:431–445, 1986

Becker JV, Kaplan MS, Tenke CE, et al: The incidence of depressive symptomatology in juvenile sex offenders with a history of abuse. Child Abuse Negl 15:531–536, 1991

Borduin CM: Multisystemic treatment of criminality and violence in adolescents. J Am Acad Child Adolesc Psychiatry 38:242–249, 1999

Bradford JM, Pawlak A: Double blind placebo crossover study of cyproterone acetate in the treatment of paraphilia. Arch Sexual Behav 22:383–402, 1993

Davis TC, Peck GQ, Storment JM: Acquaintance rape and high school student. J Adolesc Health 14:220–224, 1993

Dhawan S, Marshall WL: Sexual abuse histories of sexual offenders. Sex Abuse 8:7–15, 1996

Disher RW, Wenet GA, Paperney DM, et al: Adolescent sexual offense behavior: the role of the physician. J Adolesc Health Care 2:279–286, 1982

Dwyer SM: Treatment outcome study: seventeen years after sexual offender treatment. Sex Abuse 9:149–160, 1997

Elliott DS: The developmental course of sexual and non-sexual violence: results from a national longitudinal study. Paper presented at the annual meeting of the American Association for the Treatment of Sexual Abusers, San Francisco, CA, January 1994a

Elliott DS: Youth Violence: An Overview (Pamphlet No F-693). Boulder, CO, Center for the Study and Prevention of Violence, University of Colorado Boulder, Institute for Behavioral Sciences, 1994b

Equal Employment Opportunity Commission: Title VII Guidelines on Sexual Harassment (Rules and Regulations, 74676–74677). Federal Register 45:219, 1980

Fago DP: Evaluation and treatment of neurodevelopmental deficits in sexually aggressive children and adolescents. Profes Psychol Res Pr 34:248–257, 2003

Fehrenbach PA, Smith W, Monastersky C, et al: Adolescent sexual offenders: offender and offense characteristics. Am J Orthopsychiatry 56:225–233, 1986

Friedrich WN: Psychotherapy With Sexually Abused Boys: An Integrated Approach. Thousand Oaks, CA, Sage, 1995

Fyson R, Eadie T, Cooke P: Adolescents with learning disabilities who show sexually inappropriate or abusive behaviours: development of a research study. Child Abuse Rev 12:305–314, 2003

Gil E, Johnson TC: Sexualized Children: Assessment and Treatment of Sexualized Children and Children Who Molest. Rockville, MD, Launch Press, 1993

Grisso T: Clinical Evaluations for Juveniles' Competence to Stand Trial: A Guide for Legal Professionals. Sarasota, FL, Professional Resource Press, 2005

Hastings T, Anderson SJ, Hemphill P: Comparisons of daily stress, coping, problem behavior and cognitive distortions in adolescent sex offenders and conduct disordered youth. Sex Abuse 9:29–42, 1997

Kaemingk KL, Koselka M, Becker JV, et al: Age and adolescent sexual arousal. Sex Abuse 7:249–257, 1995

Kafka MP, Prentky R: Fluoxetine treatment of nonparaphiliac sexual addictions and paraphilias in men. J Clin Psychiatry 53:351–358, 1992

Kahn TJ, Chambers HJ: Assessing reoffense risk with juvenile sexual offenders. Child Welfare 19:333–345, 1991

Katz D: Psychopharmacological interventions with adolescent and adult sex offenders, in Sexual Aggression. Edited by Shaw JA. Washington, DC, American Psychiatric Press, 1999, pp 305–326

Kavoussi PO, Kaplan M, Becker JV: Psychiatric diagnoses in adolescent sex offenders. J Am Acad Child Adolesc Psychiatry 27:241–243, 1988

Knight RA, Prentky RA: Exploring characteristics for classifying juvenile sex offenders, in The Juvenile Sex Offender. Edited by Barbee HE, Marshall WL, Hudson SM. New York, Guilford, 1993, pp 45–83

Lewis DO, Shankok SS, Pincus JH: Juvenile male sexual assaulters. Am J Psychiatry 136 (suppl 9):1194–1196, 1979

Longo RE: Sexual learning and experience among adolescent sexual offenders. Int J Offender Therapy Comp Criminol 26:235–241, 1982

Lowenstein L: Aspects of young sex abusers: a review of the literature concerning young sex abusers (1996–2004). Clin Psychol Psychotherapy 13:47–55, 2006

Mathews R, Hunter JA, Vuz J: Juvenile female sexual offenders: clinical characteristics and treatment issues. Sex Abuse 9:187–199, 1997

McClellan J, McCurry C, Ronnei M, et al: Relationship between sexual abuse, gender, and sexually inappropriate behaviors in seriously mentally ill youths. J Am Acad Child Adolesc Psychiatry 36:959–965, 1997

McCurry C, McClellan J, Adams J, et al: Sexual behavior associated with low verbal IQ in severe mental illness. Ment Retard 36:23–30, 1998

Megan's Law, Public Law 104-145, 110 Stat 1345 (May 17, 1996)

National Task Force on Juvenile Sex Offending: Revised report. Juvenile Fam Court J 44 (suppl 4):3–108, 1993

Office of Juvenile Justice and Delinquency Prevention: Juvenile offenders and victims: a focus on violence (Summary; NCJ No 153570). Washington, DC, U.S. Department of Justice, Office of Justice Programs, 1995

Prentky R, Righthand S: Juvenile Sex Offender Assessment Protocol–II (J-SOAP-II) Manual. Washington, DC, U.S. Department of Justice, Office of Justice Programs, Office of Juvenile Justice and Delinquency Prevention, 2003

Prentky RA, Knight RA, Lee AFS: Research Report: Child Sexual Molestation: Research Issues. Washington, DC, U.S. Government Printing Office, 1997

Ryan G, Miyoshi TJ, Metzaer JL, et al: Trends in a national sample of sexually abusive youths. J Am Acad Child Adolesc Psychiatry 34 (suppl 1):17–25, 1996

Sajith SG, Morgan C, Clarke D: Pharmacological management of inappropriate sexual behaviors: a review of the evidence, rationale and scope in relation to men with intellectual disabilities. J Intellect Disabil Res 52:1078–1090, 2008

Schoor M, Speed MH, Bartelt C: Syndrome of adolescent child molester. Am J Psychiatry 122:783–789, 1966

Shaw JA: Male adolescent sex offenders, in Sexual Aggression. Edited by Shaw JA. Washington, DC, American Psychiatric Press, 1999, pp 169–194

Shaw JA, Campo-Bowen AE, Applegate B, et al: Young boys who commit serious sex offenses: demographics, psychometrics and phenomenology. Bull Am Acad Psychiatry Law 21:399–408, 1993

Shaw JA, Applegate B, Rothe E: Psychopathology and personality disorders in adolescent sex offenders. Am J Forensic Psychiatry 17:19–38, 1996

Shaw JA, Bernet W, Dunne JE, et al: Practice parameters for the assessment and treatment of children and adolescents who are sexually abusive of others. American Academy of Child and Adolescent Psychiatry Working Group on Quality Issues. Am Acad Child Adolesc Psychiatry 38 (suppl 12):55S–76S, 1999

Siegel LJ, Senna JJ: Juvenile Delinquency, 3rd Edition. San Francisco, CA, West Publishing, 1988

Snyder HN: Special Analyses of FBI Serious Violent Crimes Data. Pittsburgh, PA, National Center for Juvenile Justice, 2000

Vandiver DM, Teske R: Juvenile and male sex offenders. Int J Offender Therap Comp Criminol 50:148–165, 2006

Veneziano C, Veneziano L: Adolescent sex offenders. Trauma Violence Abuse 3:247–260, 2002

Violent Crime Control and Law Enforcement Act of 1994, Pub L 103-322, 108 Stat 1796 (September 13, 1994)

Watkins B, Bentovim A: The sexual abuse of male children and adolescents: a review of current research. J Child Psychol Psychiatry 33:197–248, 1992

Yates A: Children erotized by incest. Am J Psychiatry 139:482–485, 1982

Zgourides G, Monto M, Harris R: Prevalence of prior adult sexual contact in a sample of adolescent male sex offenders. Psychol Rep 75:1042, 1994

PART VII

Civil Litigation

Peter Ash, M.D.

Chapter 29

Civil Litigation and Psychic Trauma

Melvin J. Guyer, J.D., Ph.D.
Diane H. Schetky, M.D.
Peter Ash, M.D.

Case Example 1

LaTanya, a shy, overweight 14-year-old African American girl, was a passenger in a motorboat that collided with another boat. She was thrown overboard, became entangled in the propeller, and lost consciousness. She suffered extensive facial lacerations and nerve damage to her right arm and spent 2 weeks in the hospital. Her attorney, who is filing suit for physical damages, seeks consultation with a forensic expert to help determine if LaTanya might also have a case for psychic trauma.

Case Example 2

Robert was age 10 years when he was repeatedly fondled by a male teacher at school. Psychiatric consultation is sought 5 years later during pending litigation against the school. Questions have to do with causality, effects of the abuse, and treatment needs. Robert gives a very convincing and detailed account of the abuse. His subsequent course has been stormy, with academic failure, substance abuse, self-abuse, and conflicts around his sexual identity. His mother, who is single, portrays him as a model child prior to the abuse and minimizes the role of family or preexisting problems in Robert's current psychopathology.

Legal Issues

Tort Law

A tort is a claim of wrong done to another person that has a remedy in law, typically a monetary award to the injured party. The term derives from the Latin word *tortus*, which means twisted, and the French *torquere*, which means to torture. For an act to be a tort, it must be demonstrated that there has been a breach of a duty owed by the defendant to the plaintiff, the injured party. Further, it must be established that the plaintiff suffered compensable damage and that the damage resulted from breach of the duty. In many instances, the plaintiff may be required to show that the harm suffered was a foreseeable consequence of the breach of the duty of care (negligence) owed to the plaintiff.

Intentional Torts

An intentional tort occurs when an individual deliberately sets out to harm another through acts of omission or commission. Examples might be intentional infliction of emotional distress, slander, and, in some cases, "undue familiarity." In these cases, the plaintiff has the burden of demonstrating the intent or state of mind of the defendant. Other intentional torts may include the taking of someone's goods or property, such as when an employee or business partner wrongly takes money from the company.

Unintentional Torts

Unintentional torts include acts that are negligent but not willful, such as medical malpractice and personal injury cases. Negligence is defined as "conduct which falls below the standard established by law for the protection of others against unreasonable risk of harm" (Keeton 1984, p. 169). The standard of care is held to be that which would be expected from a reasonably careful and prudent person under the circumstances. Chapter 30, "Malpractice and Professional Liability," discusses professional malpractice in more detail.

Purpose

Generally, the sole remedy provided by a tort claim is a monetary award to the plaintiff, which is intended to compensate the victim for injuries suffered or to help restore the victim to his or her prior level of functioning. Damages may be broken down into 1) compensatory damages for pain and suffering; 2) special damages for medical and psychiatric care, property damage, and loss of income; and 3) punitive damages, which may be awarded in an intentional tort (e.g., against manufacturers of a defective product that caused harm). Compensatory damages are the most difficult to determine. How does one put a price tag on the grief and loss sustained by a child in a suit that claims wrongful death of the child's parents? Lost wages, loss of consortium damages, and exemplary damages (extra damages for aggravating circumstances) may also be awarded when circumstances require.

Comparative and Contributory Negligence

Awards may be limited if the plaintiff is found to be partially at fault, that is, has assumed unreasonable risk, contributed to his or her own injury or the negligence, or failed to mitigate his or her own damages.

Preexisting Conditions

The concept of the "eggshell skull plaintiff" deals with predisposing conditions that might render a plaintiff more vulnerable than the average person to certain stresses. Literally, it refers to a case such as a child with osteogenesis imperfecta (so-called brittle-bone disease) who suffers a skull fracture when another child at school throws a basketball at his head. Under law, the

defendant is held liable for the disproportionate harm that the eggshell skull plaintiff suffers. In other words, the defendant must take the plaintiff as he finds him. If a plaintiff has a psychological vulnerability, he or she may be entitled to recover for damages related to trauma that would not affect an ordinary person.

Evolution of Case Law

It is only recently that courts have allowed recovery for damages that are purely psychic. In the past it was feared that recovery for psychological suffering would open the floodgates to fraudulent claims. In the early twentieth century, recovery for psychic trauma was permitted for the first time—but only if there were concomitant physical losses. This then gave way to the "zone of danger" principle, which permitted recovery by plaintiffs who were at risk for physical injury owing to their proximity to a dangerous circumstance yet only suffered psychic trauma. The next extension of this was to allow recovery by a person who had a special relationship to the injured or killed party if the person witnessed the trauma but was not in the zone of danger. Thus, in *Dillon v. Legg* (1968), a mother and daughter who witnessed the negligent death of another daughter, even though they were not in danger, were allowed to recover for psychic injuries even though they suffered no physical injuries.

New Areas of Litigation

Suits Brought by Third Parties Against Therapists

One of the first suits brought by a third party against a physician occurred in the California case of *Molien v. Kaiser Foundation Hospital* (1980). The issue involved Mr. Molien's suing a physician and hospital that wrongly diagnosed his wife as having syphilis. As a result of this misdiagnosis and the suspicions it engendered, the couple divorced. The claim by Mr. Molien alleged negligent infliction of emotional distress as a result of the erroneous diagnosis. The court held that the effect on the marriage of the negligent diagnosis was foreseeable and that the physician had a duty to the husband.

The well-known case of *Ramona v. Isabella* (1994), also in California, brought the issue of third-party liability to bear on psychotherapists. Mr. Ramona sued his daughter Holly's therapist, alleging negligent and intentional infliction of emotional distress. He alleged that the therapist had suggested false memories of sexual abuse to Holly through the use of amobarbital sodium interviews and by inferring that her bulimia was caused by sexual abuse and thus was proof of sexual abuse. Mr. Ramona further alleged that the therapist encouraged Holly to confront him and that the therapist participated in this confrontation. The jury found in his favor and awarded him $500,000. It is noteworthy that Mr. Ramona was tried and convicted of a long unsolved murder based on the testimony of his daughter's recovered memory of many years ago. His conviction was later reversed, and the recovered memory testimony came under wide criticism. Mr. Ramona's suit against his daughter's therapist followed the reversal of his criminal conviction.

Another troubling case, *Althaus v. Cohen* (1998) in Pennsylvania, raised the issue of whether a treating psychiatrist has a duty to the parents of her adolescent patient. The court held that the defendant, Dr. Cohen, had a duty of care not only to Nicole Althaus, whom she was treating for alleged sexual abuse by her father, but also to Nicole's parents, who were directly affected by Dr. Cohen's alleged failure to properly diagnose and treat Nicole. Further, it held that by virtue of Dr. Cohen's involvement in related court proceedings, it was reasonably foreseeable that the Althauses would be harmed by Dr. Cohen's negligent diagnosis. Ironically, Nicole was not in her parents' custody at the time Dr. Cohen was treating her, and the parents had declined to meet with Dr. Cohen. Dr. Cohen, who had based her assessment on a prior forensic evaluation done elsewhere, did not view her role as that of an investigator or forensic psychiatrist. Nonetheless, the court faulted her for not pursuing a more vigorous investigation and for not being more skeptical of her patient's allegations. Dr. Cohen appealed the verdict but lost, and the case was then heard by the Pennsylvania Supreme Court in 1999. The Pennsylvania Supreme Court reversed the appellate court's decision and opined that a duty of care to the parents would create a conflict of interests and destroy the doctor–patient relationship (*Althaus ex rel Althaus v. Cohen* 2000; Weiss 2001).

Appelbaum and Zoltek-Jick (1996) argued that these decisions that place a burden on therapists to be detectives have a chilling effect on psychotherapy and may affect the willingness of therapists to treat alleged victims of childhood sexual abuse. They asked, "How can therapy continue when the therapist is, in effect, competing with a person outside of therapy for the allegiance of the patient?" For instance, if a therapist urges an adolescent to leave an abusive home or reports suspected abuse, will the therapist be sued for alienating the patient from his or her family? However, in most instances, mandatory reporting acts provide immunity to the reporter. Interventions by the therapist, which are outside the scope of the mandatory reporting of suspected abuse or neglect, do not enjoy the immunity that the acts provide to merely reporting. Issues of confidentiality of medical records arise if a third party brings suit and demands them as part of discovery. Note Appelbaum and Zoltek-Jick (1996); the mere threat of suit could effectively bring therapy to a halt. It should be remembered that if the patient brings a lawsuit against a third party, the patient will likely be forgoing the confidentiality of his or her treatment records, as the third party seeks discovery of any preexisting disabilities of the patient-plaintiff.

False and Repressed Memory Suits Against Therapists

The *Ramona* case has fueled subsequent claims against therapists for implanting false memories of abuse, and further momentum for these suits has come from the False Memory Syndrome Foundation. In contrast to *Ramona*, former patients who now side with their parents in saying the alleged abuse never happened have brought many of these suits. Expert witnesses may be brought into these cases to review the standard of care as well as to educate jurors on the claimed phenomenon of repression. In many instances, these cases have involved questionable therapeutic techniques used under the guise of "memory work," including guided imagery, age regression, hypnotherapy, dream work, and exposure to allegations of other "survivors" in group therapies prior to determining if indeed the patient had been sexually abused. Some therapists have erroneously attributed the absence of early childhood memory to repression of a traumatic event or attempted to attribute a host of maladies ranging from eating disorders to trouble with interpersonal relationships to repressed childhood sexual abuse. On the other hand, Brown (1998) asserted that many recanters of memories of sexual abuse have been influenced by posttherapy suggestions, such as those made by the media and false memory syndrome advocates, and that recanters are likely to be highly suggestible. The clinical field has become very polarized regarding the existence of repressed memories (McHugh 2008). The clinician needs to strive to keep an open mind regarding this issue, which has not been completely scientifically resolved. It should be noted that the American Psychiatric Association (2000b) issued a position statement addressing "Therapies Focused on Memories of Childhood Physical and Sexual Abuse" that contains cautions against relying on patients' subjective reports of abuse as a basis for concluding that abuse has in fact occurred.

Suggestibility of Child Witnesses

The 1980s saw a spate of cases alleging sexual abuse of children in day care settings. Much hysteria erupted over these cases; subsequently, there has been much criticism over how investigations were conducted and over the techniques used to interview the children involved. Subsequent sophisticated psychological research has addressed the issue of the suggestibility of children, and these studies have been used in often-successful attempts to reverse those early trial decisions that had concluded, on tainted child testimony, that abuse had occurred. Most appellate court appeals of trial court convictions, such as *New Jersey v. Michaels* (1994), have been successful, whereas a few others, such as *Massachusetts v. Amirault LeFave* (1998), have not. Judge Isaac Borenstein, who reviewed Amirault LeFave's appeal for a new trial, which was based on tainted evidence and new research findings that would show the unreliability of the children's earlier testimonies, ruled that the complainant children had been hopelessly tainted by the early investigative interviews and thus could not be witnesses in any future trial.

Judge Borenstein further held that the newly discovered evidence entitled the defendant to a new trial. Amirault LeFave, who had already served 8 years, remained free until the appellate court ruled that the issue of suggestibility had been adequately addressed in the initial trial in the 1980s and ordered her back to prison. In this case, Dr. Maggie Bruck testified about new research on the suggestibility of child witnesses and critiqued the evaluations that had been done on the young children. Dr. Diane Schetky testified as to the acceptability of the new research within the professional community. The case finally achieved some closure in 1999, when the prosecutor and defense reached an agreement that precluded further prison time in exchange for Amirault LeFave's agreement to not pursue any future claims and to avoid television interviews.

Suits Against Pharmaceutical Companies

The spread of pharmacological corporate interests into the everyday clinical practice of child and adoles-

cent psychiatry has brought with it the far-reaching and broad-based type of class-action lawsuits that previously emerged in the tobacco industry, the asbestos industry, and the silicone breast implant litigation. Claims of consumer fraud and product liability, as well as illegal collusion between drug companies and drug-testing and/or drug-promoting physicians, are increasing. These new types of legal cases typically involve large class-action lawsuits, often brought on behalf of a large plaintiff group represented by a public interest law firm or by a state public official acting on behalf of a class of patients who receive state-funded care. The remedies sought include multimillion dollar claims for the recovery of monies misspent for improper medications or medications whose benefits are fraudulently overstated and whose harms are minimized or concealed from the government, the prescribing physicians, or the patients. These latter types of claims involve failures to obtain informed consent and fraudulent misrepresentations of medication efficacy and safety.

In a current case, a federal judge issued a draft order allowing a case against pharmaceutical company Eli Lilly, which already has paid more than $1 billion to settle legal claims over the side effects of its top-selling drug, Zyprexa, to proceed to a jury trial on a claim that the company violated the Racketeer Influenced and Corrupt Organizations Act through mail fraud. The judge wrote, "There is evidence that off-label use of Zyprexa was excessive and may have been encouraged by Lilly" (*In re Zyprexa Products Liability Litigation* 2008). The draft order contained extensive discussion of expert testimony, much of it from psychiatrists.

In addition to participating in such cases as expert witnesses, child and adolescent psychiatrists may unwittingly become partners in the legal risks and civil liabilities of those corporate interests who are aggressively marketing the use of their products. Child and adolescent psychiatrists may be biased in their views as a result of undue influence by pharmaceutical representatives or speakers or by conflicts of interest with pharmaceutical companies (Schetky 2008). Thus, psychiatrists may find themselves sharing civil liability with drug companies for prescribing off-label uses of medications or for advocating through speaker bureaus or research articles untested and off-label uses of medications.

State courts and state legislators are also applying their own tort and consumer protection laws in ways that allow state actions to be brought against drug manufacturers and physicians who are the conveyors of psychotropic medications. The pharmacology industry has challenged the jurisdiction of state courts to hear tort cases relating to any of their products that have received U.S. Food and Drug Administration (FDA) approval, arguing that FDA approval of a medication creates a federal preemption of state law tort laws and bars any state court jurisdiction.

The federal preemption defense to state tort actions reached the U.S. Supreme Court in the case of *Wyeth v. Levine* (2009) and was decided in March 2009. In that case, the Court rejected Wyeth's preemption defense related to their FDA-approved antinausea medication, Phenergan. The Court, in a far-reaching decision, held that FDA approval of a medication did not preempt state courts' jurisdiction and concluded instead that state tort law is an appropriate risk management process that is complementary to the FDA's review of the safety of medications.

Thus, the preemption defense will not shield drug companies from civil liability in state courts. This assures continued negligence and product liability litigation against pharmaceutical companies as well as physicians who prescribe off-label and fail to obtain full informed consent. It can be expected that the scope of civil liability for psychiatrists arising from medication treatments will grow for quite some time.

Negligent Evaluation or Treatment of Children

Both criminal and civil lawsuits have been brought against child and adolescent therapists for failing to diagnose or erroneously diagnosing sexual abuse, for using unconventional therapy techniques, and for misusing psychiatric hospitalization. Negligent evaluation charges frequently arise in child custody and sexual abuse evaluations in which bias of the investigator is often an issue. Experts may be retained to critique these evaluations and comment on the standard of care for conducting evaluations of allegations of child sexual abuse.

Nonsexual Boundary Violations

Complaints about nonsexual boundary issues are increasing, whereas complaints about sexual boundary issues are declining. A therapist having a sexual relationship with the parent of a minor patient is also a boundary violation. Nonsexual boundary issues may involve business deals with patients, therapists pursuing social relationships with patients, or, in one case, a

psychiatrist who adopted his adolescent patient. Although, thus far, most of these complaints tend to involve adult patients, there is no reason not to encounter them with child and adolescent patients whose parents may bring complaints on their child's behalf.

Recent Developments Regarding Admissibility of Expert Testimony

The admissibility of expert testimony under *Frye v. United States* (1923) and *Daubert v. Merrell Dow Pharmaceuticals, Inc.* (1993) is discussed in Chapter 4, "Testifying: The Expert Witness in Court." As noted there, under the 1993 *Daubert* decision, the U.S. Supreme Court gave guidelines to trial judges that were to assist them in their new roles as gatekeepers over scientific opinion testimony. These included whether the opinions were derived from the use of an empirically tested methodology, known error rates, and/or other indications of the validity and reliability of the methods employed. Left unclear was the issue of how the trial courts should handle the admissibility of nonscientific expert testimony that involved specialized knowledge. However, this question was resolved in the 1999 U.S. Supreme Court decision in *Kumho Tire Co., Ltd. v. Carmichael*. This case, which involved a civil action against a tire manufacturer, alleged that a defective tire design had caused a fatal automobile accident. An issue became whether the nonscientific testimony of an expert on tire failure should be subject to a *Daubert* challenge of admissibility. The Court ruled that the various reliability factors set out in *Daubert* that applied to scientific expert testimony should also be used by the trial judge regarding the admissibility of nonscientific expert testimony.

It remains to be seen what effect this decision will have on the admissibility of mental health or psychiatric testimony. What is clear is that there will be new and more stringent challenges to the admissibility of clinical expertise, especially when it is founded on mere claims of special knowledge and experience. Opponents of such testimony will seek *Daubert* hearings, which place a burden on clinical experts to demonstrate the reliability of their methodologies and the known error rates of their predictions. Questions are likely to arise about the reliability of clinical diagnoses based on the DSM-IV-TR taxonomy (American Psychiatric Association 2000a), the efficacy of treatment interventions, and the reliability of predictions of dangerousness. The *Kumho* decision is likely to provide a legal basis to challenge the foundation of clinical judgments and, it is hoped, may serve to improve the methodologies and empirical bases from which forensic opinions are derived. In a recent review of the impact of *Daubert* on the admissibility of psychiatric testimony, it was noted that courts are conservative in applying the new strictures of *Daubert* on such testimony. They seem especially conservative when such expert testimony is offered on behalf of defendants in criminal proceedings (P. Lourgos, M.J. Guyer, and C. Lemmen, "A Decade of Daubert," unpublished manuscript, September 2003).

Issues for the Plaintiff

Statute of Limitations

The statute of limitations refers to the time period in which an action must be brought to avoid being dismissed for staleness. With a time period limit to file a complaint, the defendant is in a better position to defend himself or herself, and presumably evidence and the memories of witnesses have not yet faded. The statutory limit usually begins at the time the injury is discovered and runs until the period of limitations, which varies from state to state and with type of action, has expired. The statute is tolled for minors and in most states does not begin to run until they reach the age of majority ("tolled" means to stop the clock from running on the time allowed to file a suit). Some states have now extended the statute of limitations for cases involving alleged sexual abuse. In some jurisdictions, there is a tolling of the statute if the claim is made that memories of the abuse have been repressed and the statute begins to run only when the memories are "recovered." Other conditions that may extend or toll the statute include insanity, imprisonment, and incompetence, including being comatose.

Costs

The plaintiff who brings suit is liable for the cost of the suit, in contrast to criminal proceedings in which the state is the moving party. In many cases, plaintiff attorneys will accept a case on a contingency fee if there appears to be a good chance of recovery. In a 2007 landmark case, *Taus v. Loftus et al.* (in which one of this chapter's coauthors, M.J.G., was a codefendant), the prevailing defendants (but not Elizabeth Loftus,

who settled with plaintiff Nicole Taus) were awarded costs amounting to almost $250,000, to be paid by the plaintiff. The suit was brought by Taus claiming, *inter alia*, negligent infliction of emotional injury. Twenty of 21 of the plaintiff's claims were dismissed in pretrial proceedings; the remaining count, only against Loftus, was resolved by Loftus's settlement.

Standard of Evidence

As is discussed in Chapter 1, "Introduction to the Legal System," in civil litigation a lower standard of proof—preponderance of evidence—is used than in criminal proceedings, where the standard is proof beyond a reasonable doubt. The burden of proof lies with the plaintiff, who is obligated to prove the case he or she has brought.

Tendering Records

If a plaintiff introduces his or her mental or physical health as an issue, in most states the plaintiff waives claims of confidentiality regarding his or her medical records (the "patient-litigant exception"). The plaintiff's relevant medical records will be made available to the defendant's attorney to assist in the defense of the case.

Clinical Issues

This section focuses on clinical issues unique to civil litigation. For information on the forensic evaluation in general and the written report, the reader is referred to Chapter 3, "Introduction to Forensic Evaluations," and the American Academy of Child and Adolescent Psychiatry's (1997, 1998) practice parameters for the assessment and treatment of children and adolescents with posttraumatic stress disorder (PTSD) or who are suspected of being abused.

Questions to Be Asked

Degree of Impairment

The forensic examiner needs to determine whether the plaintiff is suffering from a mental disorder or impairment. Sometimes the effects of abuse may be subtle, such as inability to trust or feeling damaged or conflicted about sexuality. These effects taken alone do not constitute a mental disorder but may be grounds for seeking compensation. In contrast, some plaintiffs may demonstrate full-blown symptoms of PTSD, which are easily recognized following a trauma. Although easily recognized, some of these symptoms are also easily simulated as well. Inasmuch as some symptoms of PTSD are evaluated by the examiner only through a history provided by the plaintiff-claimant, the examiner must be cautious about naïve acceptance of plaintiff claims. The clinician should be mindful that many abused persons report few if any lasting negative consequences (Fergusson et al. 1996; Rind et al. 1998; Widom 1999). Lawsuits tend to lead to exaggerated symptom reports. However, the defendant's attorney may argue that these symptoms are purely subjective and imply that they could be malingered or, alternatively, that they are attributable to a trauma unrelated to the case being litigated.

Causality

If impairment is established, the next step is to determine whether there is a proximate relationship between the trauma being litigated and the symptoms reported or observed. It is useful to ask, "But for this trauma, would the patient have developed these symptoms?" Hoffman and Spiegel (1989) cautioned that the relationship between severity of trauma and ensuing harm is not necessarily linear. A severe reaction to a minimal trauma may occur if the injury is sudden and unexpected, defensive action is blocked, and the injury occurs in a safe, familiar environment. Symptoms may also be modified by constitutional factors, prior experience, the response from family and community, and the plaintiff's need to be looked after. There should also be independent and objective confirmation that a traumatic event occurred; the logical fallacy should be avoided of inferring that a traumatic event occurred based only on the presentation of PTSD-like symptoms. Many PTSD-like symptoms occur absent any traumatic event, and thus inferences of causality based on mere symptom presentation are unwarranted.

Credibility

Credibility may be affected by the plaintiff's conscious or unconscious wish for secondary gain. One may exaggerate or hold onto symptoms because they engender attention or because of the hope of financial gain. The latter is unusual for children, but they may be influenced by parental attitudes. Plaintiffs or parents may give a skewed history, minimizing the impact of other traumas or emotional problems in their life and exaggerating current claims. Hoffman and Spiegel (1989) pointed out that it is not the history of prior conditions that prejudice the plaintiff's claim so much

as it is the attempt to conceal them. Credibility is enhanced by consistency in the telling of the history over time, corroboration of findings, symptoms that seem understandable in the context of the trauma, and generally, the ability to give details. Exceptions to the last include children who undergo multiple investigatory interviews who may begin to embellish their stories or confabulate. Clinicians should recognize that credible does not mean true. Clinicians must also be keenly aware that their judgments of children's credibility are often erroneous and are frequently not better than chance (Talwar et al. 2006) (see also Chapter 16, "Reliability and Suggestibility of Children's Statements: From Science to Practice," and Chapter 17, "Interviewing Children for Suspected Sexual Abuse").

Posttraumatic Stress Disorder in Children

The diagnosis of PTSD is one of the few DSM-IV-TR psychiatric diagnoses that require exposure to a known etiologic event. Specifically, the threshold necessary to qualify for this diagnosis requires that 1) "the person experienced, witnessed, or was confronted with an event or events that involved actual or threatened death or serious injury, or a threat to the physical integrity of self or others," and 2) "the person's response involved intense fear, helplessness or horror" (American Psychiatric Association 2000a, p. 467). DSM-IV-TR does not recognize a separate category of PTSD for children, yet it notes that children with this disorder may present differently from adults. To meet the criteria for the diagnosis of PTSD, the individual must have symptoms in each of three categories: 1) reexperiencing, 2) avoidance or numbing, and 3) increased arousal. Children must have at least one reexperiencing symptom, three avoidance or numbing symptoms, and two symptoms of increased arousal (American Academy of Child and Adolescent Psychiatry 1998).

The forensic assessment of the impact of trauma in children is more complex than that in adults, for whom risk factors and damages relate primarily to the dimensions of the traumatic event and factors within the victims that affect response to the trauma. Added dimensions in evaluating children's responses to trauma include parental responses to the trauma, the impact of the trauma on the child's development, and the possibility of delayed-onset PTSD symptoms (Schetky 2003). PTSD in children may look different from PTSD in adults, and even within children and adolescents, typical symptoms vary depending on the child's developmental level. Children with PTSD are more likely than adults with PTSD to have sleep disturbances and are quite susceptible to the responses of adults around them. Somatic complaints, reluctance to go to school, and regression to younger behaviors are common following trauma. As noted by Quinn (1995), children may have more difficulty than adults in verbalizing the numbing symptoms of this disorder. Very young children may be unable to articulate any symptoms, many of which require verbal descriptions of internal states. However, children often manifest their distress in play, during which they may exhibit repetitive and monotonous acting out of the trauma to which they are not able to find resolution. Symptoms of heightened arousal, disorganization, and aggression in these children may be mistaken for attention-deficit/hyperactivity disorder or be confused with conduct disorders. Terr (1983, 1991) described cognitive and memory changes that may be associated with trauma in children, including time shortening, experiencing omens, misidentifying the perpetrator, minimizing or omitting the threat to life, and believing in a foreshortened future.

It is known that rates of PTSD are higher following traumatic acts caused by others as opposed to natural disasters (Green 1995). Separation from parents, as occurs in a kidnapping or due to physical trauma necessitating hospitalization, will heighten the child's stress and sense of helplessness. Cultural factors may also affect how PTSD is manifested (DiNicola 1996; Jenkins and Bell 1994; McGruder-Johnson et al. 2000). Debate exists as to whether children are more or less susceptible to the effects of trauma than adults. Factors that have been found to consistently mediate the development of PTSD in children include temporal proximity to the trauma and parental trauma-related distress (Foy et al. 1996). Data on severity of exposure to the trauma as a mediator of symptom formation are conflicted. Symptoms of PTSD may spontaneously remit, but for many the course may be chronic (American Academy of Child and Adolescent Psychiatry 1998).

Differential Diagnosis

In studying the source of a plaintiff's complaints, it is useful to consider other possible disorders, including the following:

Conversion disorder.   The forensic examiner needs to ask whether the child's presentation is consistent with a recognized medical or psychiatric disorder. Persons with conversion disorders are usually compliant, dependent, cooperative with evaluators, and highly suggestible. Symptoms in conversion disorders are symbolic, triggered by an unconscious psychological conflict, are not under voluntary control, and become a source of secondary gain. The picture may be complicated if the psychic trauma being litigated has triggered the conversion disorder. For instance, hysterical seizures may occur as a sequela to childhood sexual abuse, real or imagined. The important distinction to make in such a case is that the child's distress is real but is psychic not physical in origin.

Malingering.   The malingerer consciously feigns illness, often resists examination, may exaggerate symptoms or call attention to them, and is consciously using symptoms for secondary gain. Like the symptoms of persons with conversion disorders, the malingerer's symptoms often do not fit any known diagnostic entity. However, in contrast, there is no alteration in physical functioning. Typically, there will be a discrepancy between alleged complaints of functional impairment and what the plaintiff is actually able to do. Observations made by others, including detectives, may be useful in this regard.

Factitious disorder.   The patient with a factitious disorder has a need to be in the sick role and will intentionally feign symptoms or induce physical findings. In contrast to malingering, economic gain is not an issue. In Munchausen by proxy (also known as factitious disorder by proxy), a parent will induce symptoms in a child for his or her own gratification. Because these parents have a lot invested in having a sick child, they are unlikely to litigate. The forensic clinician is more likely to encounter these cases in the context of murder trials, dependency and neglect hearings, or terminations of parental rights. Children who are victims of Munchausen by proxy may go on to develop factitious disorders (see Chapter 18, "Forensic Issues in Munchausen by Proxy").

Somatoform pain disorders.   In these disorders, complaints of pain may have an important psychological basis with or without an underlying physical disorder. However, the pain is real and not feigned. For further discussion of this and factitious disorder, the reader is referred to Feldman and Eisendrath (1996).

Symptom exaggeration as a result of suggestion. While the effects of suggestion have been most studied in the context of false allegations of sexual abuse (see earlier discussion; also see Ceci and Bruck 1995; Ceci et al. 2007), suggestion can be implicated in other symptom reports as well. Suggestion often arises innocently, as when parents, physicians, or other mental health evaluators repeatedly question a child and inadvertently use methods that affect children's perceptions.

Implications of Injury on Ensuing Development

Traumas need to be understood in the context of the child plaintiff's development. For instance, a 4-year-old boy who witnesses his mother being raped is likely to confuse violence with sexuality, feel guilty about not protecting her, and perhaps develop problems separating from her because in his fantasies he imagines repeated assault. Without help, these issues may interfere with the child entering into latency, his ability to focus in school, and his development of a healthy male identity. Children who are sexually assaulted may experience reactivation of the trauma on reaching puberty when they have to deal with their own sexuality and sexual identity. Thus, some children may require therapy not only at the time of the trauma but also at subsequent critical points in their lives. There is as yet no empirical research that informs us about reactivation effects; rather, knowledge is based on clinical impressions and individual case studies.

Treatment Needs, Prognosis, and Cost

Assessing the need for treatment involves taking into consideration prior functioning; predisposing, contributing, and perpetuating conditions; the child's level of development and current functioning; the nature of the traumas; and the response from the child's environment. As noted by Quinn (1995) and found in longitudinal studies of sexually abused children (Fergusson et al. 1996), traumas that are severe in intensity, duration, suddenness, and personal impact are likely to have a more prolonged course. Chronic courses are often associated with multiple traumas and numerous losses. How supportive the child's environment is will also affect outcome. For instance, children whose mothers believe their allegations of abuse fare better than those whose mothers do not (Everson et al. 1991; Gomes-Schwartz et al. 1990). The plaintiff's strengths as well as weaknesses, diagnosis, availability of treatment, and likelihood of utilization all must be taken into consideration. Familiarity with research on effective treatments is also helpful (see reviews by Silverman et al. 2008; Stallard 2006). The cost of future therapy can be estimated based on prevailing rates in the area where the plaintiff resides, taking inflation into consideration. However, the variability among persons is so great that these estimates are necessarily speculative.

Effects of Litigation on Therapy

It is commonly believed that patients in litigation will hold onto their symptoms to gain compensation, although this notion has been challenged (Mendelson 1985). There is little evidence bearing on this issue in the child and adolescent psychiatry literature. Another concern has been that therapy might improve the plaintiff's symptoms and diminish his or her chances for recovery in court. Unfortunately, many attorneys continue to defer getting treatment for their clients until the case has been tried or settled. This does a great disservice to children and their families, many of whom cannot afford psychiatric help. Typically, years may pass before cases settle, and untreated symptoms may interfere with the child's ensuing development. A second reason for seeking therapy early on is to provide the child with support to help the child deal with the litigation and the disruptive effect it has on his or her life. For instance, a study by Runyon et al. (1988) on sexually abused children concluded that testifying in juvenile court might be beneficial to the child, whereas testifying in protracted criminal proceedings may have an adverse effect on the child. In a fairly large study, Goodman et al. (1992) found greater behavioral disturbance in children under 10 who testified compared with nontestifying children, but the effects diminished after prosecution was over. Debate continues among professionals as to whether testifying is harmful or beneficial to children, and more data are needed.

The downside to treating a patient under the shadow of litigation is that it may sidetrack therapy and prevent the child from dealing with other issues. However, the issues related to a forthcoming trial may also serve as a catalyst, because the child once again must deal with issues of trust, guilt, and lack of control over his or her life. Having to confront the alleged offender in court may exacerbate symptoms of PTSD but may also help the child begin to combat his or her fears. (This, of course, presumes that the alleged offender is actually the offender. Innocent people are sometimes tried for crimes they did not commit.) Litigation may enable the child to direct anger to where it belongs and to have his or her feelings validated. However, there is also risk that if the child's side does not prevail, the child may feel that he or she is not believed. A further risk is that the therapist may be subpoenaed to testify as to damages, thereby threatening confidentiality and trust, which are the cornerstones of psychotherapy. The child who claims damages in civil action will be subject to an independent medical examination arranged by opposing counsel.

Testifying Against Other Clinicians

Being an expert witness in a malpractice case and having to testify regarding the professional conduct of another clinician is not a comfortable position to be in, and one may even face the scorn of colleagues for doing so. However, if we fail to advocate for patients who have been mistreated by clinicians, then who will uphold the standards of practice? The expert should avoid testifying either for or against clinicians with whom he or she has any sort of professional or social relationship or with whom he or she may be in economic competition. Potential problems might arise in testifying about boundary violations of someone from a different discipline unless the expert familiarizes himself or herself with that discipline's code of ethical behavior. Malpractice litigation is discussed in more detail in Chapter 30, "Malpractice and Professional Liability."

Mass Torts

In cases involving large numbers of plaintiffs, multiple evaluators are often used by both sides.

Case Example 3

Following an explosion at an oil refinery, 125 families were evacuated from their homes in the middle of the night to safer housing. Sixty-five homes were destroyed before the fire was brought under control. The 125 families together included 273 minor children. No one in the evacuating families died, but in the ensuing class-action litigation against the oil company, plaintiffs asserted that they suffered some damage from inhaling smoke as they were evacuating and that they also suffered emotional damages from the forced evacuation, living away from their homes, and, for those whose homes were destroyed, feelings about losing all their possessions. Plaintiffs and defendants agreed on identifying 20 representative children who had not lost their homes and an additional 20 representative children whose homes were destroyed. Both plaintiff and defense attorneys wished to consult (separate) experts on structuring mental health evaluations to assess emotional damages in the representative minor plaintiffs.

In the above example, with 40 children to be evaluated, it is often useful for a team of mental health professionals to be involved and a standardized protocol to be used. For example, psychological and neuropsychological testing may be involved, in addition to a core of agreed-upon items that each interviewing clinician would address. The team would often include mental health professionals from several disciplines. While separate reports would probably be generated for each child assessed, a composite report would likely also be generated, and if the case proceeded to trial, it is likely testimony would be presented by only several of the evaluating clinicians.

Pitfalls

Failure to Consider Other Stressors

A common mistake in taking a history is to attribute all of a child's symptoms to the trauma in question without taking a thorough past history, which could unveil other sources of trauma and stress. The defense attorney will have left no stone unturned in this regard and may confront the plaintiff's expert in court with potentially embarrassing material that the expert has failed to consider. The net effect is to undermine the expert's credibility and the thoroughness of the evaluation. If confronted with new, significant information in court, the expert may need to be prepared to alter his or her opinion.

Misuse of Psychiatric Diagnoses

Inexperienced clinicians and some experts may hear a trauma history and automatically assume the patient/plaintiff has PTSD. They may also err in discounting the threshold of trauma necessary to meet the diagnosis of PTSD in DSM-IV-TR. Thus, for example, sexual harassment in school, although distressing, might not qualify as a severe enough trauma to cause PTSD. Another pitfall is when clinicians invoke syndrome testimony such as the "sexually abused child syndrome" to prove that the child was abused. Their logic tends to run along the lines that "she looks like a sexually abused child, therefore, she must be one." Such overly simplistic thinking ignores the fact that the so-called syndrome includes many nonspecific symptoms and that it is not officially recognized as a diagnosis because it lacks scientific foundation.

Failure to Consider Other Diagnoses

A forensic examiner may fail to diagnose PTSD if he or she underestimates the plaintiff's pathology or assumes it is a normal reaction to the event in question.

Inadequate time spent with the plaintiff may also result in missing the diagnosis. Another source of error is confusing preexisting psychopathology with recent-onset PTSD. As noted, heightened arousal may also be seen in children with attention-deficit/hyperactivity disorder and in children who have been exposed to domestic violence or other traumas in their lives.

Credibility

The forensic examiner needs to consider other possible explanations for a child's behavior or symptoms and to explore any contradictions in the history or the child's statements. Having done so will fortify the examiner's convictions about his or her ultimate opinion and will prepare the examiner to answer questions in court about whether he or she has considered malingering. Corroborating discovery material is important along with psychological test results to support one's findings. The forensic examiner should be proactive in seeking records and documents that will test or corroborate the plaintiff's presented history.

Subjective Nature of Posttraumatic Stress Disorder

Defense attorneys may be quick to point out the subjective nature of PTSD and suggest that it is easy to malinger this condition. This is less likely in cases involving children, as it would be difficult for them to malinger the behavioral manifestations of PTSD. Nonetheless, psychological testing may go a long way toward clarifying or fortifying a diagnosis and may be perceived by juries as more objective than the psychiatrist's findings. A number of scales have been developed for assessing PTSD (for a review, see Ohan et al. 2002). Because PTSD is, to a large extent, diagnosed by child or parental reports, independent corroboration of symptom severity and onset is even more important. Memory of symptoms readily repositions itself when litigation is pending. It is not unusual for individuals who are claiming psychic injuries to present with distorted autobiographical recollections of when their symptoms began. Thus, symptoms of long duration and problems that predated the alleged traumatic event are inaccurately recalled as having had their onset only after the event. Thus, in reconstructed memory, symptoms are wrongly ascribed as flowing from the event that is the basis of the lawsuit. Persons may report that they had no school, medical, emotional, or employment problems until the traumatic event occurred. A check of independent records may show that all of the supposedly trauma-caused problems predated the alleged trauma. One can be assured that the defense attorney in such cases will make a thorough inquiry of the plaintiff's history to see if the alleged PTSD symptoms predated the alleged trauma. The examining expert should also do so.

Issues for the Treating Therapist

Therapists of plaintiffs may be subpoenaed into court to testify concerning damages and treatment needs. How to deal with this situation is discussed in Chapter 2, "Ethics of Child and Adolescent Forensic Psychiatry," and Chapter 4, "Testifying: The Expert Witness in Court." Another peril is that in some cases of PTSD, defense attorneys have tried to attribute the plaintiff's symptoms to therapy or imply they have been induced or suggested by the treating therapist rather than to the trauma per se.

Case Example Epilogues

Case Example 1

LaTanya remained unconscious in the hospital for several days and on awakening had no recollection of the accident. Her friends and family rallied around her, and her parents noted that she seemed to be more outgoing than before her accident. Despite her nerve injury, she returned to play basketball, counter to predictions. She has been dealing well with her facial disfigurement and has decided to postpone plastic surgery. The forensic examiner found no evidence for PTSD or other symptoms of emotional distress related to the accident. She told the attorney that in the absence of memory, there is no basis for the development of PTSD symptoms and that in her opinion there is no basis for a claim for psychic trauma. The attorney agreed and did not pursue the claim for psychic trauma.

Case Example 2

It was not until his deposition that the forensic examiner learned from the defense attorney that Robert had been treated for enuresis prior to the sexual abuse and had also been diagnosed with a conduct disorder. Two siblings have substance abuse problems, an area about which the expert neglected to inquire. Although these facts did not alter his opinion about Robert's credibility, they did put more weight on a contributory role of ongoing family problems and a conduct disorder in Robert's behavioral problems.

—Key Points

— Be thorough. Shortcuts and premature conclusions can only lead to embarrassment down the line.

— Maintain objectivity. Keep an open mind, be receptive to new information, and strive for an objective stance that weighs all possibilities. Test your hypotheses throughout your work.

— Don't get too invested in the outcome. This is easier said than done when one has invested hours in a case.

— The risks of overinvolvement are those of losing objectivity and appearing on the witness stand as too much of an advocate.

— Consider the value of psychological testing to help with diagnosis and to fortify your opinions.

— Keep current with the literature. There is a burgeoning literature on PTSD, including information on neurophysiological factors that may account for the chronic and episodic nature of symptoms, as well as long-term studies. These data are relevant to diagnosis, prognosis, and treatment recommendations.

References

Althaus v Cohen, 710 A2d 1147 (Pa Sup Ct 1998)

Althaus ex rel Althaus v Cohen, 756 A2d 1166 (Pa 2000)

American Academy of Child and Adolescent Psychiatry: Practice parameters for the forensic evaluation of children and adolescents who may have been physically or sexually abused (AACAP Official Action). J Am Acad Child Adolesc Psychiatry 36:423–442, 1997

American Academy of Child and Adolescent Psychiatry: Practice Parameters for the Assessment and Treatment of Children and Adolescents With Posttraumatic Stress Disorder. Washington, DC, American Academy of Child and Adolescent Psychiatry, 1998

American Psychiatric Association: Diagnostic and Statistical Manual of Mental Disorders, 4th Edition, Text Revision. Washington, DC, American Psychiatric Association, 2000a

American Psychiatric Association: Therapies Focused on Memories of Childhood Physical and Sexual Abuse (Position Statement). 2000b. Available at: www.psych.org/Departments/EDU/Library/APAOfficialDocumentsandRelated/PositionStatements/200002.aspx. Accessed November 19, 2008.

Appelbaum P, Zoltek-Jick R: Psychotherapists' duties to third parties: Ramona and beyond. Am J Psychiatry 153:457–465, 1996

Brown D: False memory lawsuits: the weight of the scientific and legal evidence. Guttmacher Award lecture presented at the annual meeting of the American Psychiatric Association, Toronto, ON, Canada, May/June 1998

Ceci SJ, Bruck M: Jeopardy in the Courtroom: A Scientific Analysis of Children's Testimony. Washington, DC, American Psychological Association, 1995

Ceci SJ, Kulkofsky S, Klemfuss JZ, et al: Unwarranted assumptions about children's testimonial accuracy. Ann Rev Clin Psychol 3:311–328, 2007

Daubert v Merrell Dow Pharmaceuticals Inc, 113 S Ct 2786 (1993)

Dillon v Legg, 68 Cal 2d 728 (1968)

DiNicola V: Ethnocentric aspects of posttraumatic stress disorder and related disorders among children and adolescents, in Ethnocultural Aspects of Posttraumatic Stress Disorder: Issues, Research and Clinical Application. Edited by Marsella A, Friedman M, Gerrity E, et al. Washington, DC, American Psychological Association, 1996, pp 389–414

Everson M, Hunter W, Runyan D, et al: Maternal support following disclosure of incest. Am J Orthopsychiatry 59:197–227, 1991

Feldman M, Eisendrath A: The Spectrum of Factitious Disorders. Washington, DC, American Psychiatric Press, 1996

Fergusson DM, Horwood LJ, Lynskey MT: Childhood sexual abuse and psychiatric disorder in young adulthood, II: psychiatric outcomes of childhood sexual abuse. J Am Acad Child Adolesc Psychiatry 35:1365–1374, 1996

Foy D, Madvig B, Pynoos T, et al: Etiologic factors in the development of posttraumatic stress disorder in children and adolescents. J Sch Psychol 34:133–145, 1996

Frye v United States, 293 F 1013 (DC Cir 1923)

Gomes-Schwartz B, Horowitz JM, Cardarelli AP: Child Sexual Abuse: The Initial Effects. Newbury Park, CA, Sage, 1990

Goodman GS, Taub EP, Jones DP, et al: Testifying in criminal court: emotional effects on child sexual assault victims. Monogr Soc Res Child Dev 57(5):1–142, 1992

Green B: Recent research findings on the diagnosis of posttraumatic stress disorder, prevalence, course, comorbidity and risk, in Posttraumatic Stress Disorder in Litigation: Guidelines for Forensic Assessment. Edited by Simon R. Washington, DC, American Psychiatric Press, 1995, pp 13–30

Hoffman B, Spiegel H: Legal principles in the psychiatric assessment of the personal injury litigant. Am J Psychiatry 146:304–310, 1989

In re Zyprexa Products Liability Litigation, draft order issued July 2, 2008 (US District Ct E Dist of New York, Cases 04-MD-1596, 05-CV-4115, 05-CV-2948, 06-CV-0021, 06-CV-6322, 2008), p 11

Jenkins E, Bell C: Violence among inner city high school students and posttraumatic stress disorder, in Anxiety Disorders in African Americans. Edited by Friedman S. New York, Springer, 1994, pp 76–88

Keeton WP (ed): Prosser and Keeton on the Law of Torts, 5th Edition. St Paul, MN, West Publishing, 1984

Kumho Tire Co, Ltd v Carmichael, 119 S Ct 1167 (1999)

Massachusetts v Amirault LeFave, 424 Mass 618 (1998)

McGruder-Johnson AK, Davidson ES, Gleaves DH, et al: Interpersonal violence and posttraumatic symptomatology, the effects of ethnicity, gender, and exposure to violent events. J Interpers Violence 15:205–221, 2000

McHugh PR: Try to Remember: Psychiatry's Clash Over Meaning, Memory, and Mind. New York, Dana Press, 2008

Mendelson G: Compensation neurosis. Med J Aust 142:561–564, 1985

Molien v Kaiser Foundation Hospital, 27 Cal. 3d 916, 616 P. 2d 813, 167 Cal. Rptr. 831 (Cal 1980)

New Jersey v Michaels, 625 A2d 579, 642 A2d 1372 (1994)

Ohan JL, Myers K, Collett BR: Ten-year review of rating scales, IV: scales assessing trauma and its effects. J Am Acad Child Adolesc Psychiatry 41:1401–1422, 2002

Quinn K: Guidelines for the psychiatric examination of posttraumatic stress disorder in children and adolescents, in Posttraumatic Stress Disorder in Litigation. Edited by Simon R. Washington, DC, American Psychiatric Press, 1995, pp 85–98

Ramona v Isabella, 61898 Napa Cty (Cal Sup Ct 1994)

Rind B, Tromovitch P, Bauserman R: A meta-analytic examination of assumed properties of child sexual abuse using college samples. Psychol Bull 124:22–53, 1998

Runyon E, Emerson M, Edelsohn G, et al: Impact of legal intervention on sexually abused children. J Pediatr 113:647–653, 1988

Schetky DH: PTSD in children and adolescents: An overview with guidelines for forensic assessment, in Posttraumatic Stress Disorder in Litigation: Guidelines for Forensic Assessment. Edited by Simon RI. Washington, DC, American Psychiatric Publishing, 2003, pp 91–118

Schetky DH: Conflicts of interest between physicians and the pharmaceutical industry and special interest groups. Child Adolesc Psychiatr Clin N Am 17:113–125, 2008

Silverman WK, Ortiz CD, Viswesvaran C, et al: Evidence-based psychosocial treatments for children and adolescents exposed to traumatic events. J Clin Child Adolesc Psychol 37:156–183, 2008

Stallard P: Psychological interventions for post-traumatic reactions in children and young people: a review of randomized controlled trials. Clin Psychol Rev 26:895–911, 2006

Talwar V, Lee K, Bala N, et al: Adults' judgments of children's coached reports. Law Human Behav 30:561–570, 2006

Taus v Loftus et al, 40 Cal 4th 683 (2007)

Terr L: Chowchilla revisited: the effects of psychic trauma four years after a school bus kidnapping. Am J Psychiatry 140:1542–1550, 1983

Terr L: Childhood traumas: an outline and overview. Am J Psychiatry 148:10–20, 1991

Weiss K: A duty to the parents of an allegedly abused child? Althaus v. Cohen. J Am Acad Psychiatry Law 29:238–240, 2001

Widom CS: Posttraumatic stress disorder in abused and neglected children grown up. Am J Psychiatry 156:1223–1229, 1999

Wyeth v Levine, 129 S Ct 1187, 173 L Ed 2d51 (2009)

Chapter 30

Malpractice and Professional Liability

Peter Ash, M.D.

A dissatisfied patient may make a formal complaint against his or her treating clinician by filing a civil suit in court or by complaining to an administrative agency such as a state medical board, a hospital credentialing body, third-party payers, the U.S. Department of Health and Human Services, or a professional society ethics committee. All of these represent a source of potential liability to the clinician. Although a suit for malpractice is the most common type of civil suit against clinicians, clinicians may also be sued on grounds other than malpractice, such as intentional infliction of emotional distress or breach of contract. Malpractice cases generally require expert testimony to prove that the defendant clinician violated the standard of practice, and defendants generally employ forensic experts to rebut such testimony. In other types of liability cases, such as complaints to ethics committees of professional societies or state licensing boards, professionals may review the clinician's work and may be involved in the process of adjudication. This chapter focuses on the roles forensic experts take after such complaints have been filed and does not cover risk management strategies clinicians might use to avoid such complaints (for such strategies, see Ash 2002; Ash and Nurcombe 2007; Gutheil 1980; Simon and Sadoff 1992).

Malpractice Law

Negligence: The 4 D's

Professional malpractice is a type of negligence. For the plaintiff to prevail in a negligence case, he or she must prove four components, known as the 4 D's: the defendant had a *duty* of care, and there was a *dereliction* of that duty which led *directly* to *damages* (Table 30–1). The plaintiff must prove each of these by a preponderance of the evidence. Failure to prove any one element results in the plaintiff losing the case.

Duty: Doctor–Patient Relationship

A duty of care arises when a doctor–patient relationship is established. In most instances with minor patients, it is clear whether a doctor–patient relationship has been established: the minor patient has been evaluated by a clinician, and treatment has begun. Courts sometimes need to decide whether a doctor–patient relationship has been established with a minor patient before a face-to-face meeting, such as when a parent asks a clinician for advice at a cocktail party or when an appointment has been made but an adolescent commits suicide before the first appointment.

Collaborative treatment arrangements have become quite common: a psychiatrist sees a patient primarily for medication, often at a frequency of once a month or less, while a nonphysician psychotherapist

TABLE 30–1. Elements of a malpractice claim: The 4 D's

Plaintiff needs to prove:	Issue addressed:
Duty of care	Doctor–patient relationship
Dereliction of duty	Violation of the standard of care
Direct cause	Proximate cause
Damages	Money

sees the patient more frequently for psychotherapy. In the event of an adverse outcome such as a suicide, there may well be an issue of which clinician was primarily responsible. Unless there was a clear preexisting agreement, it may be difficult to apportion blame (Meyer and Simon 2006).

Because parents and other family members are often involved in treatment with a minor patient, a question may arise as to whether they, too, are patients. If the child is the index patient, poor advice given to parents may be the subject of a malpractice action brought on behalf of the child. Less clear legally is whether a parent can bring a malpractice action on the grounds that he or she, too, was a patient. There is relatively little litigation in this area, so it is difficult to know how courts will decide in a particular case. If the child is the index patient, and a mental health professional gives a family member advice—a common occurrence—the clinician might be held liable for the consequences of that advice to the family member. For example, if a therapist recommends a mother withhold visitation between the father and child out of a concern for the child's safety, and the mother then violates a court order for visitation and is later held in contempt of court and custody is changed, the mother might well have a cause of action against the therapist (see, e.g., *Montoya v. Bebensee* 1988). Some family therapy is structured such that the family, rather than any specific individual, is the patient. In such a case, it is likely that any member of the family could bring a malpractice action.

Duties to others. Because the doctor–patient relationship derives from contract law, traditionally the clinician had no duties toward third parties. In the well-known California case of *Tarasoff v. Regents of the University of California* (1976), the clinician was found to have a duty to protect others from harm when threatened by a patient. Since the *Tarasoff* decision, many other states have adopted similar rules, either by statute or by court decision. Such laws give a victim injured by a patient standing to sue the patient's clinician for malpractice. Mandatory child abuse reporting statutes also may create a duty toward a child even if the child has not been seen.

Consultation/supervision. When consulting to others, such as to schools or other physicians, the clinician's duty is typically to the consultee, such as school personnel or the referring doctor. The consultant gives advice to the consultee, who then decides whether to implement it or not. If the consultant directly prescribes treatment to the patient, then a clear doctor–patient relationship is formed. However, if no advice or treatment is given to the patient by the consulting mental health professional, many courts will not find liability to the patient.

In training programs, psychiatric residents, psychology trainees, or social work students are supervised by more senior clinicians, and a malpractice case will often include the supervisor even if he or she never saw the patient. The precise limits on when a supervisor has liability are not at all clear. Depending on the situation, the supervisor may be held liable for directing the treatment even when he or she was not informed of the data or actions that gave rise to the suit (Kachalia and Studdert 2004).

Professional liability for forensic work. A litigant who is dissatisfied with the performance of a forensic expert often has a difficult time sustaining a malpractice suit but does have open avenues of complaints to state licensing boards and professional ethics committees. Malpractice and other tort liability for forensic work has traditionally been limited under one of the following three theories:

1. A doctor–patient relationship is not usually established in conducting a forensic evaluation, so the duty of the evaluator to the evaluee is limited.
2. Testimony itself has been generally immune from suit, a longstanding rule justified by the courts' need to obtain truthful testimony from witnesses free from intimidation.
3. In evaluations conducted pursuant to a court order, the evaluator may be seen as acting as an agent of the court and so may have the quasi-judicial immunity afforded other court personnel such as judges and officers of the court.

However, liability for forensic experts has been expanding (Binder 2002), although few cases have involved psychiatrists or psychologists. In some cases, the forensic evaluation allegedly took on some aspects of a doctor–patient relationship, as occurs when a forensic evaluator gives treatment advice to an evaluee. In *Pettus v. Cole* (1996), a California case involving psychiatrists who conducted disability evaluations, the court found that a confidentiality breach occurred because the evaluators had not obtained consent to release their findings to the employer. In *Dalton v. Miller* (1999), a claim went forward on the theory that the evaluee was harmed during the course of the evaluation by the demeanor of the psychiatrist. The forensic expert also has duties to the person or agency who retained him or her and is potentially liable to the retaining party for providing poor expert consultation. Although most successful suits claimed the expert was negligent in preparing the case, in *Lambert v. Carneghi* (2008) a California appeals court found that a partisan expert (an appraiser) did not enjoy complete witness immunity but could be sued by the party who retained him for negligently providing testimony. The court did not do away with witness immunity for court-appointed experts or in suits brought by parties adverse to the expert. Whether the trend of increasing liability for forensic experts will continue is unclear.

Dereliction of Duty

In malpractice cases, the dereliction of duty is a violation of the standard of practice. While jurisdictions vary in their definition of the standard of practice, most are similar to the following: "In the absence of a special contract, physicians or other health care providers are required to possess and exercise the degree of skill and learning ordinarily possessed and exercised, under similar circumstances, by other members of their profession" (Corpus Juris Secundum [CJS] Physicians and Surgeons 1987).

Most states adopt a national standard, but some jurisdictions still use the *locality rule*, which specifies that the standard is that practiced by other members in the defendant's geographic locality. In such cases, the experts need to show they know how the profession is practiced in that locality, and it may be difficult for experts who do not practice in that state to persuade the judge they are familiar with the local standard. Because child and adolescent psychiatry is a recognized subspecialty with clearly defined training, an issue about the appropriate standard may also arise when a child is treated by a general psychiatrist. Generally, if the care is provided by a general psychiatrist in an area where child psychiatrists are available, the clinician will be held to the standard of a child and adolescent psychiatrist. However, in rural areas with acknowledged shortages of child and adolescent psy-

chiatrists, general psychiatrists treating children or adolescents may be held to a less strict standard. Because clinical psychology does not have such clear distinctions in training or board certification for those who treat children, the issue of different standards arises less often. As with most issues governed by state law, there is variation among the states in the precise definition of the standard of practice. Many states have moved from an "average practitioner" standard to a "reasonably prudent practitioner" standard, which is a higher standard. Therefore, it is important for the expert to be clear on the standards for malpractice in his or her jurisdiction.

Courts look to various sources for the standard of care (Caudill 2005), including the following:

- Statutes (such as child abuse reporting)
- Licensing board regulations or agency holdings (such as U.S. Food and Drug Administration [FDA] guidelines)
- Ethical principles of the profession (such as confidentiality)
- Case law (such as *Tarasoff*)
- Learned treatises (such as textbooks and professional articles regarding practice)
- Professional consensus of the community

Common allegations in malpractice cases are listed in Table 30–2.

When professional associations began authoring practice guidelines, there was concern among practitioners that such guidelines would establish the standard of practice and create liability. In response to this concern, such guidelines typically contain disclaimers that they do not establish a standard, and defendant clinicians have often found the guidelines useful because the guidelines typically point to a range of acceptable treatments. Applying these principles to the particulars of the case at hand becomes part of the job of the forensic expert (Recupero 2008).

Professional consensus is the least clear of these factors and the one that most requires expert testimony to establish. Deviations from the standard may encompass errors of omission or commission. Clinicians are not liable for errors of judgment, such as failing to accurately predict suicide after conducting an adequate risk assessment and formulating a reasonable treatment plan. The standard does not require the highest level of care. The fact that experts in a particular condition approach a clinical problem in a particular way does not mean that such an approach is used by the average practicing clinician. There are often several courses of accepted treatment—for instance,

TABLE 30–2. Examples of malpractice claims

Area of practice	Example plaintiff allegation
Evaluation of dangerousness	
Suicide	Weak suicide assessment documentation: "SI-" in chart of outpatient suicide
Homicide	Chart lacks violence risk assessment
Failure to protect from danger	Inpatient adolescent had sexual relationship with another patient
Failure to protect third parties	Dangerous adolescent escaped from hospital, and family and police not notified
Treatment interventions	
Failure to obtain informed consent	Risks and benefits of treatment intervention not discussed with parent(s)
Psychotherapy	Implanted memories of sexual abuse
Boundary violation	Therapist had sex with minor patient
Medication	Sodium divalproex prescribed for pregnant adolescent girl who later gave birth to baby with birth defects, and there was no determination of pregnancy status when medication was started
Ending treatment	
Negligent discharge	Patient discharged while still suicidal
Abandonment	Therapist terminated treatment without referral when parent failed to pay bill
Posttreatment	
Protection and release of information	Published case report insufficiently disguised

there are many schools of psychotherapy—and a clinician may adopt a "respectable minority" approach. Plaintiff experts testifying on the standard of care cannot reasonably criticize defendants on the ground that they would have approached the case differently; the expert needs to explain how such care is outside the mainstream of practice.

Medications.   Many medications commonly used in child and adolescent psychiatry have not received FDA approval for use in these age groups, in large part because the pharmaceutical companies have not conducted the expensive drug trials necessary for obtaining such approval. There is no formal bar to using such medications, and their appropriateness in the context of a malpractice action is a subject for expert testimony. The FDA black box warning for the use of selective serotonin reuptake inhibitor (SSRI) antidepressants in adolescents is a recent illustration of how regulatory agency actions can affect the standard of practice (Hammad et al. 2006; U.S. Food and Drug Administration 2005). The black box warning changed

practice both in how clinicians obtain informed consent and in how they monitor medications.

Managed Care.   While managed care has had a great impact on how care is delivered, the general legal rule is that the clinician, not the managed care company, remains responsible for clinical decisions. In *Wickline v. State* (1986), the court affirmed a physician's duty to provide care and suggested a duty to appeal denial of coverage by a managed care company. State legislative attempts to hold managed care companies liable have generally been thwarted by federal courts holding that the Employment Retirement Security Act (ERISA) covers insurance, which is an employee benefit. ERISA preempts state law and limits liability of the insurer to the amount of the benefit denied (see, e.g., *Pegram v. Herdrich* 2000). Thus, a patient who was improperly denied care can recover, at most, the cost of the care but cannot recover for the health damages that ensued without treatment. The ability to successfully sue a health maintenance organization (HMO) for denial of care is at the center of calls for federal "patient rights" legislation.

In practice, the existence of managed care constraints seldom arises at trial in a malpractice case. Defendant clinicians are unlikely to argue that they limited appropriate care in response to financial considerations, and plaintiff patients are unlikely to argue that they would have gladly paid for expensive care for which coverage had been denied if only the doctor had been so good as to have prescribed it.

Direct Causation

In malpractice law, the dereliction of duty must be proved to be the proximate cause of the harm. The law distinguishes between the proximate cause and the "cause in fact." The cause in fact can be defined as "that particular cause which produces an event and without which the event would not have occurred" (Black et al. 1991, p. 152). The cause in fact is often understood as the "but for" rule: the injury would not have occurred but for the action of the clinician. Proximate cause is more limited and more complex. One definition of *proximate cause* is that cause which "in a natural and continuous sequence, unbroken by any efficient intervening cause, produces the injury and without which the [injury] could not have happened, if the injury be one which might be reasonably anticipated or foreseen as a natural consequence of the wrongful act" (Black et al. 1991, p. 853). Proximate cause limits the scope of causation in two ways: 1) that there is not an intervening cause and 2) that the result is reasonably foreseeable. Consider the following sequence: an adolescent is discharged from a hospital after an adequate suicide assessment and resolution of his depressive symptoms, the next day his girlfriend unexpectedly breaks up with him, and he then goes into his bedroom and hangs himself. It is not enough for the plaintiff to argue that "but for" the discharge, the suicide would not have occurred. The defense would likely argue both that the breakup is an intervening cause of the suicide that would interrupt the causal chain flowing from the discharge and that the suicide was not foreseeable at the time of discharge.

Contributory negligence occurs when a lack of ordinary care on the part of the plaintiff contributes to the bad outcome. It plays a considerably reduced role in malpractice cases involving minor patients because minors are presumed to be less competent and less responsible than adults. States are tending to shift to doctrines of comparative negligence, in which negligence is measured as a percentage, and judgments against one party are reduced by the proportion of fault assigned to others than the defendant. Jurisdictions vary in the extent to which these defenses are available in malpractice cases, but the expert may be asked to address such issues.

Damages

If the judge or jury determines that the defendant clinician is liable, they will determine damages, measured in dollars. Most damages are compensatory damages—in theory, the amount necessary to restore the plaintiff to the position he or she was in prior to the injury. Such damages may include costs of treatment, which the forensic clinician may testify to. Other compensatory damages, such as loss of wages, loss of consortium, or pain and suffering, generally are not the province of the mental health expert. Punitive damages, damages awarded solely to punish the negligent clinician, are rare in malpractice cases. Damages in cases involving children and adolescents typically are less than damages in adult cases because economic damages (e.g., loss of future wages) are more difficult to compute (Vanderpool 2008).

Tort reform refers to statutes that make it more difficult for plaintiffs to obtain large verdicts and may include provisions that limit damages for pain and suffering (typically to a maximum of $250,000–$500,000). It may have additional hurdles, such as imposing penalties on the losing party, increasing the threshold to "gross negligence" in certain contexts, changing rules about which court will have jurisdiction, and preventing apologies by the clinician to the family from being entered as evidence of liability. Health care providers have hoped that such reform would significantly reduce malpractice insurance premiums, although whether such laws actually do so remains controversial.

Frequency of Malpractice Litigation

Members of any profession can be sued for malpractice, but child and adolescent psychiatrists seem to be at considerably greater risk for suits for malpractice compared with psychologists or social workers and pay considerably higher premiums for insurance. All payments by defendants or insurance companies to plaintiffs suing for malpractice, whether from trial verdicts or settlements, must be reported to the National Practitioner Data Bank. Analysis of malpractice payment reports to the National Practitioner Data Bank (2007) for child and adolescent patients since 2004 indicates that in the category of "Behavioral Health," there were only about a third as many claims paid for psychologists as for physicians, and only a small handful of payments for claims against social workers and counselors. This probably reflects that nonphysicians are much less involved in suits related to the use of medication, do less inpatient work, and do not have hospital admission privileges. When Bellamy (1962) surveyed appellate malpractice cases against psychiatrists in the 15 years after World War II, he found only 18 cases, none of which involved child psychiatrists. The rate rose over the next 40 years (Ash 2002), but clinicians who work with children and adolescents remain at less risk than those who work with adults.

It is difficult to obtain accurate data about the frequency of suits against child psychiatrists because insurers tend to keep such information proprietary and different insurers utilize different reporting methods. Among the most common claims are failure to protect a minor from sexual or physical assault on an inpatient unit, patient suicide, medication errors, improper touching, and failure to report child abuse (Ash 2002). The Psychiatrists' Program, the insurance program sponsored by the American Psychiatric Association, has released data regarding its claims experience for minor patients. As can be seen in Table 30–3, the types of alleged negligence (cause of loss) in child and adolescent cases are quite similar to that insurer's experience with adults. These causes of loss are similar to those reported by another insurer, the insurance program endorsed by the American Academy of Child and Adolescent Psychiatry, which found that in 2007, the top three types of claims were incorrect treatment,

suicide or suicide attempt, and improper medication (R.C. Imbert, personal communication, November 5, 2008).

The Psychiatrists' Program reported that for minor patients, 59% of cases were lawsuits, 33% of cases were administrative (including complaints to state licensing boards and ethics committees), and 8% were claims for payment. Overall, about half of the claims were for children under age 13 years, and half were for adolescents ages 13–17 years. No money was paid for 77% of claims, 20% settled, and 3% went to trial. Of those that went to trial, the vast majority of the time, the defendant doctor won (Vanderpool 2008).

Course of a Typical Malpractice Case

Filing a Case

Clinicians usually know about adverse events. Unlike cases involving adults in which confidentiality concerns may impede or delay a clinician's discussion with the family, in child cases the parents generally control record release so there are few bars to the clinician's discussing what happened with the family. Clinicians may also be concerned about saying things that sound like an apology, but in an increasing number of states, such statements are barred from being

TABLE 30–3. Cause-of-loss data from The Psychiatrists' Program,[a] 1986–2007

Primary allegation	Patients ages 1–17 years	All patients
Incorrect treatment	34%	32%
Suicide/attempted suicide	18%	15%
Drug reaction	14%	10%
Incorrect diagnosis	11%	9%
Improper supervision	8%	5%
Other	7%	16%
Unnecessary commitment	5%	5%
Breach of confidentiality	1%	2%
Vicarious liability	1%	1%
Libel/slander	1%	1%
Undue familiarity	–	4%

[a]Managed by Professional Risk Management Services, Inc.
Source.   Vanderpool 2008.

used to prove liability. Following an adverse event, most clinicians inform their malpractice insurer and, for inpatient or group practices, the risk management unit of the hospital or group. Information from mortality conferences and other peer review has generally been immune from discovery in later litigation. Recently, however, following a voter ballot constitutional amendment in Florida giving patients the right to see all health records about them, including peer review reports, the Florida Supreme Court interpreted the amendment as giving patients the right to review records created before passage of the amendment, effectively ending the confidentiality of peer review in that state (*Florida Hospital Waterman v. Buster* 2006). It is unclear whether such holdings will be replicated in other states.

Attorneys need to file a malpractice case within the statute of limitations. For adults, this is typically 2 to 5 years, depending on the state, from the time when the malpractice occurred or was discovered. However, because minors are less competent and cannot file cases themselves, the rules are different. The statute of limitations is tolled (suspended) and does not begin to run for a period of time—in most states, until the child reaches the age of majority. A clinician who treats children is therefore at extended risk for a malpractice action to be brought and so should maintain records for this longer period.

Most plaintiff attorneys take malpractice cases on a contingency basis, which means the attorney receives a percentage of any amounts paid to the plaintiff. If the plaintiff loses, the attorney gets nothing yet still has to pay expenses. To gauge the strength of a case, the attorney often asks an expert to review a case prior to filing. At this point, the expert is considered a consulting expert, and his or her opinion need not be disclosed to the other side. Once the expert's report or name is revealed on a witness list, he or she becomes a testifying expert.

To prevent frivolous cases, many jurisdictions require a plaintiff attorney to file an expert affidavit that provides an expert opinion that there is significant evidence of malpractice. Affidavits are generally considerably shorter than reports. Often, after discussing the case with an expert, the attorney will prepare a draft of the affidavit so that it will conform to the legal requirements of the jurisdiction. The expert then reviews the affidavit for accuracy, makes whatever revisions are necessary to accurately reflect his or her opinions, and provides a notarized signature. The expert who signs such an affidavit may go on to be the plaintiff's expert for the case.

Accepting a Case

When an attorney telephones or meets with a prospective forensic expert, the attorney will outline the essentials of the case and inquire as to whether the expert is interested in reviewing the relevant documents. Before experts accept cases, they should first consider whether the particular issue is in an area in which they have considerable competence, whether they have any conflicts of interest regarding the case, and whether they will be able to appear at trial if a date has been set. They should outline their fee policy, ascertain whether they are being retained as a consulting or testifying expert, and discuss what documents they will receive and review—generally everything relevant. An expert should beware if he or she is contacted shortly before the trial is set to begin, because this often indicates that other experts have already abandoned a weak case.

In most cases involving minors, the expert should ask for and review school and pediatric records, as well as medical records and other documents the attorney provides. If testimony or evaluation of a party will take place in a state where the expert does not have a license, it is prudent to seek clarification as to whether out-of-state work is a problem. Some states have physician or psychologist licensing statutes that may be interpreted to include providing testimony or conducting evaluations as the practice of the licensed profession, which raises potential problems if the expert will be testifying or evaluating parties in jurisdictions where he or she does not have a license (Simon and Shuman 1999). The American Medical Association (1998) has taken the position that physician testimony is the practice of medicine and subject to peer review. State licensing boards vary in their views as to whether out-of-state experts can testify or examine a person in their state without a license, and the expert should clarify these issues before accepting a case. Actually evaluating a person is more likely to be construed as practicing one's profession than simply providing testimony.

Reviewing Records

There are probably as many ways of reviewing records as there are forensic experts. Faced with a tall stack of paper, the expert's question is where to start. In a malpractice case, one may want to start by first reviewing the complaint and other legal documents, then the medical records that document the hospitalization or period of outpatient treatment during which the malpractice allegedly occurred, then other medical records and written documentation such as school records and pediatrician notes, and finally the depositions. If the expert is retained by the defense, he or she may want to read any available plaintiff expert reports prior to reviewing records to be on the lookout for information pertinent to specific opinions about malpractice. The expert's personal notes serve several purposes: they provide a summary and index of the record contents, help develop a timeline, and provide a structure for jotting down thoughts about the records. An expert's notes are discoverable at deposition or trial, so the expert may want to take care in writing notes about preliminary opinions so that the notes cannot be used to prove the expert is inconsistent. Taking notes on a computer allows the expert to cut-and-paste information into a more ordered structure (such as a timeline) and allows for discarding information or opinions that prove erroneous in light of later data. If the plaintiff-patient is to be interviewed, it is generally more useful to do this after the available written material has been reviewed.

Preliminary Discussion

Following the review of materials, most attorneys want to hear the expert's opinions before any report is written. Prior to that discussion, the expert may find it helpful to write a list identifying the areas in which he or she has opinions or questions. If the expert thinks that the treating doctor fell below the standard of care, the expert should also consider opinions regarding the nature of the causation between the substandard care and any harm that followed and, finally, an opinion about damages.

Providing Opinions: Reports, Deposition, and Testimony

After the expert has shared his or her opinions with the attorney and answered the attorney's questions, there will be some discussion of the next step. One decision to be made is whether the expert will be a consulting or a testifying expert. If the expert's opinion is useful to the attorney, the expert will probably be asked to write a report. General instructions for writing a forensic report are given in Chapter 3, "Introduction to Forensic Evaluations." In a malpractice case, the opinions will center on whether the standard of care was violated, whether identified violations contributed to the adverse result, and the nature of the damages. The expert should cite the bases for his or her opinions. For example, consider a case involving an adolescent who committed suicide while in outpatient treatment in which a central issue is the ade-

quacy of the risk assessment for suicide conducted at the last outpatient visit. The standard of practice for a follow-up appointment for a youth who is being treated for depression and who had some vague suicidal ideation at the previous appointment is going to be quite different from a follow-up appointment for a stable adolescent being treated for an anxiety disorder who had previously denied ever having any suicidal ideation. The plaintiff expert would want to identify the factors that put this youth at heightened risk that would necessitate a more detailed assessment than would otherwise be the case.

The expert should make sure that all of his or her main opinions are listed in the report; in some jurisdictions, opinions not listed in the report will not be admissible at trial. It is prudent to state that one's opinions are based on the evidence reviewed and to reserve the right to alter opinions if new evidence becomes available, especially if the report is prepared prior to the completion of all discovery depositions.

Discovery depositions in malpractice cases are similar to depositions in other forensic cases (see Chapter 4, "Testifying: The Expert Witness in Court"). It is important for the expert to meet with his or her retaining attorney prior to the deposition to discuss the expert's opinions and the attorney's expectations as to what areas are likely to be covered. The *voir dire* portion of the deposition will likely touch on the clinical experience the expert has had treating patients similar to the plaintiff. Lack of experience may be grounds for disqualification of the expert. It is helpful to have copies of an updated curriculum vitae to provide to each of the attorneys and the court reporter. In jurisdictions that base their rules regarding experts on the Federal Rules of Civil Procedure (2007), experts are required to provide a list of cases in which they have testified in the previous 4 years (Rule 26(a)(2)(B)(v)). If an expert has prepared a report, the expert can expect his or her expressed opinions will be scrutinized in cross-examination. At some point in the deposition, the expert will probably be asked whether he or she has any other opinions other than the ones already covered. If the expert has not prepared a report, the expert should consider preparing at least an outline of his or her salient opinions. Although such a list or a shadow report is discoverable in the deposition, it lessens the likelihood that the expert witness will leave out a key opinion. Of course, if the opinion is not asked about, the expert witness has no duty to provide it. Less experienced experts sometimes say too much at a deposition. The general rule is to answer the question asked and not go into other issues in an attempt to persuade the cross-examining attorney of the reasonableness of one's position.

Trial testimony in malpractice cases also follows the general principles for testimony discussed in Chapter 4, "Testifying: The Expert Witness in Court." Practically all plaintiffs choose a jury trial. While anticipation of cross-examination is the part that most novice experts find anxiety-provoking, direct examination is often the most difficult. If the expert does not communicate his or her opinions in a clear and credible manner to the jury, there is really nothing to be cross-examined about. The expert needs to be clear with the retaining attorney about how the direct examination will flow. Because malpractice suits are about what professionals do, it is easy to fall into using professional jargon; the expert must take care to describe professional decision making in terms understandable to the jury. Audiovisual aids can be very helpful in focusing the jury's attention. For example, many times the case will center on the professional's decision making at a critical time, such as the interview in which a medication was started or the last interview before a suicide, so it may be helpful to have a large blow-up made of the critical progress note to assist in guiding the jury through the decision-making process that was conducted—or omitted—at that time.

Hindsight bias—the tendency to overestimate what can be predicted from past events—is a powerful factor in malpractice trials. It makes the chain of causation appear to be stronger than it actually is. It can affect juries, attorneys, and forensic experts. Experts for the defense can try to overcome this bias by helping the jury see how the clinical situation appeared *before* the injury occurred (Knoll and Gerbasi 2006).

While testimony in malpractice cases involving children and adolescents is similar to testimony in cases involving adults, the fact that the patient was a minor may well color the jury's perceptions. The jury is likely to see the minor as less responsible for his or her actions, less responsible for communicating fully with the clinician, less responsible to be compliant with treatment, and so more in need of care and supervision than an adult. Further, the jury members will likely see the minor as a more sympathetic victim than they would an adult. The need by a minor for adult care will often be emphasized by the plaintiff's attorney and should be considered carefully in the presentation by the defense.

Other Tort Liabilities

While malpractice actions are the most common form of suit against clinicians, clinicians may also be sued on other grounds, including intentional torts, outrage, invasion of privacy, breach of confidentiality, and defamation. An intentional tort is one in which the clinician is judged to have intended to injure. Although expert testimony is frequently utilized in these cases, it is not required; if it can be proved that the alleged act was committed by the clinician, liability follows directly. Sex with a patient may be charged as an intentional tort, and the clinician may also be subject to criminal charges, such as child abuse. Because damages from sex with a patient are generally not covered by malpractice insurance policies, many complaints for sex with patients are worded in such a way as to not exclude malpractice coverage.

Invasion of privacy and breach of confidentiality claims arise when the clinician allegedly disclosed private information without appropriate consent, such as when a publication insufficiently disguises the patient's identity and consent was not obtained. The relatively new area of class-action litigation against pharmaceutical companies for providing inaccurate information about medications (see Chapter 29, "Civil Litigation and Psychic Trauma") raises the prospect that psychiatrists may be drawn into such litigation as codefendants either in their role as prescribers of the medications or as advocates for the use of such medications in pharmaceutical company–sponsored talks.

State Licensing Boards

Dissatisfied patients or forensic evaluees can lodge complaints with a state licensing board. This may occur in conjunction with a malpractice action. In some states, a specified number of malpractice verdicts may itself trigger a state board investigation. While most clinicians are more concerned with potential malpractice liability, in a state licensing board investigation the clinician's license to practice may be at stake. State boards are charged with protecting the public, and state boards do not need to find that poor practice actually led to damages in order to sanction the clinician. Nor is a doctor–patient relationship necessary. Complaints to state boards are also relatively common in situations in which the complainant has few other options. For example, parents dissatisfied with a court-ordered custody evaluation can challenge it during a custody trial, but they may also complain to the state board. According to Caudill (2006), 300 of 600 recent complaints against psychologists in California were for complaints about the conduct of child custody evaluations. Estimates of rates for actual sanctions against both psychologists and physicians are roughly similar and comprise less than 0.4% of licensed professionals per year (Clay and Conatser 2003; Morrison and Wickersham 1998; Van Horne 2004).

Forensic experts may get involved in state board actions in a number of ways. A large number of cases in which a practitioner is sanctioned involve a finding of substance abuse by the clinician, and in such cases, the state board may require an evaluation, a practitioner may retain an expert to help with his or her defense, a sanctioned clinician may be required to undergo monitoring, or a sanctioned practitioner may need to submit mental health evidence to have full licensure reinstated. Extensive mental health evaluation may also be requested in cases in which allegations involve boundary violations or psychotic functioning by clinicians.

Ethics Complaints

Complaints against forensic child and adolescent psychiatrists or psychologists are adjudicated according to professional ethics codes. Such complaints seldom require forensic experts for their adjudication.

Ethics complaints against forensic experts are not uncommon. Persons who have been evaluated in a civil forensic context and who are unhappy with the evaluator's opinion may see an ethics complaint as a way to fight back. While it is rare for a minor to bring an ethics complaint, angry parents, especially in a contested custody context, may do so. When the American Psychological Association (2002) revised its ethics code in 2002, it removed the specific section about forensic evaluations that had been present in the previous code and attempted to incorporate principles most germane to forensic evaluations, such as a caution about engaging in both a therapeutic and a forensic role, into principles applicable to all psychologists. The ethics code of the American Psychiatric Association (2008) also speaks in general principles to all psychiatrists. The American Academy of Psychiatry and the Law (2005) has developed an ethics code for its members but does not investigate complaints. The application of ethical principles to child and adolescent forensic psychiatry is discussed in detail in Chapter 2, "Ethics of Child and Adolescent Forensic Psychiatry."

—Key Points

- Professional liability arises in litigation contexts, especially malpractice litigation, and in other forms of complaints, for example, to regulatory agencies such as state licensing boards.

- Malpractice suits generally require expert review and testimony.

- Plaintiffs in a malpractice action must prove the 4 D's: that the clinician had a *duty* of care (generally arising out of a doctor–patient relationship), that there was a *dereliction* of that duty (a breach of the standard of care), and that the dereliction led *directly* to (was the proximate cause of) the *damages*. Expert testimony usually centers on the dereliction of duty—the violation of the standard of care—but may also address the other three points.

- Before accepting a malpractice case for review, the expert should be clear with the attorney about his or her expertise in the issue at hand, fees, availability, and scope of work. The expert should also consider whether there are any conflicts of interest in accepting the case.

- Hindsight bias is a powerful distorting factor in malpractice litigation.

- State medical boards can consider professional competence without a showing of a doctor–patient relationship or any damages.

References

American Academy of Psychiatry and the Law: Ethics Guidelines for the Practice of Forensic Psychiatry. Bloomfield, CT, American Academy of Psychiatry and the Law, 2005

American Medical Association: AMA Policy Compendium 1998: Policy H-265.993. Chicago, American Medical Association, 1998

American Psychiatric Association: The Principles of Medical Ethics With Annotations Especially Applicable to Psychiatry. Arlington, VA, American Psychiatric Association, 2008

American Psychological Association: Ethical Principles of Psychologists and Code of Conduct. Washington, DC, American Psychological Association, 2002

Ash P: Malpractice in child and adolescent psychiatry. Child Adolesc Psychiatr Clin N Am 11:869–886, 2002

Ash P, Nurcombe B: Malpractice and professional liability, in Lewis's Child and Adolescent Psychiatry: A Comprehensive Textbook. Edited by Martin A, Volkmar FR. Philadelphia, PA, Wolters Kluwer Health/Lippincott Williams & Wilkins, 2007, pp 1018–1032

Bellamy WA: Malpractice risks confronting the psychiatrist: a nationwide fifteen year study of appellate court cases, 1946 to 1961. Am J Psychiatry 118:769–780, 1962

Binder RL: Liability for the psychiatrist expert witness. Am J Psychiatry 159:1819–1825, 2002

Black HC, Nolan JR, Nolan-Haley JM: Black's Law Dictionary, 6th Edition. St. Paul, MN, West Publishing, 1991

Caudill OB: Standard of care analysis. Paper presented at the annual meeting of the American Academy of Child and Adolescent Psychiatry, Toronto, ON, Canada, October 2005

Caudill OB Jr: Avoiding malpractice in child forensic assessment, in Forensic Mental Health Assessment of Children and Adolescents. Edited by Sparta SN, Koocher GP. New York, Oxford University Press, 2006, pp 74–87

Corpus Juris Secundum: Physicians and Surgeons 70 § 64, 1987

Clay SW, Conatser RR: Characteristics of physicians disciplined by the State Medical Board of Ohio. J Am Osteopath Assoc 103:81–88, 2003

Dalton v Miller, 984 P2d 666 (Colo App 1999)

Federal Rules of Civil Procedure: Disclosure of Expert Testimony, Rule 26(a)(2)(B)(v), 2007

Florida Hospital Waterman Inc v Buster, Case No SC06-688 (Fla 2006)

Gutheil TG: Paranoia and progress notes: a guide to forensically informed psychiatric recordkeeping. Hosp Comm Psychiatry 31:479–482, 1980

Hammad TA, Laughren T, Racoosin J: Suicidality in pediatric patients treated with antidepressant drugs. Arch Gen Psychiatry 63:332–339, 2006

Kachalia A, Studdert DM: Professional liability issues in graduate medical education. JAMA 292:1051–1056, 2004

Knoll J, Gerbasi J: Psychiatric malpractice case analysis: striving for objectivity. J Am Acad Psychiatry Law 34:215–223, 2006

Lambert v Carneghi, 158 Cal App 4th 1120 (2008)

Meyer DJ, Simon RI: Split treatment, in Textbook of Suicide Assessment and Management. Edited by Simon RI, Hales RE. Washington, DC, American Psychiatric Publishing, 2006, pp 235–251

Montoya v Bebensee, 761 P 2d 285 (Colo App 1988)

Morrison J, Wickersham P: Physicians disciplined by a state medical board. JAMA 279:1889–1893, 1998

National Practitioner Data Bank: Public Data Files [author analysis]. 2007. Available at: http://www.npdb-hipdb.hrsa.gov/publicdata.html. Accessed May 22, 2008.

Pegram v Herdrich, 530 US 211 (2000)

Pettus v Cole, 49 Cal App 4th 402 (1996)

Recupero PR: Clinical practice guidelines as learned treatises: understanding their use as evidence in the courtroom. J Am Acad Psychiatry Law 36:290–301, 2008

Simon RI, Sadoff RL: Psychiatric Malpractice: Cases and Comments for Clinicians. Washington, DC, American Psychiatric Press, 1992

Simon RI, Shuman DW: Conducting forensic examinations on the road: are you practicing your profession without a license? J Am Acad Psychiatry Law 27:75–82, 1999

Tarasoff v Regents of the University of California (Tarasoff II), 551 P 2d 334, 131 Cal Rptr 14 (Cal 1976)

U.S. Food and Drug Administration: Class Suicidality Labeling Language for Antidepressants. 2005. Available at: http://www.fda.gov/cder/drug/antidepressants/PI_template.pdf. Accessed March 5, 2005.

Van Horne BA: Psychology licensing board disciplinary actions: the realities. Profes Psychol Res Pr 35:170–178, 2004

Vanderpool D: Professional liability exposure—minor patients: The Psychiatrists' Program. Paper presented at annual meeting of the American Academy of Psychiatry and the Law, Seattle, WA, October 2008

Wickline v State, 192 Cal App 3d 1630 (1986)

Chapter 31

Psychological Autopsy in Children and Adolescents

Marisa A. Giggie, M.D.

P sychological autopsy, a research tool that has been developed to evaluate the psychological circumstances of both equivocal and unequivocal deaths, has been used extensively in the investigation of pediatric suicides. The use of psychological autopsy varies, depending on the circumstances surrounding the death. If the child's death was clearly a suicide, psychological autopsy helps the family explain why the child killed him- or herself and further elucidates risk factors that can be used in preventive efforts. If the child's death was undetermined, psychological autopsy aids the medical examiner in arriving at the most probable and correct mode of death.

This chapter reviews the use of psychological autopsies in the pediatric population. The first section defines psychological autopsy, its various purposes, its use in evaluating both equivocal and unequivocal pediatric deaths, and the various methods used to conduct one. The second section reviews the epidemiology of pediatric suicide. The third section describes various types of equivocal deaths in children and adolescents, including group suicides, autoerotic asphyxia, choking game, and Russian roulette. The fourth section discusses legal issues relating to psychological autopsy, such as the admissibility of a psychological autopsy in court and types of pediatric cases that utilize psychological autopsy. The fifth and final section proposes a method to consider when conducting a psychological autopsy in children and adolescents based on the methods currently in use.

Psychological Autopsy

Psychological autopsy is a procedure used to investigate a person's death by reconstructing the person's thoughts, feelings, and actions preceding his or her death. It is also used as a research method by retrospective review of information collected concerning victims of completed suicide. The reconstruction is based on data gathered from police reports, medical and coroner's records, personal documents, and face-to-face interviews with families, friends, and others who had contact with the person before his or her death. The formalized practice of psychological autopsy arose out of the frustrations of Theodore J. Curphey, M.D., the Los Angeles coroner who was overwhelmed by a series of drug-related deaths in which the cause of death was unclear. In 1958, this frustration led Dr. Curphey to enlist the help of a team of professionals from the Los Angeles Suicide Prevention Center to aid in the investigation of these equivocal deaths (Shneidman 1981). From these investigations, the psychiatrist Edwin Shneidman coined the term *psychological autopsy* to describe the procedure he and his team of researchers developed during those investigations (Litman et al. 1963).

The psychological autopsy was originally developed to answer the following three distinct questions regarding an equivocal death: 1) Why did the individual do it? 2) How did the individual die, and why at that particular time? and 3) What were the psychological circumstances leading to the cause of death? The answers to these questions can help medical examiners and coroners make difficult determinations regarding the mode of death (circumstances surrounding a death) in equivocal demises

NASH Classification

The mode of death involves the circumstances resulting in the death and differs from the cause of death. The four modes of death are natural, accidental, suicide, and homicide, the initial letters which make up the acronym NASH (Shneidman 1981). In some cases, the cause and mechanism of death cannot be easily determined, and this is known as an *undetermined death*. The NASH classification helps death investigators decipher the circumstances surrounding an equivocal death. For example, consider a hypothetical asphyxiation from drowning (the cause of death) in a swimming pool; such a scenario gives little information regarding the circumstances surrounding the death. Did the person have a stroke while swimming and then drown (a Natural mode), did the person have an accident and struggle to stay alive (an Accidental mode), did the person drown himself (a Suicidal mode), or was the person held under water until he drowned (a Homicidal mode)? The psychological autopsy helps medical investigators connect the dots in such cases to determine the most accurate mode of death.

Purposes of Psychological Autopsy

The psychological autopsy is used for multiple purposes in the investigation of both equivocal and unequivocal deaths in pediatric and adult populations. Its primary and original purpose is to assist coroners' offices in determining the mode of death in undetermined deaths, which are estimated to be between 5% and 20% of all deaths that are investigated by medical examiners (Shneidman 1981). In both youth and adults, examples of these types of cases include drug overdoses, possible suicides, autoerotic asphyxiation, suicide by cop, vehicular suicides, school shooters/murder-suicides, and Russian roulette. In the pediatric population, further types of equivocal deaths include group suicide pacts and the choking game.

The psychological autopsy can also assist grieving families better understand the deceased's state of mind at the time of death. This is particularly useful in cases of pediatric suicide. It may be used as a post-

humous evaluation of mental, social, and environmental influences on the suicide victim, which can be therapeutic for suicide survivors (Cross et al. 2002). One example of psychological autopsy's therapeutic use in the pediatric population is in studies of suicide of academically gifted adolescents; these studies utilized the biopsychosocial approach to better clarify the psychological circumstances that contributed to the deaths of academically gifted adolescents (Cross et al. 1996, 2002). In these studies, the parents of academically gifted students who took their own lives requested a psychological autopsy to help them process their grief. In general, these families found the process of psychological autopsy was a useful means to better understand the circumstances surrounding their children's suicides (Cross et al. 2002).

Although the psychological autopsy was originally developed to study equivocal deaths, its role has expanded to analyze unequivocal suicides for research in suicide prevention. It has become a primary tool for epidemiologists and psychiatric researchers to identify risk factors for suicide, improve psychiatric care, and target youth suicide prevention efforts. For example, the psychological autopsy was used in the research phase of the Finnish National Suicide Prevention Project; its explicated aim was to reduce suicide mortality in Finland (Isometsa 2001). All suicides in Finland between April 1, 1987, and March 31, 1988 ($N = 1,397$), were recorded and analyzed using the psychological autopsy method. This study utilized face-to-face interviews of family members, usually conducted 4 months after the suicide. Also, researchers interviewed health care professionals who had treated the suicide victim within 1 year before the suicide as well as any health or social agency professionals who had contact with the victim. A multidisciplinary team also interviewed friends, relatives, and other intimates in addition to reviewing death certificates, psychiatric and medical records, police and forensic reports, and other available records on each case. In the end, a multidisciplinary team discussed the findings and generated comprehensive case reports based on the data collected.

Another example of how psychological autopsy has been used as a research tool is a large study of youth suicide in Utah. In this investigation, Utah researchers performed psychological autopsies on 51 youth ages 13 to 21 who had taken their own lives between June 1996 and November 1998 (Moskos et al. 2005). They interviewed 270 parents, siblings, friends, relatives, and other persons who had close contact with the adolescents who died by suicide. The interviews took place approximately 7 months after the suicide, and additional interviews with family, friends, and other persons (e.g., teachers, coaches, clergy) took place 9–11 months after the suicide. In the end, the researchers learned that parents and friends reported risk factors for suicide and related behaviors more often than did siblings, relatives, and other people (Moskos et al. 2005). Parents, however, more readily recognized symptoms associated with emotional problems (e.g., sadness, anger), whereas friends more often recognized risk factors associated with alcohol and drug use. This study suggested that parents and peers are the most appropriate individuals for gatekeeper training in conjunction with screening programs aimed at reducing adolescent suicide.

Another use of psychological autopsy is in litigation. Examples of types of cases in which psychological autopsy is used include life insurance claims for suicides, testamentary capacity, product liability, and malpractice.

Finally, psychological autopsies are becoming increasingly important in better understanding tragic cases involving homicide-suicides. The high-profile school shootings that have occurred in the United States over the past two decades, with the most recent episodes at Virginia Tech University and Northern Illinois University, have pushed this issue to the public forefront. Although the incidence of school-based attacks is rare, 1 in 1 million, the effects on an affected community can be devastating (Vossekuil et al. 2002). In response to the homicide–suicide attack at Columbine High School in April 1999, the U.S. Secret Service and the U.S. Department of Education initiated a study, in June 1999, to study the thinking, planning, and preattack behaviors engaged in by attackers (all under age of 18) who had carried out school shootings in the United States over the prior decades (Vossekuil et al. 2002). This joint Secret Service–Department of Education study of school shooters was a study of adolescent school shooters with the aim of identifying information that could be obtainable prior to an attack to help communities formulate policies to prevent future school-based attacks.

Researchers examined shooters' preincident thinking and behaviors in 37 incidents of targeted school violence involving 41 attackers that occurred in the United States between 1974 and June 2000. Researchers interviewed 10 surviving attackers and obtained information from primary source materials, including investigative, court, school, and mental health records. They coded information regarding the attackers' motives, preattack communications, mental health/substance use history, life circumstances, and

extensive school/relationship history. The result of this effort, similar in process to a psychological autopsy inquiry, yielded the following key findings:

- Incidents of targeted violence at school were rarely sudden impulsive acts.
- Prior to most incidents, other people knew about the attacker's idea and/or plan to attack.
- Most attackers did not threaten their targets directly prior to advancing the attack.
- There is no accurate "profile" (set of demographic traits that a set of perpetrators of a crime have in common) of students engaged in targeted school violence.
- Most attackers engaged in some behaviors prior to the incident that caused others concern or indicated a need for help.
- Most attackers had difficulty coping with significant losses or personal failures. Moreover, many had considered or attempted suicide.
- Many attackers felt bullied, persecuted, or injured by others prior to the attack.
- Most attackers had access to and had used weapons prior to the attack.
- In many cases, other students were involved in some capacity.
- Despite prompt law enforcement responses, most shooting incidents were stopped by means other than law enforcement intervention (27% apprehended by or surrendered to school staff, 22% stopped on their own or left the school, 13% killed themselves during the course of the incident, and 5% surrendered to students) (Vossekuil et al. 2002).

Conducting a Psychological Autopsy

Most psychological autopsies involve interviews of people in the life of the person who died in addition to an extensive review of medical, psychiatric, police, forensic, medical autopsy, toxicology, and other relevant records. Edwin Shneidman developed the first psychological autopsy tool in his collaboration with the Los Angeles Coroner's Office during the 1960s in which he outlined 16 content areas that should be included in such an inquiry (Table 31–1; Litman et al. 1963). Bruce Ebert, a psychologist who has worked for the Air Force and conducted multiple psychological autopsies for the military, developed a more extensive approach and has proposed that psychological autopsy should evaluate 26 content areas of an investigated person's life (Table

TABLE 31–1. Shneidman's 16 criteria

1. Information identifying the victim

2. Details of the death, including cause or method and other pertinent details

3. Brief outline of the victim's history (siblings, marriage, medical illnesses, medical treatment, psychotherapy, past suicide attempts)

4. Death history of victim's family (suicides, cancer, other fatal illnesses, ages at death, and other details)

5. Description of the personality and lifestyle of the victim

6. Victim's typical patterns of reaction to stress, emotional upsets, and periods of disequilibrium

7. Any recent—from last few days to last 12 months—upsets, pressures, tensions, or anticipations of trouble

8. Fantasies, dreams, thoughts, premonitions, or fears of victim relating to death, accident, or suicide

9. Role of alcohol or drugs in overall lifestyle of the victim and his or her death

10. Nature of victim's interpersonal relationships, including those with physicians

11. Changes in the victim before death of hobbies, habits, eating, sexual patterns, and other life routines

12. Information relating to the "life side" of the victim, like upswings, successes, and plans for the future

13. Assessment of intention (i.e., role of the victim in his or her own demise)

14. Rating of lethality (seriousness of the method used in the death)

15. Reaction of informants to victim's death

16. Comments, special features

Source.   Litman et al. 1963.

31–2; Ebert 1987). Both approaches share many similarities, with Ebert's approach focusing more on in-depth analysis of the deceased's interpersonal relationships and dissecting various motives for the death.

Methodological Considerations

In a 1990 study of psychological autopsy, Jan Beskow and colleagues evaluated methodological issues in approaching the retrospective collection of data to understand another person's death (Beskow et al. 1990). They focused less on content of material gathered than on data-gathering methods. Beskow et al. indicated that several factors must be considered before conducting a psychological autopsy: whom to interview; the qualifications, experience, and training of the interviewers; the method of the interviews; and the timing of the interviews after the death.

In most psychological autopsy studies, interviews were conducted by psychologists, psychiatrists, or specially trained interviewers (Rich et al. 1986). Beskow et al. (1990) suggested that interviewers should have clinical experience in crisis intervention because the procedure requires interviewing people in varying stages of grief and crisis. For interviews with persons in an emotional crisis, such as parents of a pediatric suicide vic-

tim, the interviewer must take into account the psychological integrity of the survivor as well as the countertransference of the interviewer. Beskow and colleagues stated that interviewers need to be flexible and adjust to the psychological needs of the interviewees. Furthermore, they recommended that the less experienced the interviewer is, the greater the need for structured interview instruments and close supervision.

Interviewers may be faced with varied reactions by interviewees during the course of conducting a psychological autopsy. Most studies report that people interviewed found the interviews therapeutic in allowing them to ventilate their feelings. For example, a 1974 British study found that a favorable response to the interview during psychological autopsy was related to better crisis outcome (Shepherd and Barraclough 1974). Another area of concern has been the timing and method of contacting informants. In studies in which informants were contacted at home without notice, few people refused to participate, whereas one-third or more refused to participate when an introductory letter was sent (Michel 1987). In a study of psychological autopsy of adolescent suicides, an initial letter was followed by a telephone call 1 week later. This method of contacting surviving family members resulted in a large refusal rate (Brent et al. 1988). Fur-

TABLE 31–2. Ebert's 26 areas

1. Alcohol history (including family history, blood alcohol levels)

2. Suicide notes (have handwriting expert review style as well)

3. Writing (including school papers, diaries, letters, journals)

4. Books (checked out of library, types of books read)

5. Relationship assessments (interview people who knew the deceased, construct level of intimacy, assess reactions to death by close ones, look for anger directed at people)

6. Marital relationship (if applicable)

7. Mood (identify mood fluctuations, symptoms of mood disorder)

8. Psychosocial stressors (e.g., losses, relationship problems, school problems)

9. Presuicidal behavior (giving away possessions, paying debts, etc.)

10. Language (any changes in language noted before suicide, such as talking more about death)

11. Drugs used

12. Medical history

13. Mental status examination of deceased's condition before death

14. Psychological/psychiatric history

15. Laboratory studies

16. Coroner's report

17. Motive assessment (make a chart divided four ways—natural, accident, suicide, homicide—and record data to support each as it is uncovered)

18. Assess feelings regarding death as well as preoccupations and fantasies

19. Military history (if relevant)

20. Reconstruction of events occurring on the day before deceased's death

21. Death history of family (suicide history in family, modes of death of family members)

22. Family history

23. Employment history (when applicable)

24. Educational history

25. Familiarity with methods of death (examine belongings for guns, knives, lethal drugs, interest in and knowledge of weapons)

26. Police report

Source. Ebert 1987.

thermore, most studies of psychological autopsies in adolescents have indicated that parents of youthful suicide victims are likely to refuse an interview if more than 6 months has transpired between the death and the first approach of the family (Beskow et al. 1990).

The time interval between the death and interview varies between studies. Most studies have shown that it is best to interview between 2 and 6 months after the death (Beskow et al. 1990). In Brent et al.'s (1988) psychological autopsy of adolescent suicides, Brent and colleagues found no differences in the reporting of key diagnostic information when interviews were per-formed between 2 and 6 months. In their study comparing 27 adolescent suicide victims with 56 adolescent suicidal inpatients, Brent et al. determined that the time interval between the death of the suicide victim (or the suicide attempt of the suicidal inpatient) and the interview had no significant effect on the informants' reports about suicide victims or suicidal inpatients. Although the interviews of parents of adolescent inpatients took place sooner than the interviews of parents of suicide victims, the relationship of postepisode interval and quality of information was not statistically significant (Brent et al. 1988).

Brent et al.'s (1988) psychological autopsy study of adolescent suicide examined the affective symptomatology of informants (mostly parents) during bereavement and how it influenced their description of the suicide victim. A concern was that parents might either idealize their child or, oppositely, exaggerate psychopathology (Barraclough et al. 1974; Brent et al. 1988). Brent et al. found that parental report did not appear to be influenced by the presence or severity of affective symptoms of the interviewee at the time of the interview. This differed from results of Griest et al. (1979), who found that mothers with affective symptoms increased reports of psychopathology in their children when evaluated in a clinic setting.

Epidemiology of Suicide in Children and Adolescents

Overall Rates of Suicide and General Statistics

Suicide is the third leading cause of death for middle and late adolescents (ages 15–19 years) in the United States, accounting for 6,313 deaths between 2002 and 2005 (crude rate of 7.6 per 100,000; Bae et al. 2005; Centers for Disease Control and Prevention 2008). Although relatively rare in young children, suicide was the fifth leading cause of death in young children and early adolescents (ages 5–14 years) between 2002 and 2005, for a total of 1,071 deaths (crude rate of 0.9 per 100,000; Centers for Disease Control and Prevention 2008).

Overall, youth suicide rates in the United States have been variable. Historical patterns show higher suicide rates for 15- to 24-year-olds during the Great Depression (1930s), lower rates during World War II (1940s), and a steady growth between the 1970s and 1990s (Cross et al. 2002). Despite this increase in youth suicide rates in the 1970s and 1980s, the past decade has seen a decrease in youth suicide in the United States (Olfson and Shaffer 2003).

Suicide completion rates increase with age and are higher for male than female adolescents; in 1999, Centers for Disease Control and Prevention surveys found male adolescents are four times more likely to die from suicide than female adolescents (National Center for Health Statistics 2003). Female adolescents, on the other hand, are three times more likely to attempt suicide than male adolescents (Canetto and Sakinsofsy 1998). Furthermore, male adolescents are more likely to use lethal methods like firearms and hanging, whereas female adolescents are more likely to overdose or cut themselves (Brent and Kolko 1990).

Historically, Native Americans have the highest rate of completed suicide, and whites have higher suicide rates than nonwhites in the United States (Gould et al. 2003). However, the gap between whites and African Americans has been narrowing because of an increase in adolescent suicides among African American males (Shaffer et al. 1994). It is interesting that risk for suicide increases with higher socioeconomic class in African American youth; this trend has been explained by increased assimilation and loss of traditional protective factors with escalation in social class (Bridge et al. 2006). Hispanic youth in the United States, on the other hand, show higher rates of suicidal ideation and attempted suicide and less suicide completion (Grunbaum et al. 2004).

Suicidal ideation and attempts are common in youth. According to the Youth Risk Behavior Surveillance System, in 2005, 17% of high school students in the United States had seriously considered suicide in the 12 months preceding the survey (Centers for Disease Control and Prevention 2006). Other research shows the prevalence of adolescent suicide attempts ranges from 1.9% to 17.7% (Bae et al. 2005).

The three leading methods of suicide completion in the United States for youth are firearms, hanging, and poisoning, whereas the leading methods in other Western nations are hanging and vehicular exhaust lead, followed by firearms and poisoning (Bridge et al. 2006). In a review of all pediatric forensic cases between 1989 and 2003 referred to the Medical University of South Carolina Forensic Pathology section, 85 youth died by suicide: 62 died by firearm (including 5 cases of Russian Roulette), 13 died by hanging, 6 died by an "other" method (bridge jumping, carbon monoxide poisoning, and self-immolation), and 4 died by drug overdose (Batalis and Collins 2005).

Risk Factors for Suicide in Children and Adolescents

Psychological autopsy studies in the pediatric population have shown that having a mental illness is the strongest known risk factor for both attempted and completed suicide, with over 90% of all completed suicides associated with psychopathology (Houston et al. 2001). A case–control psychological autopsy study of 120 of 170 consecutive suicides among youth younger than 20 years of age and 147 community age-, sex-, and ethnically matched control participants in the greater New York City area showed that more than 90% of subjects who took their own lives met criteria for at least one DSM-III psychiatric diagnosis (Gould et al. 1998). In this study, the most common diagnostic groups were mood, disruptive, and substance abuse disorders. Mood disorders were more common in female adolescent suicide completers, whereas disruptive and substance abuse disorders were more common in male adolescent suicide completers (Gould et al. 1998). Overall, a mood disorder alone or in combination with a disruptive and/or substance abuse disorder characterized most teenage suicides in this study.

Overall, depressive disorders have been consistently the most prevalent psychiatric diagnoses among adolescent suicide victims, ranging from 49% to 64% (Gould et al. 2003). Adolescents with an affective disorder are at an 11–27 times increased risk for suicide (Brent et al. 1999). Approximately one-third of male adolescents who take their own lives have a diagnosis of conduct disorder, usually comorbid with a mood, anxiety, or substance use disorder (Brent et al. 1988). Comorbid psychiatric disorders have been identified in 80% of all completed suicides (Brent et al. 1999). Multiple studies have shown that having more than one psychiatric diagnosis increases the risk for suicide fivefold (Jacobs 1999).

Substance abuse is another major risk factor for suicide, especially among older adolescent male suicide victims, with a high comorbidity with affective disorders (Gould et al. 2003). Having a substance use disorder or being intoxicated has been associated with both attempted and completed suicides in adolescents, with alcohol being the most common drug of abuse across all age groups (Gould et al. 2003). Alcohol intoxication at the time of death is highly correlative of suicide and has been found in approximately half of adolescent suicides (Shaffer 1988). Substance abuse has been associated with a greater number of suicide attempts, more serious suicidal intent, and higher levels of suicidal ideation (Jacobs 1999).

Having a prior suicide attempt is one of the strongest predictors of future suicide. In boys, it increases the risk of completed suicide 30-fold, and in girls it does so by 3-fold (Shaffer 1988). Various studies have shown that past suicide attempts increase suicidal behavior in general populations between 3 and 17 times (Pfeffer 1991).

In a psychological autopsy of adolescents and community-matched controls in New York City, suicide victims had experienced more negative stressful life events compared with community controls (Gould et al. 1996). Examples of negative events include family discord, a disciplinary crisis, a breakup with a significant other, an appearance in juvenile court, and a recent separation of parents. Other social stressors associated with youth suicide include having difficulties in school, dropping out of school, and not attending college.

Various other risk factors increase the likelihood that adolescents will engage in suicidal behaviors. These include a family history of suicidal behavior (Brent et al. 1988), older age in adolescence (Centers for Disease Control and Prevention 2006), peer suicidal behavior (Cerel et al. 2005), access to a weapon (Brent et al. 1999), physical abuse (Brent et al. 1999), sexual abuse (Fergusson et al. 1996), and adoption (Slap et al. 2001).

Types of Equivocal Deaths in Children and Adolescents

Group Suicide

Suicide clusters rarely occur in the United States, but nearly all clusters occur in adolescents and young adults (Jacobs 1999). Adolescents appear to be more influenced by what epidemiologists call *contagions*, which are exposures to suicidal behavior of others through the media, peer group, or family and which seem to increase suicide risk in some vulnerable youth (Jacobs 1999). There is a growing body of evidence that peers of suicide attempters and completers engage in more risk-taking behavior, suggesting that exposure to peer suicide increases an adolescent's own suicidal behavior (Hazell and Lewin 1993). Group suicides are reported in the media and are almost universally teenage suicide pacts.

Autoerotic Asphyxia

Autoerotic asphyxia is defined as a paraphilia of the sacrificial/expiratory type in which sexioerotic arousal and attainment of orgasm are enhanced by self-strangulation and asphyxiation up to, but not including, loss of consciousness (Uva 1995). Anthropologists have described this practice in children. For example, Eskimo children hang themselves in a sexual game (Resnick 1972), and Shoshone-Bannock Indian children play "smoke-out," "red-out," and "hang-up," which are suffocating games (Uva 1995). Almost exclusively a male phenomenon, autoerotic asphyxia accounts for between 250 and 1,000 deaths per year in the United States (Rosenblum and Faber 1979). The purpose of this activity is to increase sexual pleasure; it can be viewed as part of extreme thrill-seeking behavior commonly seen in adolescents.

The characteristics of autoerotic asphyxia death scenes include the following commonalities: 1) the victim is in a secluded or isolated location such as a basement, attic, or garage; 2) the victim's position is partially supported by the ground; 3) the injurious agent is most commonly a ligature compressing the neck; 4) a self-rescue mechanism, like a slip knot or knife for the ligature, is provided for; 5) bondage is via a physically restraining material that has sexual significance for the user; 6) sexual masochistic behavior, such as self-induced pain on genitals, nipples, or other body parts, is evidenced; 7) protective padding is found between the ligature and body part to prevent bruising; 8) attire—the male victim is occasionally dressed in one or more articles of female clothing; 9) sexual paraphernalia like dildos, vibrators, and fetish items are often found at the scene; 10) props like mirrors or erotic films are sometimes found; 11) masturbatory activity often occurs, with evidence of seminal fluid in male victims often found at the scene; and 12) evidence of previous experience is elicited from relatives and body evidence (Rosenblum and Faber 1979).

Published reports of youth found dead as a result of autoerotic asphyxia are primarily in the adolescent age group; however, there have been reported cases as young as age 11 (Herman 1974). A problem with investigating these deaths is the lack of consensus as to whether they should be classified as accidental or suicide. An argument for an accidental classification is that the deaths lack clear suicidal intent. However, an argument for a suicidal classification is that such behavior can be viewed as repetitive self-destructive behavior, similar to substance abuse (Resnick 1972). In fact, the adult bondage community has given the name "terminal sex" to sexual asphyxia. This highlights one of the differences between adolescent and adult practitioners of sexual asphyxia. Adult practitioners, in contrast to adolescents, have a clear death orientation and are depressed. Another difference between adolescent and adult practitioners is that adolescents perform the act alone and are typically heterosexual in orientation, whereas adults often practice in pairs and are primarily homosexual in orientation (Rosenblum and Faber 1979). In a study of 117 fatal cases of autoerotic asphyxia in males ages 10–56 years, Blanchard and Hucker (1991) found that as one moves from younger to older subjects, the proportion

of bondage, transvestism, or both increased; older subjects were more extensively involved in bondage during fatal asphyxia than adolescent subjects.

The Choking Game

The choking game is a dangerous activity engaged in by some youth in which blood flow to the brain is cut off by choking, hyperventilating, compressing the chest, or hanging by a rope, towel, belt, or other items (Deadly Games Children Play 2008). The purpose of this activity is to get a "high." The choking game lacks a sexual component and has been described by practitioners as initially a light-headedness due to reduced blood flow and then a powerful rush after release of pressure on the chest or neck due to a powerful surge of blood flow through carotid arteries. Youth call the choking game many other names, including "space monkey," "funky chicken," "American dream," "space cowboy," "passout," "black out," "suffocation roulette," "rising sun," "California high," "airplaning," "gasp," "tingling," and "flatliner." Most youth who die from this activity lack major psychopathology and are engaging in experimental activity (Deadly Games Children Play 2008). Some signs that suggest the choking game include bloodshot eyes, frequent unusual headaches, marks on the neck, locked doors, knots tied in a room, wear marks on bedposts or closet rods, and disorientation after spending time alone.

Strangulation is a recognized thrill-seeking behavior in youth and can be viewed as extreme risk taking. Various cases have been reported of children and preadolescents who have died from such unsafe play. One such series of case reports comes from Canada in which four boys between the ages of 7 and 12 died from hanging from continuous cloth towel dispensers in Canadian schools, and another boy nearly died the same way. Two of these cases were attributed to the choking game; in three cases the child was alone, whereas one child recovered while playing with two friends (Macnab 2001).

Russian Roulette

Russian roulette is an extreme form of risk taking in which a person aims a gun at his or her head after spinning the cylinder of a revolver with one bullet. A study of adolescents in an inpatient psychiatric group found that three of the group members reported playing Russian roulette, one member had witnessed a friend die from the game, and three had been present when the game was played (Denny 1995). The author asked the same questions of adolescents in a regional juvenile detention facility serving mostly a rural southeastern population and found that a large number of adolescents had played Russian roulette. Although most practitioners of the game were male, players of the game included both male and female adolescent offenders (Denny 1995). In Russian roulette, most adolescents play the game in the presence of others, which points to the importance of peers supporting the idea that playing the game is a way to attain social status.

Legal Issues in Psychological Autopsy

Psychological autopsy may be used in a variety of legal matters, both civil and criminal. Examples of the uses of psychological autopsy in litigation include insurance policy recovery, worker's compensation cases, medical malpractice cases against psychiatrists, testamentary capacity, and a murder victim's capacity to commit suicide when the defendant raises suicide as a defense (Biffl 1996–1997).

Regarding the admissibility of psychological autopsy into evidence, appellate court cases referring to psychological autopsies began appearing in the 1980s (Biffl 1996–1997). Many states follow the standards articulated in *Daubert v. Merrell Dow Pharmaceuticals, Inc.* (1993), in which scientific evidence must meet a general acceptance test in its professional field as well as meet standards of relevance and reliability. Based on these standards, psychological autopsy evidence will be judged on whether the method can be tested, if it has been subjected to peer review, if there are standards for the method, and if the method is generally accepted. Generally, psychological autopsy has met the *Daubert* standard for admissibility as the topic has been peer-reviewed, is generally accepted within the relevant scientific community of medical examiners and mental health professionals, and has been subject to efforts to standardize the procedure (Biffl 1996–1997).

In the Florida case of *Jackson v. State* (1989), the district court of appeals affirmed the use of psychological autopsy evidence to convict a mother of child abuse. In this case, a mother forged her daughter's birth certificate so the daughter could work at a nightclub as a nude dancer. The 17-year-old girl shot herself, and a psychiatrist testified that the mother's relationship with her daughter was a substantial contributing factor in the girl's decision to kill herself. The court held that the state had sufficient evidence to establish that psychological autopsies are accepted in the field of psychiatry as a method of evaluating suicide.

State v. Huber (1992) is another case involving child abuse and the admissibility of psychological autopsy. In this Ohio case, a father was charged with involuntary manslaughter and nine counts of sexual battery of his daughter, whom he sexually abused; she eventually killed herself. The defendant filed a motion to exclude psychological autopsy from evidence; the court ruled that the defendant could not be charged with involuntary manslaughter if he did not aid, abet, or conspire in her suicide. The court cited the *Jackson* case, saying that psychological autopsy evidence may be relevant to the charges of sexual abuse and that if the defendant were found guilty, psychological autopsy evidence could be admissible at sentencing (Biffl 1996–1997). The defendant pleaded guilty to sexual abuse the day after this ruling.

Proposed Guidelines for Conducting a Psychological Autopsy in Children and Adolescents

When Edwin Shneidman developed psychological autopsy in the 1960s, it was geared toward assessing equivocal deaths in an adult population. His work and other approaches described earlier in this chapter provide a useful framework to develop a psychological autopsy approach for the pediatric population. However, children and adolescents have unique developmental and psychosocial factors that must be considered when assessing an equivocal death. Therefore, psychological autopsy in this population requires a more developmentally based psychosocial approach. Table 31–3 highlights both the process and content issues that should be considered when conducting a psychological autopsy in a child or an adolescent.

Purpose

First and foremost, the purpose of the evaluation should be clarified before beginning a psychological autopsy of a child or an adolescent. Is the purpose of the evaluation to investigate an equivocal death, to conduct research for epidemiological purposes, to be used in a legal case, or to provide more information to survivors of an unequivocal suicide? Because psychological autopsy

---

TABLE 31–3. Psychological autopsy in children and adolescents

Process issues

Clarify purpose (e.g., investigation of equivocal death, research, malpractice case).

Select interviewers who are psychiatrists, psychologists, or other mental health professionals trained in crisis and grief intervention and interviewing of families, and provide them with supervision and support.

Contact participants in the study by telephone between 2 and 6 months after the death when possible.

Content areas

Review all available school, medical, psychiatric, police, forensic, toxicology, and other relevant records.

Review computer files (websites visited, e-mail, etc.), journal writings, letters, suicide notes, books read, music listened to, and video games played.

Interview parents/guardians, siblings, teachers, coaches or school mentors, peers, boyfriend/girlfriend, and other important people in the adolescent's life.

Review the person's mental state in the days/weeks preceding the death.

Conduct a detailed mental status reconstruction of the day and preceding day of death.

Review psychiatric, medical, family medical, family psychiatric, family death, and medication history.

Review drug and alcohol use history.

Review developmental history, including any issues of abuse/neglect.

Review family developmental history.

Review relationship history.

Review educational and legal history.

Detail other relevant history (e.g., gang involvement).

Indicate the level of access to weapons by the individual and family as well as familiarity with weapons.

Evaluate presuicidal behaviors.

Detail any psychosocial stressors.

---

is used as a tool for various purposes, it is important for the person conducting the investigation to understand its purpose in order to focus the work. For example, if the purpose is to provide more information for grieving parents on the psychosocial circumstances surrounding an unequivocal suicide of an adolescent, the investigator may decide to take a more biopsychosocial approach and utilize the format used in Cross et al.'s (2002) psychological autopsy of the suicides of academically gifted adolescents. In this approach, the investigators chronicled the suicide victims' lives based on psychosocial developmental lines in a chronological fashion on the basis of available data. In the case of litigation, the investigator may choose to take a less psychodynamic but more standardized approach that has been generally accepted by the psychiatric and forensic field so it will meet tests of admissibility in court.

Ethical Concerns

Undertaking a psychological autopsy of a suspected suicide is a sensitive endeavor and places emotional demands on the data gatherers. Therefore, the following ethical concerns should be considered before undertaking such an inquiry: level of confidence in the investigators, level of mutual respect and confidence between the examiners, informed consent, and ensuring confidentiality and anonymity (Cooper 1999). In the case of pediatric deaths, confidentiality and sensitivity to survivors' emotional state are extremely important to recognize before investigators conduct a psychological autopsy. Therefore, interviewers must be cautioned to avoid harming survivors in addition to respecting the integrity of the deceased (Beskow et al. 1990). Overall, those who conduct psychological autopsies should try to balance ethical concerns with the need to obtain information.

Interview Procedure and Time Frame

As discussed earlier, research has indicated that informants are less likely to refuse to participate in a pediatric psychological autopsy if contacted at home by telephone versus being sent an introductory letter (Barraclough et al. 1974; Brent et al. 1988; Michel 1987). Also, most studies of psychological autopsy in adolescents show that the ideal time to first approach family members is between 2 and 6 months after the death (Brent et al. 1988). Thus, based on available data and the need to balance ethical and investigatory concerns, one should ideally contact participants over the telephone and within 2 to 6 months of the death.

Content Standardization

To maintain the reliability of psychological autopsy, investigators need to use a standardized approach. Table 31–3 outlines a proposed approach for conducting a psychological autopsy in the pediatric population, addressing both process and content issues while keeping in mind that psychosocial stressors and environmental factors are extremely important to evaluate in this population.

Summary

The psychological autopsy has been used in multiple ways to better understand both equivocal and unequivocal pediatric deaths. It has applications in aiding law enforcement and medical examiners in clarifying equivocal deaths, it has helped epidemiologists better understand the risk factors inherent in pediatric suicide, it has been useful in aiding grieving survivors to process the death of a child or adolescent, and it has had multiple uses in the legal arena. Given that suicide is the third leading cause of death in adolescents in the United States, psychological autopsy has many potential public policy benefits by helping policy makers target risk factors for pediatric suicide in hopes of decreasing its incidence. Although psychological autopsy was initially created to help medical examiners better understand equivocal deaths in adults, its use has expanded in the pediatric arena, with many positive benefits.

—Key Points

— The main purposes of psychological autopsy in children and adolescents include investigating equivocal deaths, assisting grieving families to better understand the deceased's state of mind at the time of death, conducting research in suicide prevention, and litigation.

— Types of equivocal deaths more common in the pediatric than the adult population are the choking game, Russian roulette, group suicide pacts, and school shootings/murder-suicides.

— The leading methods of suicide completion in the United States for youth are firearms, hanging, and poisoning, whereas the leading methods in other Western nations are hanging and vehicular exhaust lead, followed by firearms and poisoning.

— Adult practitioners of autoerotic asphyxia differ from adolescents in the following ways: 1) adult practitioners have a death orientation and are depressed, in contrast with adolescents; 2) adults often practice in pairs and are primarily homosexual in orientation, whereas adolescents perform the act alone and are typically heterosexual; and 3) as one moves from younger to older subjects, the proportion of bondage and transvestism increases.

— Psychological autopsy has met the *Daubert* standard for admissibility in court as it has been peer-reviewed, is generally accepted within the relevant scientific community, and has been subject to efforts to standardize the procedure.

References

Bae S, Ye R, Chen S, et al: Risky behaviors and factors associated with suicide attempt in adolescents. Arch Suicide Res 9:193–202, 2005

Barraclough BM, Bunch J, Nelson P, et al: A hundred cases of suicide: clinical aspects. Br J Psychiatry 125:355–373, 1974

Batalis N, Collins K: Adolescent death: a 15-year retrospective review. J Forensic Sci 50:1444–1449, 2005

Beskow J, Runeson B, Asgard U: Psychological autopsies: methods and ethics. Suicide Life Threat Behav 20:307–323, 1990

Biffl E: Psychological autopsies: do they belong in the courtroom? Am J Criminal Law 24:123–146, 1996–1997

Blanchard R, Hucker S: Age, transvestism, bondage, and concurrent paraphilic activities in 117 fatal cases of autoerotic asphyxia. Br J Psychiatry 159:371–377, 1991

Brent DA, Kolko DJ: The assessment and treatment of children and adolescents at risk for suicide, in Suicide Over the Life Cycle: Risk Factors, Assessment, and Treatment of Suicidal Patients. Edited by Blumenthal SJ, Kupfer DJ. Washington, DC, American Psychiatric Press, 1990, pp 253–302

Brent DA, Perper JA, Goldstein CE, et al: Risk factors for adolescent suicide: a comparison of adolescent suicide victims with suicidal inpatients. Arch Gen Psychiatry 45:581–588, 1988

Brent D, Baugher M, Bridge J, et al: Age- and sex-related risk factors for adolescent suicide. J Am Acad Child Adolesc Psychiatry 38:1497–1505, 1999

Bridge J, Goldstein T, Brent D: Adolescent suicide and suicidal behavior. J Child Psychol Psychiatry 47:372–394, 2006

Canetto S, Sakinsofsy I: The gender paradox in suicide. Suicide Life Threat Behav 28:1–23, 1998

Centers for Disease Control and Prevention: —United States, 2005. MMWR Surveill Summ 55:1–108, 2006

Centers for Disease Control and Prevention: Web-based Injury Statistics Query and Reporting System (WISQARS). Atlanta, GA, National Center for Injury Prevention and Control, Office of Statistics and Programming, 2008. Available at: http://www.cdc.gov/ViolencePrevention/suicide/index.html. Accessed June 25, 2008.

Cerel J, Roberts T, Nilsen W: Peer suicidal behavior and adolescent risk behavior. J Nervous Mental Dis 193:237–243, 2005

Cooper J: Ethical issues and their practical application in a psychological autopsy of suicide. J Clin Nursing 8:467–475, 1999

Cross TL, Cook RS, Dixon DN: Psychological autopsies of three academically talented adolescents who committed suicide. J Secondary Gifted Educ 7:403–409, 1996

Cross TL, Gust-Brey K, Ball, B: A psychological autopsy of the suicide of an academically gifted student: researchers' and parents' perspectives. Nat Assoc Gifted Children 46:14–15, 2002

Daubert v Merrell Dow Pharmaceuticals, Inc, 113 S Ct 2786 (1993)

Deadly Games Children Play: About the Choking Game. 2008. Available at: http://deadlygameschildrenplay.com/en/choking.html. Accessed February 15, 2008.

Denny K: Russian roulette: a case of questions not asked? J Am Acad Child Adolesc Psychiatry 34:1682–1683, 1995

Ebert B: Guide to conducting a psychological autopsy. Profes Psychol Res Pr 18:52–56, 1987

Fergusson D, Horwood L, Lynskey M: Childhood sexual abuse and psychiatric disorder in young adulthood, II: psychiatric outcomes in childhood sexual abuse. J Am Acad Child Adolesc Psychiatry 35:1365–1374, 1996

Gould M, Fisher P, Parides M, et al: Psychosocial risk factors of child and adolescent completed suicide. Arch Gen Psychiatry 53:1155–1162, 1996

Gould MS, Shaffer D, Fisher P, et al: Separation/divorce and child and adolescent completed suicide. J Am Acad Child Adolesc Psychiatry 37:155–162, 1998

Gould M, Greenberg T, Velting D, et al: Youth suicide risk and preventive interventions: a review of the past 10 years. J Am Acad Child Adolesc Psychiatry 42:386–405, 2003

Griest D, Wells KC, Foreland R: An examination of predictors of maternal perceptions of maladjustment in clinic-referred children. J Abnorm Psychol 88:277–282, 1979

Grunbaum JA, Kann L, Kinchen S, et al: Youth risk behavior surveillance—United States, 2003. MMWR Surveill Summ 53:1–96, 2004

Hazell P, Lewin T: Friends of adolescent suicide attempters and completers. J Am Acad Child Adolesc Psychiatry 32:76–81, 1993

Herman S: Recovery from hanging in an adolescent male. Clin Pediatr (Phila) 13:854–856, 1974

Houston K, Hawton K, Shepperd R: Suicide in young people aged 15–24: a psychological autopsy study. J Affect Disord 63:159–170, 2001

Isometsa ET: Psychological autopsy studies: a review. Eur Psychiatry 16:379–385, 2001

Jackson v State, 553 So 2d 719, Fla Dist Ct App (1989)

Jacobs D: Epidemiology of Suicide: The Harvard Medical School Guide to Suicide Assessment and Intervention. San Francisco, CA, Jossey-Bass, 1999

Litman R, Curphey T, Shneidman ES, et al: Investigations of equivocal suicides. JAMA 184:924–929, 1963

Macnab A: Self strangulation by hanging from cloth towel dispensers in Canadian schools. Inj Prev 7:231–233, 2001

Michel K: Suicide risk factors: a comparison of suicide attempters with suicide completers. Br J Psychiatry 150:78–82, 1987

Moskos M, Olson L, Halbern SR, et al: Utah youth suicide study: psychological autopsy. Suicide Life Threat Behav 35:536–546, 2005

National Center for Health Statistics: National Vital Statistics System for Numbers of Deaths. 2003. Atlanta, GA, Centers for Disease Control and Prevention. Available at: http://www.cdc.gov/ncipc/factsheets/suifacts.htm. Accessed February 20, 2007.

Olfson M, Shaffer D, Marcus SC, et al: Relationship between antidepressant medication treatment and suicide in adolescents. Arch Gen Psychiatry 60:978–982, 2003

Pfeffer C: Suicidal children grow up: demographic and clinical risk factors for adolescent suicide attempts. J Am Acad Child Adolesc Psychiatry 30:609–616, 1991

Resnick H: Eroticized repetitive hangings: a form of self-destructive behavior. Am J Psychother 26:4–21, 1972

Rich CL, Young D, Fowler RC: San Diego suicide study: young vs old subjects. Arch Gen Psychiatry 43:577–582, 1986

Rosenblum S, Faber M: The adolescent sexual asphyxia syndrome. J Am Acad Child Adolesc Psychiatry 18:546–558, 1979

Shaffer D: Preventing teenage suicide: a critical review. J Am Acad Child Adolesc Psychiatry 27:675–687, 1988

Shaffer D, Gould M, Hicks R: Worsening suicide rates in black teenagers. Am J Psychiatry 151:1810–1812, 1994

Shepherd D, Barraclough BM: The aftermath of suicide. BMJ 2:600–603, 1974

Shneidman ES: The psychological autopsy. Suicide Life Threat Behav 11:325–340, 1981

Slap G, Goodman E, Huang B: Adoption as a risk factor for attempted suicide during adolescence. Pediatrics 108:1–18, 2001

State v Huber, 597 NE 2d 570, Ohio CP (1992)

Uva J: Review: autoerotic asphyxiation in the United States. J Forensic Sci 140:574–581, 1995

Vossekuil B, Fein R, Reddy M, et al: The Final Report and Findings of the Safe School Initiative: Implications for the Prevention of School Attacks in the United States. Washington, DC, U.S. Secret Service and U.S. Department of Education, May 2002

Chapter 32

Evaluations for Special Education

Jerry Wishner, Ph.D.

Case Example 1

The parents of a third grader, Josephine, who is receiving inclusive special education at her home elementary school, request an opinion by their prescribing psychiatrist to support a claim for private school tuition reimbursement. Relying on a number of parental interviews and review of unsuccessful psychopharmacological and behavioral interventions over a 3-year period, the psychiatrist sends a letter supporting the parents' claim to the school district. Overwhelming environmental conditions related to school and class size, hallway noise, use of paraprofessionals, and limited academic productivity are cited as determining factors given Josephine's mood lability and neurodevelopmental disabilities diagnosed as Asperger's syndrome. During the subsequent due process hearing, the psychiatrist is called upon to testify about his evaluation, findings, and recommendations. The psychiatrist's file is subpoenaed by the school district's counsel and is the focus of cross-examination.

Case Example 2

The recently separated parents of an eighth grader, Betty, identified as a student with a learning disability, request residential placement because of her increasing argumentativeness, work refusal, and overall defiant demeanor. Betty has stopped completing homework, has not produced written or typed work for over 3 months, but does actively participate in classroom discussions. Observed friendships have deteriorated, and Betty has become increasingly socially isolated.

She continues to read voraciously. Psychiatric evaluation is agreed upon by parents and school. After meeting with Betty and her family several times in the office, the psychiatrist observes at school and makes two home visits. The psychiatrist diagnoses an oppositional defiant disorder, narcissistic personality disorder, a specific learning disability, and very superior intelligence and recommends residential placement. The school rejects the psychiatrist's recommendation for residential placement, claiming the student's adjustment difficulties are a reaction to family dissolution and not the responsibility of the district under the Individuals With Disabilities Education Act (IDEA). The parents request a due process hearing.

Introduction

Of an estimated 49.8 million students attending public elementary and secondary school in the United States during 2008, nearly 7 million children ages 3 through 21 years received special education (Planty et al. 2008). Figure 32–1 contains a graphical depiction of the number of students receiving special education each year, and the percentage of all children, since 1976. Although special education is now regarded as a fundamental right critical to the successful development of students with disabilities, an education was not always available to the nation's children with disabilities. As recently as 1970, only one in five students with a disability residing in the United States was provided any

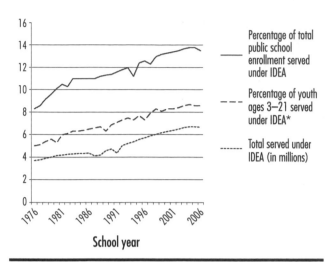

FIGURE 32-1. Numbers and percentages of children and youth ages 3–21 years served under the Individuals With Disabilities Education Act (IDEA): 1976–1977 through 2006–2007.

*Number of children and youth served as a percentage of all children and youth ages 3–21 years enrolled in early education centers and elementary and secondary schools.
Source. Data from Planty et al. 2008.

type of education at all (U.S. Department of Education 2007). At that time, many state laws still explicitly excluded children who were deaf, blind, emotionally disturbed, or mentally retarded from public school.

Today, such circumstances are unfathomable because of the 1975 enactment of federal legislation now known as the Individuals With Disabilities Education Act, or IDEA, and its ongoing enforcement (20 U.S.C. § 33: Education for Individuals With Disabilities). This landmark legislation marked the first time all children with disabilities throughout the United States were guaranteed access to special education and related services. For the first time, federal funding was provided to states to develop needed special education programs.

For fiscal year 2009, the federal budget allocated $11.3 billion to states for special education to children with disabilities, ages 3–21 years (U.S. Department of Education 2008). Though seemingly a significant contribution, the federal allocation represents only a small portion of actual state expenditures for special education. In stark contrast to pre-1975 conditions, provision of special education is now recognized as an important responsibility of government and is funded at the federal, state, and local levels. Also in contrast to pre-1975 conditions, special education is now heavily regulated. Today, federal and state laws intended to prevent recurrence of past abuses and to ensure ongoing accountability require understanding by parents and professionals to access needed opportunities. For example,

in addition to IDEA requirements, the federal No Child Left Behind Act (NCLB) of 2001 requires states to demonstrate that children with disabilities are progressing well and meeting state expectations for achievement in the same general education curriculum provided to all children. Additionally, local school districts retain accountability for students with disabilities even when placed outside the home district to receive special education. This has served to eliminate any temptation to hastily identify low-performing students as disabled and recommend out-of-district placements to avoid adverse impacts on a district's profile rather than provide effective, high-quality specialized instruction required.

Mental health professionals outside the educational setting are sometimes called upon to contribute to decisions or offer expert opinions about special education for a child. In addition to providing valuable clinical insight into a student, an understanding of the regulatory environment of special education and the conflicts parents and schools experience helps mental health professionals to be objective. When a treating or evaluating mental health practitioner is familiar with a child's school environment, that practitioner's recognition by school personnel as a credible contributor to special education decisions can be greatly enhanced. Where special education decisions are disputed and sent to an administrative and/or judicial proceeding for determination, the objective findings of a child development professional with expert knowledge of the special education environment are often very persuasive.

Legal and Regulatory Background

Since initially enacted, Congress has reauthorized and amended IDEA several times, most recently in 2004 (U.S. Department of Education 2004a). Each state interprets IDEA mandates and associated federal regulations and issues its own set of regulations for statewide implementation. In turn, school districts develop operational plans for local delivery of special education. As a result, administrative processes, eligibility criteria and procedures, delivery models, and terminology vary in different locations, requiring parents and professionals to adapt whenever interacting in different school systems. Eligibility criteria and procedures to identify a student with a specific learning disability are particularly longstanding examples of variability between school districts and the frequent change that continues today. Various approaches to the identification of learning disabilities within the schools have included ability/achievement discrepancy formulae, neuropsychological processing deficit models, and most recently, response-to-intervention (RTI) models, each with multiple procedural versions.

Despite local variability, the federal IDEA continues as the law of the land governing special education for children with disabilities, birth through age 21 years, throughout the United States. For this reason, the current discussion of mental health evaluation in special education primarily focuses on the IDEA. Mental health practitioners preparing reports for use in special education determinations will also benefit from familiarity with local school procedures and the resources in the communities they serve. Much of this information is available on the websites of local school districts and state education departments.

Mental Health Evaluation Under IDEA: Legal and Regulatory Considerations

The Special Education Process

Navigating a multistep referral, evaluation, identification, and planning process, specified in IDEA and operationally defined in local regulation, is required prior to provision of special education by a public school district. Although local procedures and terminology vary, the sequence of critical steps conforms to federal requirements and tends to be very similar among school districts. This sequence is represented in Figure 32–2.

The sequence of steps toward special education begins with concerns about a child's learning and/or school performance. Where there is evidence of difficulty, particularly when demonstrated on statewide assessments required by the NCLB, schools are expected to provide interventions and supports intended to improve student performance. Although not components of special education, such interventions are often federal mandates as well, such as the Supplemental Education Services required by NCLB. School-based RTI models similarly provide multitiered levels of support to struggling students and hope to improve performance before accessing special education.

When student difficulties are not sufficiently resolved through provision of supplemental intervention and supportive services, school professionals may request a referral for evaluation to determine if special education is needed due to a disability. Parents may refer

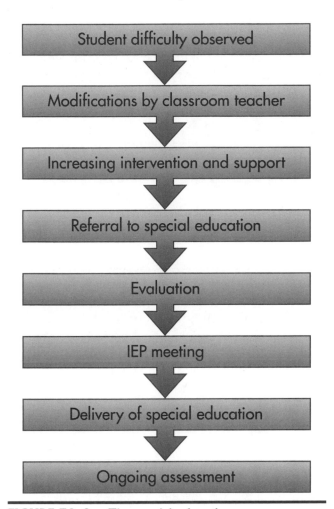

FIGURE 32–2. The special education process.
Note. IEP = Individualized Education Program.

their child for evaluation whenever they are concerned their child may have a disability requiring special education. Although schools often request an opportunity to provide supportive interventions prior to referral, and such interventions may be prudent, parents may choose to refer without delay. IDEA mandates school districts actively seek out students suspected of having a disability in "Child Find" provisions of the act.

As a next step, a school district will identify the evaluations needed to adequately examine the referral concerns expressed and request parents' consent. To determine special education eligibility, schools must provide timely, multidisciplinary evaluations in all areas of a child's suspected disability, including specialized assessments such as psychiatric evaluation, if necessary, to establish eligibility and complete educational planning. Generally, all evaluations are to be completed within 60 days.

Following completion of the school evaluations, parents may request district approval of an independent evaluation at no cost to themselves and may seek assessment by a mental health professional or other specialist. This is most often requested when parents do not believe that the findings of the evaluations provided by the school are correct. Recognizing the conflict between school and parent prior to conducting an independent evaluation under these circumstances enables the examining professional to sort out issues with parents. Explaining the range of potential outcomes of an objective evaluation is a good practice whenever parties are embroiled in a dispute. This is equally important whether retained by parents or a school district, and it helps maintain professional credibility in a community. Parents may also obtain and submit independent evaluations paid for privately that school districts are obliged to consider. Often, school districts will not forgo their own assessment procedures even when parents submit privately obtained, independent evaluations. In such situations, mental health professionals and school-based examiners may choose to consult one another to avoid repeated administration of identical instruments.

After completion of all assessments, school districts assemble a team comprised of the child's parent, teacher, and other school professionals. Required members of this team are identified in IDEA and local regulation. Parents are permitted to invite people who have knowledge of the child or special expertise. Independent mental health professionals often participate at this meeting at the request of parents. Evaluation reports and other information are reviewed, eligibility for special education is determined, and, if needed, recommendations for special education are recorded on an Individualized Education Program (IEP).

Following parental consent to IEP recommendations, provision of special education can be initiated. If parents do not agree, different forms of dispute resolution may be accessed. The IEP team may reconvene to resolve differences, the district and parents may agree to a mediation process, and/or parents may request a due process hearing, also known as an impartial hearing. Districts must convene a resolution session with parents shortly after a hearing is requested. Parental rights, including access to due process hearings, are outlined in a Procedural Safeguards Notice specified by IDEA. Impartial hearings are generally conducted in a formal, courtlike manner and are empowered to order school district actions and to award very substantial financial reimbursement to parents. Mental health professionals familiar with a child may be called or subpoenaed to testify at a hearing and, in all likelihood, be cross-examined, too. All records relating to the child or adolescent may be subpoenaed.

Individualized Education Programs

The many IEP components specified by IDEA are presented in Table 32–1. These components include descriptive information, such as present levels of performance, as well as recommendations for services, programs, placements, accommodations, assistive technology, and others. The student descriptions recorded on the IEP and the associated recommendations can be extremely important in the school life of a student. Understanding the components that describe student need for special education enables the mental health professional to prepare reports that are meaningful and useful to IEP team members making decisions. For example, the report providing a clinically rich description of a child or adolescent that is recognized by educators as information IDEA requires to determine special education eligibility is valuable. IEP teams are required to consider information about parental concerns; student strengths; cognitive ability; academic skills; functional performance at school, home, and the community; developmental differences; medical and health factors; and evaluation results. Evaluation reports that describe these factors and their impact on a student's learning experiences provide evidence of need that bears directly on eligibility and service recommendations.

Eligibility Determinations

Mental health professionals may be called upon by parents and/or schools to evaluate a child and provide expert opinion regarding disability determination, need for programs and services, and the placement the child requires to receive recommended special education. Special education and/or related services are available to children only when one or more of the 13 disabilities recognized by IDEA substantially interfere with their learning. These disability categories and their IDEA definitions appear in Table 32–2. Understanding how IDEA disability categories differ from clinical diagnostic nomenclature, including the DSM-IV-TR (American Psychiatric Association 2000) and International Classification of Disease–10 (World Health Organization 1992), enables mental health professionals to write reports suitable for use by school professionals.

To help establish special education eligibility, reports by mental health professionals that provide explicit detail about adverse educational impact are most valuable. Diagnosis of a mental disorder or disability alone, without linkage to impairment of learning, does not establish eligibility. Indeed, eligibility for special

TABLE 32–1. Major Individualized Education Program components required by IDEA, as amended in 2004

Descriptive information

Present levels:

Academic achievement

Functional performance

Developmental needs

Consideration of general factors:

Child strengths, parental concerns, test results

Recommendations

Eligibility determination:

Thirteen disability categories

Excludes as determining factors:

lack of reading and math instruction

limited English proficiency

Measurable annual goals

Progress monitoring procedures

Supplementary aids and services

Program modifications or supports for school personnel

Test accommodations

Potential special factors:

Positive behavioral supports, functional behavioral assessment, and intervention strategies

Assistive technology devices and service

Language and communication mode if deaf or hard of hearing

Braille use if blind or visually impaired

Extended school year

Special education program

Frequency, duration, and location

Related services

Frequency, duration, and location

Transition services after age 16 years

Postsecondary goals:

training, education, employment

Placement

Note. IDEA = Individuals With Disabilities Education Act.

education does not require diagnosis of a mental disorder or disability. For example, a high-functioning student with an autistic spectrum disorder may not require special education or related services to be successful, and the diagnosis of pervasive developmental disorder not otherwise specified (PDD-NOS) would not result in an IDEA disability designation as a student with autism. Another PDD-NOS student has difficulty communicating with peers in age-appropriate ways, becomes overwhelmed in the crowded lunchroom, becomes extremely agitated when classroom events do not occur as scheduled, and experiences great difficulty responding to unstructured creative writing assignments. This student may be appropriately identified as a student with autism, eligible for special education and/or related services.

In another example, a report that attempts to specify how underlying problems with attention diminish reading comprehension, impoverish note taking, interfere with the production of a well-organized essay,

TABLE 32–2. IDEA § 300.8(c) disability categories and definitions

Autism	A developmental disability significantly affecting verbal and nonverbal communication and social interaction, generally evident before age 3, that adversely affects a child's educational performance. Other characteristics often associated with autism are engagement in repetitive activities and stereotyped movements, resistance to environmental change or change in daily routines, and unusual responses to sensory experiences.
Deaf-blindness	Concomitant hearing and visual impairments, the combination of which causes such severe communication and other developmental and educational needs that they cannot be accommodated in special education programs solely for children with deafness or children with blindness.
Deafness	A hearing impairment that is so severe that the child is impaired in processing linguistic information through hearing, with or without amplification, and that adversely affects a child's educational performance.
Emotional disturbance	A condition exhibiting one or more of the following characteristics over a long period of time and to a marked degree that adversely affects a child's educational performance: (A) An inability to learn that cannot be explained by intellectual, sensory, or health factors. (B) An inability to build or maintain satisfactory interpersonal relationships with peers and teachers. (C) Inappropriate types of behavior or feelings under normal circumstances. (D) A general pervasive mood of unhappiness or depression. (E) A tendency to develop physical symptoms or fears associated with personal or school problems. (Emotional disturbance includes schizophrenia. The term does not apply to children who are socially maladjusted, unless it is determined that they have an emotional disturbance.)
Hearing impairment	Impairment in hearing, whether permanent or fluctuating, that adversely affects a child's educational performance but that is not included under the definition of deafness in this section.
Mental retardation	Significantly subaverage general intellectual functioning, existing concurrently with deficits in adaptive behavior and manifested during the developmental period, that adversely affects a child's educational performance.
Multiple disabilities	Concomitant impairments (such as mental retardation–blindness or mental retardation–orthopedic impairment), the combination of which causes such severe educational needs that they cannot be accommodated in special education programs solely for one of the impairments. The term does not include deaf-blindness.
Orthopedic impairment	Severe orthopedic impairment that adversely affects a child's educational performance. The term includes impairments caused by a congenital anomaly, impairments caused by disease (e.g., poliomyelitis, bone tuberculosis), and impairments from other causes (e.g., cerebral palsy, amputations, and fractures or burns that cause contractures).
Other health impairment	Having limited strength, vitality, or alertness, including a heightened alertness to environmental stimuli, that results in limited alertness with respect to the educational environment and that (i) Is due to chronic or acute health problems such as asthma, attention-deficit disorder or attention-deficit/hyperactivity disorder, diabetes, epilepsy, a heart condition, hemophilia, lead poisoning, leukemia, nephritis, rheumatic fever, sickle cell anemia, and Tourette syndrome; and (ii) Adversely affects a child's educational performance.

TABLE 32–2. IDEA § 300.8(c) disability categories and definitions *(continued)*

Specific learning disability	(i) *General.* Specific learning disability means a disorder in one or more of the basic psychological processes involved in understanding or in using language, spoken or written, that may manifest itself in the imperfect ability to listen, think, speak, read, write, spell, or to do mathematical calculations, including conditions such as perceptual disabilities, brain injury, minimal brain dysfunction, dyslexia, and developmental aphasia. (ii) *Disorders not included.* Specific learning disability does not include learning problems that are primarily the result of visual, hearing, or motor disabilities, of mental retardation, of emotional disturbance, or of environmental, cultural, or economic disadvantage.
Speech or language impairment	A communication disorder, such as stuttering, impaired articulation, a language impairment, or a voice impairment, that adversely affects a child's educational performance.
Traumatic brain injury	Traumatic brain injury means an acquired injury to the brain caused by an external physical force, resulting in total or partial functional disability or psychosocial impairment, or both, that adversely affects a child's educational performance. Traumatic brain injury applies to open or closed head injuries resulting in impairments in one or more areas, such as cognition; language; memory; attention; reasoning; abstract thinking; judgment; problem-solving; sensory, perceptual, and motor abilities; psychosocial behavior; physical functions; information processing; and speech. Traumatic brain injury does not apply to brain injuries that are congenital or degenerative, or to brain injuries induced by birth trauma.
Visual impairment, including blindness	An impairment in vision that, even with correction, adversely affects a child's educational performance. The term includes both partial sight and blindness.

Note. IDEA = Individuals With Disabilities Education Act.
Source. Building the Legacy: IDEA 2004, Regulations. Washington, DC, U.S. Department of Education, 2004b.

and hamper management of school materials will be far more helpful to an IEP team than a clinical note stating a student has been prescribed medication for attention-deficit/hyperactivity disorder (ADHD). In the first instance, eligibility as a student designated "other health impaired" may receive serious consideration; in the latter instance, the note provides little help in establishing eligibility. When members of an IEP team understand how a diagnosed condition impedes learning and achievement, determining eligibility for special education is significantly enhanced.

Emotional Disturbance

Mental health professionals frequently offer opinions to establish eligibility for special education for students with emotional disturbance. Knowledge of the term *emotional disturbance* as defined in IDEA is essential, as is recognition of defining differences in eligibility used by the Center for Mental Health Services and the Social Security Administration. Because of the longstanding variability among criteria for designation as a student with an emotional disability in different educational locations, mental health professionals also need to be familiar with local school practices for establishing eligibility.

In some states, children and adolescents diagnosed with conduct disorders have been excluded from eligibility for special education as students with emotional disturbance if they are not also identified with coexisting disorders. This exclusion of conduct disorders was based on the IDEA definition of emotional disturbance and its exclusion of social maladjustment when an emotional disability is not also present. Consistent with the very high rate of comorbid conditions among children and adolescents with disabilities, many believe there are insufficient empirical grounds for conceptualization distinguishing social maladjustment and emotional disturbance.

As is true for all IDEA disability categories, mental health reports describing the characteristics adversely affecting education are likely to be the most helpful when eligibility as a student with an emotional disturbance is considered. If a conduct disorder is reported, careful identification of coexisting disorders (e.g., anxiety disorder, mood disorder) should be included.

When a student diagnosed with a conduct disorder does not meet sufficient criteria for a coexisting disorder, detailing past and present symptomatology can be helpful to establishing eligibility.

In some cases, court decisions have upheld denial of eligibility due to social maladjustment when it was distinguished from an emotional disturbance by evaluating clinicians, but in other cases other courts were not particularly concerned about the diagnosis of a conduct disorder or the etiology of aberrant behavior, only whether it hampered learning over a long period of time (e.g., *Mrs. B. v. Milford Board of Education* 1997; *Muller v. East Islip UFSD* 1998; *Pinn v. Harrison* 2007).

Learning Disabilities

The recent changes to school procedures for identification of specific learning disabilities required by IDEA amendments (2004) and subsequent federal regulations (2006) are noteworthy examples of the potential discrepancy between clinical diagnosis and special education designation. Although the IDEA definition of a specific learning disability has remained unchanged since 1977, identification procedures no longer require demonstration of a severe discrepancy between ability and achievement, as in the past. Instead, new regulations encourage use of evaluation procedures designed to determine if a student responds to a series of increasingly intensive, individualized interventions that are described as scientific and research based. Such approaches are commonly known as response-to-intervention, or RTI, models, and they represent the emergence of a transactional disability conceptualization rather than one based on student deficits alone.

Currently, there is no formal definition of RTI in regulation, nor is there a consensus in the educational and research communities. RTI models at present vary widely, as do the multitiered, high-quality individualized services critical to effective implementation and successful outcomes for all students. The regulatory and educational trends toward RTI models for identification of specific learning disabilities are, nevertheless, important to psychiatrists and other mental health professionals evaluating student eligibility for special education. Current DSM-IV-TR definition and diagnostic criteria for learning disorders (315.00 Reading Disorder; 315.1 Mathematics Disorder; 315.2 Disorder of Written Expression) include a substantial ability/achievement discrepancy no longer required under IDEA and do not address issues of student responsiveness to instruction. The distinction reflects IDEA regulatory expectation for evaluations that are instructionally relevant to support recommendations for special education eligibility.

Recommendations for Related Services and Programs

Perhaps the best known IDEA mandates require schools to recommend and provide a free appropriate public education (FAPE) in the least restrictive environment (LRE) to all eligible students with disabilities. FAPE and LRE are important standards for all special education decisions and recommendations. Besides eligibility, mental health professionals sometimes offer recommendations about the type of special education programs and related services needed by a student. IDEA identifies different types of special education and related services along a "continuum of alternative services." This continuum sequences programs by their level of restrictiveness. Under IDEA, programs are regarded as more or less restrictive based on degree of meaningful access to nondisabled peers. Operationally, restrictiveness is determined by the extent a student with a disability is integrated with nondisabled peers for instruction in addition to the typical opportunities for lunch, recess, and physical education. Proximity to the local school the child would attend if not disabled is also an appropriate consideration.

Level of restrictiveness does not necessarily correspond to the level of intensity of recommended services. For example, a very significant level of special education support may be recommended to permit a student with disabilities to remain at the local school, integrated with nondisabled peers. The extent to which school districts provide special education in this manner varies considerably and is related to resource allocation, as well as the local model for service delivery. Despite the potential recommendation of intensive special education supports, districts and/or parents may feel an appropriate education is not available at a given location, and this can become a source of contention. When mental health professionals from outside the school system are familiar with local educational practices and resources, as well as the source of parent–school conflict, meaningfulness of recommendations is strengthened.

School districts are obligated by IDEA to recommend an appropriate special education in the LRE. The continuum of service depicted in Figure 32–3 can serve as a reference when considering the level of restrictiveness of local school district programs. Familiarity with the continuum of service outlined in IDEA and understanding what is meant by "restrictive" will

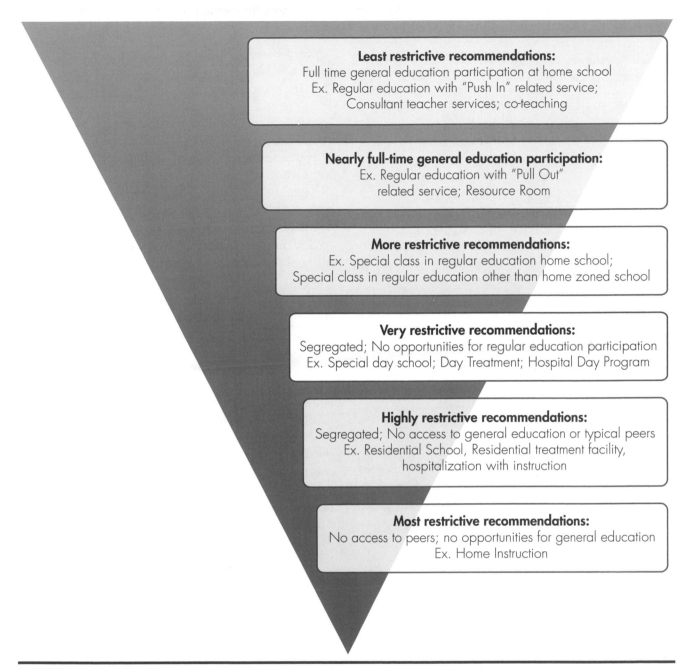

FIGURE 32–3. Continuum of special education services.

be important to psychiatrists and others offering opinions about appropriate special education recommendations. A list of related services currently identified in IDEA is presented in Table 32–3.

Inclusive special education programs are increasingly recommended by school systems in the form of a coteaching program. Coteaching programs provide both a general and a special education teacher in a classroom for some portion of the day who share instructional responsibilities for all students. Special education recommendations such as coteaching and consultant teacher services are provided to students with disabilities in their general education classrooms. Compared with resource room service or special class placement, these services are provided in a less restrictive environment. Efficacy studies of more restrictive placements, such as special classes, have often not found the student success and outcomes anticipated (Bunch 1997; Cartledge 2005; Rea et al. 2002; U.S. Department of Education 1998; Wagner et al. 1993). Inclusive special education recommendations have also been encouraged by federal regulations intended to remedy the disproportionality of racial and ethnic subgroups in restrictive and segregated special education settings.

TABLE 32–3. IDEA-related services § 300.34

Speech–language pathology and audiology services

Interpreting services

Psychological services

Physical and occupational therapy

Therapeutic recreation

Counseling services, including rehabilitation counseling

Orientation and mobility services

Medical services for diagnostic or evaluation purposes

School health services

School nurse services

Social work services

Parent counseling and training

Recreation, including recreation therapy

Transportation

Other IDEA services, from sections as noted:

Assistive technology service § 300.6

Travel training § 300.39 (2) (ii)

Transition services § 300.43

Note. IDEA = Individuals With Disabilities Education Act.
Source. Building the Legacy: IDEA 2004, Regulations. Washington, DC, U.S. Department of Education, 2004b.

Functional Behavioral Assessment, Behavior Intervention Plans, and Discipline

IDEA requirements address the behavioral challenges students with disabilities may exhibit. Functional behavioral assessment (FBA) is required whenever behavior is observed to interfere with learning. FBAs record systematic measurement of targeted behavior and the environmental contingencies present in specified settings. FBAs are intended to be context specific. Relying on information gathered through direct observation, interviews, and review of records, school personnel attempt to determine the underlying purpose of the exhibited behavior or the "function" it serves. Because exhibited behaviors may be symptoms associated with psychopathology rather than a purposeful response to the environment, mental health assess-

ment may be an important component to fully understanding the behavior exhibited. Those findings may suggest distinctly different interventions than those suggested from recorded observation alone.

The Behavior Intervention Plan (BIP) developed from the FBA may be multifaceted or limited in scope. Based on obtained data and the functional purpose supposed, interventions might include the following: introduction and rehearsal of adaptive behaviors, explicit teaching of deficient social or coping skill, manipulation of situational consequences that may be reinforcing the targeted maladaptive behavior, elimination or modification of situational antecedents believed to be eliciting the targeted behavior, and provision of additional resources to modify the student's experience, and others, in any appropriate combination. Monitoring behavior change and the plan's effectiveness is accomplished by ongoing FBA procedures and revisions. A mental health professional participating in the assessment and planning might suggest additional therapeutic interventions unavailable to school personnel.

While FBAs and BIPs are educational interventions, Manifestation Determination Reviews are a component of disciplinary procedures related to school suspensions. IDEA provides students with disabilities particular rights during disciplinary proceedings. If misconduct is shown to be related to a student's identified IDEA disability, the duration of suspensions and/or a change of placement may be limited. At manifestation determination meetings, schools must also demonstrate provision of FAPE and use of FBAs and BIPs. Parents and/or school officials may seek mental health recommendations for a student with disabilities under certain disciplinary circumstances.

The 2004 amendments to IDEA also introduced an explicit prohibition on mandatory medication. Schools are not permitted to require a student with a disability to take medication as a condition to attend, to be evaluated, or to receive services. Consulting and/or evaluating psychiatrists commonly review current medication regimens of referred students, as well as the history of past trials and their outcomes. In other instances in which a student has not been treated pharmacologically, a consulting psychiatrist may discuss its appropriateness with parents. When employed or contracted by a school district, a consulting psychiatrist should exercise caution if exploring and commenting on medication. A parent and/or teacher may misinterpret any such discussion by a psychiatrist retained by a district as a school-imposed requirement to medicate. In most cases, school districts are not seeking a medication consultation from evaluating psychiatrists.

Mental Health Evaluation Under IDEA: Clinical Considerations

Evaluation Procedures and Program Recommendations

Assessment that fully considers the child's needs in the context of home, school, and community provides the strongest rationale for specific recommendations of special education schools and/or programs by examining psychiatrists and mental health professionals. Rarely can such information about student need for support in different settings be acquired sufficiently in just one or two office visits. In addition to parent, child, and family interviews, school visits, observations, and interviews with teachers are almost always necessary to offer informed conclusions about a child's experience, needed interventions, and appropriate special education recommendations. Occasionally, a home visit may be very useful as well.

Classroom observation of a student is a required component of the multidisciplinary assessment mandated by IDEA. Generally, a school-based professional other than the child's classroom teacher completes this type of required observation. In addition to information about the student and family, the examining mental health professional intending to offer special education recommendations will also require information about settings, instructional environments, and the student's interactions. The psychiatric observer assessing the appropriateness of an educational setting for a student may appropriately focus on schoolwide characteristics and their impact on a student. Salient information about building size, student population, average class size, support personnel, available technology, student schedules, special programs, and teacher training can generally be obtained through interview and consultation. Other types of clinically important information related to the social milieu is best acquired through direct observation and include factors such as school climate, orderliness, noise level, teacher expectations, teacher–student communication, sensitivity toward differences, and parent–school relationships (Brookover et al. 1979; Ysseldyke and Christenson 2002). Visiting a school and observing in the halls, lunchroom, playground, and classrooms are among the best ways to learn about a school's social milieu (American Academy of Child and Adolescent Psychiatry 2005).

The observing mental health clinician may find a rich description of the social milieu a determining factor when recommending a placement appropriate for the particular vulnerabilities of a student with a disability. For example, the large, noisy, and sometimes chaotic middle school may not be an appropriate placement for the young adolescent student with Asperger's syndrome because of the student's idiosyncratic hypersensitivities and rigid need for routine. On the other hand, creative accommodations (e.g., use of a different entrance) and modifications (e.g., an altered schedule of class changes) may sufficiently ameliorate vulnerabilities and enable the student to remain at the home school.

Similar to the examination of a school's social milieu, parent and family interviews can include examination of home support for learning when conducted as part of an evaluation for special education. A parent's experiences seeking assistance and services at school; level of school involvement and value on education; understanding of a child's disability, homework routines, books, and reading at home; attribution of student difficulties and successes, expectations, and aspirations; and manner of discipline have been linked to student achievement and can be assessed (Ysseldyke and Christenson 1993). These areas of inquiry may also indicate the need for parent counseling as an IEP-related service.

Eligibility and Program Recommendations

Although IDEA defines 13 disability categories to establish eligibility for special education, identification procedures vary widely in schools. Students referred for special education evaluation often do not fit into a single IDEA disability category. A variety of problems coexist for many children and adolescents. A significant body of research has found that the academic performance of students identified by schools with emotional disturbance frequently meet the eligibility requirements for identification of learning disabilities (Mattison et al. 2002; Nelson et al. 2004). Researchers studying students with learning disabilities who are unresponsive to educational interventions have identified considerable overlap of emotional disorders (Connor et al. 2003). The matter is further complicated when considering the presentation of students with ADHD frequently identified under IDEA as "other health impaired" students. Connor et al. (2003) identified great overlap among children with ADHD, learning disability, and emotional disturbance.

Considerable school resources are expended for identification of one or more of the IDEA disability categories to establish eligibility. Similarly, the efforts for differential diagnosis by mental health practitioners consume significant time and effort. Ironically, much of special education across the United States is delivered in noncategorical formats. The majority of special education programs and services are recommended based on functional needs, generally not a disability designation. As a result, students with diverse disability designations but similar academic, social, and functional needs are often enrolled side by side in many special education programs (Buvinger et al. 2007).

Test Accommodations

Mental health professionals are often called upon to recommend appropriate test accommodations for eligible students. In the current competitive environment of high-stakes testing, the importance of recommendations for test accommodations has been heightened for many parents, students, and schools, and these test accommodations have come under increased scrutiny by state departments of education and other institutions (Camara and Schneider 2000; Franek 2006; Gross 2002). When examining the impact of test accommodations provided to students with disabilities, Elliott et al. (2001) found evidence of the intended outcomes not only for students with disabilities but also many nondisabled students seeking test accommodations.

IEP recommendations for test accommodations generally apply to statewide testing programs required by NCLB and other tests administered under the authority of a school, local district, or state education department. Accommodations may be available to eligible students for college entrance examinations, to young adults for graduate school entry exams, and later on for professional licensing examinations. Entitlement is considered by the appropriate agency (e.g., state licensing board, the College Board) under Section 504 of the Rehabilitation Act and/or the Americans With Disabilities Act of 1990. A history of IEP recommendations may be helpful to such requests but does not ensure they will be granted. Consistent use of IEP recommended test accommodations is often necessary to substantiate the need for continued entitlement.

Recommendations for test accommodations are intended "to level the playing field" for students with disabilities whose test performance may be unfairly impeded by the disability and/or unfairly judged when compared with others. Accommodations in the manner tests are administered or the manner in which a

student responds are designed to enable students with disabilities to demonstrate their mastery without being impeded by their disabilities. Appropriately selected test accommodations do not, however, compromise the construct tested (Koenig and Bachman 2004). A list of commonly selected test accommodations is presented in Table 32–4. In addition to the equitable assessment of an individual student with a disability, test accommodations have been important to the inclusion of students with disabilities in state assessment programs and the availability of associated high-quality educational opportunities.

An important distinction between accommodations and modifications has emerged in education literature devoted to the issue of valid and appropriate accommodations. Unlike accommodations, modifications typically alter the content of tests, thereby mod-

---

TABLE 32–4. Sample test accommodations

Test presentation

Additional examples of directions provided

Braille

Directions read aloud

Enlarged print

Increased spacing: reduce visual print per page

Questions read aloud

Prompt on-task focusing

Repeat oral instructions

Sign language administration

Student response

Access to word processor, with or without spell and grammar check

Adaptive writing devices

Adaptive seating

Allow student to answer in test booklet

Calculator

Dictate response to a scribe; may require oral spelling and punctuation

Schedule over multiple days

Student breaks

Time extensions

Test environment

Separate location

Small group

Study carrel

ifying the construct tested. Although used interchangeably elsewhere, the U.S. Department of Education and state education departments are steadfast in distinguishing accommodations and modifications. Permitting accommodations while eliminating modifications is an attempt to ensure students with disabilities are provided the same curriculum as nondisabled peers and educator accountability is maintained. If mental health professionals are consulting about the selection of appropriate test alterations for a child with a disability, appreciating the accommodations-modifications distinction, preserving the construct to be tested, and using correct terminology will strengthen their recommendations.

At IEP meetings, introduction of recommendations for instructional accommodations linked to a student's disability tends to be far less controversial than requests for test accommodations. While the former is often recognized as a legitimate need for effective instruction, the latter often elicits concerns for equity and fairness. As a result, it is sometimes possible to avoid or limit such concerns by establishing the need for instructional accommodations prior to recommendations for test accommodations. The face validity of recommended test accommodations is heightened when they resemble the instructional accommodations recommended. For example, instructional accommodations such as preferential seating may help establish the need for a special location when a student is taking a test. The need for additional wait time during instruction may correspond to the need for time extensions during tests.

Transition Services

The 2004 IDEA amendments strengthened school district mandates to provide transition services to children with disabilities 16 years and older, or younger if appropriate. These services are designed to "facilitate the child's movement from school to postschool activities, including postsecondary education, vocational education, integrated employment (including supported employment), continuing and adult education, adult services, independent living, or community participation." Highlighting this provision here is important for several reasons. Many school districts are relatively new to offering transition services that may have been provided by adult service agencies and other government agencies in the past. As students with significant disabilities continue to experience greater success and access new opportunities, new transition services will be needed. For example, greater numbers of

individuals with autistic spectrum disorders are entering college than ever before. New services will be needed to support these new transitions. School collaborations with psychiatrists and related mental health professionals experienced in treating adolescents and young adults with significant disabilities can be instrumental to the development of needed services. IEP recommendations may be part of that collaboration.

Parent–School Conflicts: Clinical Considerations

Parents' role to advocate and acquire needed resources for their child with a disability and a school district's responsibility to manage limited resources often thrust parties into conflict. Elsewhere, discussions of outcomes for children commonly refer to maximizing potential, yet the standard for special education determinations embedded throughout IDEA is "appropriate education." Nearly from the outset, implementation of federal special education law and special education decision making in schools has been rife with conflict and controversy, often followed by litigation.

The nature of parent–school conflicts about special education recommendations varies. In many situations parents may argue for services and resources not recommended, believing financial considerations, not the child's needs, took precedence. In other circumstances, parents may reject recommended services, fearing their child has been unfairly identified as a student with a disability and will be stigmatized. In another situation, a parent may resist a recommendation for coteaching as an attempt by the school district to deny the special school placement really needed. Yet another parent may resist the recommendation for a special school placement, feeling her child is the victim of discrimination and will be harmfully segregated and excluded. Confounding matters further, the same child presenting in different school districts may receive very different recommendations.

Objective evaluation can help resolve conflict by providing a full description of the child and current functioning, identifying the types of instructional interactions needed, and determining the appropriate resources and level of service to provide that instruction. Reserving judgment about specific educational recommendations until parents and school officials consider how and where the identified instructional experience can be provided may help reestablish some level of cooperation among disputing parties. Even when collaborative resolution is not readily available, discussion and exploration of the conflicting ideas expressed by parents and school officials provide important assessment information. Because mental health examiners are often recruited by a family or school after a conflict has arisen, there is a potential risk to objectivity in favor of the recruiting party's position. It is in everyone's best interest to reserve judgment and develop an explicit plan for evaluation with explanation of how and when recommendations will be made. When working for a local school, the district has an obligation to provide the written report of findings and recommendations. Ideally, the examining professional reviews the report with the family. When the examining professional is employed by the family, the report is only released with the consent of the parents.

Mental Health Professionals and Special Education Dispute Resolution

When parents disagree with school district recommendations for special education, IDEA requires provision of specified dispute resolution procedures to parents. Resolution of disputed recommendations is available through various means, including local mediation, "last chance" resolution meetings, due process or impartial hearings, administrative state review, state and federal courts, and, in some instances, the U.S. Supreme Court. Testimony from professionals educating, treating, and/or evaluating a student is routinely sought by schools and parents during dispute resolution at the level of an impartial hearing and usually not at subsequent proceedings. In addition to teachers and other educators, sources of important testimony often include psychiatrists, psychologists, social workers, therapists, and counselors, whether employed by a school or parent. The records of an evaluating or treating psychiatrist, or other mental health professional, may be requested by attorneys representing parents or a school district and subpoenaed by an empowered hearing officer or judge.

Special educational due process hearings are structured to provide opportunities for disputing parties, parents, and school districts to present their opposing position and argue about its legitimacy. The proceedings are adversarial and can sometimes be embroiled in impassioned accusations and heated exchanges, particularly when testimony is cross-examined.

Mental Health Evaluation Under Section 504 of the Rehabilitation Act of 1973

In addition to IDEA, civil rights statutes such as Section 504 of the Rehabilitation Act of 1973 and the Americans With Disabilities Act of 1990 (ADA) also influence school practices for students and others with disabilities. Section 504 is not education law, as is IDEA; rather, it is civil rights legislation—applicable to all schools and agencies receiving any form of federal funding—intended to ensure that students with disabilities have full access to school activities and opportunities equivalent to those of their nondisabled peers. All public schools, as well as other entities receiving federal funds, are covered by Section 504. In practice, recommendations for students identified as eligible under Section 504 are most often for reasonable classroom and school accommodations to prevent discrimination within a general education environment. Although Section 504 requires districts to provide FAPE, including needed general and special education, as well as related aids and services, IDEA is almost always the vehicle for recommending special education program and services. IDEA provides funding to school districts for provision of special education and related services; Section 504 and ADA do not.

In its earliest application at schools, barriers to physical accessibility were addressed by provision of ramps, handrails, adapted bathroom facilities, and the like. Since that time, students with other types of disabilities in need of accommodation in the regular education classroom have increasingly been identified. Students with attentional disorders may require brief breaks during instructional activities and testing. Students with a history of dysgraphia may require access to word processing for note taking and essay examinations. As the emphasis on competitive performance on standardized tests has grown in recent years, so too have requests under Section 504 for extended time accommodations during tests. At this time most college websites include instructions for requesting and documenting the need for such accommodations.

Schools and other institutions often ask just a few questions to determine eligibility for reasonable accommodations. Generally, these broad questions closely resemble the language of the act; for example, Is there a mental or physical impairment? Is a major life activity substantially limited? Interpretation of these seemingly straightforward questions often proves to be far more complex than may have been anticipated. For example, which tasks are regarded as major life activities, and which are not?

Effective January 2009, amendments to ADA and Section 504 broadened interpretation of eligibility. Recent amendments expanded recognized major life activities. This category now includes (but is not limited to) caring for oneself, performing manual tasks, walking, standing, lifting, bending, seeing, hearing, speaking, breathing, learning, reading, concentrating, thinking, communicating, and working.

If eligibility is established, a Section 504 plan specifying the reasonable accommodations should be drafted. Reasonable accommodations are identified to prevent or eliminate discrimination and to ensure that the needs of students with disabilities are met, as well as the needs of other students. It should be noted that diagnosis of a disability does not in itself automatically generate Section 504 protections. Observation of a substantial limitation on a major life activity is also a determining factor. and guides development of specific recommendations. (See Chapter 5, "Special Education: Screening Tools, Rating Scales, and Self-Report Instruments," for additional information.)

Case Example Epilogues

Case Example 1

During the impartial hearing, the treating psychiatrist testified that he believed Josephine's overall third-grade experience was poor, that her behaviors worsened, and that she became increasingly sad and hopeless throughout the year. He also noted that Josephine's behavior and social experience improved greatly as she began to attend the private school where she was placed unilaterally. He testified the program recommended by the school district was inappropriate and that Josephine would not benefit there. Upon cross-examination, the psychiatrist explained the basis of his professional opinions about Josephine's work productivity and academic success were reports from the father throughout the year and that he had not visited the school, consulted with any teachers, or reviewed Josephine's work products. The psychiatrist did not discuss these topics with Josephine directly, nor did his treatment notes indicate such discussion. Talk therapy had stopped by mid-year when the psychiatrist viewed it as unproductive. Also during cross-examination, the psychiatrist reported that his familiarity with the recommended placement was based on a long history treating other children in the community. In the hearing officer's decision for the school district, he cited the voluminous student work Josephine's teacher had retained and had entered into evidence during the hearing and that the IEP team's recommendations were "reasonably calculated to enable Josephine to receive educational benefits," the standard established through precedent, although he believed the private school was likely to provide even greater benefit.

Case Example 2

In the hearing officer's decision for the parents, she noted that since the residential program was needed by Betty to benefit from instruction, it is the school district's obligation under IDEA. Although Betty was not diagnosed with depression at this time, the hearing officer concluded there was sufficient evidence of a "generally pervasive mood of unhappiness over a marked period of time" and that, considering the entire record, Betty exhibited "inappropriate types of behaviors and feelings under normal circumstances." Several of the criteria for designation as a student with an emotional disturbance were satisfied.

—Key Points

— Psychiatric and mental health evaluation may be requested by parents or school officials as a necessary component of the multidisciplinary assessment required by federal law to determine a child's potential need for special education. Parents are also entitled to present reports of psychiatric evaluations completed independently of schools.

— Prior to initiating assessment requested by school officials for special education considerations, the mental health evaluator needs to inform the parent of planned evaluation procedures (e.g., professional consultations, observations, interviews), explain the purposes of the evaluation, describe how obtained information will be used, discuss whether any information will be confidential, and identify to whom the report will be released. A signed written consent agreeing to the evaluation activity described, indicating consent is granted voluntarily and may be revoked, is required by federal special education law (IDEA). Most school districts have a standardized form available for this purpose.

— Because mental health evaluations are frequently sought after conflict has emerged, objectivity may be risked in favor of the referral source's position. It is in everyone's best interest for the mental health professional to reserve judgment, outline evaluation procedures, and discuss how different potential findings may lead to different recommendations.

— In addition to parent, child, and family interviews, assessment by a mental health expert is intended to provide meaningful special education recommendations and should include consultation with teachers and therapists, review of records, and multiple observations of the child in diverse school settings (e.g., classrooms, lunchroom, playground, hallways).

— Reports of expert mental health assessment can be most useful for special education planning when diagnosed disorders are described within the context of school, learning, and interactions with others. Information from responses to the following types of questions can be particularly useful when IEP teams are planning special education: How does the described disorder impede learning? How will the child's performance on typical classroom tasks or during school activities be affected? What types of instructional interventions are needed? What special environmental conditions may be needed? How is the child's behavior and social-emotional development affected? What management techniques will be helpful? What are regarded as some of the most important goals for the child?

— To establish eligibility for special education, the mental health clinician needs to identify diagnosed mental disorders as one or more of the current IDEA disability categories and describe fully the significant impairment to learning.

— Recommendations for placement in a selected special education setting by an examining mental health expert are most appropriate when the special needs of a child with a disability are fully identified, the current program is observed to be inadequate, and the recommended setting is well known to the psychiatric examiner.

— Following completion of evaluation procedures, the mental health expert should review findings with parents and school personnel and submit a final written report. The clinician should not submit a draft report for approval or agree to requested revisions other than correction of factual error.

— When parents dispute school recommendations for special education, the examining and/or treating mental health clinician may be called to testify at a due process hearing, and records may be subpoenaed.

References

American Academy of Child and Adolescent Psychiatry: Practice parameters for psychiatric consultation to schools. J Am Acad Child Adolesc Psychiatry 44:1068–1084, 2005

American Psychiatric Association: Diagnostic and Statistical Manual of Mental Disorders, 4th Edition, Text Revision. Washington, DC, American Psychiatric Association, 2000

Brookover WB, Beady C, Flood P, et al: School Social Systems and Student Achievement: Schools Can Make a Difference. New York, Praeger, 1979

Bunch G: From here to there: the passage of inclusion special education, in Inclusion: Recent Research. Edited by Bunch G, Valeo A. Toronto, ON, Canada, Inclusion Press, 1997, pp 9–23

Buvinger E, Evans SW, Forness SR: Issues in evidence-based practice in special education for children with emotional or behavioral disorders, in Advances in School-Based Mental Health Interventions, Vol 2. Edited by Evans SW, Weist MD, Serpell ZN. Kingston, NJ, Civic Research Institute, 2007, pp 19-1–19-13

Camara WJ, Schneider D: Testing with extended time on the SAT I: effects for students with learning disabilities (College Board Research No RN-08). New York, College Entrance Examination Board, 2000

Cartledge G: Restrictiveness and race in special education: the failure to prevent or to return. Learning Disabilities: A Contemporary Journal 3(1):27–32, 2005

Connor DF, Edwards G, Fletcher KE, et al: Correlates of co-morbid psychopathology in children with ADHD. J Am Acad Child Adolesc Psychiatry 42:193–200, 2003

Elliott SN, Kratochwill TR, McKevitt BC: Experimental analysis of the effects of testing accommodations on the scores of students with and without disabilities. Journal of School Psychology 39(1):3–24, 2001

Franek M: Time to think. New York Times, March 29, 2006, Op-Ed

Gross J: Paying for a disability diagnosis to gain time on College Boards. New York Times, September 26, 2002

Individuals With Disabilities Education Act (IDEA), Pub. L. No. 101-476, 104 Stat. 1142 (October 30, 1990)

Koenig JA, Bachman LF (eds): Keeping Score for All: The Effects of Inclusion and Accommodation Policies on Large-Scale Educational Assessment. National Research Council. Washington, DC, National Academies Press, 2004

Mattison RE, Hooper SR, Glassberg LA: Three-year course of learning disorders in special education students classified as behavioral disordered. J Am Acad Child Adolesc Psychiatry 41:1454–1461, 2002

Mrs B v Milford Board of Education and Mary Jo Kramer, 103 F 3d 1114 (1997)

Muller v East Islip UFSD, 145 F 3d (1998)

Nelson JR, Benner GJ, Lane K, et al: Academic achievement of K–12 students with emotional and behavioral disorders. Except Child 71:59–73, 2004

No Child Left Behind Act of 2001, 20 USC § 6311, Pub. L. No. 107-110

Pinn v Harrison, 473 F Supp 2d 477 (2007)

Planty M, Hussar W, Snyder T, et al: The condition of education 2008 (NCES No 2008-031). Washington, DC, U.S. Department of Education, National Center for Education Statistics, Institute of Education Sciences, 2008

Rea PJ, McLaughlin VL, Walter-Thomas C: Outcomes for students with learning disabilities in inclusive and pull-out programs. Except Child 68:203–222, 2002

U.S. Department of Education: To assure the free and appropriate public education of all children with disabilities: 20th annual report to Congress on the implementation of the Individuals With Disabilities Education Act. Washington, DC, U.S. Government Printing Office, 1998

U.S. Department of Education: Assistance to States for the Education of Children With Disabilities and Preschool Grants for Children With Disabilities: Final Rule (Fed. Reg. 34 CFR Parts 300 and 301). Washington, DC, U.S. Government Printing Office, 2004a

U.S. Department of Education: Building the Legacy: IDEA 2004, Regulations. Washington, DC, U.S. Department of Education, 2004b

U.S. Department of Education: To assure the free appropriate public education of all children with disabilities: 27th Annual Report to Congress on the Implementation of the Individuals With Disabilities Education Act. Washington, DC, U.S. Government Printing Office, 2007

U.S. Department of Education: Fiscal Year 2009 Budget Summary, Section II B: Special Education and Rehabilitative Services. Washington, DC, U.S. Government Printing Office, 2008

Wagner M, Blackorby J, Cameto R, et al: The Transition Experiences of Young People With Disabilities: A Summary of Findings From the National Longitudinal Transition Study of Special Education Students. Menlo Park, CA, SRI International, 1993

World Health Organization: International Statistical Classification of Diseases and Related Health Problems, 10th Revision. Geneva, World Health Organization, 1992

Ysseldyke JE, Christenson SL: The Instruction Environment System II. Longmont, CO, Sopris West, 1993

Ysseldyke JE, Christenson SL: Functional Assessment of Academic Behavior: Creating Successful Learning Environments. Longmont, CO, Sopris West, 2002

Chapter 33

Clinical and Forensic Aspects of Sexual Harassment in School-Age Children and Adolescents

Praveen Kambam, M.D.

Elissa P. Benedek, M.D.

Behaviors that may constitute sexual harassment have a history as long as that of the workplace. Legal definitions of sexual harassment in the workplace have developed only over the past few decades, whereas the definition of sexual harassment in schools is still unclear. The parameters of the definition of sexual harassment vary, depending on U.S. Supreme Court decisions, and the rather fluid status of sexual harassment as it applies to children and adolescents is reflected in the number of recent court decisions.

Since the U.S. Supreme Court decision in *Davis v. Monroe County Board of Education* (1999), the number of requests made to child and adolescent psychiatrists for forensic assessment of children, adolescents, and their parents who allege sexual harassment in the classroom has increased dramatically. Roles of the forensic psychiatrist may include directly evaluating an alleged victim, testifying as an expert, and consulting to educational institutions.

In 2008, the U.S. Supreme Court issued two new important decisions in retaliation claims filed by current and former employees (*CBOCS West, Inc. v. Humphries* 2008; *Gomez-Perez v. Potter* 2008). Courts continue to grant new rights to employees claiming retaliation based on sex, race, or age. How these new decisions may be applied to students is yet to be determined.

Legal Issues

Definitions and Basis of Sexual Harassment Claims

Legally, sexual harassment is considered to be a form of sex discrimination. Current definitions of sexual harassment are derived from Title VII of the Civil Rights Act of 1964 and Title IX of the Education Amendments of 1972. Title VII states that it is "illegal to discriminate against employees on the basis of race, color, religion, sex, or national origin." Interestingly, the inclusion of sex-based discrimination in Title VII may have been accidental, because it was the result of an amendment by a legislator hoping to make the act so unacceptable that it would be defeated (Shrier 1996).

In 1972, the Equal Employment Opportunity Act was passed establishing the role of the Equal Employment Opportunity Commission (EEOC) in enforcing Title VII. The EEOC issued the first guidelines on sexual harassment in the 1980s, establishing harassment on the basis of sex as in violation of paragraph 703 of Title VII (Equal Employment Opportunity Commission 1980a, 1980b). The Equal Employment Opportunity Commission (1988) also provided the first formal definition of sexual harassment: unwelcome sexual advances, requests for sexual favors, and other verbal or physical conduct of a sexual nature constitute sexual harassment when

1. Submission to such conduct is made, either expersonally or impersonally, a term or condition of an individual's employment;
2. Submission to or rejection of such conduct by an individual is used as the basis for employment decisions affecting an individual; and/or
3. Such conduct has a purpose or effect of unreasonably interfering with an individual's work performance or creating an intimidating, hostile, or offensive working environment.

Courts recognize two categories of sexual harassment in the workplace. *Quid pro quo* harassment is harassment that links a condition of employment to a supervisor's receipt of sexual favors from a subordinate. *Hostile work environment* harassment occurs in a work environment that is permeated with discriminatory intimidation, ridicule, or insult that is sufficiently severe or pervasive to alter the conditions of the victim's employment and create an abusive working environment (*Harris v. Forklift Systems, Inc.* 1993).

Title IX prohibits sex discrimination in educational programs that are recipients of federal monies. Prior to 1992, Title IX was primarily used in lawsuits to challenge discriminatory practices in athletic programs and admission policies. Since the Supreme Court's decision in *Franklin v. Gwinnett County Public Schools* (1992), Title IX has been used to financially compensate recipients of sexual harassment in school environments.

Categories of sexual harassment in schools are based on categories of sexual harassment in the workplace, that is, quid pro quo and hostile environment. In its 1997 release of a report titled "Sexual Harassment Guidance: Harassment of Students by School Employees, Other Students, or Third Parties," the Office of Civil Rights expanded and adapted the EEOC definition to expressly apply it to the school environ-

ment. Hostile environment harassment was defined to include "unwelcome sexual advances, requests for sexual favors, and other verbal, non-verbal, or physical conduct of a sexual nature by an employee, by another student, or by a third party" that is "sufficiently severe, persistent, or pervasive to limit a student's ability to participate in or benefit from an education program or activity or to create a hostile or abusive educational environment" (U.S. Department of Education 1997, p. 12038).

Key Cases

In *Franklin v. Gwinnett County Public Schools* (1992), a high school student alleged that she had been sexually assaulted and harassed by her teacher, that her public school was aware of and took no action to halt the harassment, and that the school discouraged her from pressing charges. The U.S. Supreme Court, drawing an analogy to harassment in a workplace situation, ruled that the student was entitled to monetary compensation under Title IX for the school district's intentional discrimination as evidenced by failure to stop the teacher's known sexual harassment of the plaintiff.

In a 5–4 decision regarding school districts' strict liability for teacher–student harassment, the Supreme Court in *Gebser v. Lago Vista Independent School District* (1998) set what it considered a high hurdle for students to meet in successfully suing school districts for teacher–student harassment. In that case, a teacher was sexually involved with a student, and the school was held liable for the teacher's behavior because the Court stated, "a teacher's sexual overtures toward a student are always inappropriate." The Supreme Court held in *Gebser* that a school can be held liable for monetary damages if a teacher sexually harasses a student and a school official with actual knowledge of and authority to address the harassment is deliberately indifferent in responding.

After *Franklin*, which was a case of teacher–student harassment, several lawsuits were filed to obtain monetary compensation for student–student harassment. Because of wide variation in the courts regarding liability and compensation for student–student harassment, the U.S. Supreme Court heard the appeal of LaShonda Davis in *Davis v. Monroe County Board of Education* (1999). Briefly, the facts of the case were that LaShonda Davis, a fifth-grade student, alleged that over a 6-month period, a male classmate taunted, fondled, and rubbed against her. He also attempted to fondle LaShonda's breast and genital areas and asked for sex in explicit and offensive terms. Despite repeated complaints by LaShonda's mother, the school did not intervene and even declined LaShonda's request to reassign seats so that the two would no longer be sitting next to each other. The family pressed criminal charges and the boy pleaded guilty to sexual battery in juvenile court. Subsequently, the family sued the school board under a Title IX claim. However, the lower federal court held that Title IX did not apply to student–student sexual harassment.

On appeal, the U.S. Supreme Court held, in a 5–4 decision, that schools may be held liable for peer sexual harassment. The Court ruled that Title IX funding recipients are liable only where they know of the sexual harassment and respond with "deliberate indifference." The Court essentially amplified the decision in *Gebser*, announcing that a school also may be liable for monetary damages for student–student sexual harassment in the school's program if the conditions of *Gebser* are met. The Court differentiated school and workplace environments because students may still be learning how to interact appropriately with peers and thus limited liability to behavior "so severe, pervasive, and objectively offensive that it denies the victims equal access to education" and excluded ordinary acts of "teasing and name calling among school children." The Court further limited liability to situations in which the funding recipient exercises control over both the harasser and the context in which the harassment occurs.

Controversies

Justice Anthony Kennedy authored a vehement 34-page dissent, taking issue with the majority's premise that "sex discrimination" and "sex harassment" were the proper ways to describe what he called at various points "immature, childish behavior" and "inappropriate behavior by children who are just learning to interact with their peers." Kennedy stated, "The norms of the adult workplace…are not easily translated to peer relationships in schools" where "teenage romantic relationships and dating are part of everyday life." He added, "A teenager's romantic overtures to a classmate (even when persistent and unwelcome) are an inescapable part of adolescence."

Public reaction to the ruling has been mixed. Concerns have been raised of schools overreacting to avoid liability in response to trivial transgressions, such as the case of a North Carolina school district's decision to suspend a 6-year-old boy for kissing a 6-year-old girl on the cheek. On the other hand, the National School Board Association supports the Supreme Court's decision, noting that it set a high liability standard and that many schools already had sexual harassment and discrimination policies in place.

Schools and courts will likely continue to face significant litigation over liability for peer sexual harassment under Title IX because many questions regarding application of Title IX in these circumstances remain unanswered. There were no clear guidelines specifying when peer sexual harassment becomes known to the school; what type of school employee must know about the harassment; what behaviors are considered sufficient to be called severe, pervasive, and objectively offensive enough; and what interventions would discharge deliberate indifference. Continued debate over analogies between workplace and school settings will also likely contribute to continued litigation.

Other Overlapping Claims

Definitions of school sexual harassment overlap somewhat with criminal definitions of sexual assault (e.g., fondling, grabbing, pulling clothing off, and forcing unwanted kisses) and may blur the boundaries between harassment and criminal behavior, allowing for prosecution under criminal law. Moreover, crimes committed in the course of sexual harassment may include rape, sodomy, and sexual battery.

Claims may be brought under the area of assault and battery. For example, in one case, a school district was asked to defend an assault case against a coach who routinely patted male football players on the buttock. The coach defended his behaviors, stating that such encouragement was common in his field, and the case against the school district was dismissed.

A plaintiff may proceed with claims under state law rather than pursuing Title VII litigation. The restriction of complaints being brought to federal court only after all EEOC remedies have been tried and exhausted does not apply to litigation under state law. Thus, a case may be brought to a state court in a variety of ways. Claims are often filed in conjunction with Title VII claims to potentially obtain unlimited compensatory and punitive damage remedies.

Some of the most common tort claims include intentional infliction of emotional distress or the tort of outrage. For example, in a recent case, a 17-year-old girl named Sally was in treatment for severe depression. She reportedly lost 15 pounds and her school grades declined precipitously. Sally reported to her psychiatrist and subsequently to her parents that she was involved in a sexual relationship with her math teacher under the guise of after-school tutoring. She stated that she enjoyed the relationship but felt guilty, ashamed, and saddened by it. Her parents consulted an attorney, who recommended filing litigation alleging intentional infliction of emotional distress. The claim was upheld by the court because reasonable people would consider the teacher's behavior as outrageous and Sally's psychological distress was precipitated by her relationship with the teacher.

Brief Review of the Literature

After bringing the subject of unwanted sexually oriented behavior and teasing occurring in school-age populations to the fore by a national survey published in 1993, the American Association of University Women (AAUW) published a second national survey in 2001 that yielded similar results on the extent of such behaviors in students in grades 8 to 11 (American Association of University Women 1993, 2001). Approximately 81% of the respondents reported having been subjected to what the study defined as sexual harassment. Slightly more girls (83%) than boys (79%) reported being harassed, and the behavior occurred most often during the middle of school or junior high years. The percentage of boys reporting harassment slightly increased between surveys (49% vs. 56%). The large numbers of students who report that school employees harass students declined slightly from 44% to 38%. Interestingly, slightly over half of the students said that they had also harassed others.

Attention was further directed to this issue by papers published by the Wellesley Center for Research on Women (e.g., Stein et al. 1993), which has also published guides for schools regarding policy-making and prevention issues (e.g., Stein and Tropp 1994). These studies obtained similar results to the AAUW surveys, finding that, of 342 urban high school students, 87% of girls and 79% of boys also reported harassing others. They found that girls are more often subject to more overt forms of harassment and that boys more often use sexually harassing behaviors. Girls perceived being sexually harassed as more threatening than did boys. The authors indicated that the incidence of peer harassment is so pervasive that it appears to be the norm. When defining sexual harassment, the studies have included a broad range of behaviors, such as sexual comments and looks; showing sexually oriented pictures or notes; "mooning" someone; touching or brushing up against someone in a sexual manner; pulling down, snapping, or grabbing clothing; and forcing unwanted kisses or other behavior.

In the above studies, reported negative impacts on students experiencing sexual harassment centered on school performance and other psychosocial effects. School performance impacts include finding it hard to pay attention in school, not wanting to go to or talk in school, absenteeism, and truancy. Depression, anxiety, and stress-related symptoms such as loss of appetite; nightmares or disturbed sleep; loss of interest in regular activities; social isolation; loss of friends; and feeling sad, upset, afraid, threatened, or embarrassed were also reported.

There is little literature on the clinical assessment of children who complain of having been sexually harassed and particular characteristics these children might show. The AAUW (1993, 2001) studies indicated that girls were more likely than boys to report school impacts from harassment and specific educational repercussions. Girls were more likely to report feeling upset, ashamed, embarrassed, or self-conscious. This higher likelihood of reporting found in the AAUW studies may be bias (i.e., boys may want to appear "tough" or be affected by societal pressures related to gender roles). Students who experienced harassment with physical contact, compared with those who experienced nonphysical harassment, were more likely to report emotional and behavioral reactions, although some nonphysical harassment was particularly upsetting, such as spreading rumors or being called gay or lesbian. Literature on disabled or sexual-orientation minority students is limited but indicates that students with disabilities experience more peer sexual harassment than nondisabled peers and that lesbian students experience more peer sexual harassment than heterosexual female peers (Fineran 2002a, 2002b).

Studies of college students who have been harassed have been reviewed (e.g., Paludi 1990). In one study (Houston and Hwang 1996), 80 female college students were asked about their experiences of sexual harassment in high school. Women who reported few positive behaviors between their parents, having unwanted sexual contact during childhood, and having an overprotective mother reported a greater number of sexual harassment incidents compared with women who had not experienced any of these problems.

If an adult (e.g., a teacher) is the harasser, the behavior may fall into the category of sexual abuse or assault, and thus the literature on sexual abuse of children by adult authority figures is relevant. While the literature regarding the effects of sexual harassment on adults may be pertinent (e.g., O'Donohue 1997), this literature generally indicates that adults have a broad range of responses to sexual harassment instead of displaying a "typical" pattern.

Other than this, we know little about such questions as what type of harassment causes the most severe problems, what type of adolescents are most likely to be significantly affected by harassment, and whether harassment causes any particular symptoms more often than others.

Cyberbullying and Cyberharassment

With the advancement and proliferation of information technologies, new venues for sexual harassment are emerging. One consequence of this advancement is cyberbullying and cyberharassment. Stopcyberbullying.org defines a cyberbullying situation as when a child or adolescent is "tormented, threatened, harassed, humiliated, embarrassed or otherwise targeted" by a child or adolescent "using the Internet, interactive and digital technologies, or mobile phones" (http://www.stopcyberbullying.org). If the perpetrator is an adult, the behaviors are instead called cyberharassment or cyberstalking. The four categories of cyberbullies described are 1) Vengeful Angel; 2) Power-Hungry, or Revenge of the Nerds; 3) Mean Girls; and 4) Inadvertent Cyberbully, or "Because I Can." Of all teenagers who use the Internet, 32% reported that they have been targets of cyberbullying behavior (Lenhart 2007). Although cyberbullying represents a broad category of online bullying behaviors, a subset of behaviors may involve behaviors constituting sexual harassment. For example, a "Mean Girls" cyberbully may film a victim using the restroom and post the video on *YouTube.com* or post rumors on social networking sites about the victim being a "slut."

There is no established case law in this new area. However, school liability concerns could be raised when cyberbullying or cyberharassment is occurring through a school district Internet system or via a cell phone on campus. Interestingly, in 2005, in an effort to prevent students from exposure to or engagement in inappropriate online activities, a private Catholic high school in New Jersey, Pope John XXII Regional High School, banned its students from using *MySpace.com* and *xanga.com* even if accessed from their home computers. Civil litigation (e.g., intentional tort litigation) may be brought against a cyberbully and the parents of the bully based on intentional infliction of emotional distress, negligent supervision of a child, defamation, or invasion of privacy. Criminal claims may also be filed (see Chapter 19, "Forensic Issues and the Internet").

Clinical Issues

Forensic clinicians will most often encounter sexual harassment of school-age children and adolescents when approached by attorneys representing parties in civil suits. The clinician will typically be asked to assess the presence and extent of psychological and emotional damage sustained by the plaintiff, and sometimes by his or her family, as a result of alleged sexual harassment. Concerns may be raised about problems characteristic of psychopathology, such as depressive or anxious behavior, social or emotional withdrawal, parasuicidal behaviors or suicide attempts, drug and alcohol abuse, eating disorders, risky sexual behavior, and other acting-out behaviors. The clinician is asked to determine whether any of these conditions exist and to what extent they may be related to the sexual harassment alleged in the lawsuit. Clinicians may also be asked to speak to developmental issues regarding the nature and impact of the harassment.

Case Example

Amy, an eighth-grade student in a public middle school, is sent to a forensic psychiatrist for evaluation after reporting to her parents that she was teased by male peers calling her "slut, prostitute, whore, and weenie." She reports that she believes her older brother is jealous of her academic performance and has started a rumor that she eats "Weenies" (penises). She states that at first she was only teased by her brother's circle of friends, but now, at all school athletic events, a large group of students yell, "Weenie," make obscene hand gestures, and "roll their tongues in their mouths" when she passes by. Her mother complains that in response to her complaints, the school administrator advised her, "Boys and girls just do that kind of thing." The administration has taken no action and states it has no future plans to address the issue.

The conduct that Amy alleges appears to meet the Office of Civil Rights definition of sexual harassment, because it includes verbal and nonverbal harassment by peers. In examining Amy's school record, the forensic expert noted there was a drop in her grades between the seventh and eighth grades and that there was a connection between the drop in her grades and the behavior she alleged. There were no other confounding variables. The forensic psychiatrist could not opine on the credibility of Amy's complaints, emotional condition, and the relation between Amy's anxiety and depression and the behavior of her classmates in this case. However, the expert recommended a course of treatment for Amy's depressive disorder. Although the forensic psychiatrist had no opinion on the credibility in this case, in other cases he did offer an opinion, suggesting that if the complaints were found to be credible by the court or jury, such conduct might be responsible for symptoms or aggravation of preexisting symptoms.

Developmental and Social Context

As noted earlier, cases of teacher–student harassment are often indistinguishable from cases in which an adult sexually assaults a minor. Liaisons between a female teacher and male student excite widespread media publicity and public interest and have been the focus of recent books and movies (e.g., the 2008 movie *After School*, the 2000 movie *All American Girl: The Mary Kay Letourneau Story*, and the 1999 book *Un Seul Crime L'amour* [Only One Crime, Love]). Some cases of allegations of sexual harassment by a school employee may be more verbal in nature and consist of grossly inappropriate or unwanted sexually oriented comments, in or outside of the classroom, or of pervasive "put-downs" or displays of favoritism toward one gender. The courts have yet to fully define where such behavior crosses into the realm of harassment, but the clinician should be aware that he or she may need to understand how a school setting can be made a hostile environment by responsible adults.

One of several issues to consider in the clinical evaluation of cases of alleged peer sexual harassment is developmental context. Sexually oriented teasing, touching, and taunting as well as other kinds of teasing and bullying are extremely common in adolescent groups. Rumors may circulate regularly, and there are "in groups" and "out groups." Some of these behaviors may be defined as inappropriate, be potentially harmful, and require intervention by school personnel and parents. However, especially in younger adolescent groups such as middle school populations, these behaviors are closely intertwined with development. Early adolescence is a time when sexual development proceeds at a fast pace when young teens may be extremely aware of their own and others' sexual maturation, yet lack the emotional maturity to avoid inappropriate language and behavior. Additionally, heightened self-consciousness may leave early adolescents quite vulnerable to comments aimed at their sexuality or body.

In a legal case, although controversy regarding specifics of assessing the issue remains, whether a particular behavior reaches the level of sexual harassment is a question of fact. According to the courts, what does set it apart is behavior, based on a student's gender, that is objectively offensive to the student and severe and pervasive enough to interfere with the student's ability to participate in school.

Similar to standards in adult cases of harassment, in child and adolescent cases, whether a particular behavior is considered harassment by the courts depends on the behavior being both subjectively and objectively offensive—that is, the behavior must be offensive to both a reasonable person (objective) and the plaintiff (subjective). For example, if a plaintiff complains of being told offensive dirty jokes but his classmates report that he is a storehouse of such jokes and tells them all the time at parties, his complaints may be found meritless since they do not meet the subjective test. Likewise, if a student has adopted the mores of her extremely sexually conservative parents and is offended by very mild language, her complaints may be found meritless since they do not meet the objective test.

The impacts of behaviors potentially constituting harassment are modulated by developmental considerations. Thus, the clinician must attempt to understand the behavior of the alleged harasser and peer target with knowledge of child and adolescent development and understanding of the context in which the harassment occurs.

Diagnostic Issues

Awareness of typical child and adolescent behavior is important in assessing claims for compensation of damages associated with peer sexual harassment. For example, a middle school child may commonly cry in his or her room or have emotional outbursts, even if that child had not behaved in this way before; however, symptoms such as escalating problems with appetite, sleep, and destructive temper tantrums that significantly impair the child's ability to carry out daily activities are another matter. Each case must be evaluated with consideration of the cognitive, temperamental, emotional, and sexual maturation of the parties involved, as well as the context and pervasiveness of the behavior and response of the social environment.

The diagnosis of posttraumatic stress disorder (PTSD) has become a common consideration when evaluating children who complain of mental and emotional damage resulting from traumatic events. Commonly used threshold criteria for a PTSD diagnosis require that the trauma must be quite severe, involving actual or threatened death or serious injury or a threat to the physical integrity of the child, and that the response to the threat must be extreme, involving intense fear, helplessness, or horror. Given these threshold criteria and the pervasiveness of sexually harassing behaviors in everyday adolescent life, it would likely be rare that a diagnosis of PTSD would be appropriate in a peer sexual harassment case. However, a broad range of other diagnostic possibilities, including anxiety, adjustment, disruptive behavioral, depressive, eating, or substance use disorders, as well as no diagnosis, should be considered.

Forensic clinicians frequently must deal with controversial social issues in their practice, and they must be aware of and combat against forces of bias. The clinician who fails to seriously consider an allegation of sexual harassment with the excuse that "boys will be boys" or "all adolescent girls are seductive" will likely be unable to perform an objective evaluation. The clinician who fails to seriously consider an allegation of peer sexual harassment with the view that "sexual behavior between adolescents is unavoidable" or that all alleged harassment is merely immature behavior will also be likely unable to perform an objective evaluation. Likewise, the clinician who fails to understand the complexity of such behaviors in the context of a developmental context and assumes all behaviors are harassment will have a similar problem. Lastly, it is important to be aware of and guard against societal biases that male students sexually harassed by female school employees are less affected than female students harassed by male school employees.

Components of Assessment

The assessment of a child who alleges that he or she has been sexually harassed should be conducted in a manner similar to any other child and adolescent forensic evaluation. A thorough review of all case documents, reflecting both sides, should be made, including case pleadings, depositions, school and medical records, and all electronic communications, such as e-mails and communications on social networking sites such as *MySpace, Facebook,* or *Friendster.* Interviewing a child or adolescent's parents may assist in obtaining accurate information about the child's developmental history and temperament as well as information that an adolescent may hesitate to reveal or minimize.

Careful attention should be paid to the cultural and ethnic background of the child and his or her family and how these factors affect the perception and reaction to sexual harassment.

Both parents and the child should be asked for a full developmental history, including a sexual history. The quality of the marriage and the manner in which the parents relate to each other as well as parental history of sexual abuse or harassment should be assessed. Data on parenting styles and sibling relationships should be obtained. Information gathered on peer relationships should include when, whether, or how the child has been teased and how the child has responded, including being the perpetrator of bullying or teasing of others and under what circumstances this has occurred. The child's basic temperament should be assessed, including areas such as reaction to change, emotional responsiveness, activity level, and sociability. Information about typical coping responses to social and emotional problems is helpful in determining possible deviance from "normal" adolescent coping mechanisms. The developmental history should include exploration of the child's move from latency into adolescence, where the child is in developmental maturity, and how the child and the parents have handled these transitions. An understanding of the child's concept of his or her own body image and any discomfort is helpful. History of previous traumas, harassment, or abuse should be thoroughly assessed.

A report by the child about what happened should be taken in as much detail as possible so that full understanding of the event(s) and context is obtained. Interview of both parents and child about how the alleged harassment has affected the child is essential and should include questions about psychiatric symptoms, day-to-day behavior changes, and any changes in areas such as school attendance and participation in school and social activities. Data should be gathered on how parents, peers, and school personnel have responded to the situation. Overreacting or underreacting by parents may affect the child's ability to cope with the situation, and overreacting or underreacting by school administration may contribute to the problem. For example, after an adolescent boy complains to his mother of sexual harassment by members of his football team, she tells the vice principal in charge of discipline, the school investigates by questioning the coach and disciplining some members of the team, and subsequently the boy does not receive fair playing time from his coach and is beaten up by his team members.

Psychological testing may be used as an added source of data regarding issues of personality and psychopathology (see Chapter 6, "Psychological Testing in Child and Adolescent Forensic Evaluations"). A thorough mental status and symptom history should be obtained from both child and parents. The symptoms history should include questions about all characteristic adolescent pathological behaviors, such as problems with appetite, mood, sleep, or drugs or alcohol. A thorough assessment will provide the clinician with a full picture of the child and his or her environment, both before and after the alleged incidence of harassment, thus allowing for informed expert opinion on the presence and extent of any damages sustained and exacerbating or mitigating factors to the damages.

Forensic Assessment

It is critical to remain objective in evaluating a child for sexual harassment. The conduct of the teacher or peer harasser as described may appear to be clearly egregious. However, it is important for the evaluator not to become too empathic with the child or too angry at the alleged harasser.

After a careful clinical evaluation requested by attorneys, the forensic expert may be asked to testify either on behalf of a child, adolescent, or school or as an expert designated by the court. Prior to undertaking the forensic evaluation, the evaluator should clarify and understand what his or her role will be and what types of questions he or she might be asked to answer. The evaluator should clarify the limits of potential testimony, beyond questions of psychiatric or psychological conditions, treatment considerations, prognosis, and other areas of expertise, such as a school's response, in cases where there is an allegation of sexual harassment.

The trier of fact will decide the ultimate issue. The forensic evaluator can shed light on the emotional condition of the child or adolescent who alleges harass-

ment, not on the ultimate issue of whether the harassment did or did not occur or whether the report of the child or adolescent is credible. There are differing levels of comfort between experts on offering further expanded opinions on the casual nexus between the plaintiff's complaints and current symptoms. Drawing on collateral data, such as statements from individuals other than the plaintiff, depositions, EEOC findings, and school records, experts comfortable offering such opinions can address issues related to and factors suggesting credibility (e.g., consistency with other data and apparent malingering). The expert may also give an opinion that, assuming certain facts to be true, the alleged behaviors have caused new symptoms or aggravated preexisting symptoms. The forensic evaluator can also shed light on possible confounding variables and whether the alleged damages are related to the alleged sexual harassment or other confounding issues in the child's or adolescent's history or present life.

Table 33–1 presents consolidated guidelines for evaluating school-age youth for the presence and extent of psychological and emotional damage sustained as a result of alleged sexual harassment.

Consultation to Schools

From elementary school to universities and vocational schools, sexual harassment is a serious problem for students at all educational levels. Students are often too frightened or too embarrassed to report sexual harassment. The number of requests made to child and adolescent psychiatrists for forensic consultation with regard to children, adolescents, and their parents who allege sexual harassment in the classroom has increased dramatically since the Supreme Court decision in *Davis*.

TABLE 33–1. Guidelines for clinical forensic assessment of alleged sexual harassment

Take a complete sexual history from parents and child.

Review school documentation (e.g., grades, counselor reports) and all prior mental health reports.

Explore broader contexts of alleged behaviors (e.g., developmental, cultural, social contexts).

Depending on comfort level, consider limiting forensic reports to diagnosis, treatment plan, and psychiatric/psychological issues versus expanding opinion to include factors related to veracity of allegations of harassment.

Be mindful of forces of bias.

Obtain psychological tests if appropriate.

Seek consultation if findings are unclear.

The revised sexual harassment guidelines issued by the U.S. Department of Education Office for Civil Rights offer clinicians some help in consultation to schools (Revised Sexual Harassment Guidance 2001). The guidelines note there may be several correct ways for school administrators to respond to allegations of harassment but the important thing is for school employees to pay attention to the school environment and not hesitate to respond to sexual harassment in the same reasonable, commonsense manner as they would to other types of serious misconduct. The guidelines also note that it is a school's responsibility to respond to sexual stereotyping by gender, covered by Title IX, if it is sufficiently serious to deny or limit a student's ability to participate in or benefit from a school program. The guidelines emphasize that Title IX "does not extend to legitimate non-sexual touching or other non-sexual conduct" and gives examples of a high school athletic coach hugging a student who made a goal, a kindergarten teacher's consoling hug for a child with a skinned knee, or a student's sports maneuver requiring contact with another student as not being considered sexual harassment. However, should nonsexual conduct take on sexual connotations and rise to the level of sexual harassment, these behaviors would be covered by Title IX.

The guidelines provide explicit information in determining a school's responsibility.

1. The school must determine the degree to which the harassing conduct affected the education of one or more students.
2. The school must determine if the conduct in question is welcome or unwelcome. For example, if the conduct is between a school's employee and its student (in particular an elementary school student), it can never be considered consensual. In secondary school students, there is strong presumption that the sexual conduct between an adult school employee and a student is not consensual. In cases involving older secondary students, a number of factors should be considered, including a student's age, possible disability, and the degree of influence of the adult over the student.
3. The school has a responsibility to address the harassment and to respond promptly and effectively to any allegation of sexual harassment, in particu-

lar if the school determines that the alleged harassment occurred in the context of an employee's provision of aid, benefits, or services to a student.
4. The school is also required to adopt and publish grievance procedures and to alert students and parents of avenue for informal and formal action, including a description and explanation of grievance procedures.
5. It may also be appropriate for a school to take interim measures in the investigation of a complaint. For example, if a student alleges that he or she has been sexually assaulted by another student, the consultant may suggest placing the students immediately in separate classes or in different housing arrangements on a campus, pending the school's investigation. Similarly, if the alleged harasser is a teacher, allowing the student to transfer to a different class may be an appropriate suggestion.
6. In cases involving potential criminal conduct, the consultant may need to emphasize the responsibility of the school to determine if an appropriate law enforcement authority should be notified.
7. In all cases, the school should make every effort to prevent disclosure of the names of all parties involved unless necessary to carry out an investigation.
8. If the school determines that sexual harassment has occurred, it must take reasonable, timely, age-appropriate, and effective corrective action, including steps tailored to the specific situation. School personnel may need to counsel, warn, or take disciplinary action against a harasser based on the severity of the harassment or any records of prior incidents. Schools may be required to provide other services to the student who was harassed, such as counseling or tutoring. For example, in a recent clinical situation an instructor gave a student a low grade because the student failed to respond to sexual advances. The school was advised to make arrangements for an independent reassessment of the student's work and change the grade accordingly. Similarly, the school was counseled to take steps to prevent any further harassment and to prevent any retaliation against the student who made the complaint (and was the subject of the harassment).

—Key Points

— Legally, sexual harassment is considered a form of sex discrimination. Claims for compensation typically derive from Title IX of the Education Amendments of 1976, which prohibits sex discrimination in educational programs that are recipients of federal monies.

— The broad scope of behaviors that may be defined as sexual harassment allows additional avenues for filing claims such as criminal and tort claims and claims under state law.

— Categories of sexual harassment in schools parallel adult workplace harassment categories (i.e., quid pro quo and hostile environment harassment).

— The *Franklin v. Gwinnett County Public Schools* (1992) ruling held that a student was entitled to monetary compensation under Title IX for a school district's intentional discrimination as evidenced by failure to stop a teacher's known sexual harassment of the plaintiff (teacher–student harassment).

— The *Davis v. Monroe County Board of Education* (1999) ruling held that a school may be held liable for monetary compensation under Title IX for student–student harassment if the school is aware of such harassment and responds with deliberate indifference.

— Consideration of developmental, cultural, and social context is critical in evaluating claims of sexual harassment in children and adolescents.

References

American Association of University Women: Hostile Hallways: The AAUW Survey on Sexual Harassment in America's Schools. New York, Louis Harris and Associates, 1993

American Association of University Women: Hostile Hallways: Bullying, Teasing, and Sexual Harassment in School. Washington, DC, American Association of University Women Educational Foundation, 2001

CBOCS West Inc v Humphries (No 06-1431), 474 F 3d 387 (2008)

Civil Rights Act of 1964 (Title VII), 42 USC § 2000-2(a) (1964)

Davis v Monroe County Board of Education, 526 US 629 (1999)

Equal Employment Opportunity Commission: Guidelines on Sexual Harassment, 29 CFR § 1604.11(B) (1980a)

Equal Employment Opportunity Commission: Title VII Guidelines on Sexual Harassment, 45 Fed Reg (219: Rules and Regulations):74676–74677 (1980b)

Equal Employment Opportunity Commission: Equal Employment Opportunity Commission Guidelines, 29 CFR § 1604.11(A)(a) (1988)

Fineran S: Sexual harassment and students with disabilities. Paper presented at the annual meeting of the Society for the Study of Social Problems, Washington, DC, August 2002a

Fineran S: Sexual harassment between same-sex peers: the intersection of mental health, homophobia, and sexual violence in school. Social Work 47:65–75, 2002b

Franklin v Gwinnett County Public Schools, 503 US 60 (1992)

Gebser v Lago Vista Independent School District, 524 US 27-4 (1998)

Gomez-Perez v Potter (No 06-1321), 476 F 3d 54 (2008)

Harris v Forklift Systems Inc, 114 S Ct 367 (1993)

Houston S, Hwang N: Correlates of objective and subjective experiences of sexual harassment in high school. Sex Roles 34:189–204, 1996

Lenhart A: Cyberbullying and Online Teens: Pew Internet and American Life Project. June 27, 2007. Available at: http://www.pewinternet.org/pdfs/PIP%20Cyberbullying%20Memo.pdf. Accessed July 25, 2008.

O'Donohue W: Sexual Harassment: Theory, Research and Treatment. Boston, MA, Allyn & Bacon, 1997

Paludi MA (ed): Ivory Power: Sexual Harassment on Campus. Albany, NY, SUNY Press, 1990

Revised Sexual Harassment Guidance: Harassment of Students by School Employees, Other Students, or Third Parties, Title IX January 2001. Washington, DC, U.S. Department of Education Office for Civil Rights, 2001

Shrier DK (ed): Sexual Harassment in the Workplace and Academia. Washington, DC, American Psychiatric Press, 1996

Stein N, Tropp L: "Flirting or Hurting": A Teacher's Guide on Student-to-Student Sexual Harassment in Schools. Wellesley, MA, Center for Research on Women, 1994

Stein N, Marshall N, Tropp L: Secrets in Public: Sexual Harassment in Our Schools. Wellesley, MA, Center for Research on Women, 1993

U.S. Department of Education, Office of Civil Rights: Sexual Harassment Guidance: Harassment of Students by School Employees, Other Students, or Third Parties (62 Federal Register 12034, March 13, 1997). Washington, DC, Office of Civil Rights, 1997

Index

*Page numbers printed in **boldface** type refer to tables or figures.*